T0297652

SECOND EDITION

Occupational Therapy Interventions

Function and Occupations

SECOND EDITION

Occupational Therapy Interventions

Function and Occupations

AUTHORS

Catherine Meriano, JD, MHS, OTR/L
Professor of Occupational Therapy
Quinnipiac University
Hamden, Connecticut

Donna Latella, EdD, OTR/L
Professor of Occupational Therapy
Quinnipiac University
Hamden, Connecticut

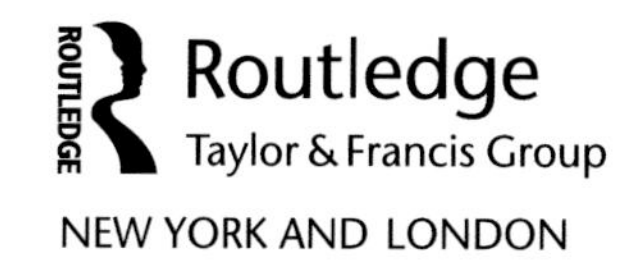

NEW YORK AND LONDON

Instructors: *Occupational Therapy Interventions: Function and Occupations, Second Edition Instructor's Manual* is available. Don't miss this important companion to *Occupational Therapy Interventions: Function and Occupations, Second Edition*. To obtain the Instructor's Manual, please visit www.routledge.com/9781617110559.

First published in 2016 by SLACK Incorporated

Published 2024 by Routledge
605 Third Avenue, New York, NY 10017
4 Park Square, Milton Park, Abingdon, Oxon OX14 4RN

Routledge is an imprint of the Taylor & Francis Group, an informa business

Library of Congress Cataloging-in-Publication Data

Names: Meriano, Catherine, editor. | Latella, Donna, editor.
Title: Occupational therapy interventions : function and occupations /
[edited by] Catherine Meriano, Donna Latella.
Description: Second edition. | Thorofare, NJ : Slack Incorporated, [2016] |
Includes bibliographical references and index.
Identifiers: LCCN 2016004160 | ISBN 9781617110559 (alk. paper)
Subjects: | MESH: Occupational Therapy--methods | Occupational
Therapy--psychology
Classification: LCC RM735 | NLM WB 555 | DDC 615.8/515--dc23 LC record available at http://lccn.loc.gov/2016004160

ISBN: 9781617110559 (pbk)
ISBN: 9781003525325 (ebk)

DOI:10.4324/9781003525325

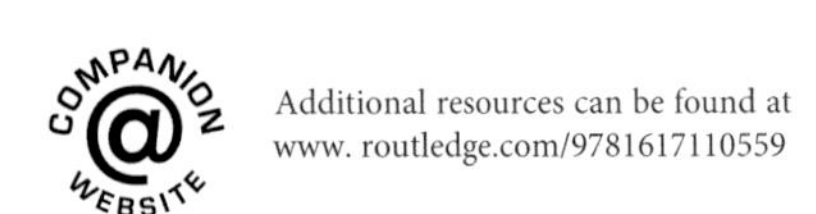

Additional resources can be found at
www. routledge.com/9781617110559

Dedication

We wish to dedicate this text to our families: John, Kathleen, and Jay Meriano and Domenic, Kristy, and Dylan Latella. Your support and patience through the writing of this updated text was greatly appreciated. This is also dedicated to the talented faculty and students of the Occupational Therapy Department of Quinnipiac University, as well as all of our former clients and their families, who have assisted in teaching us about the intervention process.

Contents

Instructors: *Occupational Therapy Interventions: Function and Occupations, Second Edition Instructor's Manual* is available. Don't miss this important companion to *Occupational Therapy Interventions: Function and Occupations, Second Edition*. To obtain the Instructor's Manual, please visit www.routledge.com/9781617110559.

Acknowledgments

We would like to than Brien Cummings, of SLACK Incorporated for his ongoing support of occupational therapy and this project. We would also like to thank Pam Hewitt for her support in researching evidence.

About the Authors

Catherine Meriano, JD, MHS, OTR/L is a tenured Professor of Occupational Therapy at Quinnipiac University, Hamden, Connecticut. Her clinical background is in acute care, outpatient rehabilitation, and nursing home practice. Catherine is received her certification in Advanced Online Teaching from the Online Learning Consortium and teaches in both the Post-Professional Occupational Therapy Doctorate program, which is online, and the traditional entry-level Masters of Occupational Therapy program. Her teaching responsibilities include Legal and Ethical classes in both programs, Problem-Based Learning, Documentation of practice and Administration. Her publications and presentations have included topics such as evaluation of the upper extremity, dysphagia, academic integrity, legal issues in health care and legislative advocacy for occupational therapy. Catherine enjoys spending time in the clinic, traveling with her family, and spending time with her husband and two children.

Donna Latella, EdD, OTR/L is a tenured Professor of Occupational Therapy at Quinnipiac University, Hamden, Connecticut. Her clinical background is in acute care, outpatient rehabilitation, homecare, and nursing home practice. Presently, Donna's clinical practice is spent between homecare, outpatient, as well as working as a Registered Therapist in Hippotherapy and a Certified Therapeutic Riding Instructor. Her teaching responsibilities include Research, Adult Interventions, Health Conditions, Problem-Based Learning, Capstone Graduate Project, and Service Learning. Donna volunteers with her certified therapy dog, pot-bellied pig and horses providing animal-assisted therapy in reading programs, hospitals, and day centers. Her publications and presentations have covered topics such as evaluation of the upper extremity, dysphagia, leadership, service learning, animal-assisted therapy, educational malpractice, and learning styles. Donna enjoys jogging, horseback riding, and boating with her husband, two children, and many pets.

Contributing Authors

Amy P. Burns, JD, MOT, OTR/L (Appendix B)
Associate Center Director
Cooperative Studies Research Coordinating Center
Department of Veterans Affairs
West Haven, Connecticut

Marilyn B. Cole, MS, OTR/L, FAOTA (Chapter 7)
Professor Emeritas
Quinnipiac University
Hamden, Connecticut

Margo Ruth Gross, EdD, LMFT, LMT, OTR/L (Chapter 8)
Assistant Professor
Sacred Heart University
Fairfield, Connecticut

Kimberly D. Hartmann, PhD, MHS, OTR/L, FAOTA (Chapter 5)
Professor of Occupational Therapy
Director of the Center for Interprofessional Healthcare Education
Quinnipiac University
Hamden, Connecticut

Deanna Proulx-Sepelak, MHA, OTR\L (Chapter 2)
Clinical Associate Professor of Occupational Therapy
Quinnipiac University
Hamden, Connecticut

Martha J. Sanders, PhD, MSOSH, OTR/L, CPE (Chapter 6)
Assistant Professor of Occupational Therapy
Quinnipiac University
Hamden, Connecticut

Francine M. Seruya, PhD, OTR/L (Chapter 10)
Clinical Associate Professor
Quinnipiac University
Hamden, Connecticut

Peter Tascione, OTR/L (Chapter 8)
Occupational Therapy Supervisor
Connecticut Valley Hospital
Middletown, Connecticut

Roseanna Tufano, LMFT, OTR/L Chapter 9)
Assistant Professor of Occupational Therapy at Quinnipiac University
Hamden, Connecticut

Tracy Van Oss, DHSc, MPH, OTR/L, FAOTA (Chapter 4)
Associate Clinical Professor
Quinnipiac University
Department of Occupational Therapy
Hamden, Connecticut

Robert Wright, OTR/L (Chapter 6)
Wright2Work
Colchester, Connecticut

Preface

In 2002, the American Occupational Therapy Association created the Occupational Therapy Practice Framework (Framework) that replaced the medical terminology used by many clinicians. This new document re-emphasized the role of occupational therapists working with clients to improve or maintain skills in functional activities, both in institutional settings and community settings. Since then, the document has been updated to a 2nd edition in 2008 and most recently to a 3rd edition in 2014. This practice framework was designed to clearly delineate the evaluation and intervention processes, as well describe all of the factors that impact functional activities. While the main focus is these functional tasks, or occupations, the foundational skills required for these tasks have also been addressed. These foundational skills include motor skills and processing skills. In addition, the client's patterns of activity have also been addressed.

This text has been created to blend the Framework with the entry-level clinical skills in use today for the intervention of adults with physical disabilities. In addition, this text will assist more experienced clinicians to integrate the Framework terminology and its purpose into practice. There are several interventions which are discussed only briefly as these are not typically entry-level skills. These are interventions that require advanced training, such as advanced dysphagia techniques, aquatics, the use of physical agent modalities, driver training, etc. Resources for additional education can be found in the Appendix at the end of the text.

As students emerge from universities well-versed in the Framework document, they will need tools which discuss intervention using the most current terminology. As well, experienced clinicians also require these same tools to remain current and grow with the field of occupational therapy.

An instructor's manual in the form of a class syllabus has also been included in the materials. The syllabus is designed to follow the format of the text and the newest edition of the OTPF. The syllabus is designed broad enough for professors to tailor it to the needs of their own curriculum and teaching/learning style.

Introduction

This text will begin with a thorough review of the Occupational Therapy Practice Framework: Domain and Process. (3rd Ed) (Framework) (AOTA, 2014). Following this, Chapter 2 will discuss the foundational skills required for all areas of occupation. While the Framework document is a very thorough document, it does not include every aspect of clinical intervention. When an area requires further definition, such as in perceptual skills, other references will be utilized to supplement the Framework document. The Foundational Skills chapter is primarily discussing remediation techniques for these skills. Once the foundational skills have been reviewed, each area of occupation—activities of daily living (ADL), instrumental activities of daily living (IADL), work, retirement/volunteer, education, leisure, and social participation—will be discussed. While information regarding evaluation is contained within these chapters, with a sampling of evaluation provided in Appendix B, the primary focus of the text is intervention. Remediation, adaptation/compensation, and maintenance are addressed in the chapters. Because much remediation focuses on practicing a task, the emphasis in these chapters is on adaptation/compensation. Wellness will be addressed in Chapter 9 regarding education to address both disability prevention and health promotion.

Throughout these chapters, information more specific to the topic will be provided regarding frames of references, pathologies, psychosocial considerations, the role of the OTA, safety, and more. Chapter 1 provides a general overview of these topics, and reference back to this first chapter is often recommended.

The chapters that cover more traditional areas of occupation for adult interventions have similar formats. These chapters are Foundational Skills for Functional Activities, Activities of Daily Living, and Instrumental Activities of Daily Living. The remaining chapters—Education, Work, Retirement/Volunteer and End-of-Life Issues, Leisure, Social Participation, and Wellness—cover much of the same information as the Framework document, but in a more narrative and general format.

At the end of many chapters, a case study is presented. Appendix A, at the end of the text, is a resource guide compiled from all of the chapters. This contains useful web resources, ordering information, and continuing educational opportunities (for more advanced skills training). Appendix B is a grid that provides information pertaining to a sampling of evaluations.

It should be noted the term *occupational therapist, occupational therapy practitioner*, or *therapist* throughout the text does not indicate OTR only. It is important to emphasize the collaborative relationship that exists between the registered occupational therapist (OTR) and the occupational therapy assistant (OTA). According to AOTA, both OTRs and OTAs are responsible for providing quality occupational therapy services including direct intervention with clients (AOTA, 2015). The focus of this text is intervention, and therefore, the majority of the information can apply to both types of practitioners. Some information related to non-standardized evaluation and specialized topics may pertain to the OTRs; however, standardized evaluations, as well as collaboration, on the part of the OTA are vital in establishing intervention plans.

Bibliography

American Occupational Therapy Association. (2014). Occupational therapy practice framework (3rd ed.). *American Journal of Occupational Therapy, 68*(Suppl. 1), S1-S48.

American Occupational Therapy Association. (2015). *The reference manual of the official documents of the American occupational therapy association* (19th ed.). Bethesda, MD: AOTA.

1 Introduction

Catherine Meriano, JD, MHS, OTR/L
Donna Latella, EdD, OTR/L

Chapter Objectives

By the end of this chapter, the student will be able to do the following:

- Comprehend the domain and process of the Occupational Therapy Practice Framework as it relates to occupational therapy's focus on occupation and daily living skills.
- Comprehend related occupational therapy models/frames of reference.
- Comprehend the impact of modes of injury upon occupational performance.
- Describe and give examples of the specific categories of the Occupational Therapy Practice Framework, including occupations, performance skills, performance patterns, context and environment, activity demands, and client factors.
- Describe the evaluation process and its components as related to engagement in occupation.
- Describe the intervention process and its components as related to engagement in occupation.
- Comprehend occupational therapy intervention approaches, and recognize the differences between them, in order to establish an appropriate intervention plan.
- Comprehend the types of occupational therapy interventions.
- Describe and understand the outcome process as it relates to successful engagement in occupation.
- Understand and apply specific documentation skills to occupational therapy intervention.
- Understand the role of the family/caregiver during the intervention process.
- Understand the importance of evidence-based practice in occupational therapy practice.

Meriano C, Latella D.
Occupational Therapy Interventions: Function and Occupations, Second Edition (pp 1-34).

Occupational Therapy Framework Domain and Process: Domain of Occupational Therapy

The Occupational Therapy Practice Framework: Domain and Process (American Occupational Therapy Association [AOTA], 2014) guides the core concepts and constructs of occupational therapy practice. The Framework was created in order to evolve with the current needs of the profession. The purpose of the Framework is to describe the domain of human activity as well as the process of occupational therapy evaluation and intervention as they relate to occupation. Specifically, it guides the profession of occupational therapy to focus on the individual client's engagement in daily occupations throughout the evaluation and intervention processes. In addition, the third edition emphasizes the "client" also as an organization or population (AOTA, 2014).

The domain of occupational therapy sets the stage for, and encompasses, the evaluation and intervention processes. It focuses on the client's ability to engage in meaningful and purposeful daily activities, or occupations, in whatever context is appropriate for those occupations. Each aspect of the domain is seen as equally important in the occupational therapy process. For example, evaluating the motor skills of a client who has sustained a wrist fracture is considered to be as important as evaluating the client's ability to perform daily routines. Occupations are "everything we do in life, including actions, tasks, activities, thinking, and being" (Law, Baum, & Dunn, 2005, p. 6). The multiple occupations of every individual are unique, each with its own context and meaning to a particular client. Therefore, how will the working mother who enjoys yoga continue her meaningful occupations and roles with an upper extremity injury?

According to the Framework document, the domain of occupational therapy consists of occupations, which are made up of performance skills, performance patterns, and client factors that are impacted by the context and environment, as well as activity demands (AOTA, 2014). Figure 1-1 depicts this information visually, and each term is defined below.

Occupations

The occupational therapy practitioner must first examine the individual client's occupations. These are general categories of areas in which individuals typically perform activities or occupations that are meaningful to them. For the adult population, these areas include the following (AOTA, 2014):

- Activities of daily living (ADL)
- Instrumental activities of daily living (IADL)
- Rest and sleep (Note: Rest and sleep will be integrated within the discussions of the applicable chapters rather than in a separate chapter.)
- Education
- Work
- Play (Note: Because the adult population is the focus of this text, there will not be a chapter on play.)
- Leisure
- Social participation

Within occupational therapy practice, the therapist considers the many occupations, as above, in which the individual or group may engage. Occupational therapy then addresses the performance issues affecting the individual's or group's abilities to perform these occupations. In order

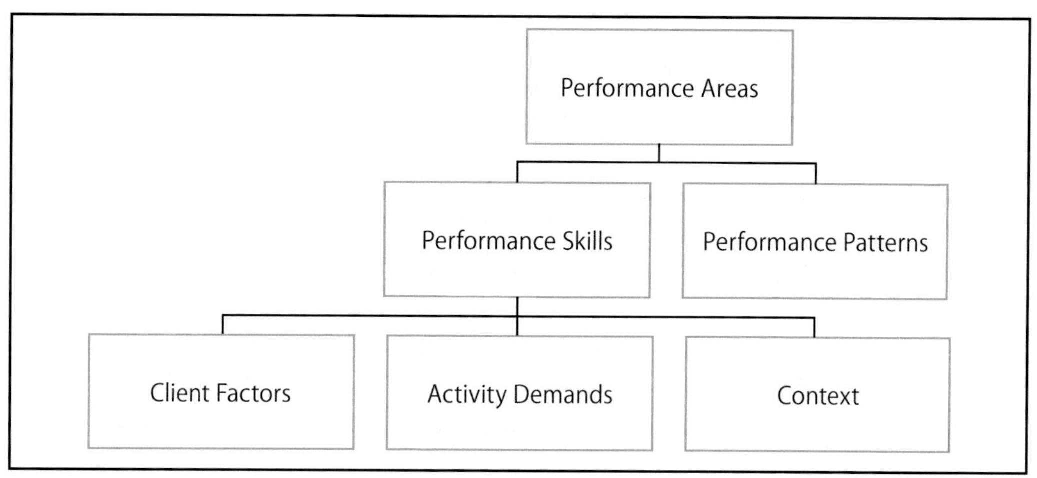

Figure 1-1. Domain of occupational therapy. (Adapted from American Occupational Therapy Association. (2014). Occupational therapy practice framework (3rd ed.). *American Journal of Occupational Therapy, 68*(Suppl. 1), S1-S48.)

to work on performance issues, the occupational therapist must know which performance skills and patterns are needed for the specific areas addressed, as follows:

Performance skills	Performance patterns
Motor skills	Habits
Process skills	Routines
	Rituals

Social Interaction Skills

Because skills are small components of performance and have functional purposes, they must be analyzed for their effectiveness, or lack of effectiveness, during performance. Motor skill examples include aligning, stabilizing, positioning, bending, gripping, manipulating, and coordinating. Using the example of the client with the wrist fracture, a motor skill deficit may be decreased ability to perform bilateral fine motor tasks because the client's affected upper extremity may be immobilized in a cast. Manipulating small items such as a key may be a difficult fine motor task. Social interaction skills include interacting with not only others but the environment as well. A client who typically uses upper extremity gesturing to communicate may be significantly limited while immobilized in a cast. Performance skills are impacted, but not dictated, by context, activity demands, and client factors (AOTA, 2014). As another example, a client may have limited body function but may have learned to compensate for this limitation and still be able to complete necessary motor skills in a particular activity. In this example, the unusual method of attaining motor skills may impact performance but will not necessarily dictate a new method.

Performance patterns of a person, group, or population include: habits, which are automatic behaviors; routines, which are established sequences of occupations/activities that provide daily structure; and roles, which are a set of socially accepted behaviors. The performance patterns are activities that we do on a frequent basis until they become a common behavior in our daily tasks (AOTA, 2014). Therefore, how will the working mother who does yoga on a daily basis perform her daily routines, roles, and responsibilities after sustaining a wrist fracture? How can occupational therapy support the rituals and routines of a specific group's customs or cultural practices in daily living skills?

Table 1-1

Context, Activity Demands, and Client Factors

Context	Activity Demands	Client Factors
Cultural	Objects used and their properties	Body functions
Physical	Space demands	Body structures
Social	Social demands	
Personal (age, gender, education, socioeconomic status)	Sequencing and timing	
Spiritual	Required actions	
Temporal (day/year, stage of life)	Required body functions	
Virtual	Required body structures	

Adapted from American Occupational Therapy Association. (2002). Occupational therapy practice framework. *American Journal of Occupational Therapy, 56*(6), 609-639.

These performance patterns are influenced by context and environment (AOTA, 2014). Contexts are interrelated internal or external conditions that are within and surround the individual and influence performance. The environment is the external physical and social factors that occur in the client's daily life. Context includes the cultural, personal, temporal, virtual, physical, and social influences impacting the individual's functions on a daily basis. In addition, the individual's personal data (age, socioeconomic status, etc.) and temporal information (when activity is performed, stage of life, etc.) must be reviewed. Virtual contexts occur when a client is surfing the Internet, taking an online course, or using email. The occupational therapist considers specific contexts that may influence the performance of a specific activity or occupation (AOTA, 2014). Consider the social context of an adult who has attended a bridge game at a friends house as a daily routine for many years. This is a meaningful activity for the client, although the routine may be limited after a cerebral vascular accident, particularly if the client is no longer able to drive. How might this contextual limitation be evaluated and adapted for this client? The occupational therapist must also assess the activity demands placed on an individual in order to partake in a particular occupation (AOTA, 2014). Activity demands are unique to each activity completed by the client, whereas context may be similar for a group of activities. An example of activity demands is as follows: Once the dilemma of transporting the client to a friend's home is solved, the space demands and required actions for accessibility into and around a friend's home may be additional issues. Lastly, the occupational therapist assesses the client factors such as values, beliefs, spirituality, body functions, and body structures that may influence performance. Specifically, illness, disease, and disability may affect an individual's ability to engage in chosen occupations such as the mental, sensory, and movement-related functions of visiting a friend. Specifically, a client may not have sufficient memory after a cerebral vascular accident to participate in a game of bridge as he or she did in the past. In addition, how might vision and endurance limitations affect ability to participate in this meaningful activity? (AOTA, 2014). Table 1-1 summarizes these areas.

The Process of Occupational Therapy

The process of occupational therapy begins with evaluation of the client's occupational needs, issues, meaningful activities, and desires. The results determine intervention strategies that focus on engagement in occupations. These intervention strategies are then assessed in the outcome process to determine whether appropriate outcomes have been achieved (AOTA, 2014).

Evaluation Process

The evaluation process of occupational therapy is aimed at assessing a client's goals and needs, as well as barriers to performance. The evaluation process focuses on the entire domain of practice (as above) and how each area may influence client performance. The occupational therapist uses skilled observation and applicable assessment tools in order to determine a problem list. The process has the following two steps:

- Step One: The occupational profile determines the client's needs, problems, and concerns about daily performance of occupations. This process includes the clients' history, background, values, and priorities in terms of his or her occupations.
- Step Two: The evaluation of occupational performance focuses on identifying specific issues and evaluating those that may affect performance.

It is important to note that the client's input, priorities, and goals guide the evaluation process (AOTA, 2014). Specifically, when evaluating occupational performance, the therapist should ask the client questions such as the following: What are your goals in the recovery process? What do you do for fun? What is important to you during the recovery process or upon discharge from therapy?

Step One: The Occupational Profile

As stated previously, the occupational profile is completed to determine the client's interests and goals. The profile can also assist the therapist when determining what forms of intervention to use. Therefore, if a client is having difficulty completing ADLs because of decreased fine and gross motor coordination, the therapist can certainly practice ADLs with him or her. Typically, however, clients dress only once per day, and in settings such as hospitals clothes may not be available. To allow for additional coordination training, the therapist could pull out the pegs and Theraputty (CanDo), which would probably result in a bored client. On the other hand, if the therapist knows from the occupational profile that this client enjoys painting, then the therapist has an activity for therapy that will engage the client while improving coordination.

Step Two: Analysis of Occupational Performance

Each of the chapters in this text will discuss the evaluation of occupational performance specifically for the chapter's topic: Foundational Skills, ADL, IADL, Rest and Sleep, Education, Work/Retirement, Leisure, Social Participation, and Wellness. In addition, Appendix B provides a sampling of evaluations.

Intervention Process

AOTA (2014) separates the intervention process into three substeps: intervention plan, intervention implementation, and intervention review.

The intervention plan is based on the results of the evaluation process. It guides the intervention process and is designed to enhance participation in occupations and activities. The intervention plan is created in collaboration with the client, taking into consideration the following (AOTA, 2014):

1. Client goals, beliefs, values, and health as determined by the occupational profile and the medical history.

2. Performance skills, performance patterns, and client factors, which are influenced by context/environment, activity demands, and factors determined by the evaluation process.
3. The setting or circumstance surrounding the interventions, including any limitations on intervention imposed by the setting or the payment source.
4. Applicable theories or models/frames of reference.
5. The appropriate approach (i.e., create, promote, establish, restore, maintain, or modify).
6. The interaction with family and caregivers.
7. Evidence-based research.

In addition, the occupational therapist uses the knowledge of occupation, human performance/development, and the effects of disease and disability as a guide to the intervention process. Each of the topics listed will be discussed later in this chapter.

Intervention implementation puts the plan into action in order to enhance client performance. It involves a skilled process that includes collaboration with the client in order to enhance occupation and activity participation. Interventions focus on changing the context and environment, activity demands, client factors, and performance skills or patterns, as appropriate. Change in one area usually affects another, resulting in a dynamic process. For example, interventions that involve increasing functional mobility (ADL area) will enhance the client's return to independent performance patterns (e.g., habits, routines, rituals, and roles). Outcomes are identified and documented throughout interventions while clients are continuously reassessed through this dynamic interrelationship (AOTA, 2014). The role of the occupational therapist may also change as this dynamic intervention process continues. The process includes the therapeutic use of occupations and activities, preparatory methods and tasks, education and training, advocacy, and group interventions (AOTA, 2014).

Therapeutic use of occupations is not unique to occupational therapy; however, with the holistic rather than the medical model of intervention, occupational therapists have multiple opportunities to utilize this skill. Occupational therapists provide interventions regarding such personal issues as bathing, toileting, and sexual activity, as well as individual interests of leisure, social participation, and work. In these sessions, therapists have the opportunity to "develop a collaborative relationship with clients to understand their experiences and desires for intervention (AOTA, 2014, p. S12). In addition, therapists working in the area of adult physical dysfunction include psychosocial issues in the intervention plan, not just physical issues. Lastly, behavioral issues may also require intervention, and modeling of proper behaviors by the therapist is an essential component of the intervention plan. For example, this form of intervention may be required following a cerebral vascular accident or a traumatic brain injury with clients who have impaired mental/cognitive functions such as thought, personality, or temperament issues.

As therapists utilize the skill of therapeutic use of occupations, they must be aware of their own attitudes, beliefs, and values. Clients may have different ways of completing occupations or have different attitudes regarding an occupation. For example, therapists and clients may differ in terms of beliefs and values regarding "appropriate" forms of sexual activity, cultural emphasis on food and acceptance that feeding may be unsafe, a family's unwillingness to take a parent home, and what constitutes appropriate attire for work or leisure. In all of these situations, the therapist must acknowledge his or her own beliefs and values, but not impose them on the clients or caregivers. Chapter 8 offers a more in-depth discussion of therapeutic use of occupations, as well as the therapeutic use of self.

According to the Framework, therapeutic use of occupations or activities can include occupation-based and purposeful activities or preparatory methods (AOTA, 2014). Throughout this text, occupation-based and purposeful activities will be described together as functional activities. Preparatory methods are described as foundational skills. One of the determinations an occupational therapist must make is whether to begin intervention with these foundational skills or through the use of functional activities. According to Zoltan (2007), these forms of intervention are called a top-down or bottom-up approach. With a top-down approach, the occupational therapist adjusts the activity or occupational performance with the goal of promoting independence with the use of adaptive and compensatory techniques. Consider the client with memory function deficits, who may need to use a planner as a compensatory technique to complete a daily routine or schedule. Conversely, the bottom-up approach addresses underlying dysfunction in the foundation skill areas and assumes the client will improve in functional ability as a result. This indicates that foundational skills are the building blocks for the functional activities. With some clients, it will be necessary to work on these skills in isolation, prior to beginning or in conjunction with functional activities. With other clients, intervention of functional activities will also improve foundational skills through their incorporation in the functional activities. For example, the client with a memory deficit may initially work on memory activities before or while attempting the above compensatory technique. While the beginning of this text reviews the remediation of foundational skills, the majority of the text will concentrate on the remediation, adaptation/compensation, and maintenance of functional activities.

The top-down approach has been refined by Fisher in the Occupational Therapy Intervention Process Model (Fisher, 2002). In this model, Fisher has further divided the top-down approach into "simulated occupation" and "restorative occupation," finding that the interventions utilizing actual activities were preferred over the simulated situations. While simulations offer some benefit, the client will find greater meaning completing actual activities, thus improving carryover (Fisher, 2002).

While the most common settings for consultation are in the areas of work/volunteering and adult education, it can occur in any setting. According to the Framework, consultation occurs when the therapist collaborates with the client to identify problems and possible solutions. Because the expertise of therapists is so varied, consultation can be requested of therapists in community, educational, vocational, medical, and many other environments. Consider the therapist who may evaluate the client's home environment and make recommendations for accessibility and safety but does not implement them. The therapist is functioning as a consultant in this example.

Education, on the other hand, should occur in all environments. Even though the Framework defines education as "activities involved in learning and participating in the educational environment" (AOTA, 2014, p. S20), this does not mean that education should occur on a limited basis. Education regarding the purpose of occupational therapy, the occupations of individuals, and the importance of purposeful activity is ongoing for most therapists in all settings. Consider the therapist who provides in-service programs regarding the role of occupational therapy to new medical interns every year in a hospital setting. It is also important to note that while AOTA has distinguished education in this manner, most settings and payers acknowledge, and require documentation for, ongoing education regarding the completion of functional activities with clients.

The second portion of the intervention implementation process is to monitor the client's response and progress through continuous assessment. The intervention review process continually assesses the effectiveness and progress of the plan by reviewing the actions and/or interventions that were completed and the outcomes that were achieved, were not achieved, or are no longer a priority for the client. The intervention plan is adjusted accordingly in collaboration with the client. The intervention review process also includes a determination and recommendations for discharge, additional referrals, or continuation of services as appropriate (AOTA, 2014).

Performance Skills and Patterns

Prior examples illustrated how performance skills can impact an individual's function. Throughout this book, the emphasis of intervention will be on functional activities. As occupational therapists, however, we utilize the task analysis process to break down these functional activities into performance skills, performance patterns, and client factors and view how context/ environment and activity demands impact these functional tasks. This means that goals associated with performance skills (e.g., coordination) are acceptable as long as they lead toward a functional goal, as in ADLs.

The intervention plan may also have goals specifically related to performance patterns, context, activity demands, and client factors, provided that these relate back to the occupations of interest for the individual client.

The Setting

If a client's performance skills and performance patterns will be impacted by the context and environment where the functional activity occurs, the client's actual context would appear to be the ideal setting for intervention. Unfortunately, this is not always possible, particularly given the vast institutional and community programs in which occupational therapists practice. This forces many therapists to simulate the context and activity as much as possible.

However, some of these settings further limit the simulation for safety, insurance, or financial reasons. For example, using a cooking task may be limited by safety concerns or structural issues. While working at an adult day care center on a wellness program, clients may not be allowed to put food into or take food out of the ovens because the director may have concerns about the clients' safety. In a prison system, there are restrictions regarding the use of sharp cooking utensils. A hospital setting may include a kitchen, but it is not tailored to simulate each client's home kitchen.

Financial concerns also play a role in settings, particularly in clinics that receive Medicare funds, private insurance, or workers' compensation. The caseworker often is not an occupational therapist but can limit the number of visits allowed for occupational therapy. The ongoing Medicare caps have at times resulted in clients receiving less care than recommended by the therapist.

Lastly, the setting itself can limit the context of therapy. For example, hospital-based therapists may be able to complete home visits, but typically this is to gather information for clinic simulations and to prepare for discharge. The client does not usually attend these visits to practice any skills in his or her home.

Introduction to Occupational Therapy Models and Occupational Performance

Occupational therapy is rooted in a client-centered focus in order for the practitioner, client, and caregivers to participate in the therapeutic process (Schell, Gillen, & Scaffa, 2014). Intervention is in collaboration with the client to facilitate occupational engagement (AOTA, 2014).

Specific concepts of humanism are attributed to Carl Rogers and Abraham Maslow. Rogers believed that the client should be allowed to set his or her own goals, direct therapy, and find solutions to problems. Maslow believed that the client should be viewed as the expert of his or her own life and that the therapist should guide the client to self-actualization through the use of genuineness, nonjudgmental acceptance, and understanding (Cole, 2011). Today, components of the humanistic approach are seen in many of the client-centered theories that will be discussed in this section.

The occupational therapy models discussed subsequently are intended to provide the backdrop or framework for the assessment and intervention processes. The first section includes examples of frames of reference or models that are client-centered and have been chosen because they are collaborative in nature and, according to Law (1998), are more likely to engage clients in the occupational therapy process. In turn, this engagement has been shown to increase satisfaction, success in therapy, and positive outcomes. In addition, Christiansen, Baum, and Bass (2015) discuss the importance of client-centered models involving the activities, tasks, and roles of the individual. The second section includes examples of systems models that are holistic and include the interaction of systems inside, as well as outside of, the client. Systems models focus on occupational function/dysfunction and everyday routines that may be impacted (Bruce & Borg, 2002). Other chapters throughout the text will also discuss frames of reference or models that are appropriate to the specific chapter.

Section 1: Client-Centered Models

Client-Centered Approach

The client-centered approach involves the therapist working with the client in order to decide which areas of occupational performance should be addressed. Depending on their ability to participate, clients will contribute to the decision-making process and make choices. If the client is cognitively unable to participate, then the family-centered therapy approach is attempted, with the family representing the client.

The client-centered approach to occupational therapy practice focuses on the respect for, and collaboration with, the individual receiving services. This approach, then, facilitates the client to find meaning in his or her own daily occupations. The ultimate goal of the client-centered approach is to empower clients by allowing them to direct the course of intervention and contribute to the process. For example, part of their contribution may include looking at their own strengths and areas of limitations, in order to prioritize the intervention plan. Through person-centered communication, the therapist facilitates and enables the client to be responsible for decision making. In order for this approach to be successful, the therapist must have a good understanding of the client. The environment in which this empowerment occurs must be caring, respectful, visionary, and supportive (Law, 1998, 2002).

The Person-Environment-Occupation-Performance Model

The person-environment-occupation-performance (PEOP) model was first described in 1991 (Christiansen et al., 2015) and has been updated over the years in order to meet the growing needs of occupational therapy practice. The model focuses on health, participation, and well-being of individuals, groups, and populations. As occupational therapists, we understand the significance of a person engaging in an occupation within a specific environment. The interactive and interdependent effect of these three variables leads to occupational performance. PEOP defines occupational performance as "the doing of meaningful activities, tasks, and roles through complex interactions between the person and environment" (Christiansen et al., 2015, p. 40). As a systems-based approach, PEOP emphasizes the complexities of a client-centered focus and the impact of motivation in determining occupational performance outcomes (Christiansen et al., 2015).

Christiansen et al. (2015) state that the PEOP model focuses on elements that describe what individuals do in their daily lives, what motivates them, and how their personal characteristics interact with occupations that are undertaken to influence occupational performance. The model suggests that individuals are naturally motivated to explore, master, and succeed in the environment for positive adaptation. Adaptation describes how well individuals are able to meet their daily challenges in everyday life through achieving set goals. The model also addresses the belief that individuals are motivated to face new challenges with increased confidence when they are in a setting that encourages success. In addition, a sense of fulfillment and a development of identity come from feelings of mastery and accomplishment of goals within everyday occupations. As a result of these meaningful experiences, individuals begin to understand who they are and their place in the world. Pertinent issues regarding the elements of the model are discussed below.

According to the PEOP model, occupational performance depends on (1) the nature of the task, (2) the role to be performed, (3) the characteristics of the individual person, and (4) the supportive environment. These critical factors must be aligned for successful performance, which in turn leads to healthy participation and positive well-being (Christiansen et al., 2015). A client's narrative or personal story, which includes past, current, and future perceptions, choices, interests, goals, and needs, is a relevant starting place for determining occupational performance outcomes. This holistic approach allows for collaborative goal-setting and intervention planning (Christiansen et al., 2015).

The PEOP model is based on three primary factors as described below.

Person Factors

Every person comprises six interrelated components. PEOP lists these components as cognitive, psychological, physiological, sensory, motor, and spirituality. The occupational therapist begins with an assessment of these person components to determine capacity and one's ability or inability to participate in occupations. Motivation is a key factor to engagement in occupations. The intrinsic aspect of motivation includes a person's internal drives and needs, which occur as a result of free choice and without external reward. For example, a person with an intrinsic desire for self-fulfillment on the job is motivated to go to work each and every day regardless of how much he or she makes or whether the boss acknowledges his or her performance. Extrinsic factors also influence a person's motivation and need to be assessed in each person's environment. External rewards such as a paycheck or external praise such as achievement awards are significant to sustaining one's performance. Extrinsic factors can have both a positive and/or negative impact on occupational performance. Cognitive theories of motivation help us to understand how people motivate themselves through setting goals, planning actions, and achieving goals. Cognition helps us to explain why we seek gratification and how we determine personal expectations and goals (Christiansen et al., 2015).

Self-efficacy is a psychological factor that is critical to sustaining occupational performance even under adverse conditions. Self-efficacy allows a person to view him- or herself as competent. This element is vital for success in occupational performance tasks because an individual's feelings of competence directly influence the outcome. Other psychological factors impacting occupational performance include a person's self-concept, self-esteem, self-identity, metacognition, self-awareness, and emotional state. In addition, factors that involve the senses can affect the person and occupations (Christiansen et al., 2015).

Environmental Factors

PEOP identifies six key components within one's environment: (1) culture, (2) social determinants, (3) social support and social capital, (4) education and policy, (5) physical and natural context, and (6) assistive technology.

The environment has both a direct and indirect impact on occupational performance. The occupational therapy assessment process seeks to understand the client's environmental factors that may present as barriers or positive contributors to occupational performance (Christiansen et al., 2015).

Occupation Factors

PEOP identifies three key components to every occupation: (1) roles, (2) activities, and (3) tasks. Occupations need to be understood from the client's perspective (i.e., what a person wants and needs to do). Christiansen et al., (2015) describe occupational performance as the "doing" aspect of occupation and as complex: "The PEOP model is transactional, in that it views everyday occupations as being affected by and affecting both the person factors and the environments that characterize a client's home, work/school, and community life" (p. 50).

Within the PEOP model, the occupational therapist will consider these factors and apply them within a client-centered focus. The client and therapist work together to identify issues related to living skills and performance of occupations. The two will collaborate on appropriate goals, intervention, and outcomes of therapy.

The Person-Environment-Occupation Model

The person-environment-occupation (PEO) model focuses on occupational performance and its link to people, occupation, roles, the environment, work, and play as a dynamic, interwoven process. The approach to occupational therapy also acknowledges the importance of context, temporal conditions, physical and psychological aspects, and influences of behavior. Because the environment is always in flux, individuals need the behaviors necessary to shift while working toward goals.

The PEO model makes the following assumptions (Law, Cooper, Strong, Stewart, Rigby, & Letts, 1996):

1. The person is a unique being who has many roles that are dynamic and variable across time and context, duration, and importance.
2. Within this model, the environment includes cultural, socioeconomic, institutional, physical, and social aspects.
3. Occupation is considered to be self-directed, functional tasks and activities engaged in over a lifetime.
4. Occupational performance is the dynamic experience and outcome of the interaction between the person, environment, and occupation. It involves meaningful, purposeful activities and tasks in which an individual engages over a lifetime.
5. The model assumes that the person, environment, and occupation interact continually over time and space. Occupational performance is optimized when these are considered compatible.

When following the PEO model, the focus of the occupational therapy evaluation and intervention should be to elicit change and facilitate improved occupational performance. This occurs by collaborating with the client, involving his or her occupation, and considering the environment specific to the individual.

Occupational Adaptation Model

First introduced by Schultz and Schkade (1992a, 1992b), this model encourages the therapist to assist the client to identify occupations to which he or she is interested in returning. Based equally on the individual, the environment, and the client's interactions, this model emphasizes the use of meaningful occupations to allow the client to experience adaptation. When the client responds to the challenges, adaptation occurs and leads to mastery. Because the client is completing tasks that hold meaning, internal motivation is present. While foundational skills, such as range of motion (ROM) and edema are addressed, they are focused toward the activity that the client desires to complete. Gibson and Schkade (1997) later found that occupational therapy intervention focused on the roles and contexts that were identified as important by the clients resulted in higher levels of independence and less restrictive discharge environments.

Section 2: Systems Models

The Model of Human Occupation

Kielhofner and Burke (1980) described the Model of Human Occupation (MOHO) as an open or dynamic system that influences occupational behavior in individuals. "Being engaged in occupation means doing culturally meaningful work, play, or daily living tasks in the stream of time and in the context of one's physical and social world" (Kielhofner, 1995, p. 3). Occupation, according to Kielhofner and Burke (1980), is the action or doing in which humans occupy their world. Occupational behavior occurs when one makes choices and takes action. Humans are occupational by nature, and thus need to be active.

MOHO describes the human open system as a cycle that influences occupational behavior. According to this systems theory, information coming into the human being is input. This information is internally processed as throughput. Based on how an individual processes and forms beliefs about this information, he or she will perform behavior or react emotionally. This response is called output. Lastly, information that comes back into the system from the environment is called feedback (Kielhofner & Burke, 1980).

This model emphasizes how individuals continuously engage in this feedback loop. Information is processed (step two of the cycle) via three subsystems:

1. The volition subsystem consists of three components: personal causation, valued goals, and interests. These components influence behavior and are differentiated out of an individual's innate urge to explore and master the environment. Individuals also incorporate information from experience to form internal symbolic representation. The enactment of occupational behavior and performance is guided by these components (1980).
2. The habituation subsystem consists of habits and roles. Habits guide human automatic behavior and do not always require conscious attention (1980). According to Bruce and Borg (2002), many people find security in their habits and may feel uncomfortable when changing them. Kielhofner (1995) explains how roles are images individuals keep regarding the positions held in various social groups and of the obligations with those positions.
3. Performance is responsible for influencing occupational behaviors via skills and the constituents of skills. Skills are further defined as perceptual motor skills, process skills, and communication/interaction skills (Kielhofner & Burke, 1980). Bruce and Borg (2002) also state that this subsystem is constantly interchanging information between the constituents and the environment in the processing of information during problem solving and actions.

The environment significantly impacts an individual's behavior by providing feedback about the output, or actions taken. The environment is believed to be composed of components: objects, tasks, social groups, and culture (Kielhofner, 1995). Objects are used by individuals to perform tasks. Tasks are used for performance in the environment. Social groups are natural collections of individuals such as clubs or families. Culture refers to the values and technology that can affect an individual's performance.

Kielhofner (1995) discussed an individual's functional status as being in order or disorder. Order connotes a state of health with positive feedback loops and successful performance of daily living tasks. To explain this concept further, the term occupational function has also been used to suggest that the individual is able to choose, organize, or perform occupation without difficulty

(Bruce & Borg, 2002). The individual is able to meet social demands with positive feedback from the environment. Disorder connotes the inability to perform occupational tasks, decreased or absent role performance, and the inability to meet role responsibilities (Kielhofner, 1995). Bruce and Borg (2002) discussed the concept further using the term *occupational dysfunction* to reflect impaired occupational performance. Dysfunction occurs when an individual has difficulty performing, organizing, or choosing occupations or when occupational behavior results in a decreased quality of life. Occupational dysfunction can impact the cycle negatively including one's habits, volition, performance, and the ability to negotiate in the environment.

MOHO looked at the development of occupation as a lifelong process, which includes changes in the individual as well as the environment. As developmental changes naturally occur, the human system must learn, relearn, and adapt in order to respond to, and maintain, an appropriate level of function. Occupational development is a process of transformation with periods of stability followed by transition and then, eventually, a new order of behavior.

The Ecology of Human Performance

The Ecology of Human Performance is based on the premise of how human behavior and task performance are affected by the interaction between a person and the context (or the ecology). In turn, the person, the context, and task performance affect each other through the transactional process of human performance. A specific transaction will affect an individual's performance as the person, context, or performance range are changed by the actual experience. Within this model, the occupational therapy intervention process is designed to improve the client's performance by changing variables such as the person, the context, the task, or the transaction between them. The intervention process involves the client, the family, and the occupational therapist in collaboration (Schell et al., 2014).

Within this model, occupational therapy intervention strategies may include the following (Schell et al., 2014):

1. Establishing or restoring an individual's abilities/performance in a specific context.
2. Changing the context or task.
3. Modifying or adapting the contextual characteristics and task demands to reflect performance in context.
4. Preventing barriers to performance in context.
5. Designing interventions to enhance performance.

The Ecology of Human Performance model has four basic assumptions (Law, 1998):

1. Persons and contexts are unique and dynamic.
2. Natural contexts are not the same as contrived contexts.
3. Occupational therapy involves improving self-determination and inclusion of individuals with disabilities in any context.
4. Contextual supports are included when achieving independence. Definitions include the following (Schell et al., 2014):
    - Person: An individual with unique abilities, experiences, and needs, such as cognitive and psychosocial. A person is not predictable, because everyone is unique and complex. The meaning attached to a person's tasks and contexts influences performance.
    - Occupations or tasks: A set of behaviors needed to reach a goal. Tasks are influenced by a person's roles.

- Performance: Includes the process and results of interactions within the context when engaging in a task.
- Environment/context: Includes the temporal and environmental aspects.
- Temporal aspects: Include an individual's age, developmental stage, place in life phases, and disability status.
- Environmental aspects: Include physical, social, and cultural aspects.
- Person-context-task transaction: The major variable that affects performance.

In summary, when the occupational therapy evaluation and intervention process are considered within the Ecology of Human Performance model, the variables of person, context, and task performance have an affect on, and are affected by, human performance.

The Approach

The Framework delineates five intervention approaches: create, restore, maintain, modify, and prevent (AOTA, 2014). The first two categories (create and restore) involve changing the individual's environment including physical, social, and institutional issues, as well as technological strategies such as devices and aids. The third category (maintain) focuses on the person and on the approaches to recovery/adaptation of neurological, sensory, and motor issues. The last two categories (modify and prevent) involve the delivery of services and the strategies the occupational therapist will use to facilitate changing attitudes, policies, and laws that affect the rehabilitation process. For the purposes of this text, the five intervention approaches have been modified slightly. Chapter 9 will focus on creation (health promotion) and prevention (disability prevention), Chapter 2 will focus on remediation (restore), and the remaining occupational area chapters will discuss remediation (restore), compensation/adaptation (modify), and maintenance of each occupational area.

The occupational profile will tell the therapist which approach the client is interested in. This approach should be a starting point. However, if a client has a progressive disease, such as Parkinson's disease, and the client's desire is to address only remediation of skills, the therapist has an obligation to educate the client/family about the disease process and attempt to combine some remediation along with environmental adaptations and other compensatory strategies.

Within these approaches, there are general principles that require definition and discussion. Grading of activities in these approaches, carryover/generalization by the client, and the purchase of adaptive or durable medical equipment are three such topics.

Grading of activities is more commonly used in the remedial approach but can also be utilized at times when using the adaptive/compensatory approach. Grading reflects how an activity is paced depending upon the needs and abilities of the client in order to achieve success in occupations (Pendleton & Schultz-Krohn, 2013). As a client gains skill in a particular foundational task or occupational task, the expectations will increase. Grading can include asking the client to complete more of the task, complete the task with higher quality, complete a task with greater complexity, or complete a task with less time allotted. Because a comprehensive task analysis is completed prior to initiation of intervention, the therapist has a clear understanding of what components of a task can be graded as improvement is noted. A specific example of grading is as follows:

Upon discharge from a rehabilitation facility, the client must independently make his or her own lunch each day. The intervention may begin with the client preparing a light meal of a cold cheese, lettuce, tomato, and mayonnaise sandwich. After this goal has been achieved, meal preparation may be upgraded to making a grilled cheese sandwich or a cheese omelet. In the event that the initial light meal was unsuccessful, the activity may be downgraded to one step (e.g., of just adding one ingredient, such as the cheese).

One form of grading is referred to as *chaining*. Backward chaining is when a therapist begins a task and then asks the client to complete the task (Pendleton & Schultz-Krohn, 2013). This allows the client a sense of accomplishment when he or she finishes a task. As the client demonstrates improvement, the therapist completes less and less of the task, eventually requiring the client to complete the entire task independently. Forward chaining can also be used. This is when the client begins the task and the therapist steps in to complete it once the client is unable (Radomski & Latham, 2014). As improvement is noted, the therapist will offer assistance later and later in the process. While both of these methods offer grading, forward chaining can often lead to a feeling of failure for the client because he or she had to be "saved" by the therapist. For this reason, backward chaining is preferred. A typical example of grading involves tying shoes. This multistep, cognitive, and fine motor task may be broken down by either forward- or backward-chaining the activity. Cuing can also be used as grading. The amount of cues, either visual or auditory, should be decreased as the client's skills improve. If cues are required after discharge, they become a maintenance tool.

Whether or not grading of activities is required, the occupational therapist is observing for carryover and generalization during ongoing sessions. While these terms are similar, they are not identical. Carryover, as defined by the *American Heritage Dictionary* (2000), is "something transferred or extended from an earlier time or another place." Relating this definition to occupational therapy, instructions given or tasks learned will be repeated at later sessions of therapy or by the client in a setting similar to the original setting of instruction. This alone will not allow a client to be independent, because settings often change for the client. Because of this, generalization is required. While most individuals think of generalization as making a general statement, as in the *American Heritage Dictionary*'s (2000) definition of "a principle, statement or idea having general application," occupational therapists think of generalization as the ability to complete carryover in a variety of settings. According to Jacobs and Simon, the occupational therapy definition is "applying previously learned concepts and behaviors to a variety of related situations, skills, and performance in applying specific concepts to a variety of related solutions" (2015, p. 120). Therefore, successful occupational therapy intervention requires not only carryover but also generalization. Toglia (1991) has taken this concept even further by defining levels of generalization as near, intermediate, far, or very far depending on the degree of change from the original task to the new task. If the new task is similar to the one already mastered, then the generalization is near. Likewise, if there is a great deal of difference between the two tasks, the generalization is very far. The characteristics of the tasks that are changed are referred to by Toglia (1991) as *surface characteristics*, such as variations in size, directions given or how a task is presented, or underlying concepts, such as a change in the planning required by the client in order to complete the task. The further down the continuum of Toglia's generalization, the further away from simple carryover the client moves. It is the responsibility of the occupational therapist to move the client from simple carryover to generalization.

The third general topic is adaptive equipment/durable medial equipment (DME). Mann, Llanes, Justiss, and Tomita (2004) asked more than 1,000 elderly people what their most important assistive device was, and the top five (when controlled for number of people using the devices) were oxygen tanks, dentures, three-in-one commodes, computers, and wheelchairs. This same study states that the participants had an average of 14 pieces of equipment and used 12 (2004). This suggests that while adaptive equipment/DME may not be on the top of all clients' lists of favorites, they are utilizing the equipment for the most part. It also demonstrates that clients have a different definition of "assistive device" than most therapists. This is an important consideration when educating clients regarding equipment.

When suggesting equipment to a client, the following considerations must be reviewed with the client:

- Prospective use of the equipment: required frequently or on rare occasions?
- Desire of the client: does he or she want this or do you, as the therapist, think he or she needs it?
- Cost of the equipment: adaptive equipment and bathroom DME generally are not covered. Is there an alternative that is available in the general population?
- Functionality: is the piece of equipment going to be functional in all appropriate environments for the client?

Modes of Injury

While this text is not a pathology manual, prior examples have demonstrated that knowledge of pathology and the anticipated course of illness is important when determining the most appropriate intervention approach. The occupational therapist must utilize his or her knowledge of human performance/development and the effects of disease and disability when determining which approach to utilize with a particular client. Examples of pathologies will be mentioned throughout the book, but a general review is provided here for reference in all chapters. Wellness, by definition, does not focus on injury and will not be reviewed.

Nearly all injuries/illnesses will result in limitations of at least one foundational skill. As discussed later in this chapter, these skills can be addressed individually or during functional activities. Chapter 2 will emphasize the remediation of each skill, while other chapters will address the foundational skills in relationship to the occupation. The modes of injury for foundational skills are addressed throughout Chapter 2 as each skill is addressed. While these skills are addressed individually, it is important to note that many clients have deficits in multiple areas, and overlap of deficits will also occur, such as decreased ROM secondary to edema of the hand.

Modes of Injury for Occupations

While modes of injury for specific skills can be delineated, occupationally based deficits can relate to a large number of injuries. Often, clients do not have just one diagnosis that is impacting the occupations but a few to several. In addition, an original injury may result in future diagnoses such as chemical dependency, depression, etc. Someone who is diabetic may experience sensory, visual, and cardiac symptoms, while someone with a spinal cord injury may have depression along with all of the other medical complications associated with this diagnosis. Nearly any injury or illness can result in a limitation to occupations; however, minor injuries, such as a well-healing hand fracture, can be easily overcome without the intervention of occupational therapy. When skilled intervention is required, the injuries or illness are usually more significant. The most common injuries/illnesses fall into two categories: orthopedic and neurological. Common orthopedic injuries are lower extremity fractures, joint replacements, amputations, or spinal surgeries. Upper extremity fractures and joint replacements can also indicate the need for occupational therapy.

Neurological injuries can result from trauma, such as spinal cord injuries or brain injuries, or from nontraumatic events such as cerebral vascular accidents, brain aneurysms, or cancer. Specific neurological diseases can also impact function, such as Parkinson's disease, Guillain-Barré syndrome, amyotrophic lateral sclerosis, multiple sclerosis, etc.

Many of the orthopedic injuries and some of the neurological illnesses will have a typical course that includes improvement in function. For these individuals, a remedial approach or a combination of remediation and adaptation will be appropriate. Some of these illnesses, however, will be progressive in nature, in which case less remediation is typically appropriate while greater emphasis is placed on adaptation and maintenance of skills.

Interaction With Family and Caregivers

As mentioned previously, the family and caregivers will impact the intervention plan. If working with an older adult, the caregivers should be involved throughout the process of intervention planning, as they will be completing many tasks at home with the client. When working in adult settings, the anticipated support of the family after discharge can impact the intervention plan significantly. In addition, it is essential to know how much time and interest family members and caregivers have for training by the occupational therapist.

Evidence-Based Practice

The process of evidence-based practice involves the use of research studies in order to select the most clinically and cost-effective approaches to evaluation and intervention. This approach to practice may also enhance clinical reasoning skills, particularly through the evaluation of the evidence and the appropriate application/integration into therapy.

Evidence-based practice also allows the occupational therapy practitioner to educate the client regarding the effectiveness of the evaluation and intervention processes chosen. Specifically, it involves informing the client of the intervention's benefits and risks, as well as positive and negative implications. This further enhances the client-centered environment by allowing the client to make informed decisions about the services provided (Law, Baum, & Dunn, 2005).

Law et al. (2005) discuss three challenges of evidence-based practice: the responsibility of the therapist to keep up on current literature, to develop good communication skills, and to understand how to evaluate the evidence within the literature.

In addition, Christiansen et al. (2015) identify the challenges of evidence-based practice as being able to access, evaluate, and interpret the literature; collect data to support intervention recommendations; and communicate possible outcomes to the client.

Law and MacDermid (2014) emphasize the need for occupational therapists using evidence-based practice to become reflective practitioners. Reflective practice involves the use of clinical reasoning skills and self-assessment for decision making. Law and MacDermid suggest the following five steps as a process for evidence-based practice (2014):

1. Pose a clinical question
2. Search for the evidence
3. Appraise the literature
4. Make a decision
5. Assess the effectiveness of the intervention and proficiency with the process of evidence-based practice

Law and MacDermid (2014) also emphasize that in the evidence-based practice process, evidence should not be considered alone. A competent therapist should consider all of these factors before making recommendations.

Outcome Process

While the intervention review is completed informally on an ongoing basis, the outcome process measurement is a formal reassessment of the progress toward the anticipated outcomes. The outcome process involves choosing a measurement for each anticipated outcome and then measuring the progress toward achieving the outcomes. The therapist should choose outcomes and measures such as those related to occupational performance, improvement, enhancement, prevention, health and wellness, quality of life, participation, role competence, well-being, and occupational justice of life (AOTA, 2014). It is important to create outcome measures early in the process because this will help to define the focus of intervention. These outcome measures should be valid, reliable, sensitive to client change, match targeted outcomes, and be selected to complement the client goals. It is also important to review the ability of an outcome measure to predict future outcomes (AOTA, 2014).

Once outcome measures have been determined, it is just as important to utilize this information appropriately. Therapists should compare progress to the targeted outcomes throughout the intervention process and assess the outcomes results in order to adjust the intervention plan. Figure 1-2 summarizes the occupational therapy process in the form of a decision tree for therapists.

Documentation in Intervention

Documentation in occupational therapy intervention involves the practitioner's contribution to the client's record. It is a method of communication of services provided for the health care team as well as third-party payers. Whether documentation is collected and presented through a medical record or any other form of record-keeping, it remains a vital component of the intervention process. This important component requires appropriate terminology and professionalism, which in occupational therapy is driven by the Occupational Therapy Practice Framework (AOTA, 2014), as well as the Guide to Occupational Therapy Practice (Moyers & Dale, 2007; Sames, 2014).

Purpose of Documentation

Through the use of written words, documentation is completed as a chronological record of the client's progress or story that serves as a basis for clinical reasoning, decision-making effectiveness of intervention, and need for occupational therapy services (Sames, 2015).

AOTA (2014) describes the following general purposes of documentation:

1. A communication tool for the health care team, client, and family.
2. A means of providing facts about a client from an occupational therapy perspective.
3. Justification or rationale for occupational therapy services, outcomes, clinical reasoning, professional judgment, and reimbursement.
4. A chronological record of client care and status regarding occupational therapy services.

Additional, specific purposes of documentation are the following:

- Accountability for actual intervention and time spent with client
- A method of recording results of evaluation, intervention, and re-evaluation
- A method of recording and measuring progress, status of client's condition, and response to intervention
- A required legal document that may be used as evidence in court cases

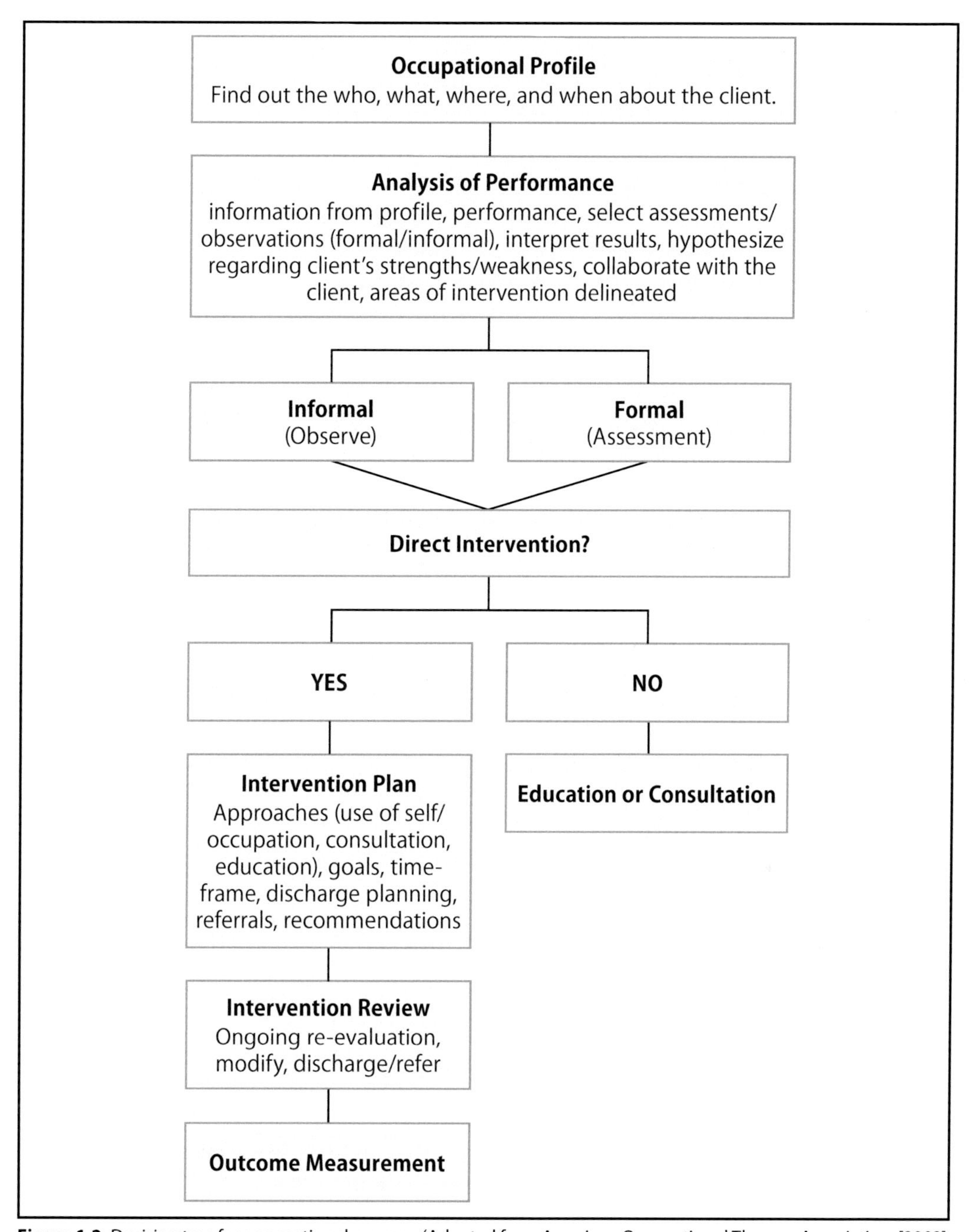

Figure 1-2. Decision tree for occupational process. (Adapted from American Occupational Therapy Association. [2002]. Occupational therapy practice framework. *American Journal of Occupational Therapy, 56*(6), 609-639.)

- A requirement in order to see progress and validate reimbursement by third-party payers
- An ethical responsibility of health care professionals
- Documents a baseline of function

- Provides continuity of care
- A permanent record of occurrences
- Allows for emphasis on observable, measurable changes in progress
- May communicate meaningful and functional outcomes
- Informs other team members of the specifics of each intervention session and allows a smooth transition into the next session, particularly in the event that the assigned therapist is unable to work with the same client
- Demonstrates the effectiveness of occupational therapy intervention
- Provides data for research and education

Important Considerations of Documentation

Good documentation skills require good writing skills and reflect the language specific to occupational therapy practice (Sames, 2015). Developing good writing skills is a process and requires close supervision and training from fieldwork training onward. It is important to consider who will read documentation. Therefore, words must be chosen carefully (Sames, 2015). Potential audiences may include the following:

- Other team members
- Peers
- Peer reviewers
- Accrediting agencies such as Joint Commission on Accreditation of Health care Organizations (JCAHO) and Commission on Accreditation of Rehabilitation Facilities (CARF)
- Insurance companies and third-party payers
- Clients and their family members
- Administrators
- Lawyers
- Researchers
- Any other chart reviewers

General Guidelines for Documentation

Documentation should be completed in a timely manner, not only because it is easy to forget the details of every client on a caseload, but also to provide up-to-date information on the client. For example, the client may have demonstrated new safety issues or recent progress in therapy. The next individual working with the client needs to know this information for safe and appropriate interventions and interactions. The therapist must demonstrate good time management skills, allowing for appropriate documentation time for each client. The time required for documentation depends on the type, which may include a daily note, initial evaluation, weekly reassessment, and/or discharge summaries. Typically, documentation is entered into the progress section of the client's chart or medical record.

Additional general documentation guidelines include the following:

- Be accurate and collect accurate information
- Be complete
- Use proper spelling and grammar

- Be concise and clear
- Avoid jargon. Jargon includes words that are typically understood by one discipline or group of professionals such as *compensatory techniques* or *minimal setup*. Unacceptable abbreviations should also be avoided (Sames, 2015)
- Avoid arrows, hyphens, etc.
- Be careful with buzzwords and "red flag" words. Buzzwords are considered to be popular or currently used words such as *collaborative* and *community*. The problem is that these terms may be unfamiliar to some audiences and may become unpopular over time. Red-flag words are terms that may, for example, put reimbursement of services in jeopardy. These words include *maintain* and *continued* (Sames, 2015)
- If it is not documented, it did not happen or does not exist
- Be timely for accuracy of memory and to not take away from time with client
- "Paint a verbal picture" (Sames, 2015)
- Focus on function, underlying cause, progress, and safety
- State expectations for progress, slow progress, or lack of progress
- Summarize need for skilled services

When to document:

- Upon admission
- Daily
- Weekly
- Monthly formal re-evaluation
- When change occurs, with progress or lack of progress
- Medical changes or complications or when client is placed "on hold" for therapy
- When physician needs information

Considerations for documentation:

- Discharge summary: show barriers to progress or effectiveness of intervention.
- Think about what you will write before doing it (students should do rough drafts on fieldwork until cleared by supervisors)
- Sign and date
- Check for grammatical/spelling errors
- Use blue/black pen—no erasing
- Cross errors out neatly with a single line and write "error," initials, and date next to the error
- Limit use of abbreviations; only use accepted ones
- Write legibly, including signature (or print name underneath or beside the signature)

General Documentation Standards

- Client identification: This includes the client's name and medical record number on each page of documentation.
- Date and type of contact: Each type of documentation should always be dated. Occasionally, it is also required to state the time of day and length of session provided. A heading should be given for the type of contact, such as a screening or evaluation.

- Type of documentation: The name of the department (e.g., Occupation Therapy/Rehabilitation) and the type of documentation (e.g., SOAP note) should be clearly delineated.
- Signature/countersignature: The practitioner must legibly sign his or her name, followed by the professional title (e.g., OTR/L). Room must be left for any required countersignatures, such as students. Signatures should be placed at the end of the documentation.
- Terminology: Only facility-accepted, professionally recognized terminology and abbreviations should be used.
- Corrections: Errors should be corrected by drawing a line through the word(s), initialing next to the error, and indicating the date. Only blue or black ink should be used. No erasable pens or correction liquid should be accepted.
- Confidentiality and handling of records: All official rules and regulations for confidentiality, storage, and disposal of records must be followed (AOTA, 2014).

Documentation Process

1. Client identification: referral/MD orders and contact note
2. Screening: chart review and actual screen
3. Initial evaluation process: use of assessment tools such as interview/Occupational Profile, observation, standardized/nonstandardized formats, and Analysis of Occupational Performance
4. Intervention process: intervention plan, setting of collaborative goals, select approaches, methods, tools, and strategies
5. Intervention implementation: how intervention is delivered and carried out
6. Intervention review: monitoring progress, targeting outcomes, and re-evaluate and adapt plan

Types and Formats of Documentation

The type and format of documentation used will depend on the setting in which the services take place. For example, many community-based settings do not have formal client charts or computerized systems of documentation. The facility may only have a folder that is considered the client's record. The documentation approach may also vary, depending on the team approach. For example, with a transdisciplinary approach to intervention in which the health care team's responsibilities are blurred, the contributors to the documentation process may not be the same with each session. This documentation may take a very formal format, such as a daily subjective, objective, assessment, and plan (SOAP) note or a less formal approach, such as a weekly narrative note, depending upon the third-party payer. The multidisciplinary approach to documentation typically involves standardized forms with Medicare as an example. For the most part, the type of documentation used is driven by the third-party payer, the intervention setting, and the client population, which are all considered the documentation "audience" (Schell et al., 2014).

Specific Types of Documentation

Screening Note

A screening note is a brief chart review, interview, and observation of the client in order to determine whether full evaluation is needed. No referral or billing is required. A brief contact note or specific screening form should be documented to either state that further evaluation is not recommended or to request a referral and evaluation.

Contact Note

A contact note is a brief narrative note containing the time spent with the client, the reason, and the type of screening, such as the following:

- Communicate that the referral was received, evaluation/discharge note was completed, or the reasons why it was not completed
- Document screenings
- Document all contacts with client and family
- Indicate missed sessions and refusals
- State that the evaluation was completed
- Indicate equipment given or splint fabricated and instructions issued
- Document any other pertinent issues that may occur between intervention sessions (e.g., if a client is observed to have a significant safety issue, such as a fall when a practitioner happens to be walking by the room, documenting the details of the event and how it was handled; Sames, 2015)

General Documentation Categories

- Initial evaluation report: After the physician referral is received, the therapist may be begin the process of gathering data through documentation review, observation, interview, and full hands-on assessments. Data is interpreted and documented, goals are set with time frame, and intervention plan/recommendations are communicated. Precautions and contraindications are highlighted along with the client's goals/expectations. The report is documented on an evaluation form specific to the facility or third-party payer (Sames, 2015).
- Intervention/progress note: The documentation of the actual intervention session may take many forms, as discussed later in this section. The practitioner will also objectively discuss the amount of assistance required to complete tasks, as well as the instructions and cuing needed. The assessment of the session may include documentation of the client's response to intervention and overall participation in therapy. A summary of progress toward goals with updates of goals and plan are documented (Sames, 2015).

  Typical components of the intervention note may include the following:

  - The date
  - Type of interventions: The practitioner will list the methods, modalities, group/individual, strategies, activities, adaptive equipment and/or techniques used during the session.
  - Length of session
  - Progress toward goals with updates and changes, as appropriate
  - Client's response to intervention
  - Comparison with previous reports and status
  - Time frame changes and recommendations
  - Equipment recommendations
  - Home program
  - Caregiver instruction
  - Plan/discharge recommendations with revised goals and plan, as appropriate

- Re-evaluation report/note: As evaluation is an ongoing process, it is very much interwoven within each intervention session. As such, the practitioner is informally re-evaluating on a continuous basis. Formal re-evaluations, and the forms used to complete them, will be conducted according to the facility's policy, as well as third-party payer needs. Re-evaluations may include the following:
    - Data recorded and reported regarding reassessment
    - Comparative analysis of findings and summary
    - Modification of goals
    - Update plan
    - Need for discharge
- Discharge note/discontinuation of service: Discharge from therapy may be due to the client achieving set goals, lack of progress, maximum benefits of therapy, insurance caps, or the client refusing to participate in therapy. The discharge note includes information to summarize the assessment, interventions, and outcomes of service. It may take various formats including a specific discharge form that may be created by the facility/program. The documentation summarizes the client's evaluation/intervention processes from beginning to end (Sames, 2015).

  Components of a discharge note should include the following:
    - The beginning and ending date of services
        - Related diagnosis
        - Precautions
        - Reason for occupational therapy referral
    - The therapy process/summary of intervention strategies
    - Re-evaluation, goal status, attainment, progress in therapy, reason why goals not achieved
    - Functional outcome of services
    - Number of completed sessions
    - Home programs, maintenance programs, and caregiver instructions
    - Recommendations/equipment needed
    - Follow-up plans and/or referrals for continued occupational therapy as well as other services in the continuum of care (Sames, 2015)
- MD report: Often reports are sent to the physician regarding the client's progress either on a monthly basis or with each scheduled visit. The format of the report depends on where the client is within the intervention process. For example, if the client is seeing the physician at a time for re-evaluation, this format may be used. If the client is close to discharge time, the particular note may be used. Physicians may have a specific format that they require or desire.

Computer-Based Documentation

Client documentation is rapidly shifting to a computer-based record and is often referred to as an *electronic health record* (EHR) or *electronic medial record* (EMR). Computerized systems are an alternative to paper charts or files, are more accessible to the health care team, and are an efficient means for recording and storing client data. In addition, physician referrals and communication between the health care team are more timely, therefore enhancing client care as well as third-party payment and billing procedures. Other benefits of using an EHR system include enhanced confidentiality, decreased medical errors (e.g., through eliminating handwriting legibility problems), cost-effectiveness (after initial implementation), assisting with client scheduling, decreasing the need for paper use and storage, ease of use and access, and overall efficiency of service delivery. Potential barriers to EHR use may include the cost of adopting and maintaining a computerized system, staff resistance to change from paper documentation, time and cost for training staff, availability of Internet access in some areas, and ongoing technical support of the electronic system (Sames, 2015).

Formats of Documentation

Any of the formats listed below may be included when creating computer programs for documentation.

SOAP Note

The SOAP note is a very well-known form of progress note. The acronym represents the four components of the note: the subjective, objective, assessment, and plan. This format provides a consistent structure for all disciplines to follow. The format also allows for a quick review of the client's status prior to intervention. The structure allows the therapist to follow trends and patterns that may occur during the intervention process, which makes the SOAP format very inter-disciplinary in nature.

Details of a SOAP Note

- S = Subjective: This is the client's report/perceptions of the problem, often documented as a quotation such as, "Client stated . . ." or "Client reported . . . ."
- O = Objective: The objective section consists of factual or professional information that is confirmed or validated by the therapist. Baseline data and/or progress on goals, observations, and client performance may be included. The information is often presented in a chronological or story format. The data is not interpreted here. The objective section may begin with "Client was seen for . . ." or "The intervention consisted of . . . ." A chronological listing of the interventions participated in follows.
- A = Assessment: The assessment is directly related to the subjective and objective sections. The therapist's professional opinion and analysis are documented. This analysis includes clarification of client goals and problems and the therapist's ratings of client progress. In this section, the subjective and objective data may be interpreted and a prioritized list of problems to be addressed may be developed.
- P = Plan: The plan section specifies the type, frequency, and duration of interventions to use in next session and/or in response to progress or lack of. Updated goals may be listed here. This section also includes discharge plans and home programs as appropriate. Specifically, this section should provide enough information for a substituting therapist to take over the next session, if needed.

Example of a SOAP Note

- S: "My right shoulder hurts only when I sleep on it."
- O: Intervention consisted of heat pack to right shoulder for 10 minutes; bilateral assistive active range of motion (AAROM) exercises including towel and dowel exercises, 15 repetitions/2 sets; client donned bra and shirt with moderate assist for right upper extremity (RUE). Client replaced clean clothes on low shelves of closet with minimal assist, ice pack placed on right shoulder for 5 minutes at end of session. During activity, client's pain assessed at right shoulder: 6/10 (on a scale of 0 to 10).

- A: Despite level of pain, client appeared happy with today's progress with AAROM and ADLs. Client seems to have a high tolerance for pain and occasionally requires cues to not push herself too hard.
- P: Educate client on pain management techniques such as visualization. Educate client on alternative positioning when sleeping to decrease shoulder pain. Increase AAROM to 20 repetitions, as tolerated. Attempt above ADL activities with no assistance, as tolerated.

DAP Note

The DAP note format is very similar to the SOAP note. The acronym represents the three components of the note: description, assessment, and plan. This format also provides a consistent structure for all disciplines to follow, although it is not used as frequently. Similarly to the SOAP note, the interdisciplinary format also allows for a quick review and the ability to follow trends and patterns.

Details of a DAP Note

- D = Description: This is the findings section of the note, which combines the subjective and objective components of the SOAP note. This section documents quotes or paraphrases regarding the client's perceptions, description of the session, observations, results/findings, and facts.
- A = Assessment: This section documents exactly the same information as in the assessment section of the SOAP note.
- P = Plan: This section documents exactly the same information as in the plan section of the SOAP note.

Example of DAP Note (adapted from above SOAP note)

- D: "My right shoulder hurts only when I sleep on it." The intervention consisted of heat pack to right shoulder for 10 minutes; bilateral AAROM exercises including towel and dowel exercises, 15 repetitions/2 sets; and client donned bra and shirt with moderate assist for RUE. Client replaced clean clothes on low shelves of closet with minimal assist, ice pack placed on right shoulder for 5 minutes at end of session. During activity, client's pain assessed at right shoulder: 6/10 (on a scale of 0 to 10).
- A: Despite level of pain, client appeared happy with today's progress with AAROM and ADLs. Client seems to have a high tolerance for pain and occasionally requires cues to not push herself too hard.
- P: Educate client on pain management techniques such as visualization. Educate client on alternative positioning when sleeping to decrease shoulder pain. Increase AAROM to 20 repetitions, as tolerated. Attempt above ADL activities with no assistance, as tolerated.

Narrative Note

Narrative notes do not have a specific structure as do SOAP and DAP notes. This format typically begins with objective data, follows with interpretive/assessment information, and ends with a review of objectives met as well as plans for the next session. This narrative note also tells a story that allows for more flexibility in communicating information. The writer is responsible for including all information in a smooth, flowing note, with as much detail as needed. The SOAP or DAP note can be easily converted to a narrative format (Sames, 2009).

Table 1-2

Sample Documentation Form

Client Name	Date	Date	Date	Date
Heat Pack	Time and body part			
Therapeutic Exercise	Body part(s), exercises, repetitions, sets			
Physical Agent Modalities	Modality used, intensity, duration, other settings			
ADL activities	Activity, level of assistance needed, adaptive equipment			
Client Education	Topic and materials issued			
Ice Pack	Time and body part			

Adapted from American Occupational Therapy Association. (2002). Occupational therapy practice framework. *American Journal of Occupational Therapy, 56*(6), 609-639.

Example of Narrative Note (adapted from above SOAP note)

Today, the client stated she is experiencing pain when sleeping on her right shoulder. She was seen for heat pack to right shoulder for 10 minutes; bilateral AAROM exercises including towel and dowel exercises, 15 repetitions/2 sets; and client donned bra and shirt with moderate assist for RUE. The client replaced clean clothes on low shelves of closet with minimal assist, ice pack placed on right shoulder for 5 minutes at end of session. During activity, the client was assessed for right shoulder pain: 6/10 (on a scale of 0 to 10). Despite her level of pain, the client appeared happy with today's progress with AAROM and ADL. She seems to have a high tolerance for pain and occasionally requires cues to not push herself too hard. The next session should provide client education on pain management techniques such as visualization and on alternative positioning when sleeping to decrease shoulder pain. If tolerated, increase AAROM to 20 repetitions. Also, if tolerated, attempt above ADL activities with no assistance.

Flow Sheet/Checklist

There are several advantages to using flow sheets when documenting. They offer a concise format for tracking progress and allow for a quick look at the documentation, much data to be compiled in a small space, and easy coverage of the client's care, if needed. Flow sheets may also include formatting data with graphs, tables, and charts.

The disadvantages of a flow sheet/checklist primarily include the limited space for documenting any psychiatric issues, descriptions, or client reactions that are necessary for holistic client-centered interventions. This format cannot replace progress notes, which should be completed on a weekly, biweekly, or as-needed basis. A basic example of a flow sheet for an outpatient setting (based on the earlier example) can be found in Table 1-2.

Documentation Examples

- Screening: contact, SOAP note, DAP note, narrative note, or screening form created.
  Frequency: typically one time with possible follow-up as needed.
- Contact: narrative note, checklist/flow sheet.
  Frequency: depends on purpose of note.
- Evaluation: standardized/nonstandardized forms.

Frequency: one formal evaluation.

- Intervention: SOAP note, DAP note, narrative note, flow sheet/checklist.
  Frequency: depends on format(s) used; may be daily, weekly, or monthly.
- Re-evaluation: standardized/nonstandardized forms, SOAP note, DAP note, or narrative note.
- MD Report: SOAP note, DAP note, narrative note, or re-evaluation format.
  Frequency: written on appointment basis, monthly, or upon discharge.
- Discharge summary: discharge summary form, re-evaluation form, narrative note.
  Frequency: upon discharge.

Writing Goals

Effective goal writing is a vital component of the evaluation and intervention processes. It is a collaborative process that includes the therapist, occupational therapy assistant, client, and family/caregivers. The purpose of goal setting is to measure the effectiveness of the chosen interventions (Sames, 2015). In addition, goal writing serves to indicate changes in baseline skills that are expected to occur as a result of the intervention plan.

The specific goal-writing methods used depend on the models or frames of reference chosen, the intervention setting, the types of outcomes anticipated (Sames, 2015), and the intervention approach in the Framework (AOTA, 2014). This section will discuss these specifics mentioned above.

Considerations when writing goals:

- Goals should be created in collaboration with client/family.
- Consider the client's present condition or diagnosis.
- Consider the client's limitations and strengths.
- Does the client have any complications secondary to his or her conditions?
- Client's medical history, precautions, and prognosis.
- What is the facility, environment, or setting in which therapy will occur?
- What is the client's discharge environment?
- What is the timeline for therapy?
- Are there any clinical pathways , standards, protocols when working with this client?
- What frames of reference will be followed?
- Does the client have insurance? What is the client's insurance? Are there any insurance limitations? Is the client paying?
- What are the desired outcomes of therapy?
- What is the predicted length of stay for this client?
- What are the considered continuum of care and discharge plans/options for this client?
- What are the client's/family's needs and goals?

General Types of Goals

Remediative/Restorative/Rehabilitative

This type of goal is used when a client no longer can perform tasks due to an illness or injury. The goals are written to change a functional level or achieve a stated function. For example, within 2 weeks, the client will toilet herself independently while using the dominant upper extremity (Sames, 2015).

Habilitative

This type of goal attempts to teach a client new skills that were never taught previously. Often, this type of goal is used with clients who have developmental delays. For example, by the end of the school year, the client will be able to participate in physical education for 15 minutes at a time (Sames, 2015).

Maintenance

This type of goal is used when the client has not demonstrated further progress in therapy. Maintenance attempts to sustain the client at the present level of function without losing gains. This approach to goal writing is typically used in long-term settings and on discharge from therapy. For example: Upon discharge from therapy, the client will continue to be independent in her assisted living situation (Sames, 2015).

Modification/Compensation/Adaptation

This type of goal adapts the context, environment, or the tools regarding the activity, instead of changing the client's abilities. For example: Within 1 week, the client will independently don socks with the use of a sock aide (Sames, 2015).

Preventative

This type of goal addresses potential "at risk" issues with occupational performance. For example, the client will demonstrate three proper body mechanic techniques when caring for her child, within 3 weeks (Sames, 2015).

Health Promotion

This type of goal may be used more frequently in emerging practice areas. The emphasis of this approach is on enhancing contexts and activities in order to maximize occupational participation. Goals may be addressed with clients individually or in a group, community, or organization. For example, within 1 month, all students of Anytown Elementary School will be educated by the occupational therapist in proper body mechanics when wearing backpacks (Sames, 2015).

These types of goals actually parallel the Occupational Therapy Intervention Approaches, as listed in Table 7 of the Framework document (AOTA, 2014). Therefore, the goal-writing process will guide the choice and process of the interventions. Before beginning intervention, it is important to consider the goal-writing and intervention approaches.

Formats and Methods of Goal Writing

There are many formats or guides for writing goals. Generally, goals involve the "who, what, where, and when" approach. The who is typically the client and/or caregiver involved in the goal/intervention. The what is the occupational performance skill or behavior to be addressed. The where may be included to state the environment in which the behavior or skill will occur. The when may be included to address the time of day when the skill or behavior will be addressed.

Action words or verbs should be used when writing goals to describe the client's behavior or skill to be addressed. Action words include *bathes, dresses, eats, walks, reaches,* and *zippers.*

Goals must be measurable, observable, and functional. They must describe a change in the client's occupational performance skill or behavior, how much (measurably) the behavior will change, and how this behavior will be measured. The ultimate intent in goal writing is to measure to show progress.

When considering the functional aspect or outcomes of goal writing, it is important to consider relating the goal to meaningful, purposeful aspects of the client's life. This is achieved through a collaborative approach with the client. Functional goals may include those that enhance occupational performance, improve skills, improve role performance, promote health and wellness, prevent dysfunction, and/or improve quality of life.

Types of Outcomes

1. Occupational performance
2. Prevention
3. Health and wellness
4. Quality of life
5. Participation
6. Role competence
7. Well-being
8. Occupational justice (AOTA, 2014)

More specifically, there are several formal methods that guide goal writing. One will be described in the following section.

ABCD Method

The ABCD method of writing goals was developed by Ginge Kettenbach (1990). Each letter describes a specific component included in each client-centered goal.

- A: The audience is typically the client, although in certain circumstances, the goal may be specific to the caregiver. (This text refers to the audience as the *client*. Depending on the facility/environment, the audience may be referred to as the *patient, consumer,* or *student.*)
- B: The behavior is specifically what is expected of the audience. Sames (2009) describes the behavior as something that is seen, heard, done, or said. The behavior represents an action such as dressing, bathing, eating, speaking, or walking. The choice of words in the goal writing should represent these actions.
- C: The conditions are specific circumstances under which behavior must occur, support the behavior, clarify the goal, or state how much cuing or assistance is needed (Sames, 2009). For example, the client may need minimal assistance to feed himself or maximal verbal cuing for safety in the shower.
- D: The degree represents the measurement component of the goal. In order for a goal to be measurable, it must include a realistic, specific time frame and a duration, frequency, percentage, or degree that quantifies the amount of function the client will attempt to achieve.

Sample Goal Using ABCD Method

Within 2 weeks (degree), the client (audience) will independently (degree) feed herself (behavior) using an adapted fork and spoon (condition).

Specific Types of Goals

The two specific types of goals are long-term goals (LTG) and short-term goals (STG). LTGs tend to be more global in nature and generally address occupational performance. Most often, only one LTG is written in order to set the stage for the STGs. The duration of an LTG is typically set to discharge time or the time when therapy will end. Although LTGs are measurable, observable, and functional, they again tend to be more general in nature.

Examples:

- Client will achieve full independence in order to be discharged to live alone at home in 4 weeks.
- Client will complete a 4-hour workday, independently, within 4 weeks.

STGs are often referred to as objectives. The duration of STGs is typically shorter and they are very specific in nature, particularly in terms of being measurable, observable, and functional. STGs address occupations and are written in order to be up- or downgraded as the client's functional abilities change. Typically, multiple STGs are written that directly relate back to the LTG. STGs should also have functional outcomes.

Examples:

- Client will attend to a group task for 30 minutes with only one verbal cue for redirection in order to prepare for return to work within 2 weeks.
- Client will complete upper extremity (UE) dressing with minimal assistance using reacher and sock aide within 2 weeks in order to live alone.
- Client will increase RUE shoulder flexion by 40 degrees within 2 weeks in order to complete ADLs.
- Client will ambulate to bathroom, using rolling walker and contact guard within 2 weeks in order to return home.

Progress Levels

- Total assistance (dependence) = client does 0%
- Maximum assistance = client does 1% to 24% of task
- Moderate assistance = client does 24% to 75% of task
- Minimum assistance = client does 75% or more of task
- Standby assistance = client does 100% and has supervision
- Independent status = (I)
- Contact guard
- Close supervision/Standby
- Distant supervision/Standby
- Setup
- Adaptive equipment
- Different types of cuing (Sames, 2015)

Legal Considerations

- Accuracy
- Completeness
- Timeliness
- Gaps in documentation/blanks
- Objectivity
- Corrections/erasing
- Negative statements
- Sufficient MD orders
- Possible denials of payment
- Tamper-free
- Client can see records
- Unalterable
- Include date and time
- Legible signature
- Confidentiality
- Health Insurance Portability and Accountability Act (HIPAA)
- Abbreviations
- Document correspondence and teaching sessions
- Grammar/spelling
- Fraud/plagiarism

Confidentiality Issues

- Not taking home paperwork bearing client's name
- Permission from client to use/share
- Right to see
- HIPAA
- Family Educational Rights and Privacy Act (FERPA)
- Storage of documents

Common Mistakes in Documentation

- Failure to state affected body part or side of body
- Failure to state actual motion
- Failure to state in measurable terms

- Failure to attach time frame
- Failure to use functional outcome
- Failure to include functional activities

Summary Questions

1. Describe the Occupational Therapy Practice Framework as if to another health care professional.
2. Name and discuss the components of the evaluation and intervention processes.
3. Discuss the general differences between the approaches to intervention.
4. Discuss the components of the documentation process in occupational therapy intervention.
5. Discuss the "bottom-up" approach to intervention.

References

American heritage dictionary of the English language (4th ed.). (2000). Boston, MA: Houghton Mifflin.

American Occupational Therapy Association. (2010). Standards of practice for occupational therapy. *American Journal of Occupational Therapy, 64*(Suppl.), S10-S11.

American Occupational Therapy Association. (2013). Guidelines for documentation of occupational therapy [Supplemental material]. *American Journal of Occupational Therapy, 67*(6), S32-S38.

American Occupational Therapy Association. (2014). Occupational therapy practice framework (3rd ed.). *American Journal of Occupational Therapy, 68*(Suppl. 1), S1-S48.

Bruce, M. A. G., & Borg, B. A. (2002). *Psychosocial frames of reference* (3rd ed.). Thorofare, NJ: SLACK Incorporated.

Christiansen, C., & Baum, C. M. (1991). *Occupational therapy: Overcoming human performance deficits.* Thorofare, NJ: SLACK Incorporated.

Christiansen, C., Baum, C., & Bass, J. D. (2015). *Occupational therapy: Performance, participation, and well-being* (4th ed). Thorofare, NJ: SLACK Incorporated.

Cole, M. (2011). *Group dynamics in occupational therapy* (4th ed.). Thorofare, NJ: SLACK Incorporated.

Fisher, A. G. (2002). A model for planning and implementing top-down client-centered, and occupation-based occupational therapy interventions. Short course presented at University of New Hampshire.

Gibson, J. W., & Schkade, J. K. (1997). Occupational adaptation intervention with patients with cerebrovascular accident: a clinical study. *American Journal of Occupational Therapy, 51*(7), 523-529.

Jacobs, K., & Simon, L. (Eds). (2015). *Quick reference dictionary for occupational therapy* (6th ed.). Thorofare, NJ: SLACK Incorporated.

Kettenbach, G. (1990). *Writing SOAP notes.* Philadelphia, PA: F.A. Davis.

Kielhofner, G. (1995). *A model of human occupation: Theory and application* (2nd ed.). Baltimore, MD: Williams and Wilkins.

Kielhofner, G., & Burke, J. P. (1980). A model of human occupation, Part 1: Conceptual framework and content. *American Journal of Occupational Therapy, 34*(9), 572-581.

Law, M. (1998). *Client-centered occupational therapy.* Thorofare, NJ: SLACK Incorporated.

Law, M., Baum, C., & Dunn, W. (2005). *Measuring occupational performance* (2nd ed.). Thorofare, NJ: SLACK Incorporated.

Law, M., Cooper, B., Strong, S., Stewart, D., Rigby, P., & Letts, L. (1996). The person-environment-occupation model: A transactive approach to occupational performance. *Canadian Journal of Occupational Therapy, 63,* 9-23.

Law, M., & MacDermid, J. (Eds). (2014). *Evidence-based rehabilitation: A guide to practice* (3rd ed.). Thorofare, NJ: SLACK Incorporated.

Mann, W. C., Llanes, C., Justiss, M. D., & Tomita, M. (2004). Frail older adults' self-report of their most important assistive device. *Occupational Therapy Journal of Research, 24*(1), 4-14.

Moyers, P. A., & Dale, L. M. (2007). *The guide to occupational therapy practice* (2nd ed.). Bethesda, MD: AOTA Press.

Pendleton, H. M., & Schultz-Krohn, W. (2013). *Pedretti's Occupational Therapy Practice Skills for Physical Dysfunction* (7th ed.). St. Louis, MO: Elsevier.

Radomski, M. V., & Trombly Latham, C. A. (2014). *Occupational Therapy for Physical Dysfunction* (7th ed). Philadelphia, PA: Lippincott Williams & Wilkins.

Sames, K. (2014). *Documenting occupational therapy practice* (3rd ed.). Upper Saddle River, NJ: Pearson Education, Inc.

Schell, B. A., Gillen, G., & Scaffa, M. E. (2014). *Willard and Spackman's occupational therapy* (12th ed.). Philadelphia, PA: Lippincott Williams & Wilkins.

Schultz, S., & Schkade, J. K. (1992a). Occupational adaptation: Toward a holistic approach for contemporary practice, part 1. *American Journal of Occupational Therapy, 46*(9), 829-837.

Schultz, S., & Schkade, J. K. (1992b). Occupational adaptation: Toward a holistic approach for contemporary practice, part 2. *American Journal of Occupational Therapy, 46*(10), 917-925.

Toglia, J. (1991). Generalization of intervention: A multicontext approach to cognitive perceptual impairment in adults with brain injury. *American Journal of Occupational Therapy, 45*(6), 505-516.

Yerxa, E. J. (1998). Health and human spirit of occupation. *American Journal of Occupational Therapy, 52*, 412-418.

Zoltan, B. (2007). *Vision, perception, and cognition* (4th ed.). Thorofare, NJ: SLACK Incorporated.

2 Foundational Skills for Functional Activities

Deanna Proulx-Sepelak, MHA, OTR/L

Chapter Objectives

By the end of this chapter, the student will be able to do the following:

- Comprehend the underlying or foundational skills an individual requires to successfully engage in functionally meaningful tasks.
- Describe specific theories/frames of reference as related to foundational skills.
- Comprehend safety issues as related to foundational skills.
- Delineate between the role of the occupational therapist and the occupational therapy assistant as they pertain to foundational skills.
- Comprehend and identify psychological implications as related to impairments in foundational skills.
- Comprehend the impact of modes of injury on foundational skills.
- Identify restorative techniques for impairments in specific foundational skills.
- Identify maintenance strategies for general activities of daily living (ADLs) that incorporate foundational skills.
- Identify general precautions and contraindications for various foundational skill interventions such as physical agent modalities (PAMs) and therapeutic exercise.

Chapter Overview

The goal of this chapter is to outline the underlying skills that an individual requires to successfully engage in functionally meaningful tasks. These foundational skills, in the order that they are presented within this chapter, include client factors of pain and edema, sensation, joint range of motion (ROM), strength, endurance, coordination, muscle tone, and skills of cognition and perception. Material within this chapter will highlight restorative or remedial approaches in these skill areas. Subsequent chapters within the text will then analyze the adaptive/compensatory approaches as related to the specific areas of occupation outlined by the Occupational Therapy Practice Framework document (American Occupational Therapy Association [AOTA], 2014).

Meriano C, Latella D.
Occupational Therapy Interventions: Function and Occupations, Second Edition (pp 35-136).

As a precursor to this chapter, it is important to reiterate the collaborative relationship that exists between the registered occupational therapist and the certified occupational therapy assistant. As health care becomes increasingly driven by the efficient utilization of resources, many rehabilitative establishments are trending toward the use of registered occupational therapists as evaluative administrators and occupational therapy assistants as both collaborators in developing the client-centered intervention plan and actual facilitators of that plan, given appropriate supervision. This chapter is written using *occupational therapist* as a general term and with full reference to both occupational therapists and occupational therapy assistants as vital components of the rehabilitative team.

How do restorative approaches differ from those with an adaptive or compensatory focus? Restoration, per the Framework document, is "an intervention approach designed to change client variables to establish a skill or ability which has not yet developed or to restore a skill or ability which has been impaired" (AOTA, 2014, p. S33). This definition is further simplified in *Taber's Cyclopedic Medical Dictionary* (2009) as those techniques implemented with the "intention of remedy" or to "cure and relieve disease (or illness)." In general, approaches considered restorative are those that occupational therapists implement to enhance or improve an underlying impairment, while those approaches considered compensatory in nature are implemented by occupational therapists with the intent to adapt for an underlying condition or deficit that has been deemed long-standing.

According to Zoltan (2007), intervention takes one of two forms: a top-down or bottom-up approach. With a top-down approach (refer to Chapter 1), the occupational therapist adjusts the activity or occupational performance with the goal of promoting independence by using adaptive and compensatory techniques. Conversely, a bottom-up approach addresses underlying dysfunction in the foundation skill areas and assumes that the client will improve in functional ability as a result. An example of the concept of restoration is as follows: The occupational therapist may conduct an ADL session with a client who demonstrates deficits in the areas of coordination, strength, ROM, and cognition. Here, the occupational therapist is fostering improvement in the foundational skills through repetition in a familiar task, not adapting the task as one would in a compensatory or top-down approach. It is important to note that this concept has been simplified here for clarity and that in most circumstances occupational therapists will combine top-down and bottom-up approaches in order to maximize individualized outcomes (Zoltan, 2007).

Occupational therapists emphasize the importance of the client-centered or client-driven approach and formulate intervention with clients, not for clients. To do so, the occupational therapist recognizes and respects all clients as individuals with a unique set of factors, performance skills, patterns, contexts, and priorities that guide their engagement in meaningful occupation. This principle is outlined more specifically in Chapter 1 and is re-emphasized here to underscore the significance of maintaining a client-centered approach even when focusing on foundational skill areas. Furthermore, the occupational therapist must consider clients' safety, their psychosocial adaptation to the given illness or injury, and their individual perception of pain. A clear respect for these individual attributes not only supports the overall well-being of a client but also directly contributes to the degree of therapeutic rapport needed during the ever-critical, initial stages of intervention and healing.

All clients are individuals with their own personal means of coping and adaptation to a life-altering event such as illness or injury. This process occurs at differing levels and time frames for each client. As outlined by Falvo in *Medical and Psychosocial Aspects of Chronic Illness and Disability* (2009): "Some actively confront their condition, learning new skills or actively engaging in intervention to control or manage the condition. Others defend themselves from stress and the realities of the diagnosis by denying its seriousness, ignoring intervention recommendations, or refusing to learn new skills . . . Still others cope by engaging in self-destructive behavior . . . (that) has detrimental effects on their physical condition" (p. 12). In all, occupational therapists must respect that this process of acceptance is occurring throughout the intervention process, must be sensitive to it, and whenever possible provide education and advocacy in support of clients and their families or caregivers.

The occupational therapist will then work to develop the intervention plan both in collaboration with the client and with careful attention paid to the specific aspects of any given activity that enables success in the execution of occupation. The Framework (AOTA, 2014) identifies this as activity demands. Of significance to the discussion on foundational skills for functional activity is the manner in which aspects of activity demands are categorized. This includes such items as required actions and performance skills, body functions, and body structures. Required actions and performance skills are further defined by the Framework as "actions required by the client that are an inherent part of the activity" (2014, p. S32). These include motor, process, and social interaction skills. Required body functions are defined as "the physiological functions of body systems . . . required to support the actions used to perform the activity" (2014, p. S32). And required body structures are "anatomical parts of the body such as organs, limbs, and their components (which support body function)" (2014, p. S32). In essence, these three aforementioned aspects of activity demands per the Framework (AOTA, 2014) specifically identify those underlying foundational skills necessary for the engagement in all meaningful activity and will serve as the focus of this chapter.

Each foundation skills subsection within this chapter specifically presents any applicable and related definitions, potential modes of injury or illness that may lead to a deficit in that foundation skill area, and typical occupational therapy restoration techniques for improving that skill. Diagrams, figures, and tables are provided as a means of summarizing data within each subsection. In addition, special considerations and possible maintenance program components have been included.

Restorative Techniques for Pain and Edema

The consideration of individually perceived pain for each of our clients is critical to the success an occupational therapist will have during the restorative or healing stage of recovery. In most cases, the degree of perceived pain will present as either one of the greatest enablers or barriers to the degree of success a client will experience during the rehabilitative process. Restorative intervention generally begins just after an injury or onset of illness, and as a result, much of our intervention choices may further aggravate the degree of discomfort our clients experience. Therefore, the occupational therapist must prioritize pain management within the development of the intervention plan, making it a foundational skill for functional activity within the context of this textbook.

Pain is notoriously difficult to measure accurately. This is due to the subjective nature in which our clients report it: a symptom experienced internally that may not necessarily be observed externally. Although clients may be asked to report their pain using the traditional rating scale method, it is the therapist's ethical duty to establish priority of that identified pain and infuse strategies that address it in daily, weekly, or even monthly intervention sessions. These strategies should not only allow clients an avenue to openly express perceived pain, but also to include techniques within the realm of occupational therapy that allow for the effective management and relief of the pain.

Definitional Analysis

Pain is defined by the Framework (AOTA, 2014) as a body function specific to sensation. For further analysis, pain is described in *Taber's Cyclopedic Medical Dictionary* (2009) as "an unpleasant sensory and emotional experience arising from actual or potential tissue damage or described in terms of such damage. Pain includes not only the perception of an uncomfortable stimulus but also the response to that perception" (p. 1680). Through these definitions, one is better able to appreciate pain, not only as a basic body function, but also as a foundational skill required for the successful engagement in all meaningful occupation. For example, the perception or fear of exacerbating pain may inhibit a client's ability to sleep sufficiently (area of occupation), to attend to others (specific mental function), or to produce efficient movement (neuromusculoskeletal and movement-related functions). A client's pain may then affect his or her performance skills including motor skills, process, and social interaction skills (such as gesturing, posturing, engaging, or expressing oneself). It is through analyzing the specifics of this definition that we are able to recognize the true, potentially devastating effects of our clients' experiences with pain.

Modes of Injury or Illness

A review of the typical modes of injury or illness is not and should not be emphasized when discussing pain specifically. Again, pain is a subjectively perceived sensation with potentially profound effects on a client's ability to succeed with occupational therapy intervention. What is of importance is not necessarily the mode from which the pain occurs, but rather, the existence of it.

Pain may exist secondary to a very wide array of health conditions. In many cases, pain perceived by a client is not in isolation, but secondary to another cause such as an injury to the body. Therefore, when considering effective restorative techniques to address pain, the occupational therapist will also employ methods that address any potential underlying causes for the pain. This includes attention to the physiological response of the body to injury or insult (e.g., inflammation or edema).

Restorative techniques for addressing pain and edema are appropriately selected given careful attention to the natural healing process of the human body. As described by Starkey (2013), injuries to tissues require the body system to initiate a repair response. This response calls upon both the vascular and immune systems to reduce loss of blood, accumulate leukocytes and lymphocytes as protective mechanisms, and begin the process of tissue regeneration. This repair response occurs over the period of days to months and directly dictates the type of methods that are appropriate and effective for the occupational therapist to implement. The initial phase, or inflammatory phase of healing, begins immediately following the injury and is characterized by erthromatosis (condition of redness) or cyanosis (blueness of skin), warmth, swelling, and pain at the site of injury. "Inflammation has a bad reputation as an unwanted and unneeded part of the body's response to injury. Nothing could be further from the truth. Inflammation is a necessary part of the healing process. However, if the duration or intensity of the inflammation is excessive, the process becomes detrimental" (Starkey, 2013, p. 14). This quotation clearly demonstrates the purpose of edema, however when this edema persists, appropriate intervention method selection when addressing pain and edema in conjunction with the biological healing process must be addressed (Starkey, 2013).

Conditions typically related to the sudden, or acute, onset of pain and localized edema include fractures, sprains, strains, tears, lacerations, arthritides, and musculoskeletal disorders such as exacerbated lateral epicondylitis or carpal tunnel syndrome. In addition, neurological damage resulting in a lack of motor function may also contribute to edema and pain. Refer to Table 2-1 for a summary of restorative techniques in both the acute and subacute phases of healing as they relate to addressing pain and Table 2-2 for those related specifically to edema.

When symptoms of pain and edema last for greater lengths of time following the onset of injury, they are often considered chronic in nature. Pain or edema that has not been properly addressed in the acute phase, or that is minor enough to avoid detection for a prolonged period of time, or is further exacerbated by such factors as prolonged immobility and general deconditioning, is often

Table 2-1

Remedial Pain Techniques of the Biomechanical Theory According to Phase of Healing

Health Condition	Remedial Techniques per Phase of Healing
Pain, including soft-tissue injuries, fractures, lacerations, sprains, strains, tears, arthritides, musculoskeletal disorders	Acute phase: Cold thermal modalities, nonthermal ultrasound, splinting for protection, passive range of motion (PROM), active assistive range of motion (AAROM), active range of motion (AROM), iontophoresis Subacute phase: Hot and/or cold thermal modalities, ultrasound, PROM, AAROM, AROM, manual therapies, phonophoresis, aquatic rehabilitation

Table 2-2

Remedial Edema Techniques of the Biomechanical Theory According to Phase of Healing

Health Condition	Remedial Techniques per Phase of Healing
Edema, including soft-tissue injuries, fractures, lacerations, sprains, strains, tears, arthritides, musculoskeletal disorders	Acute phase: Cold thermal modalities, nonthermal ultrasound, compression garments, compression pumps, compression wrapping, elevation, PROM, AAROM, AROM Subacute phase: Hot and/or cold thermal modalities, thermal ultrasound, compression garments, compression pumps, compression wrapping, retrograde massage, elevation, PROM, AAROM, AROM, aquatic rehabilitation, manual lymph drainage

associated with the development of chronic conditions (Starkey, 2013). Conditions that may result in chronic pain or edema include cancers, amputations, fibromyalgia, complex regional pain syndrome, and nerve injuries or entrapments. Longer-term symptoms associated with multiple exacerbations of arthritis and musculoskeletal disorders, such as lateral epicondylitis or carpal tunnel syndrome, may also be considered chronic in certain circumstances. Therefore, a discussion as to techniques used by occupation therapy for addressing chronic pain and edema (see Table 2-5) can be found later in the "Maintenance" subheading of this section.

Intervention choices for edema are based not only on whether it is acute or chronic in nature but also on other contributing factors. As described by Artzberger and White (2011), these factors include the cause of the edema. It can be from a single injury such as trauma or from a systemic diagnosis such as stroke. Other contributing factors, such as blood clots, lymphatic function, and cardiac function must also be considered. The cause of the edema itself will dictate whether the intervention approach is localized or generalized and is executed with careful attention paid to potential contributing factors. For a complete list of precautions, see Table 2-22.

Restorative Techniques: Biomechanical Frame of Reference

Restorative strategies for pain (see Table 2-1) and edema (see Table 2-2) are guided by the tenets found in the biomechanical frame of reference that applies principles of physics to voluntary human movement (Cole & Tufano, 2008). Methods typically identified with this frame include both range of motion and the use of PAMs.

Physical Agent Modalities

It is important to note that the use of PAMs by occupation therapists is often regulated by state-specific legislation and licensure laws. This legislation is enacted as a means of protected clients from the array of potential contraindications that may arise secondary to the implementation of a PAM. Refer to Tables 2-21 through 2-24 for a summary of the potential indications and contraindications of PAMs most readily employed by the occupation therapist. These regulations vary from state to state; some require continuing education or certification beyond the competency level required for registration, while others require the prescription of the medical doctor. It is the occupation therapist's responsibility to be readily aware of their own governing state's legislature regarding the use of modalities as well as the AOTA's position paper on the use of PAMs in general. The AOTA position paper regarding the use of PAMs is available for purchase from the AOTA (refer to Appendix A for additional contact information). PAMs, as discussed in the content of this chapter, will be outlined in general to accurately illustrate this point.

Superficial thermal modalities include the use of heat and/or cold for their counteractive effects on injury. Cold modalities, including ice packs, ice massage, and vapocoolant sprays, are implemented for the purpose of desensitizing pain receptors and minimizing edema in the acute stages of healing. In general, prefabricated gel-based ice packs are cooled to approximately 0°C to 18°C (32°F to 65°F) and applied for 20 to 30 minutes. Starkey recommends application directly to the skin for the most benefit and to wrap the pack in order to compress skin tissue, again increasing the depth of the modality (2014). In practice, however, most clients tolerate the modality better with a light pillowcase wrapped around the cold pack to buffer the skin slightly. This is also beneficial for infection control reasons. Ice massage is a technique in which frozen water in the form of a popsicle is applied in a rubbing fashion directed to the inflamed and/or painful area for 5 to 10 minutes (Starkey, 2013). Vapocoolant sprays are also utilized for short-term relief pain caused by muscle spasms and trigger points. When utilizing vapocoolant sprays, a client is typically positioned with the identified muscle on passive stretch or lengthened state. The spray is applied two to three times in a rhythmic, sweeping, unidirectional manner along the length of the muscle while producing a passively progressive stretch (Houglum, 2010). The stretch is then released in a smooth and gradual manner. It should be noted that if either the client or therapist is pregnant, this modality is contraindicated.

Heat modalities tend to be strictly contraindicated in the acute phase, but are implemented widely in the subacute and chronic phases of the healing process. The occupational therapist may use commercial hot packs, paraffin wax baths that provide circumferential heating to all surfaces (very common in subacute arthritis), fluidotherapy (Chattanooga Group) units in which the extremity is placed while warmed air (also has a nonheated setting) circulates grated corn husks within the enclosure, or ultrasound at a continuous setting to produce the desired effects of heat on subacute or chronic pain and edema. Each of these identified PAMs is applied for approximately 15 to 20 minutes, with the use of a protective barrier for the skin, to promote tissue healing (Cameron, 2009; Starkey, 2013).

Iontophoresis (Figure 2-1) is indicated to promote healing, decrease pain, and minimize edema. Under the direction of a physician, this PAM uses low-amplitude electric currents to deliver prescription medications such as corticosteroids (anti-inflammatory) or analgesics transdermally to

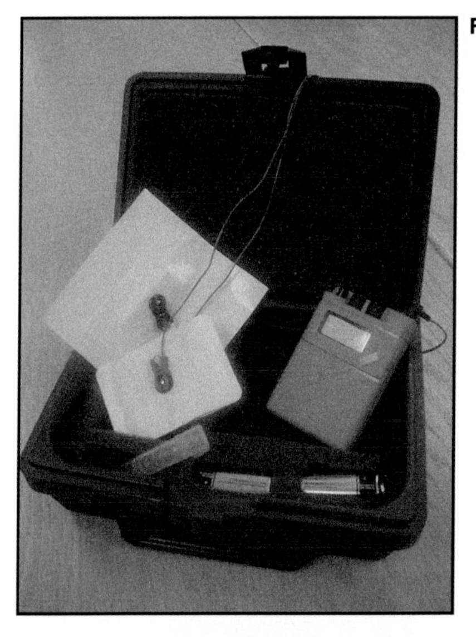

Figure 2-1. Iontophoresis unit.

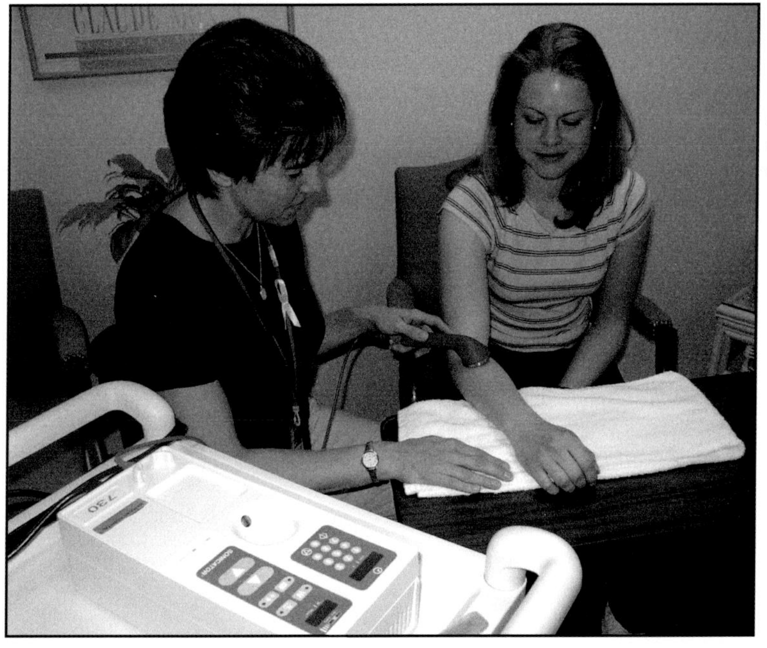

Figure 2-2. Demonstration of ultrasound application with prescribed medication, formally termed *phonophoresis*, as an intervention for pain and edema associated with subacute lateral epicondylitis.

the direct site of injury. This restorative pain and edema technique is found to be very effective for many clients (Cameron, 2009; Starkey, 2013). However, careful attention must be paid by the occupational therapist to the precautions and contraindications (see Table 2-21) inherent to the use of this PAM and to the client-specific tolerance of an electrical modality.

Ultrasound, briefly mentioned previously, can also be implemented with the use of medication to produce a similar response to that of iontophoresis. When ultrasound is used in this manner, it is called *phonophoresis* (Figure 2-2). This process uses transcutaneous prescription medications, such as corticosteroids, which permeate through the skin and directly to the site of injury via sound waves. The sound waves provided by the ultrasonic transducer are set to a nonthermal or

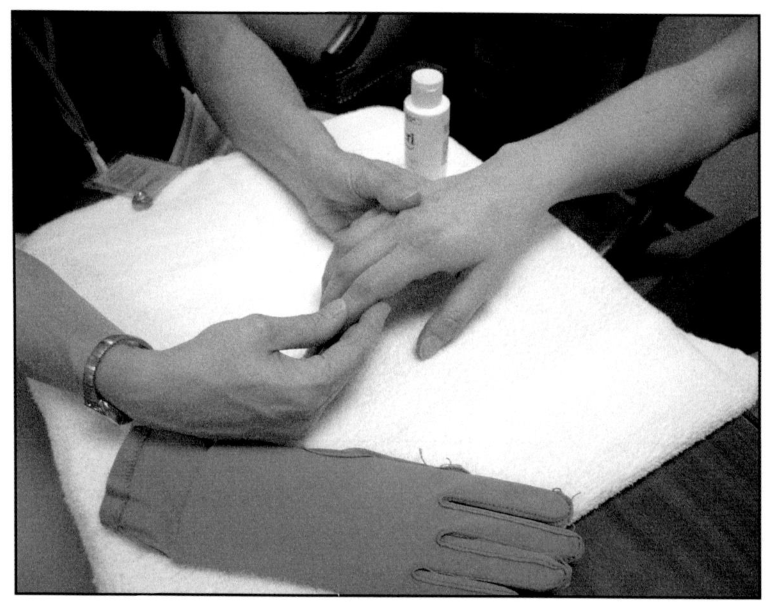

Figure 2-3. Demonstration of massage technique for subacute edema within the hand. Massage is performed in a distal to proximal direction using a lanolin-based lotion. Also pictured is a compression glove that provides circumferential compression to the hand during continuous wear outside of the occupational therapy session as is tolerated.

pulsed level of delivery in this application. "The nonthermal effects are used primarily for altering membrane permeability in order to accelerate tissue healing" (Cameron, 2009, p. 181). This process includes the removal of excess fluids seen in edema and is most commonly implemented in the subacute phases of healing.

Transcutaneous electrical nerve stimulation (TENS) is another type of therapeutic electrical modality implemented with the goal of interrupting the physiological pain cycle (Cameron, 2009; Starkey, 2013). In contrast to those previously described, the TENS modality is frequently reserved for use in conditions characterized by long-term pain or chronic pain, as seen for example in nerve entrapments, rotator cuff tears, and complex regional pain syndromes (Vance, Dailey, Rakel, & Sluka, 2014).

Compression techniques may also be implemented by the occupational therapist to promote a mechanical decrease in acute, subacute, or chronic cases of edema. The underlying theory for compression-related techniques is to facilitate the return of edematous fluids to the heart for efficient removal by the circulatory system (Cameron, 2009). Techniques as simple as elevating an affected area above the heart allow for gravitational forces to facilitate removal of excess fluids in acute and subacute stages. In addition, aquatic rehabilitation techniques recruit the principles of hydrostatic pressure to circumferentially compress affected areas to achieve the same outcome in mostly subacute or chronic situations (Aquatic Exercise Association, 2010). Bandage wrappings, garments such as fitted gloves (Figure 2-3), or electric pumps that provide timed, intermittent, and circumferential compression via filling a plastic sleeve that encloses the affected area with air are all flexible enough in nature to be implemented in either acute, subacute, or chronic stages of recovery. These types of strategies generally require high intensity and frequency, often considered a laborious process due to the natural accumulation of fluids from upright posture rather than from gravity alone. Careful attention must be paid to ensure adequate circulation is maintained within the extremity during any mechanical compression techniques.

Splinting is also a restorative technique used as a means to protect from further injury and to foster rest during the acute healing process. It is critically important in this application that the occupational therapist provides education to the clients and caregivers as to the appropriate wear schedule for the splint. This wear schedule must be designed to balance rest and use in accordance with the recommendations of the physician and based on the type of injury in order to avoid fostering disuse of affected muscles and joints. Prolonged disuse will promote the shortening of muscle tissue and potentially cause further disability. Therefore, the use of the splint should be implemented by the occupational therapist in conjunction with a program promoting joint ROM within the limits presented by the acute injury.

Retrograde massage techniques facilitated manually by the occupational therapist provide temporary compression to the tissues affected by edema. With firm-pressure massage specifically, the therapist provides manual compression (using a lanolin-based lotion to decrease friction) along the affected extremity and in the direction of the heart, where excess fluids are then removed. Refer to Table 2-22 for a general outline of this procedure. This technique is provided in conjunction with appropriate positioning against gravity, as was discussed previously. This form of massage is specifically reserved for the subacute stage in order to avoid any possibility of further injury to susceptible tissues during acute healing. Another form of massage, manual lymph drainage, is used in cases of chronic edema specifically. Here, the therapist manually performs techniques designed to elicit a release of "trapped" lymph within the system. Lymph is produced when excess fluids, as seen with edema, permeate into the interstitial space at the cellular level (Cameron, 2009). The lymphatic system attempts to remove these fluids through its circulation and expel them via the kidneys. In lymphedema, there tends to be a blockage or overload in this system, which in turn causes an abnormal accumulation of the lymph fluid. The etiology may be congenital factors, trauma, pregnancy, and cancers or cancer-related treatment (Beers, Porter, Jones, Kaplan, & Berkwits, 2006). Lymphedema is a specialty area within occupational therapy and requires additional training for proficiency. Appendix A offers more information and resources on lymphedema training.

Range of Motion

In accordance with the individualized injury and precautions set by the physician, the occupational therapist may utilize passive range of motion (PROM), active-assisted range of motion (AAROM), and active range of motion (AROM) regimes as additional restorative techniques to address acute pain and edema. As a natural reaction to discomfort, clients tend to avoid use of the affected joints, thereby fostering the accumulation of added fluids that can impede the healing process. The "healing" fluids are composed of proteins and cells necessary for preventing infection and, when left in a static state, create damage surrounding tissues and can prohibit available range of motion (Starkey, 2013). This illustrates the significance of edema as a potential complication in healing and, therefore, the importance of implementing restorative techniques for effective management. Gentle muscle contraction, as seen with ROM, acts as a vasopneumatic pump to encourage return of the excess fluids to the heart, prevent the adhesion of surrounding tissues, and minimize resulting discomfort in the acute stage of healing. Occupational therapists progressively encourage this process by means of teaching ROM programs, such as tendon gliding exercises for edema accumulating in the hand (Figure 2-4). Tendon gliding exercises specifically are completed at the intensity of five repetitions twice daily at regular intervals, until the edema has diminished (Prosser & Conolly, 2003).

Manual Techniques

Manual therapies is a collective term describing restorative techniques implemented by the occupational therapist that require the use of therapeutic touch. Lymphedema techniques, described previously, are also categorized here in addition to craniosacral, myofascial release, and

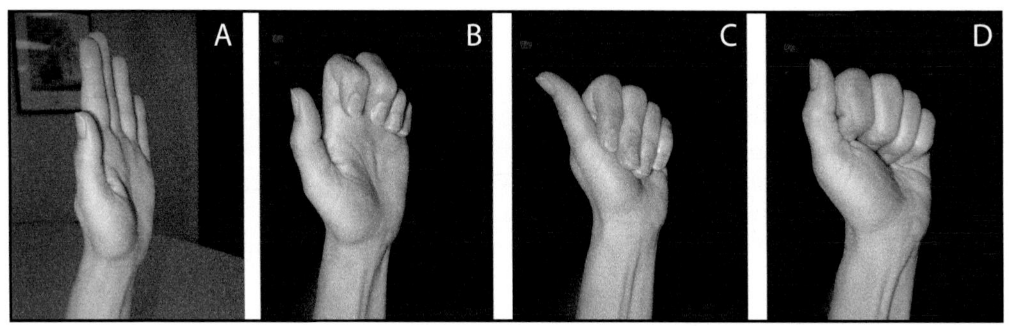

Figure 2-4. Flexor tendon gliding exercises implemented to maintain smooth motion among tendons of the hand in the presence of edema. (A) All joints of digits 2 to 5 are in extension. (B) Distal interphalangeal (DIP) and proximal interphalangeal (PIP) joints are flexed while metacarpophalangeal (MCP) joints remain extended. (C) MCPs move into flexion while DIPs become extended and PIPs remain flexed. (D) All DIPs, PIPs, and MCP joints are flexed.

Table 2-3

Remedial Techniques for Pain

• Superficial thermal modalities • Iontophoresis • Joint ROM and positioning • Phonophoresis	• TENS • Manual therapies • Aquatic rehabilitation techniques

techniques of strain counterstrain. Though each has its own unique approach, collectively these techniques are founded on the belief that dysfunction arises from tensions occurring within the fascia layer of the body and are implemented to restore uniformity throughout that system. They are all purely manual or hands-on techniques and are therefore typically contraindicated in the acute healing stages and more commonly used in the subacute and chronic phases. Due to the potential of hands-on techniques to further aggravate painful tissues, they are often used in conjunction with other pain-minimizing PAMs such as superficial heat vapocoolant sprays. Given the specialized nature of these techniques, continuing education is required to ensure safe and successful implementation. Refer to Appendix A for additional information and resources on these specialized technique options.

Techniques at a Glance

Refer to Table 2-3 for pain-specific techniques and Table 2-4 for edema-specific techniques, as well as the summary provided in Table 2-21 that outlines general procedures and precautions.

Special Considerations

As stated earlier in this section, when indicating the use of PAMs, it is the responsibility of the occupational therapist to be both knowledgeable about the specific modality and well aware of state licensure and legislation governing implementation. This procedure is recommended as a safeguard to clients and therapists alike as a result of the delicate contraindications and precautions their use presents in each individual application. "Although a number of conditions, including pregnancy, malignancy, the presence of a pacemaker, impaired sensation, and impaired cognitive status indicate the need for caution with the use of most physical agents, the specific contraindications and precautions for the specific agent being considered and the specific (client)

Table 2-4 Remedial Techniques for Edema	
• Massage • Compression garments • Compression wraps and pumps • Positioning/splinting	• Elevation • Joint ROM • Manual lymph drainage • Aquatic rehabilitation techniques

situation must be evaluated before an intervention may be used or should be rejected" (Cameron, 2003, p. 423). For example, fractures or tendon lacerations are situations in which the use of heat modalities is traditionally contraindicated due to the potential effect they may have on the healing tissues. However, over the last 25 years, there is increasing evidence that low-dose ultrasound can actually accelerate the healing of bone (Cameron, 2009). Additionally, heat modalities are strictly contraindicated in arthritis when symptoms are of an acute exacerbation; however, the literature recommends their use in the subacute and chronic stages (Cameron, 2009). Overall, the occupational therapist must carefully consider all of these issues when evaluating the use of PAMs as restorative techniques to address pain and edema on a case-by-case basis.

An additional consideration lies in the effectiveness of a multidisciplinary approach to the restoration of pain specifically. For example, the physician is ideally prescribing pharmaceutical agents designed to diminish the perception of the client's pain, psychology and social work departments are providing support systems to the client as avenues of coping with the pain, and rehabilitative services are implementing restorative approaches to address the underlying causes for the pain. It is only through this collaboration of professionals that pain can be effectively addressed.

Thermal injuries (or burns) were intentionally omitted from this discussion of pain. Pain is a critical issue for any client who has sustained a thermal injury and is directly related to the degree and extent of the burn itself. In many cases, high-dose medications are the primary and most effective means of controlling pain associated with burns over the duration of the healing process, and the presence of edema from direct trauma to the tissue itself may be minimal compared to edema from the impact of the injury/disuse of the limb. Occupational therapists may implement the longer-term techniques described in the management subsection that follows. However, here the desired outcome becomes maintaining versus restoring. It is because of these and other unique situations presented by thermal injuries that it is discussed here generally and not in the context of other restorative strategies for addressing pain and edema.

Maintenance Programs

Discussion of conditions that cause chronic pain and edema was deferred to this portion of the subsection because techniques implemented by the occupational therapist in cases of chronic pain and edema are employed to maintain rather than restore an underlying health condition. The intended outcome of using maintenance strategies is to enable clients to effectively cope and manage chronic symptoms while engaging in meaningful daily activity. These techniques are summarized in Table 2-5.

Occupational therapy intervention for chronic pain heavily emphasizes education in a variety of alternative coping methods. Biofeedback techniques provide clients with a visual or auditory cue to effectively change various physiologic functions of stress or discomfort including muscle tension, perspiration, heart rate, and blood pressure (Schatman, 2009). Imagery is often facilitated by the therapist in a controlled environment, guiding client's attention away from uncomfortable symptoms. Participation in complementary and alternative therapies may also be encouraged by

Table 2-5

Management Techniques for Managing Chronic Pain and Edema

Health Condition	Management Techniques
Pain including cancers, amputations, fibromyalgia, complex regional pain syndrome, arthritides and musculoskeletal disorders, and nerve injuries	Biofeedback, TENS, imagery, reiki, yoga, tai chi, ai chi
Edema including cancers, arthritides, and congestive heart failure	Ai chi, compression garments, compression pumps

the occupational therapist and includes reiki, yoga, and tai chi, again as methods of promoting wellness and healthy coping in the presence of chronic pain (Stoney, Wallerstedt, Stagl, & Mansky, 2009). Ai chi has also become a more common recommendation because it combines the therapeutic effects of tai chi and warmth as a means to manage pain. Ai chi is essentially tai chi performed in a warm water pool (Bottomley, 2009). While all of these techniques have an impact, it is best to review the occupationally-based interventions; however, there is limited evidence to support this for occupational therapy (Robinson, Kennedy, & Harmon, 2011).

As for management techniques in cases of chronic edema, the delineation from methods for restoration becomes less obvious. Management tools are the very same as those implemented in the subacute stages of recovery or healing. However, in this application, they are intended for long-term use. Predominantly, occupational therapists recommend the use of compression garments or intermittent pumps to clients experiencing long-term issues with fluid accumulation. Aquatic interventions are again mentioned here due to the mechanical principles that directly aid in the return of excess fluids to the heart—chiefly, hydrostatic pressure. The importance of traditional elevation must also be emphasized to clients and carried over whenever possible as an effective method for the management of chronic edema.

As discussed earlier, the efficacy of acute, subacute, or chronic pain and edema techniques require aggressive intensity to yield efficient results. This requires the occupational therapist to educate clients on the importance of carrying over strategies throughout the day outside of the occupational therapy session and within the context of everyday life. The effective implementation of PAMs in occupational therapy intervention requires the occupational therapist to also create an individualized program for clients to carry out independently in order to achieve the overall treatment goal. Also of consideration is that many of these clients are discharged from occupational therapy services early in the healing process, further emphasizing the importance of a well-developed and understood individualized maintenance program. For example, clients receiving cold modalities for pain and edema while in the occupational therapy session should also be educated and deemed safe to independently follow an individualized home program with that modality. Similarly, those receiving massage should be taught self-massaging techniques. In addition, to ensure successful execution of either technique used above as examples, the occupational therapist must consider the intensity or frequency expected of the client and the tools available to the client for effective execution (e.g., recommending the use of a bag of frozen vegetables rather than the purchase of commercially available and often costly cold packs before and after each meal daily). Overall success is best achieved when working within the context of the client.

Restorative Techniques for Sensation

Definitional Analysis

Sensation is categorized by the Framework (AOTA, 2014) as a client factor under sensory functions, which include vision, hearing, vestibular functions, taste, smell, proprioception, touch, pain, and sensitivity to temperature and pressure. For the purposes of this section, a further subdivision of sensation will be delineated into two distinct categories: those sensory functions obtained via the peripheral nervous system (PNS), including pain and temperature, and those functions obtained via the central nervous system (CNS), including discrimination of touch or the integration of righting reactions required for postural control. Sensation, or lack thereof, holds a vital role in overall intervention planning of occupational therapy. As discussed in the previous subsection, continuous sensory signals of pain can impede a client's ability to engage in personally meaningful occupations. This principle also hold true for a client who has diminished sensation. This subsection describes the restorative approaches occupational therapists commonly implement to address both exaggerated and diminished sensory responses.

Modes of Injury or Illness

Sensation is affected primarily by two modes of injury or illness: those affecting the CNS and those affecting the PNS. This delineation assists in discussing the typical modes of injury or illness that yield sensory disturbances.

The CNS receives sensory messages by way of receptors located throughout the body. These receptors convey messages directly to the brain regarding characteristics of touch, temperature, taste, vibration, sound, position, and pain. Sensibility, or the ability to interpret sensory stimuli, is a result of the accurate interpretation of these stimuli within the brain, which, in turn, results in our ability to respond accordingly. Sensation serves many other functions as well. These include protective responses to noxious stimuli and the ability to recognize familiar touch, smells, and tastes. Therefore, sensation is considered a body function per the Framework, specific to the sensory receptors that are located throughout the body or as part of the PNS. However, the ability to accurately interpret those senses and execute appropriate responses is a function of cognition occurring within the CNS.

The CNS, including the brain and spinal cord, is responsible for interpreting sensory information. The brain and spinal cord are vulnerable to an array of illnesses or injuries manifested either internally, such as stroke, meningitis, abscesses, and tumors, or externally, such as with traumatic brain injury (TBI) or spinal cord injury (SCI). Each portion or lobe of the brain harbors its own unique contributions to the body as a whole. Specifically, the parietal lobe houses the primary somatosensory cortex where the receptor information from throughout the body is deduced. Therefore, trauma, either internal or external to the parietal lobe or surrounding area of the brain, may affect sensory interpretation. Likewise, a condition that causes degeneration of this critical area of the brain, such as multiple sclerosis (MS), would produce similar results. Degenerative types of sensory disturbances vary greatly in both extent and intensity from client to client regardless of diagnosis; one person may have a complete loss of sensation on the left side of the body, another in both lower extremities, while another only in the right arm. Also, degenerative CNS conditions tend not to follow a specific dermatome distribution, as is typically the case with PNS injuries or illnesses.

Most sensory information travels to the CNS for interpretation via the PNS or sensory receptors throughout the body. The only exception is in reflexive responses to noxious stimulus that harbor the explicit purpose of protection by way of reflexes at the spinal level. Injury or illness affecting sensation may therefore occur at the level of the PNS, sparing the CNS, and present with

<table>
<tr><th colspan="2">TABLE 2-6
REMEDIAL SENSIBILITY TECHNIQUES OF THE COGNITIVE PERCEPTUAL THEORY ACCORDING TO ORIGIN OF INJURY OR ILLNESS</th></tr>
<tr><th>Origin of Injury or Illness</th><th>Remedial Techniques</th></tr>
<tr><td>CNS impairment such as seen with traumatic brain injury, stroke, spinal cord injuries, or brain tumors with generalized effects</td><td rowspan="2">• Sensory retraining program
• Desensitization programs with dowels and/or immersion bins
• Pressure garments
• Massage techniques
• Fluidotherapy at a nonthermal setting</td></tr>
<tr><td>PNS impairment in sensation such as seen with neuropathies, impingements, burns, and tumors located outside of the CNS with localized effects</td></tr>
</table>

sensory deficit in specific dermatomes areas. This can also result secondary to trauma or degenerative diseases of the peripheral nerves themselves. Trauma affecting the PNS is most commonly the result of direct nerve damage, as can be the case with fractures, edema, burns, lacerations, or impingements that thereby halt the sensory messages sent to the brain. The conduction of sensory information via the PNS can also be impeded by illnesses such as diabetes, neuropathies, Guillain-Barré syndrome, post-polio syndrome, systemic sclerosis, and tumors within the PNS. Multiple sclerosis (MS) may also cause PNS deficits if the characteristic plaques form along the peripheral nerves specifically.

Disruption of the sympathetic nervous system may also contribute to disturbances of sensation. Complex regional pain syndrome (CRPS) is a health condition characterized by pain, vascular changes, abnormal hair growth and/or nail growth, muscular weakness and atrophy, as well as changes in the overall degree of sensitivity of the affected extremity. Though etiology is unclear, much of the literature indicates that symptoms develop secondary to preexisting conditions and are linked with sympathetic nervous system dysfunction or the control center for vasomotor activity and sweat gland functions within the body (Sebastin, 2011). Occupational therapists regularly implement desensitization programs for clients experiencing symptoms of CRPS; however, much emphasis is also placed on the management of chronic pain symptoms. These desensitization programs are briefly outlined in Table 2-5 and are further explored in a compensatory framework within the remaining chapters of this text.

Restorative Techniques: Dynamic Interactional Approach

Restorative techniques for sensation are based primarily within Joan Toglia's dynamic interactional approach (Cole & Tufano, 2008) and are summarized in Tables 2-6 and 2-9. Sensation must first be perceived and accurately interpreted to respond accordingly through motor output. It is through the sensory perceptions that one is able to interact with the environment efficiently.

Restorative techniques include providing clients with an array of opportunities to provide engagement in familiar sensory experiences of all types. The following example illustrates this in the context of an everyday task. While at a restaurant, a man orders a root beer float that arrives at the table in a frosty mug. He then reaches for the mug to take a refreshing sip and the root beer spills down his front and onto the tabletop. What has happened? Misinterpretation of a sensory experience: what appeared to be a frosty glass mug was actually a plastic rendition weighing much less than anticipated based on a subconscious recollection of similar sensory experiences. Therefore, the motor response was miscalculated and too forceful for a plastic mug, causing it to spill. The inaccurate perception caused an inaccurate response.

Table 2-7 Hierarchy of Sensory Recovery
S0: Absent Sensory Functions
S1: Deep Pain
S1+: Superficial Pain Sensibility
S2: Pain and Mild Touch Sensibility
S2+: Pain and Touch Sensibility With Moderate Hypersensitivity
S3: Pain and Touch Sensibility With Mild Hypersensitivity, Static 2-Point Discrimination to 15 mm
S3+: Localization of Touch, Static 2-Point Discrimination 7 to 15 mm
S4: Complete Recovery of Sensibility
Note: A client may begin intervention for a sensibility impairment at any point along this continuum. Symptoms of sensory impairments are case-specific. Adapted from Spicher, C., Kohut, G., & Miauton, J. (1999). At which stage of sensory recovery can a tingling sign be expected? *Journal of Hand Therapy, 12*(4), 305.

Restorative techniques for impaired sensibility take the form of either re-education of receptors (in cases of a loss or decrease in sensation) or desensitization (in cases of heightened sensory responses). Depending on the mode of injury or illness, as well as the extent of that injury or illness, all clients will present individually and with highly variable levels of hypersensitivity or hyposensitivity. With this said, the following discussion of restorative techniques is intended to represent a general overview; much of the specifics are determined by the occupational therapist given a particular case with independent indicators of sensory dysfunction.

Sensory Retraining Techniques for Hyposensitivity

When hyposensitivity or anesthesia (lack of sensation) is present, the occupational therapist typically will implement a sensory training or retraining program. This is defined as a "general term for therapy aimed at enabling a person to regain contact with his or her environment [via sensory input and] . . . includes . . . body awareness exercises and sensory activities utilizing objects" (Jacobs & Simon, 2015, p. 268).

When considering the use of sensory retraining techniques, it is also important to discuss the typical pattern of recovery with regard to sensibility following injury or illness to the CNS or PNS. This process is summarized in Table 2-7 and is very case specific; this table represents only a generalization. Some clients may never experience a complete absence of sensation, while others may never achieve a full recovery of sensation. Some may have maximal degrees of impairment involving all senses, while others may only have select loss of only thermal or light touch receptors leaving all else intact.

In cases of sensory loss, restorative techniques of retraining are intended to provide the body with experiences that will remind the system of how everyday items and movements feel. Tasks of retraining may include an array of activities such as a fine motor task in identifying coins by touch alone (stereognosis) to those of a gross motor nature such as moving the arm above the head to successfully brush one's hair. Emphasis is not so much placed on the type of item or movement, but rather on the recruitment of other perceptions such as vision in retraining the "sense" of the particular task. Therefore, the occupational therapist must use skills of grading activity, or adjusting the degree of difficulty a given task presents, to provide challenge yet allow success. For example, the occupational therapist may encourage the client's use of vision to identify common everyday items by touch, then grade the task over time by occluding vision, thereby placing the demands of identification solely on the interpretation of touch. This can be achieved by beginning with the identification of large, textured items of different shape, and then grading to those that are small, nontextured, and of similar shape. See Table 2-8 for examples of textures that may be used; however, many occupational therapy clinics create textured items from simple materials purchased at local merchants. The rate of gradation will depend on the client, the degree of sensory loss, and the individual rate of recovery.

Desensitization Techniques for Hypersensitivity

Clients experiencing hyperesthesia (increased sensitivity) or paresthesias (abnormal or misinterpreted sensation) benefit from restorative techniques focusing on the desensitization of sensory receptors. These symptoms can be seen in either PNS or CNS disturbances. The occupational therapist will initiate an individually appropriate program of restoration using dowels (or sensory wands) and immersion bins that provide graded exposure to various textures. Figure 2-5 provides illustrations of these techniques. Table 2-8 depicts this concept of techniques as specifically outlined by Barber (1990); however, the textures used may vary depending on manufacturer. Additionally, a third phase may be employed in this process, whereby vibration is introduced to provide a more vigorous sensation than that of phases one and two described previously (Waylett-Rendall, 2002). Refer to Appendix A for a listing of rehabilitation equipment manufacturers' websites and information on obtaining product catalogs. Some occupational therapy clinics, as mentioned previously, will autonomously create their own desensitization programs using textures readily available at local merchant stores. Occupational therapy intervention is initiated by having the client organize the sensory stimulation bins or dowels in a sequence of least to most abrasive, then begin with stimulation via the texture that is most tolerated for 10 minutes, three to four times per day as a home program, applied directly to the affected area (Waylett-Rendall, 2002). Graded progression to increasingly more abrasive textures is then guided by the therapist with particular attention to the client's personal level of tolerance.

Physical Agent Modalities for Hypersensitivity

Occupational therapists may also use sensory experiences, such as continuous pressure by way of pressure garments, massage techniques, or fluidotherapy at a nonthermal setting, in an effort to desensitize. These techniques are employed to further amplify the bombardment to sensory receptors and regain accurate perception and are typically used in conjunction with the more traditional desensitization program. Note, fluidotherapy is also a modality of sensory bombardment at a nonthermal setting only given to the contraindication of using a heat setting in the presence of abnormal sensation. Without a reliable sensory feedback system, all other PAMs are contraindicated secondary to the potential for injury to tissues. Refer to Table 2-22 for contraindications of PAMs in general.

Quantifying Sensory Restoration Techniques

Also illustrated in Table 2-7 is the mention of static, two-point discrimination measures. This is included as a method of objectively measuring sensation. This sense is of particular importance in that two-point discrimination (in contrast to one-point) requires collaboration of multiple senses to interpret accurately. Hence, improvement in a client's performance with two-point discrimination translates to improved sensibility. This is noted as a means of illustrating the efficacy of both desensitization and sensory re-education techniques. However, it is also vital to mention that restoration can be directly influenced by the client's level of motivation as well as by the degree of severity in sensory impairment. This concept will be further explored as a special consideration

TABLE 2-8

SENSORY TRAINING SAMPLES

SAMPLE TEXTURE PROGRAM	
Dowel or Wand Techniques	**Immersion Bin Techniques**
Moleskin (Dr. Scholl's)	Cotton
Felt	Terrycloth
Foam padding	Dry rice
Velvet	Popcorn
Semi-rough cloth	Lima beans
Velcro loop	Macaroni
Hard foam	Plastic wire insulation pieces
Burlap cloth	Small beads
Rug backing	Large beads
Hook-and-loop fastener	Hard plastic cut-outs

Adapted from Barber, L. (1990). Desensitization of the traumatized hand. In J. Hunter, L. Schneider, E. Mackin, & A. Callahan (Eds), *Rehabilitation of the hand* (3rd ed., pp. 721-730). St Louis, MO: Mosby.

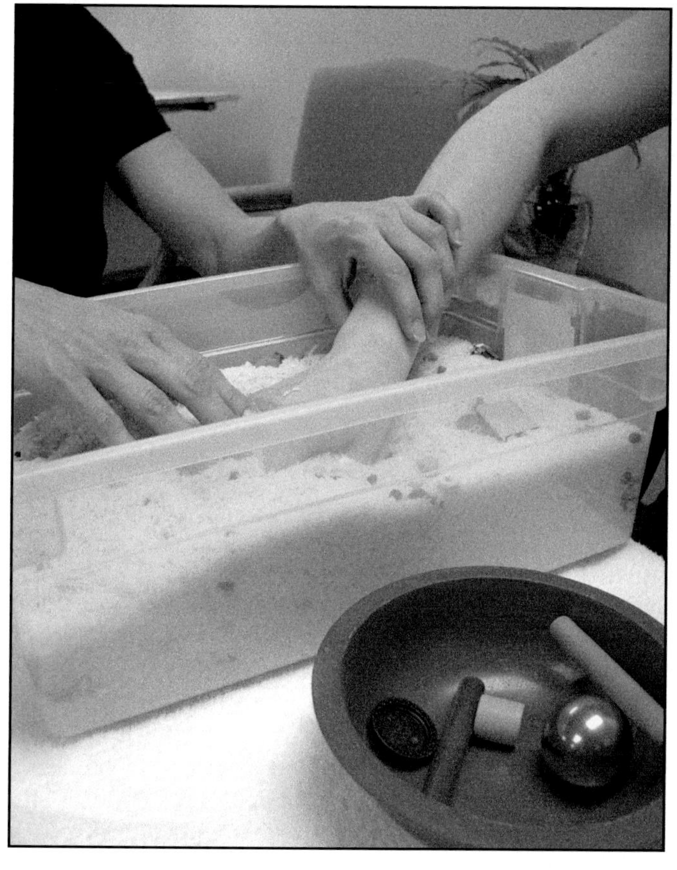

Figure 2-5. Demonstration of the use of immersion for desensitization. In this example, small items are placed in a bin of rice, and the client is being asked to retrieve the items. The rice medium provides extra sensory input to the receptors as tolerated by the client. Many therapists also choose to use immersion as a sensory retraining method in situations of decreased sensibility again asking the client to locate items within the immersion bins without using the adaptation of vision.

Table 2-9 Remedial Techniques for Sensibility
• Nonthermal or electrical physical agent modalities • Sensory retraining emphasizing the graded use of vision • Desensitization provided via immersion bins or sensory wands (dowels)

with regard to the potential comorbidity of cognitive compromise in CNS injuries and the resulting barriers it poses to addressing sensory disturbance.

Techniques at a Glance

Tables 2-9 and 2-22 illustrate the most commonly implemented techniques of restoration for sensibility in general.

Special Considerations

The issue of safety is vital when discussing intervention for a client experiencing compromised sensibility. Education for the client and caregivers is required to minimize the possibility of injury given the nature of impairment. In the absence of accurate sensory input, the body is subject to an array of injuries including burns, cuts, and decubiti, as examples. The occupational therapist must emphasize to clients and caregivers alike that sensation is a protective response for the body system and when absent the client must use added caution in all tasks of daily life (e.g., not reaching blindly into a utensil drawer in the kitchen or testing the temperature of the running water prior to entering the bathtub). The client should be educated to rely on the visual sense as a compensatory measure to promote safety until accurate sensory responses can be re-established. This concept is further discussed in Chapters 3 and 4 as techniques of adaptation and compensation.

Occupational therapists must also recall that each client coming to therapy in need of sensory restoration does so as an individual with his or her own set of previously acceptable and unacceptable sensory experiences. Some may have strictly avoided certain textures such as woolen garments, tight socks, or even caps that cover the ears. Others may be entirely unbothered by these sensory experiences. In all, it is the duty of the occupational therapist to create an individualized program that considers not only the client's current level of tolerance but also the prior level of tolerance before the onset of sensory impairment.

Of equal importance to the prior considerations is a client's cognitive status. Many of the underlying modes for compromised sensibility are a result of trauma to the CNS. Therefore, the occupational therapist must assess the client's cognitive status and adjust methods accordingly. For example, a client unable to respond accurately to a simple question, such as gender or name, may be experiencing impaired attention or even a barrier in communication, such as aphasia. Given these points, the client cannot be expected to partake in a sensory program without concern for potential safety issues arising secondary to the cognitive disability alone. It is imperative that the occupational therapist assess the cognitive status of any client with a sensory impairment in order to ensure general safety and optimal outcomes.

As a final consideration, the degree to which a sensory program is successful relies heavily on frequency. The occupational therapist should enable the carryover of clinic-based techniques into the client's everyday life to allow for continuous sensory input both within and outside of the clinic. As in a desensitizing program, clients may be provided with a scrap of denim, a piece of moleskin, or an illustration of massage procedures, for example, and then be educated as to the procedure of providing the stimulus. With sensory retraining, clients should be encouraged to actively engage in daily routines, while recruiting vision as a measure of safety in order to expose the area of impairment to as many traditional sensory experiences as possible. This frequently represents a key factor in the overall success of treatment.

Maintenance Programs

As mentioned in the previous section, it is important to engage clients in their individualized sensory programs outside of the occupational therapy clinic. The general time frame in which nerve regeneration occurs is challenged regularly by clients who regain function in weeks, months, and even years beyond the original onset of sensory impairment. Therefore, those who have not reached full recovery at the time of discharge should be encouraged to continue techniques of sensory remediation as tolerated. The maintenance program should also specifically outline any potential safety issues the client must continue to observe in the future given their status at time of discharge. Complementary therapies, such as participation in reiki, tai chi, ai chi, and yoga, may also be recommended to foster holistic health and wellness while also drawing exaggerated attention to the sense of body position. This provides an excellent opportunity for sensory retraining by means of active engagement in meaningful leisure tasks that can be inherently motivating for the client. In addition, aquatic techniques are growing in popularity as a measure of restoration due to the compressive forces of hydrostatic pressure. This force, inherent to a water environment, also provides an opportunity for sensory bombardment and an additional intervention option for desensitization (Sinclair, 2008).

Restorative Techniques for Range of Motion

Definitional Analysis

ROM is defined by the Framework (AOTA, 2014) as a subcomponent of client factors in the category of neuromusculoskeletal and movement-related functions. This subcomponent elaborates on the definition, adding that ROM is also a function of joints and bones, including the mobility of joints structures, the stability of joint structures, and the mobility of skeletal bones.

Mobility of joints refers to the biomechanical roots of arthrology, the composition of joint structure and functions as they relate to a "junction or pivot point between two or more bones" (Neumann, 2010, p. 28). Neumann goes on to describe how the nature of normal aging, long-term immobilization, trauma, or disease processes all potentially affect the structure and therefore function of our joints. This statement then considers other potential factors such as the integrity of articular bone surfaces, synovial membranes, intra-articular fluids, and the bursa. Illness or injury may compromise these components as is seen in osteoarthritis, rheumatoid arthritis, and gout.

In considering the stability of joints, one must recall the integral nature of capsular ligaments and muscle integrity. For example, muscles lacking in sufficient tone, such as is commonly seen in neurological conditions, will often impede ROM due to poor joint stability. An illustration can briefly be made by the condition of a subluxation in the shoulder joint. Here, the head of the humerus is displaced downward from the glenohumeral cavity as a result of decreased tension in the proximal shoulder musculature. Without the underlying structural integrity of the shoulder joint itself, range of motion is hindered and can even be harmful due to the increased potential for soft tissue impingement.

The mobility of our bones can be classically portrayed by the scapulohumeral rhythm or interplay between the scapula and humerus during glenohumeral motions above 90 degrees. For example, in analyzing glenohumeral abduction to a maximum of 180 degrees ROM, upward rotation of the scapula is responsible for 60 degrees, while humeral abduction is responsible for the remaining 120 degrees of the total movement. An illness or injury resulting in compromised motion at the scapula would then affect the overall ROM available at the shoulder joint due to immobility of bone alone.

Modes of Injury or Illness

Many modes of injury or illness exist that either primarily or secondarily affect ROM. This section presents an overview of the more commonly recognized injuries and illnesses for which restorative approaches are implemented.

Primary modes of injury or illness are described as "first in time or order" (Venes, 2009, p. 1892). Therefore, the injury itself is the reason for the limitation observed in ROM. These include such health conditions as bone fractures; spinal cord injuries; muscular or soft tissue injuries including a rotator cuff tear, simple sprain, or tendon lacerations; and inflammation of the joint cavity as seen with arthritic conditions.

Secondary modes of injury or illness are considered to be those "produced by a primary cause" (Venes, 2009, p. 2091). These health conditions that secondarily affect range of motion can include all types of acquired brain injuries, such as external trauma, cerebrovascular accidents (CVA), brain abscesses or tumors, or neurologically based infections (e.g., meningitis). Also included as a potential secondary mode are the degenerative diseases, such as MS, amyotrophic lateral sclerosis (ALS), Guillain-Barré syndrome, and myasthenia gravis (MG), where general debility gives rise to prolonged immobility of joints. Prolonged immobility impedes range by means of adhesion or contracture formations and though mentioned here can often cause permanent limitation in available ROM. This is discussed further in the Special Considerations segment of this subsection.

Restorative Techniques: Biomechanical Frame of Reference

In most cases, issues of ROM are addressed by occupational therapists under the biomechanical frame of reference as discussed earlier in this chapter. Refer to Tables 2-10 and 2-23 for a summary of the restorative techniques most frequently implemented by occupational therapy to address limits in ROM.

So often, the lingering barrier clients continually face in their recovery from illness or injury is the functional significance found in ROM and strength. Therefore, the facilitation of repetitive range through the available arc of motion is a commonly used restorative strategy across diagnoses or health conditions. The main goal of this technique is to maintain or increase the ROM as well as prevent contractures or adhesions that can potentially form secondary to immobility.

Range of Motion

As a technique, ROM itself is broken into three main types: PROM, AAROM, and AROM. The type of range elicited as an intervention approach depends heavily on the client's physical status at the given point in time. For example, a client with little or no active range would then require the therapist to passively move the joint through its full arc of motion, termed *PROM*. Also included here would be the implementation of pendulum exercises, designed to facilitate PROM using gravity as the passive force, rather than that of the therapist. In addition, a client can be taught techniques of using an unaffected extremity to passively guide the affected limb through its arc of motion. This technique is referred to as self-ROM, commonly executed in cases of hemiparesis. This may be further encouraged through the use of a dowel, a cane, or by an overhead pulley system to recruit both the affected and unaffected extremities simultaneously. Refer to Figure 2-6 for an illustration of commonly implemented self-ROM motion exercise. The occupational therapist may also employ techniques of AAROM in which the therapist or assistive device (e.g., pulleys) works collaboratively with the client, sharing effort as necessary to achieve full ROM. Figure 2-7

Table 2-10

Remedial Range of Motion Techniques of the Biomechanical Theory According to Health Condition

Health Condition	Remedial Techniques
Fractures Soft-tissue injury including tears, sprains, tendon lacerations, etc.	Subacute phases of recovery: PROM, AAROM, self-ROM, AROM
Spinal cord injuries Acquired brain injury including TBI, CVA, brain cancers, abscesses, meningitis, etc. Degenerative diseases including MS, ALS, Guillaine-Barré, and MG	PROM, AAROM, self-ROM, AROM

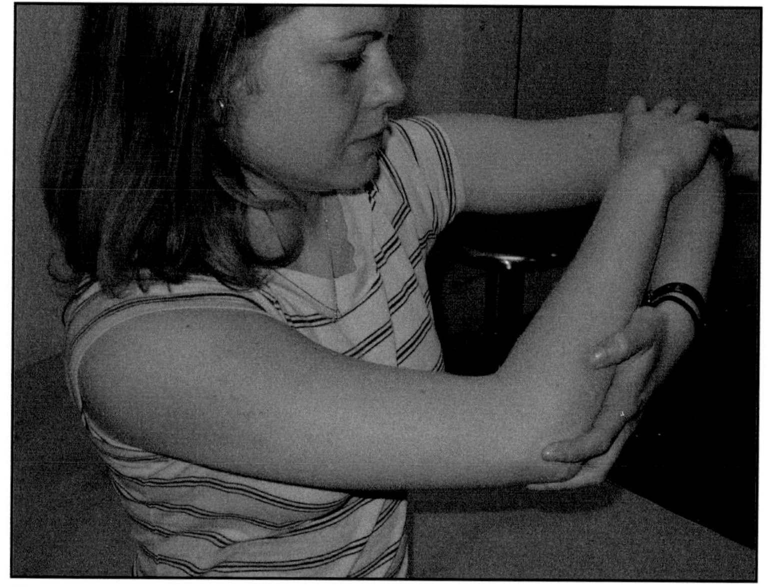

Figure 2-6. Demonstration of a self-ROM exercise wherein the most mobile extremity supports and assists movement in the least mobile joints through the entire arc of horizontal abduction and adduction at the shoulder joint.

provides an illustration. Finally, AROM is implemented once clients are able to move their joints through the arc of motion independently against gravity. Here, the occupational therapist will create a client-specific program to be executed independently to enhance or maintain available AROM. Prefabricated card file systems are used frequently to facilitate this goal. These tools are readily available through manufacturers (listed in Appendix A) and provide a wide array of simply illustrated and narratively described active-, passive-, and self-assisted exercises in the form of a 3×4-inch card—one designated for each exercise. This allows the therapist to select appropriate exercises for the client, compile them in a page format, photocopy (copyright provided with purchase), and then insert recommended intensity (repetitions and sets) to foster independence in the overall exercise program. See Figure 2-8 for a sample of this type of program. Computer-based

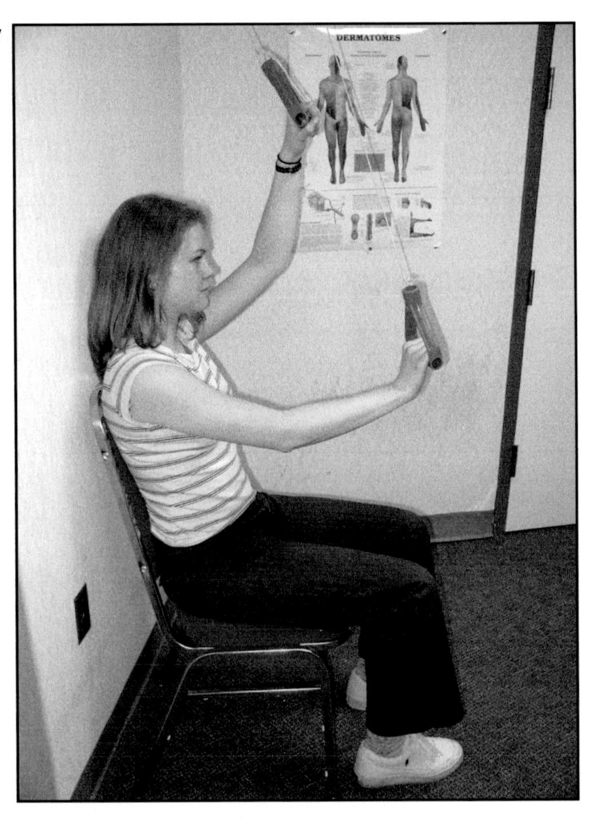

Figure 2-7. Demonstration of pulleys commonly considered either a technique of PROM or AAROM.

or Web-based services are becoming more readily available to support therapists with crafting individualized home exercise programs. If available, occupational therapists can also video-record clients completing a home program with a tablet or phone and email the video to clients for future reference.

Typical intervention strategies to facilitate increased AROM or AAROM can also include pulley exercises, wall-mounted shoulder wheels, arm ergometers, or the various tool attachments in work simulators such as the Baltimore Therapeutic Equipment (BTE) PrimusRS (Figure 2-9). Additional information about the BTE and other work simulators can be found in Appendix A. Though these techniques are not necessarily based in function, they are commonly employed as adjunctive methods and are proven strategies of restoration for addressing deficits in ROM. With added occupational focus, the therapist may employ activity analysis to foster these same biomechanical approaches in a functional context, such as having clients reach to hang clothes on a clothesline or replace dishes in upper kitchen cabinets to address decreased glenohumeral flexion. Here the focus remains on restoration while employing creativity in the use of strategies that actively engage participation in personally meaningful activities.

Physical Agent Modalities

Per state-specific guidelines, superficial heat modalities are frequently used as a preparatory method to techniques for ROM. The purpose here is to promote tissue elasticity in preparation for the stretch associated with range exercises. Moist heat packs, thermal (continuous) ultrasound, and fluidotherapy represent the most commonly used methods for this purpose and, as indicated previously, are implemented for a duration of 15 to 20 minutes to achieve desired thermal effects

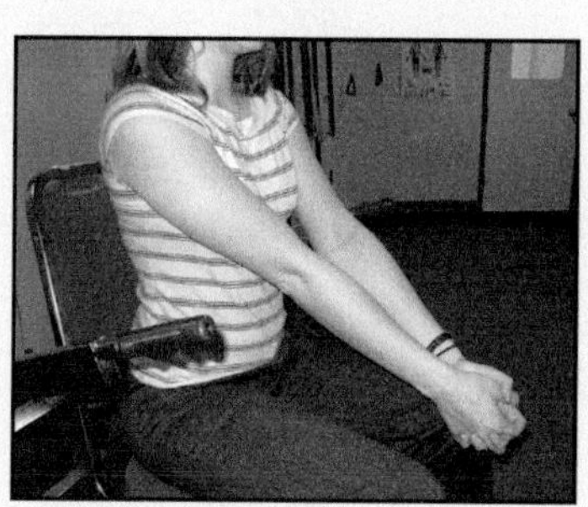

1. Grasp a ___ pound weight. Hold firmly in palm, but do not squeeze with fingers.
2. Begin with your elbow straightened out in front of you and resting on a supportive surface (see left).
3. Gently raise the weight by bending at the elbow only in a direction towards your shoulder (see right).
4. Complete _____ repetitions.
5. Complete _____ sets in all.

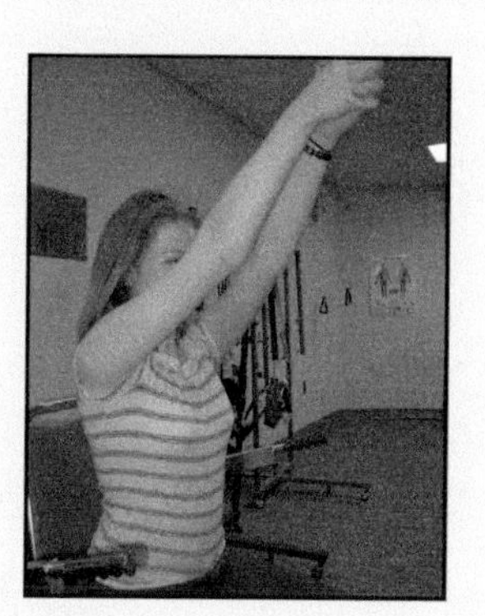

Remember to use breathing techniques taught in the clinic and stop immediately in the event you experience any pain or discomfort.

Figure 2-8. Sample card program for ROM. The therapist then simply fills in the blanks according to the individual's needs and tolerances as part of the maintenance program.

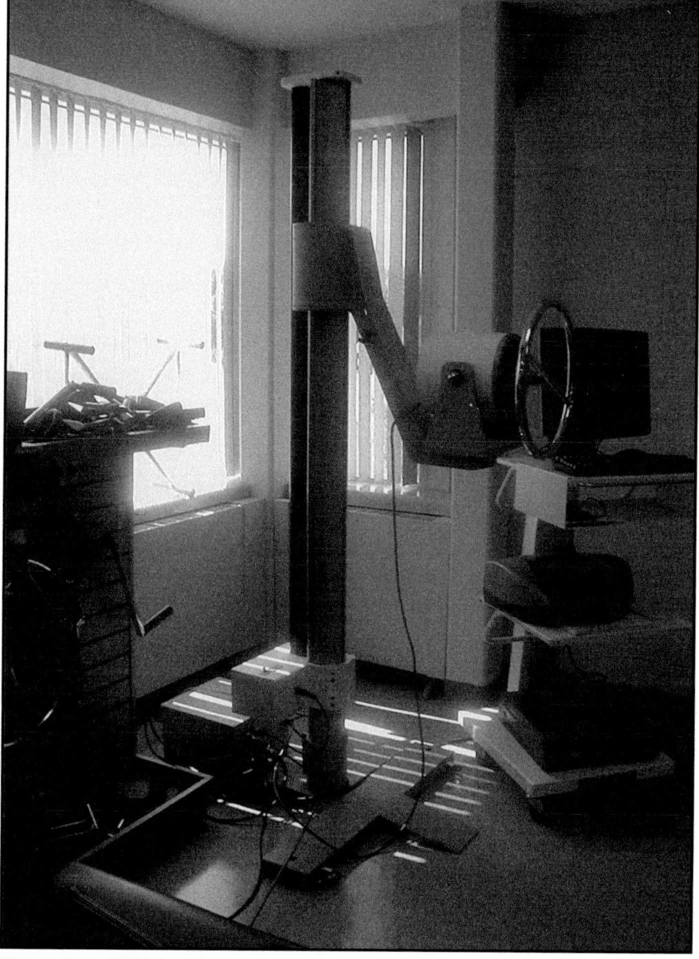

Figure 2-9. BTE PrimusRS.

Table 2-11 Remedial Techniques for Range of Motion
• PROM: Pendulum exercises and therapist-facilitated techniques • AROM: BTE, wall mounted shoulder wheels, card style programs, use of functional activity engagement • Physical agent modalities: Including moist heat, ultrasound, or fluidotherapy • AAROM: BTE, pulleys, shoulder wheels, card style programs • Self-ROM: Pulleys, dowel, or cane exercises

(Cameron, 2009). Again, careful attention must be paid to any conditions that may contraindicate the use of therapeutic heat. Refer to Table 2-24 for a review of indications and contraindications.

Techniques at a Glance

Refer to Table 2-11 and 2-23 for a general outline of restorative techniques commonly employed by the occupational therapist to address deficits in ROM.

Special Considerations

When restorative intervention strategies are implemented with the intent of increasing available ROM at an affected joint or joints, the therapist must consider inherent precautions or contraindications specific to the underlying mode of injury or illness. An example can be found in weight-bearing precautions commonly put in place by the physician after acute fractures to allow undisturbed time to support the natural healing process. Also, the occupational therapist must be aware of any preexisting range of motion limitations by prompting the client to report a history of prior injuries, fractures, or joint disorders, such as arthritis.

Clients should also be informed of the necessity for proper positioning. Here, occupational therapists will provide education to clients emphasizing that a position of comfort may also lead to deformity via the shortening of soft tissues. Family members and caregivers should also be oriented to proper positioning and the potential ramifications of prolonged immobility. This includes the use of splinting techniques, briefly described earlier in the pain and edema subsection of this chapter.

The efficient management of pain and edema are also vital components in optimizing ROM. Full ROM can be significantly impeded by the presence of pain and edema. Hence, it is important to ensure that these issues are addressed simultaneously, using the appropriate combination of aforementioned techniques, in order to optimize the ROM that a client is able to regain overall.

Maintenance Programs

A key component to maximize the outcome of restorative ROM treatment is the carryover of a maintenance program. Here, it is the role of the occupational therapist to create an individually meaningful exercise program that addresses client-specific needs, adheres to the condition-specific precautions, and is easily understood in both technique and relevance to the healing process. With ROM, maintenance programs commonly consist of fostering active engagement in typical, everyday activity, such as dressing, grooming, washing, as well as specific exercise programs to promote additional PROM, AAROM, or AROM. As mentioned earlier, occupational therapists can create written recommended maintenance programs with the use of card-style systems, computer-based programs, or virtual technology. Typically, a well-rounded maintenance program also emphasizes a balance between straightforward biomechanical exercise and the engagement in meaningful activities that specifically recruit ROM in a targeted joint or joints.

Restorative Techniques for Strength

Strength plays an integral role in resuming independent engagement in meaningful activity following injury or illness. Of significance to note is the interrelationship between ROM and strength against gravity. Without strength, one will not be able to achieve full active ROM against the force of gravity.

The significance of gravity in the physical environment is often taken for granted until one is faced with an injury or illness that limits strength capacity. It then becomes more evident that active motion can be limited by decreased strength alone. For example, a manual muscle test of the biceps muscle in elbow flexion yields a strength rating of "poor." This indicates that the client is unable to achieve full active ROM in a gravity plane but successfully can in a gravity-eliminated or -supported plane. Hence, without the required strength from the muscle to move the limb segment into flexion against gravity, the client then too has limits in ROM. Therefore, restorative approaches for addressing strength vary greatly depending on the degree of limitation. In this "poor" elbow flexor example, simply to promote full active range against gravity alone would be a plausible and credible restoration technique. Resistance would then be graded, beyond that of the gravitational force, once improvement is noted. Conversely, a client exhibiting full ROM in all planes could then move to more aggressive restorative methods such as progressive resistive exercise (PRE) programs.

Definitional Analysis

Per the Framework (AOTA, 2014), strength is defined as a foundational skill or client factor specific to "neuromusculoskeletal and movement-related functions" of the body (p. S23). It is further categorized as a function of muscle power. With attention paid to general performance, strength is required to execute motor skills such as including bending, reaching, positioning, and the overall calibration of human movement "as the person effectively interacts with and moves objects and self around the task environment" (AOTA, 2014, p. S25). Strength is also required to convey intentions and needs through the physicality of communication. In all, this foundational skill is vital in one's ability to successfully engage in many aspects of meaningful occupation.

Modes of Injury or Illness

Strength, as a foundational skill, is affected by a wide array of health conditions. Primary modes of injury or illness, as they relate to strength, include those directly affecting the integrity of the soft tissue including muscle tearing or tendon evulsions. These conditions directly compromise the length-tension relationship of musculature and therefore the ability to produce maximal muscle force (Neumann, 2010).

Secondary causes are far more commonly seen and frequently are characterized by conditions that result in prolonged immobility. Here, the lack of physical movement creates an opportunity for muscle wasting and/or the formation of contractures and adhesions among muscular structures. Examples can be found in degenerative conditions including MG, ALS, Guillain-Barré syndrome, MS, or even conditions resulting from major multiple trauma to the body as is seen often in high-velocity collisions. Of added importance is the significance of prognosis in the underlying condition. For example, both ALS and Guillain-Barré syndrome cause progressive muscle weakness yet

Table 2-12
Remedial Strength Techniques of the Biomechanical Theory According to Health Condition

Health Condition	Remedial Technique
Soft tissue injuries including tears, sprains, tendon lacerations, etc. Prolonged immobility Degenerative diseases including MS, ALS, Guillain-Barré, and MG	Therapeutic exercise programs designed to address the client's specific needs and interests, progressive resistive exercise (PRE), neuromuscular electrical stimulation, work simulators, aquatic rehabilitation techniques

harbor distinctly different prognoses. The occupational therapist must consider each of these facts to create an intervention plan that is both individualized and effective to achieve optimal outcome.

Restorative Techniques: Biomechanical Frame of Reference

As was the case with restorative ROM techniques, the intervention strategies used to address the underlying causes of decreased strength are fundamentally based in the biomechanical frame of reference as discussed in the beginning of this chapter. These commonly implemented techniques are summarized in Tables 2-12 and 2-24.

Therapeutic Exercise Programs

The most commonly implemented restorative technique for addressing strength is the use of therapeutic exercise programs designed specifically to meet a client's needs. This technique offers much flexibility based on the degree of strength limitation each client experiences. This method has been viewed as controversial in the occupational therapy community that ascribes to functional activity engagement (Breines, 2013) over traditional strengthening programs. However, given that strength is a foundational skill to successful engagement in functional activity, occupational therapists must address this specifically to foster maximal return to occupational independence.

All clients must be physically able to endure a therapeutic exercise regime or deemed medically stable with regard to respiratory and cardiovascular functions prior to engaging in a strengthening program (refer to Special Considerations section). Given this point, the occupational therapist should have immediate access and ability to use assessment tools including a stethoscope, blood pressure cuff, and a pulse oximeter (oxygen saturation measurement device) in order to closely monitor a client's tolerance of treatment.

Occupational therapists create therapeutic exercise programs to improve strength specifically using items such as free weights or barbells, BTE PrimusRS, wrist weights, hand grippers, TheraPutty (North Coast Medical), and/or TheraBand (Hygenic Corporation). Skills of gradation are infused to provide enough challenge yet avoid over-fatigue of the muscle tissue. Gradation is achieved with the use of varied repetitions and sets of exercise unique to the capabilities of each client as well as with the use of graded resistance items. For example, TheraBand, TheraPutty, or hand grippers can be purchased from manufacturers as color-coded sets, illustrating to the therapist and client alike the idea of graded resistance (Figures 2-10 through 2-12). For example, TheraPutty is available in yellow as the least resistive compound, followed by red, green, and blue. This same progression is available in TheraBand products. A more current product on the market is Progressive Putty (Sammons Rehab). With this product, provided additives allow the therapist to increase the

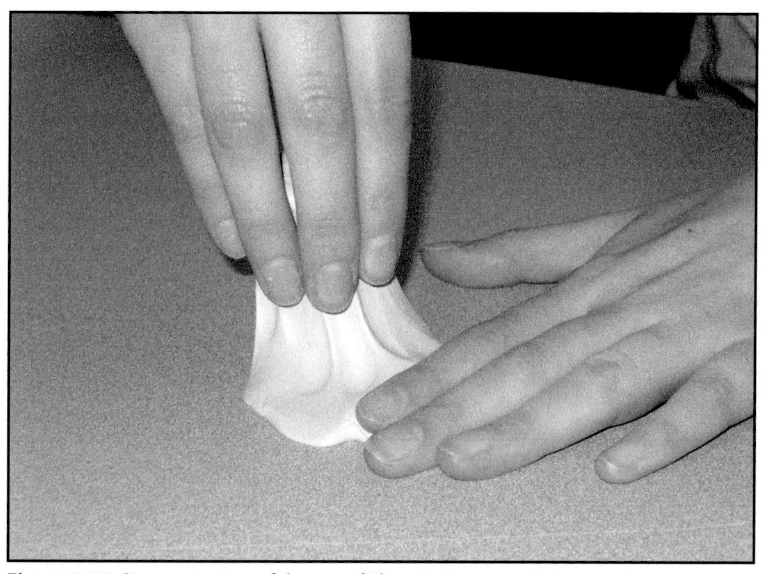

Figure 2-10. Demonstration of the use of TheraPutty as a resistive exercise to promote increased strength in the finger flexors.

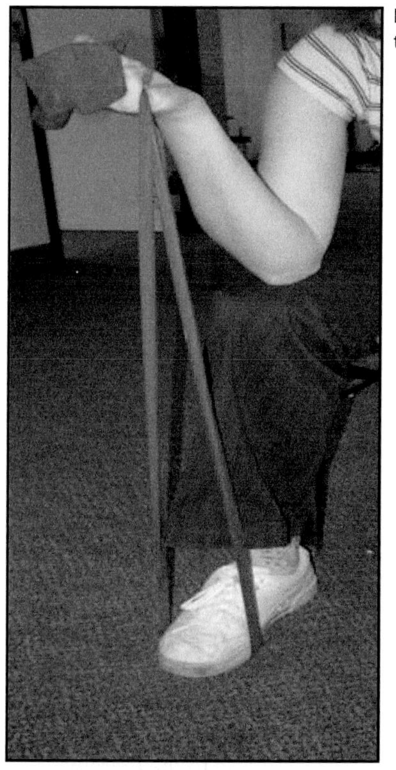

Figure 2-11. Demonstration of the use of TheraBand as a resistive exercise to promote strength in the elbow flexor musculature.

resistive qualities of the same compound rather than purchasing various compounds. Refer to Appendix A for more information on obtaining catalogs that offer an array of strengthening tools.

Another technique for grading the resistance of strength exercises is to adjust the type of muscle contraction required of the client. Isometric muscle contractions do not produce limb movement,

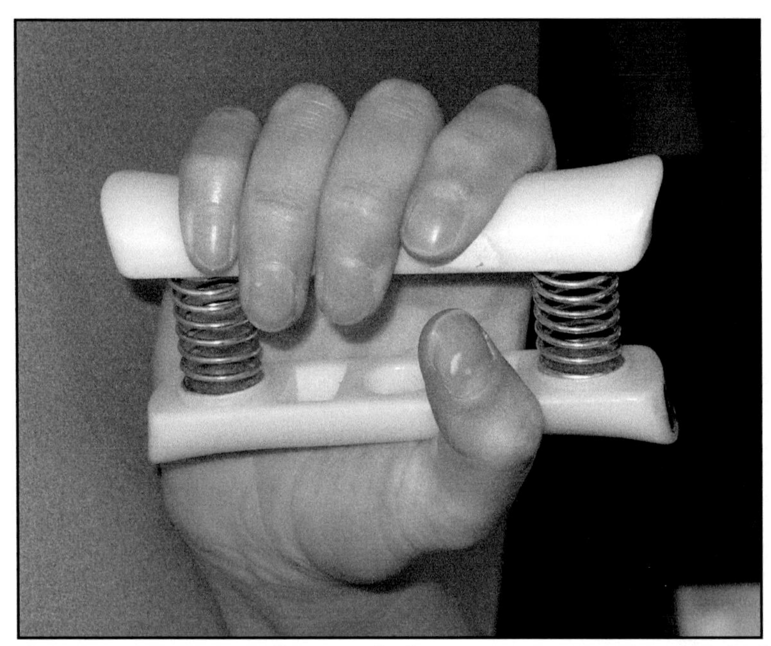

Figure 2-12. "Grippers" are effective methods to increase gross grasping strength of the hand.

for example. This type of static contraction is commonly the first in the progressive exercise regime for cases of maximally compromised strength; contraction without movement eliminates the need to produce force against gravity. This technique is also implemented in cases in which joint structure is compromised since strengthening can be fostered without eliciting potentially damaging movement among the joint structures. Isometric exercise, however, is contraindicated in cases of cardiac compromise due to the increased demand this type of contraction places on the heart.

Isotonic or concentric muscle contractions are facilitated by promoting a shortening in the length of a muscle against gravity. For example, an isotonic or concentric contraction of the biceps muscle would produce a shortening of that muscle and, therefore, elbow flexion. This exercise is commonly referred to as a *bicep curl*. With isotonics, motion against the force of gravity is recruited in an upright position, further increasing the demands for muscle strength. This can be graded to meet individual needs by adjusting the direction of movement produced, the weighted resistance, the speed of movement, the number of repetitions, and the number of sets required of the exercise program.

Conversely, the therapist may choose to foster eccentric muscle contractions or activation of muscle fibers as the muscles lengthens rather than shortens. This type of contraction can be achieved by using simple free weights. For example, a client with his or her arm fully extended overhead and grasping a 2-pound weight is then asked to bend at the elbow while maintaining full flexion at the shoulder so as to "touch" the back of their head. This would then facilitate a lengthening, or eccentric, contraction of the triceps muscle as the limb moves downward with gravity. For eccentric contraction, the therapist often recruits the assistance of a mini-gym or workout station, because resisted lengthening is inherently difficult to achieve in a gravity environment.

Finally, the therapist may choose to foster isokinetic contraction of muscles. This technique allows for a more functional approach by eliciting reciprocation among the agonist and antagonistic muscles similar to that of movement required to interact with one's environment. Tools of isokinetics are often equipment-based and employ technology to simplify the process of providing

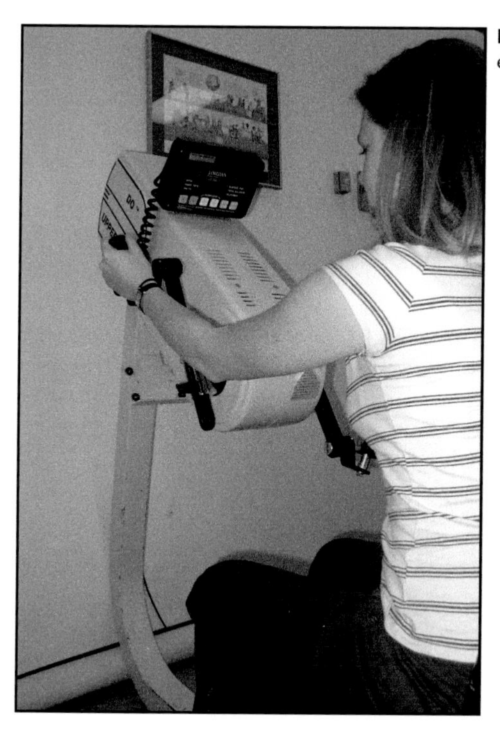

Figure 2-13. Demonstrations of the therapeutic use of an arm ergometer.

graded resistance. An example is found in the use of an arm ergometer that allows the speed of revolution to be mechanically controlled (Figure 2-13). This equipment requires the strength of reciprocating muscles groups, yet more importantly allows ease of gradation via limits placed on duration or speed of movement. Regardless of the amount of effort applied by a client, the ergometer will only allow the preset number of revolutions.

Of note, many occupational therapists will choose to address strength in the context of engaging in meaningful activity versus that of pure biomechanical exercise. For example, the therapist may engage the client in a desired leisure task while wearing 1-pound wrist weights. This is a beneficial approach in working with individuals who do not typically engage in or find purpose in engaging in a traditional weight-lifting program. This then offers occupational engagement while also creating enough resistance to foster improved muscle strength.

Neuromuscular Electrical Stimulation: A Physical Agent Modality

Neuromuscular electrical stimulation (NMES), also referred to as *functional electrical stimulation* (FES), is a method used to externally elicit active muscle contraction and therefore secondarily promote muscle strength. These terms are erroneously used interchangeably given the preparatory method of NMES is not always implemented in a manner that embeds function. It is only when this method is used in conjunction with functional activity that it is then accurately deemed FES. NMES is provided via electrode placement over given motor points located along a weakened muscle's length. The electrical impulse causes a concentric contraction of the designated musculature and is considered restorative in nature when implemented in cases of temporary muscle weakness. This includes health conditions such as incomplete SCI, acquired brain injury, and shoulder subluxation. Bellew (2012) indicates that the use of NMES as a modality to promote strength has been well studied, but most have focused narrowly on the quadriceps muscle alone. These studies have demonstrated strong efficacy for NMES as a strengthening technique in both healthy and weakened musculature when implemented in the early stages of the rehabilitation process. NMES is a physical agent modality that requires additional training to safely and effectively administer. Again, regulations on the use of PAMs vary from state to state, and it is the responsibility of the therapist to be aware of governing legislation.

Work Simulators

Work simulators, such as the BTE PrimusRS (discussed previously) and the ERGOS II Work Simulator (Simwork Systems), present another option for providing muscular resistance to develop strength. These equipment-based options offer greater control in grading resistance provided to muscle groups during simulated functional activity. For example, the BTE PrimusRS offers an array of attachments designed to simulate particular movements required of a given activity including driving, golfing, or opening a jar. The integrated software program allows the therapist to easily grade resistance that is then recorded as part of a digitalized exercise program tailored to meet the individualized needs of each client. The customized computer screen also offers graphics that allow clients to visualize contractile strength and see progress over time.

Progressive Resistive Exercise

PREs are derived from the DeLorme method (Dutton, 2012). According to DeLorme, muscles must be taxed beyond everyday activity in order to promote the remediation of strength. Hence, the therapist must first identify the maximal capacity of a client, or the maximum weight a person can lift through the full arc of motion times 10 repetitions (Dutton, 2012). Once identified, the therapist will then prescribe resistive exercise: 10 repetitions at 25% the determined maximal capacity, 10 repetitions at 50%, and 10 repetitions at 100% capacity. The program is completed once per day, 4 to 5 days per week. As maximal capacity increases, resistance should also be increased. This is a formal program designed to increase strength; oftentimes the occupational therapist will employ less formal variations of this original program. Refer to Table 2-24 for an outline of the PRE method.

Aquatic Rehabilitation Techniques

Aquatic rehabilitation approaches may also be employed for the restoration of strength. Though aquatic rehabilitation does not currently require specific certification to implement, continuing education within this domain is recommended as a means of understanding the therapeutic advantages of treatment in water. Water inherently provides an environment that is free of gravitational force. The simple elimination of this force presents an ideal opportunity to foster strength while also engaging in a leisure activity. Strength is promoted via the viscosity properties of water, or the tendency of water molecules to adhere to one another (Schrepfer, 2007).

The force required to separate molecules of water far exceeds that of air molecules. Therefore, resistance to the simple activity of walking in water requires greater muscle strength than when walking on ground and without the application of additional weights. The resistance is upgraded by increasing the depth of water or by the strategic incorporation of floatation devices that further enhance the resistive properties of water (Schrepfer, 2007). Though this is an incredibly valuable option, the occupational therapist must again use his or her skills in client-centered intervention to ensure the successful use of an aquatic technique; not all individuals enjoy the thought of swimming, and precautions must be taken in situations of open wounds, conditions of heat or fatigue sensitivity, and cardiac or respiratory compromise.

Techniques at a Glance

Refer to Tables 2-13 and 2-24 for a summary of restoration techniques commonly used to address issues of strength.

Table 2-13 Remedial Techniques for Strengthening
• PREs • Work simulators • PAMs: NMES • Aquatic rehabilitation techniques • Traditional Exercise: TheraPutty, TheraBand, grippers, free weights

Special Considerations

When using restorative techniques to address strength, the occupational therapist must be readily aware of the client's medical status and the presence of any possible contraindications or precautions. For example, physicians may contraindicate the use of exercise for clients with certain cardiac conditions or may put in place precautions, such as avoiding resistive exercise above 90 degrees of shoulder ranges of motion. Other common contraindications include conditions of general debility or acute exacerbations of disease. When implementing therapeutic exercise with any client it is imperative that the occupational therapist be able to recognize signs of not only fatigue but also of distress, such as excessive perspiration, labored or rapid breathing, or changes in facial skin color (very pale or red). As to minimize the potential for these events, the occupational therapist should observe all governing guidelines for the use of exercise as a therapeutic intervention. These guidelines are summarized in Table 2-14 and emphasize the use of a phased approach including warmup, stretching, strengthening, and relaxation portions during every exercise session.

As mentioned earlier in this section, the occupational therapist also must be considerate to the underlying cause for muscular weakness. For example, an individual with a progressive degenerative health condition would be particularly sensitive to over-fatigue of muscle tissue. Such a circumstance may even potentially set the client's progress back in the continuum of recovery. Therefore, this point is repeated to emphasize the attention a therapist must pay to both diagnostic and prognostic indicators in an effort to foster maximal recovery of muscle strength.

Maintenance Programs

To achieve an overall increase in strength, the frequency in which the program is completed often warrants execution both within and outside the occupational therapy clinic (i.e., two to three times per day). Therefore, the therapist may initiate the actual program in the clinic, train the client on proper completion of each component, and then recommend completion as part of the home program. Figure 2-14 provides a sample of this type of program. Frequently, clients are instructed to substitute traditional free weights or hand grippers with more common everyday items such as cans of vegetables, a foam "squish" ball (often marketed for stress relief or in the children's section of local retail stores), or even by carrying everyday weighted items such as bags of groceries or baskets of laundry. In addition, occupational therapists who have successfully integrated the use of aquatic techniques and established safe independence in pool-based exercise may consider encouraging clients to actively participate at community-based pools and aquatic centers. This allows the therapist to encourage engagement in meaningful activity while still focusing on the restoration of strength.

Table 2-14

General Guidelines for Engagement in Therapeutic Exercise Programs: A Phased Approach

1. Request that the client report how he or she is feeling in general. Is there any report of pain or discomfort or other contraindicating symptoms such as nausea, dizziness, excessive fatigue, or shortness of breath (SOB)? Outside of the initial therapeutic exercise session, always request that the client report the tolerance of exercises performed in the previous session.
2. Obtain a baseline pulse rate, blood pressure reading, and baseline oxygen saturation, if indicated. Normal pulse rates at rest generally lie within the range of 60 to 100 beats per minute (BPM). Normal blood pressure at rest is under 140/90 mm Hg and normal oxygen saturation is 90% to 100%.
3. In the absence of any abnormalities previously identified, exercise should begin with a general warm-up activity such as taking three deep, cleansing breaths followed directly by AROM, as tolerated, among all joints of focus for that session's exercise elements.
4. Proceed to verbally instruct and demonstrate to the client elements of stretching muscle fibers as a preparatory technique for resistive exercise. Again, focus on muscle groups intended to be active during the session.
5. Provide the client with clear directions and demonstration of the exercises he or she is expected to perform. For example, to activate the biceps, the therapist should demonstrate a traditional biceps curl while also pointing out proper positioning and joint alignment throughout each repetition.
6. Walk the client through each set of exercises. For example, have the client complete one set of five repetitions of biceps curls with a 1-pound weight. Re-evaluate client tolerance as outlined in guideline 1. This is the step where the occupational therapist will individually upgrade or downgrade the exercise by adjusting the number of repetitions or sets. At the client's initial exercise session, expectations should be minimal so as to have the opportunity to evaluate tolerance not only during the exercise program but also at the subsequent session.
7. Monitor the client as he or she performs the recommended repetitions and sets at each of the designated joints. Be attentive to any signs or symptoms of poor tolerance as outlined briefly in guideline 1. In the event that poor tolerance is suspected, cease all exercises and obtain a pulse and blood pressure reading. Clients who have been inactive as a result of illness or disability should not have greater than a 20 to 30 BPM increase, with the systolic blood pressure reading remaining relatively stable with the established baseline and no more than a 10 mm Hg increase from resting in the diastolic reading. In the presence of SOB, the occupational therapist may also obtain a pulse oximetry reading. These readings should then be shared with medical personnel or emergency services who can further assess the client. Always err on the side of caution and ask for assistance to evaluate a client when any suspicion arises.
8. Given good tolerance, also provide the client with ample rest opportunities, particularly in the initial session. This may be as frequent as between each set of exercise completed. Ensure that the client has access to hydration and be aware of any potential swallowing precautions such as those seen in acquired brain injuries and some degenerative diseases.

(continued)

Table 2-14 (continued)

General Guidelines for Engagement in Therapeutic Exercise Programs: A Phased Approach

9. Following completion of the recommended exercise program, take a pulse reading and guide the client through a relaxation exercise. For example, the client may be requested to again take deep, cleansing breaths, or the therapist may facilitate a simple guided imagery technique. This provides the body system with the time required to return to the resting point.
10. Following relaxation, obtain a pulse reading. The client should have returned to the resting pulse level following the relaxation phase. Monitor the client until pulse returns to normal relative to the initial reading.
11. Within a short time period, clients are generally able to demonstrate independence with safely and effectively executing many aspects of the individualized program. The occupational therapist should always monitor the client's participation directly to assess tolerance levels.
12. All exercises should be immediately ceased and medical assistance called for any clients complaining of "chest pain or pain referred to the teeth, jaw, ear, or arm; excessive fatigue; light-headedness or dizziness; nausea or vomiting; SOB; or unusual weight gain of 3 to 5 pounds in 1 to 3 days" (Trombly & Radomski, 2002, p. 1078).

Adapted from Huntley, N. (2002). Cardiac and pulmonary diseases. In C. M. Trombly & M. V. Radomski (Eds.), *Occupational therapy for physical dysfunction* (5th ed., p. 1078). Philadelphia, PA: Lippincott Williams & Wilkins.

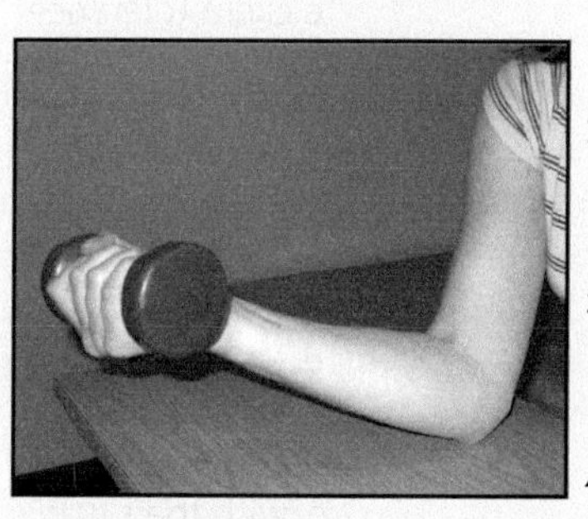

1. Grasp a ___ pound weight. Hold firmly in palm, but do not squeeze with fingers.
2. Begin with your elbow straightened out in front of you and resting on a supportive surface (see left).
3. Gently raise the weight by bending at the elbow only in a direction towards your shoulder (see right).
4. Complete _____ repetitions.
5. Complete _____ sets in all.

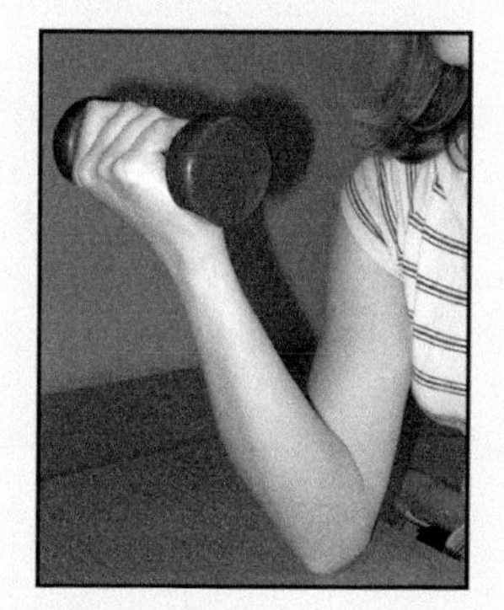

Remember to use breathing techniques taught in the clinic and stop immediately in the event you experience any pain or discomfort.

Figure 2-14. Sample card program for strength. The therapist then simply fills in the blanks to create an individualized program that best meets the needs of the client as part of the maintenance program.

Restorative Techniques for Endurance

Definitional Analysis

Muscle endurance is categorized as a client factor per the Framework (AOTA, 2014) and is further defined as a function of the neuromusculoskeletal and movement-related functions as well as cardiovascular and respiratory functions. It is also considered a function of the muscles and of exercise tolerance, including aerobic capacity, stamina, and fatigability.

Jacobs and Simon (2015) reflect the above definition as "sustaining cardiac, pulmonary, and musculoskeletal exertion over time; ability to sustain effort over time" (p. 97). This is an important aspect of endurance; without the ability to sustain effort over time, a client's engagement in meaningful occupation is left compromised.

Modes of Injury or Illness

In essence, any and all events of injury or illness can potentially affect one's endurance. A simple bout with the 24-hour flu can cause one to feel tired for a few days afterward. Magnify those consequences with such events as pneumonia, respiratory failure, or having sustained an acquired brain injury, all of which are commonly associated with prolonged immobility and bed rest. This analogy allows us to better illustrate the substantial effect a decrease in endurance can have on functional performance and illustrates the most evident reason or mode for it: a lack of engagement in routine, everyday physical activity.

Any condition resulting in the inability to engage in daily activity for a prolonged period of time will result in debility, also known as decreased endurance. In its simplest form, endurance is then better categorized by the degree of impairment rather than mode of injury or illness. Many situations of mildly compromised endurance go without formal intervention and are addressed simply by re-engaging in normal daily routine as tolerated. These also tend to be situations characterized by short hospital stays of a few days or less with discharge back to the home setting. In the event that occupational therapy is required following discharge, intervention is commonly performed in the outpatient clinic or in the home with a focus on the primary diagnosis, not the secondary limitation of endurance. On the contrary, a client requiring a lengthy hospital stay, complicated by a subsequent visit to a subacute care or rehabilitative hospital setting, represents the most common scenario associated with a moderate to maximal compromise in endurance.

Modes of moderate to maximal level of impairment in endurance may include a client recovering from a fractured hip complicated by a deep vein thrombosis requiring anticoagulation therapy and bed rest for the period of several days to a week. It may include a client with Guillain-Barré syndrome resulting in temporary paralysis for weeks or possibly a client who has sustained an acquired brain injury or exacerbation of chronic obstructive pulmonary disease (COPD) resulting in the need for mechanical ventilation. Each plausible scenario presented will certainly yield significant impairment of a client's ability to endure personally meaningful activity.

Restorative Techniques: Biomechanical Frame of Reference

As is the case with most restorative strategies that address physically based foundational skills, the biomechanical frame of reference supports the most diverse array of methods commonly employed by the occupational therapist to address compromised endurance and is summarized in Table 2-15.

Promotion of Activity Engagement

As occupational therapists, we historically embrace the therapeutic value of engagement in purposeful activity as well as the power of motivation and interest on the healing process. Therefore, occupational therapists will interview the client as to their interest, leisure pursuits, or hobbies and infuse those identified as methods for addressing issues of endurance. The occupational therapist implements his or her skills in gradation to provide the ideal challenge while avoiding over-fatigue and minimizing frustration. These measures can take any form, depending on the level of impairment presented by the client. For example, a session may be conducted in which a client engages in painting while seated in a high-back chair with armrests and using a lap tray for 10 minutes.

Table 2-15

Remedial Endurance Techniques of the Biomechanical Theory

- Active engagement in graded functional activity engagement designed to address the client's specific needs and interests.
- Exercise programs with no or low weight, low repetitions, and high number of sets.
- Arm ergometers at a client-specific frequency and duration.
- Pulley programs at a client-specific frequency and duration.

The sessions would then progress to standing at an upright easel for 30 minutes, thereby fostering sustained activity over time. An additional technique commonly employed is forward or backward chaining. The occupational therapist may also elicit chaining as a means of ensuring motivational success for clients. As detailed in Chapter 1, the occupational therapist will break down a functional task into its component parts and then grade the level of assistance provided in completing the task with the client. In backward chaining, the occupational therapist begins the task and the client completes it. This technique then promotes client confidence in his or her skills by avoiding a sense of failure inherent in being unsuccessful in an attempt. The therapist then decreases the assistance while the client continues to gain skill and confidence, eventually becoming independent with the entire task (Woodson, 2014). If the therapist is unable to decrease assistance, then restoration is no longer an appropriate approach. An example can be found in the use of cooking as a strategy to improve endurance. With backward-chaining a cooking task, the occupational therapist will begin the task by setting out all of the required supplies, while the client is responsible for actual preparation only. This would then be graded accordingly, allowing the client to complete all required facets of the task successfully. In general, clients tend to truly enjoy activity-based interventions and, by infusing personal interest, are better motivated to actively participate and improve their level of endurance.

Traditional Exercise Programs

Another popular approach to restoring endurance is exercise with no or low weights and high repetitions; a process that fosters physical endurance over muscle strength. Examples of these include the use of pulley exercises, work simulators, and arm ergometers all previously described in detail amid the ROM and strength subsections of this chapter.

Techniques at a Glance

Table 2-15 outlines the most implemented restorative techniques for issues of endurance.

Special Considerations

Again, as was the case with strength, the occupational therapist must pay close attention to how a client is tolerating interventions designed to foster increased endurance. Frequently, clients underestimate the effect that decreased endurance has on their ability to engage in routine, often simple daily tasks. The signs and symptoms requiring attention include diaphoresis, shortness of breath, pallor of skin, and/or complaints of faintness, dizziness, or even nausea. In some cases, endurance may be so compromised that the simple act of sitting up to the edge of the bed will elicit these signs. In this scenario, the occupational therapist and physical therapist may work collaboratively to address a goal such as tolerating upright positioning while seated at the edge of a bed for 5 minutes. Small gains such as this over time will improve endurance to a point where intervention goals can include bedside ADLs and eventually showering as the client and therapist work together to restore daily roles and routines.

Also of consideration in this area is the psychosocial well-being of the client. The most severe cases of compromised endurance occur secondary to prolonged immobility, and that immobility is typically the result of a very serious illness or injury, possibly with a complicated recovery. It is important that occupational therapists use their background in mental health to acknowledge a client's feelings, empower self-advocacy, and refer to ancillary services within the team as necessary.

Maintenance Programs

Overall, a maintenance program designed to foster optimal endurance should emphasize graded re-engagement in those activities a client would characterize as constituting a typical daily routine prior to the onset of the illness or injury. Careful attention should also be placed on the active and independent execution of work simplification and energy conservation techniques during the tasks of everyday living and are explained in further detail in Chapters 3 and 4 of this text.

Restorative Techniques for Coordination

Definitional Analysis

Coordination is categorized per the Framework document (AOTA, 2014) under body functions/ neuromuscular and movement-related functions as "control of voluntary movement" (p. S23). For the more specific purposes of this section, Venes (2009) defines coordination as "the working together of various muscle to produce certain movements .... Coordinated movement requires sequencing of muscle activity and stability of proximal musculature" (p. 523). Therefore, coordination is requiring of both the somatosensory system and the neuromusculoskeletal system, working together to allow for refined movement, as presented in the Framework (AOTA, 2014). Movement-related functions, such as eye-hand coordination or bilateral integration, require the subconscious integration of reflexes and righting reactions, in addition to accurate interpretation of sensory/perceptual information, that then enable one to successfully interact with the external environment.

Coordination is further delineated into the categories of fine and gross motor skills (AOTA, 2014). Fine motor skills are those movements controlled by smaller or more precise joints and musculature, whereas gross motor skills refer to those generated by larger musculature producing larger ranges of movement, such as at the shoulder and hip joints (Thomas, 2012). The ability to coordinate both fine motor and gross motor movement relies heavily on accurate interpretation of sensory information and the ability to control resulting movement. "Within the individual, movement emerges through the cooperative effort of many brain structures and processes . . . including those that are related to perception, cognition, and action" (Shumway-Cook & Woollacott, 2012, p. 4). Given coordination is the product of an interaction among a variety of complex body systems, a wide array of illnesses and injuries may impede this foundational skill.

Modes of Injury or Illness

Neurologically based impairments of coordination, otherwise known as ataxia, are seen typically as secondary symptoms of an illness or injury. As is the case with many other foundational skills covered within the contents of this chapter, ataxia can occur as a result of a wide array of neurological conditions. Many of these types of conditions fall under the category of acquired brain injuries (ABI).

Injuries to the brain, and specifically to the cerebellum, include trauma by means of an external force (TBI), aneurysms, infections, abscesses, tumors, or CVA caused by hemorrhage, ischemia, or infarct. Each of these injuries may potentially affect the coordination centers of the brain and result in ataxic or uncoordinated movement patterns.

Degenerative disorders of the central and/or peripheral nervous systems may also represent the underlying cause for ataxia, dystonia, or dyskinesia. Dystonia is defined as "prolonged involuntary muscle contractions that may cause twisting (torsion) of body parts, repetitive movements, and increased muscular tone" (Venes, 2009, p. 712). This symptom is commonly seen in illnesses such as Parkinson's, Huntington's, and Creutzfeldt-Jakob diseases, as well as in disease-related dementias. Dyskinesia is defines as "a defect in the ability to perform voluntary movement" (Venes, 2009, p. 706), thus directly affecting the ability to perform coordinated movement. Some illnesses causing dyskinesia can include MS, Parkinson's disease, post-polio syndrome, myasthenia gravis, ALS, or even peripheral neuropathies in general.

Therefore, overall, the mode of illness or injury responsible for a deficit in coordination can be quite inclusive, ranging from acute trauma to degenerative disease processes. However, the mode of injury or illness is of significance due to the impact it has on the choice of intervention strategy. This concept will be explored further in the Special Considerations portion of this subsection.

Restorative Techniques: Motor Control and Motor Learning Frames of Reference

When addressing coordination issues, restorative strategies applied tend to be grounded in a combination of theories grouped by Cole and Tufano as "Motor Control and Motor Learning Frames" (2008) and are specifically summarized in Table 2-16. The shared basic tenet of these theories is found in the concept of the brain's ability to reorganize following neurological insult, commonly referred to as the principle of neural plasticity.

"Plasticity or neural modifiability, may be seen as a continuum from short-term changes in the efficiency or strength of synaptic connections to the long-term structural changes in the organization and numbers of connections among neurons" (Shumway-Cook & Woollacott, 2012, p. 84). Essentially, this principle asserts that the brain is able to regenerate neural pathways damaged by illness or injury through sprouting or regrowing alternate pathways that then allow for the recovery of motor control. An analogy can be found in the image of a collapsed bridge along an interstate highway. Immediately following the "collapse," traffic may be backed up for miles and chaos ensues as vehicles scramble to locate alternate routes to their ultimate destinations. Though the alternate route may not be the most efficient means to get where one needs to go, it serves an important purpose in allowing the required time for "reconstruction" at the bridge site. Once reopened, the repaired bridge will again allow for the passage of vehicles as it did in the past, though never the same as it once had prior to the event. This premise applies when considering the effect of injury or illness on the neural pathways of the brain. In neural plasticity, the collapse of one pathway will cause the diversion of impulses to alternate routes in order to reach their final destination. Though the diverted routes may never be as efficient as the original paths, nonetheless they meet an important interim purpose. To enhance the efficiency in rebuilding neural pathways, repetition is believed to have significant value. Hence, this principle also emphasizes the repetition of normal movement patterns as a means of shaping the regeneration process.

The theoretic bases from which approaches are divided in the realm of motor control and motor learning are classified by Almhdawi, Mathiowetz, and Bass (2014) as either neurophysiological or system-based and task-related. This classification is the result of the growth in understanding the complexity of human movement by scientists and clinicians alike through investigative research and practice. The conventional neurophysiologic (neurodevelopmental) approaches

Table 2-16

Remedial Coordination Techniques of the Motor Learning and Neurodevelopmental Theories According to Health Condition

Mode of Injury	Remedial Technique
Acquired brain injuries including TBI, stroke, meningitis, abscesses, and tumors	Motor learning approaches: • Task-oriented approach • Carr and Shepherd approach • Constraint-induced approach • Graded, functionally oriented tasks • Backward chaining of functionally oriented tasks OR
Degenerative diseases including Parkinson's, Huntington's, MS, ALS, and post-polio	Traditional sensorimotor approaches of... • Bobath/NDT: Weight-bearing, weight shifting, key points of control • Proprioceptive neuromuscular facilitation (PNF): Diagonal movement patterns, multisensory cueing, kinesthetic feedback • Rood: Muscle co-contraction, multisensory cuing

include Rood's sensorimotor approach, Kabat and Knott's proprioceptive neuromuscular facilitation, Brunnstrom's approach, and Bobath's neurodevelopmental treatment, all of which share in the reflexive and hierarchical model of motor control (Almhdawi et al., 2014; Shumway-Cook & Woollacott, 2012). Very popular in use among the occupational and physical therapy domains, these approaches prevailed as the strategy of choice for many years in the restoration of normal movement patterns after neurological impairment. The contemporary, task-oriented approaches are based on a systems model of motor control and motor learning that emphasizes repetitive engagement in functional activity as a restorative method for motor dysfunction (Almhdawi et al., 2014).

In the current rehabilitative era, Rao (2011) brings eloquent clarity to the shift from the use of traditional neurophysiologic approaches to that of the contemporary task-oriented approaches. Describing the phenomena as "paradigm shifts" related to the treatment of and restoration of neurologic dysfunction (2011, p. 94), Rao concludes: "The evidence reviewed . . . based on the results of randomized controlled trials, clearly demonstrates (at a grade A level) (supported by at least one level 1 study) that neurotherapeutic (neurodevelopmental) approaches are at best no more effective than traditional therapy and in fact are inferior to training based on a task-oriented approach" (2011, pp. 95 & 100). Therefore, the task-oriented approaches will be reviewed first and followed by those of the neurophysiologic classification. Although lacking in evidence, as is summarized by Rao (2011) and reproduced with permission in Tables 2-17 through 2-19, neurophysiologic approaches harbor clinical significance in shaping the profession as it stands today and are therefore included in this subsection of the text.

The Task-Oriented Approach

The task-oriented/related approach described by Horak (1991), Almhdawi et al. (2014), and Shumway-Cook and Woollacott (2001) emerged following review of the most current research on motor behavior, control, and development in conjunction with motor learning theories. The task-oriented approach also shares a foundation in neural plasticity but uniquely recognizes the significance of client-centered intervention or the individual with unique interests, experiences, desires, and motivators. Hence, the return of coordinated movement within this approach is a result of repetitive engagement in personally preferred movement patterns occurring within the natural environment.

The onset of illness or injury disrupts the preferred motor patterns that enable successful activity engagement. This approach requires the occupational therapist to analyze the component parts of completing the preferred task, identify the physical barriers to engaging in those tasks (such as a lack of coordination), and facilitate successful re-engagement in that task by means of grading and chaining the client's participation in context accordingly. Rao (2011), in review of current efficacy studies, states that there is substantial evidence to suggest that task-oriented training leads to improved functional outcomes in both level of impairment and activity engagement.

The Carr and Shepherd Approach

Carr and Shepherd, Australian physical therapists, have applied motor control and learning principles to occupational therapy interventions for motor difficulties occurring secondary to CNS dysfunction. This approach, referred to as the *motor relearning programme* (MRP), very closely resembles the task-oriented approach given the emphasis of clients to engage in personally preferred tasks, but differs in that intervention is implemented with the goal of motor recovery and not actual completion of the task itself (Shapero & Sabari, 2008). Carr and Shepherd, therefore, use the engagement in functional activity for the powerfully motivating factors it elicits within a client alone. Here, it is through engaging repetitively in motor tasks that neural plasticity can be best facilitated.

The Carr and Shepherd approach uniquely harbors a biomechanical component given a foundation in human kinesiology and specifically the analysis of kinematic and kinetic requirements for completing functional tasks. This approach sees the therapist as a coach whose primary role in intervention is to provide education to clients by means of verbal and nonverbal communication techniques (Ivey & Mew, 2010), again similar to the task-oriented approach. The secondary role is then to manually guide normal movement patterns and/or minimize abnormal movement patterns during activity engagement that arise commonly after neurological insult. As in other motor learning theories, Carr and Shepherd place much emphasis on the use of repetitive practice to elicit the efficient return of coordinated motor performance. Overall, the method is one in which the client is actively learning principles to optimize normal movement patterns, as guided by the therapist, during engagement in a preferred personal activity. In 2010, Langhammer and Stranghelle published the results of a second study conducted to re-examine their early findings on the efficacy of Carr and Sheppard's MRP approach versus that of the Bobath approach, also known as the *neurodevelopmental (NDT) approach*. After a review of the outcome measures, Langhammer and Stranghelle (2000, 2010) reconfirmed and strengthened the earlier findings that when compared to the traditional techniques of Bobath (NDT), MRP techniques are preferable in both the capacity and the quality of movement for clients in the acute rehabilitation setting after stroke.

The Constraint-Induced Movement Therapy Approach

Recently, more attention is being drawn to the constraint-induced movement therapy (CIMT) approach as the rehabilitative field continues to move toward evidence-based practice models. With related publications dating back to the 1960s, E. Taub and colleagues began by conducting experiments on primates in which a single forelimb was deafferented surgically through dorsal rhizotomy (Rao, 2004). After the procedure, the primates tended to disuse the affected (deafferent) limb. Taub, Uswatte, and Pidikiti (1999) suggested that this was a learned behavior in which the

Table 2-17

Evidence for Effectiveness of Neurotherapies

Authors and Year	Aims/Rationale	Design and Subjects	Intervention and Outcome Measures	Results	Comments	Rating
Basmajian et al. (1987)	Compare two PT approaches: Behavioral (including biofeedback) and Bobath in subacute stroke stage	RCT 29 subjects Training 3 times a week for 5 weeks Pre-testing and post-testing; 9-month follow-up Subjects with first MCA infarcts	*Behavioral group*: Electromyographic biofeedback through conceptualization, skill learning, rehearsal, and transfer *Bobath group*: Facilitation with controlled sensory input 1. Upper Extremity Function Test 2. Health Belief System 3. Beck's Depression Inventory 4. 16 PF (for mood and affect)	Both groups improved; no differences were seen between groups Bobath treatment was not superior to behavioral treatment	Small sample size Good study	II
Mudie et al. (2002)	Compare task-related, Bobath, and feedback approaches for training weight symmetry in subacute stroke stage	Double-blind RCT 40 subjects Training 5 times a week for 2 weeks; assessment 1 week before study and 2 and 12 weeks after study	*Feedback group*: Provided visual feedback of symmetry via monitor during reach *Task-related group*: functional reach in various directions and distances *Bobath group*: Increasing range of motion, normalize tone, improve balance during reach *Control group*: Standard occupational therapy and PT 1. Weight distribution in sitting 2. Weight distribution in standing 3. Barthel index	Bobath group was better at sitting symmetry at 2 weeks; feedback and task-related groups were better at 12 weeks; feedback group was better at standing symmetry at 2 weeks; task-related group was better than Bobath group; and task-related group was better in functional gains	Good study Small sample size	II

(continued)

Table 2-17 (continued)

Evidence for Effectiveness of Neurotherapies

Authors and Year	Aims/Rationale	Design and Subjects	Intervention and Outcome Measures	Results	Comments	Rating
Pollack et al. (2002)	Test effect of independent sitting balance as adjunct to standard therapy based on Bobath approach in subacute stroke stage	RCT with blocked randomization with 2:1 ratio 28 subjects Training 5 times a week for 4 weeks; assessment at start at end of training and 2 weeks after training	*Experimental group*: Construction tasks that encouraged balance 1. Proportion of patients achieving normal symmetry of weight distribution during standing, sitting, rising to stand, sitting down, and reaching	No differences were seen across groups	Unequal groups Small sample size One outcome measure	II
Lord & Hall (1986)	Compare NDT to traditional therapy	Retrospective study of 39 subjects	ADL scale	No differences across groups	Unequal groups	IV
Wagenaar et al. (1990)	Compare NDT and Brunnstrom approaches in acute stroke stage	Case series Alternating treatment design 7 subjects with MCA stroke Training for 5 times a week for 21 weeks; each phase lasted 5 weeks	1. Action Research Arm Test 2. Walking velocity over 8 m 3. Barthel index 4. VROPSOM List (Dutch version of the Depression Adjective Checklist) 5. Neuropsychological tests	Walking speed was better for only one patient during Brunnstrom treatment; all patients showed some recovery in the first 8 to 10 weeks	Small sample size No true control group	V

(continued)

Table 2-17 (continued)

Evidence for Effectiveness of Neurotherapies

Authors and Year	Aims/Rationale	Design and Subjects	Intervention and Outcome Measures	Results	Comments	Rating
Hesse et al. (1994)	Test the effect of an NDT-based in-patient program on gait in subacute stroke stage	Case series 148 subjects who could walk 20 m independently Training 5 times a week for 4 weeks; assessment at beginning and at 4 weeks	All patients received occupation therapy, speech therapy, and neuropsychological training as needed 1. Gait measures (peak vertical ground reaction force, loading and deloading rates, time to peak force) 2. 10-m walk 3. Walking endurance 4. Stair climbing	Time for walking and climbing improved, but no endurance; stance duration and symmetry improved	No control group	V

Reprinted with permission from Rao, A. K. (2011) Approaches to motor control dysfunction: An evidence-based review. In G. Gillen (Ed.), *Stroke rehabilitation: A function-based approach* (3rd ed., pp. 117-155). St Louis, MO: Mosby.

Table 2-18
Evidence for Task-Oriented Approach

Authors and Year	Rationale	Design and Subjects	Intervention and Outcome Measures	Results	Comments	Rating
Dean, Richards, & Malouin (2000)	Test the effect of task-related circuit training	RCT pilot study 2-month follow-up 9 subjects Exercise for 1 hour, 3 times a week for 4 weeks	*Experimental group*: Strengthening and functional activities *Control group*: Functional activities 1. Walking speed and endurance 2. Vertical ground reaction force 3. Step test	Experimental group performed better on walking speed and endurance and on force production	Small sample size Study only tested added influence of strength training	II
Nelles et al. (2001)	Test brain plasticity after task-related training in early stroke stage	RCT 10 subjects after first stroke; early subacute stroke stage Training 4 times a week for 3 weeks	Task oriented functional reach in different directions and distances *Control group*: Stretching, ROM 1. Positron emission tomography scan	After training, task-oriented group showed activation of contralateral sensorimotor cortex and bilateral activation of the inferior parietal cortex; control group showed weak activation of only the inferior parietal cortex	Good study Small sample size	II
Malouin et al. (1992)	Test application of a task-oriented treatment in improving gait after acute stroke stage	Case series design 10 subjects 2 sessions/day, 5 days/week for 8 weeks	Early standing, weight-shifting, isokinetic exercises and treadmill training 1. Treadmill velocity 2. Training duration	Treadmill velocity and training duration increased	Small sample size No control group Double the typical treatment time in PT	V

(continued)

Table 2-18 (continued)

Evidence for Task-Oriented Approach

Authors and Year	Rationale	Design and Subjects	Intervention and Outcome Measures	Results	Comments	Rating
Smith et al. (1999)	Test a task-oriented treadmill exercise program in chronic stroke stage	Case series 14 subjects Training 3 times a week for 3 months	Reflexive and volitional torque generated by dynamometer at different velocities	Torque production for concentric and eccentric contractions increased	Small sample size No control group	V
Monger, Carr, & Fowler (2002)	Test a task-specific home exercise program in chronic stroke stage	Pretest, post-test case series design 6 subjects, 1 year after stroke 3-week home exercise program	Intervention was based on motor learning; sit-to-stand and stepping was practiced at different seat heights, speeds, and repetitions 1. Motor Assessment Scale (MAS) 2. Vertical ground reaction force 3. Walking speed over 10 m 4. Grip strength	Scores on the MAS, vertical ground reaction force, and walking speed improved for experimental group; grip force did not improve	No control group; small sample size Good pilot study	V
Bassile et al. (2003)	Test effect of a task-related obstacle training program in chronic stroke stage	Case-series Pre-training and post-training; 1 month follow-up 5 subjects Training 2 times/week for 5 weeks	Subjects walked along a 10-m walkway over obstacles on two thirds of the trials 1. MAS walking section 2. 6-minute walk distance 3. Walking velocity 4. SF-36	Improvements seen in walking velocity, 6-minute walk distance, MAS, and SF-36	Good pilot study Small sample size No control group	V

Reprinted with permission from Rao, A. K. (2011) Approaches to motor control dysfunction: An evidence-based review. In G. Gillen (Ed.), *Stroke rehabilitation: A function-based approach* (3rd ed., pp. 117-155). St Louis, MO: Mosby.

Table 2-19
Evidence Table for Constraint-Induced Movement Therapy

Authors and Year	Rationale	Design and Subjects	Intervention and Outcome Measures	Results	Comments	Rating
Van der Lee et al. (1999)	Evaluate the effectiveness of forced use therapy; compare CIMT with Bobath therapy in chronic stroke stage	RCT 60 subjects Experimental group: immobilization and training Control group: bimanual training based on NDT Training was 6 hours/day 5 days/week for 2 weeks Follow-up for 1 year	*Experimental group*: Splint worn for most of the day; training of functional activities *Control group*: Bimanual activities 1. Rehabilitation Activities Profile 2. Action Research Arm Test (ARAT) 3. Fugl-Meyer Assessment 4. Motor Activity Log (MAL)	CIMT group performed better on ARAT and arm use 1 week after training; gains on ARAT were maintained after 1 year CIMT group had greater amount of arm use, but did not maintain in the long term	Good study CIMT group performance better at start of training Modest benefit of CIMT over Bobath approach	I
Taub et al. (1993)	Test whether forced use of the impaired limb counteracts learned nonuse in chronic stroke stage	RCT 9 subjects in chronic stroke stage Experimental group (4): restraint of the unimpaired limbs for 23 hours; therapy for 6 hours/day 5 days/ week for 2 weeks	Limb restrained for 23 hours/day for experimental group Control group asked to focus on use of impaired limb 1. Emory Motor Function Test 2. ARAT 3. MAL 4. Passive range of motion	Performance time was quicker for restraint group; quality of movement and functional ability were better for restraint group	Small sample size Experimental group had much more training Training massed over 2 weeks No comparison with traditional rehabilitation	II

(continued)

Table 2-19 (continued)

Evidence Table for Constraint-Induced Movement Therapy

Authors and Year	Rationale	Design and Subjects	Intervention and Outcome Measures	Results	Comments	Rating
Dromerick, Edwards, & Hahn (2000)	Compare CIMT with OT in the acute stage	RCT 20 subjects Experimental group (11): Mitten worn 6 hours/day, plus OT and CIMT training 2 hours/day for 5 days/week for 2 weeks Control group (9): Standard OT and circuit training	Mitten worn 5 hours/day for 14 days 1. ARAT 2. Barthel index 3. Functional Independence Measure (FIM)	CIMT group had better total ARAT scores and upper extremity FIM scores No other differences were seen	Little support for benefit of CIMT approach Small sample size	II
Page et al. (2002)	Test the efficacy of a modified CIMT protocol in subacute stroke stage	RCT 14 subjects Modified CIMT group: half hour PT and OT 2 times a week for 10 weeks	*Modified CIMT group*: Restraint for 5 hours/day; training 1 hour/day *Traditional group*: PNF therapy 1. Fugl-Meyer Assessment 2. ARAT 3. MAL	No change was seen in traditional and control group Modified CIMT group improved on Fugl-Meyer Assessment, ARAT, and MAL	Small sample size	II
Wolf et al. (1989)	First study to test CIMT in chronic stroke age	Case series Pretreatment and posttreatment 21 subjects Restraint and training, 3-month follow-up	14 days of restraint and 10 days of training 1. Wolf Motor Function Test (WMFT)	Arm function improved following restraint and training	No control group Small sample size, limited outcome measures	V

(continued)

Table 2-19 (continued)

Evidence Table for Constraint-Induced Movement Therapy

Authors and Year	Rationale	Design and Subjects	Intervention and Outcome Measures	Results	Comments	Rating
Kunkel et al. (1999)	Replicate findings of Taub et al.	Case series design Pre-treatment and post-treatment 5 subjects in chronic stroke stage 3-month follow-up	Limb restrained for 23 hours a day for 14 days 1. MAL 2. WMFT 3. ARAT	Restraint improved MAL, WMFT, and quality of movement	No control group Small sample size	V
Blanton & Wolf (1999)	Test the effectiveness of CIMT in subacute stroke stage	Case report Pretreatment and post-treatment 3 month follow-up 14 days of restraint and 10 days of training	Hand constrained in a mitten for 23 hours a day 1. WMFT 2. MAL	Completion time improved on the WMFT; improvement seen on self-report (MAL)	Single patient; limited generalizability	V
Miltner et al. (1999)	Replicate earlier findings on the benefit of CIMT	Case series 15 subjects in chronic stroke stage Sling on arm for 90% of waking time for 12 days Training for 7 hours/day for 8 days 6-month follow-up	Restraint and shaping with familiar household objects 1. MAL 2. WMFT 3. ARAT	Actual amount of use and quality of movement; functional ability improved and was retained over 6 months	No control group Small sample size Massed practice	V
Page et al. (2001)	Test the efficacy of a modified CIMT protocol; compare CIMT embedded in therapy with therapy and no therapy in a subacute outpatient setting	Case series 6 subjects 2 subjects: OT/PT 3 times/week for 10 weeks plus sling and mitt for 5 hours/day 5 days/week 2 subjects: OT/PT for 10 weeks 2 subjects: no therapy 10-week follow-up	CIMT and traditional group received 30 minutes of training 3 times a week 1. Fugl-Meyer Assessment 2. ARAT 3. WMFT 4. MAL	CIMT group performed better on Fugl-Meyer Assessment, ARAT, WMFT, and MAL	Small sample size No statistical analysis of useful modification CIMT approach to outpatient therapy	V

primates preferred the positive reinforcement obtained through coordinated use of the unaffected limb over the negative experiences resulting from the attempted use of the affected limb.

As the studies of Taub et al. (1999) continued to analyze this "learned nonuse" (p. 239) of the affected limb, the group discovered that after a device that physically constrained the movement of the unaffected or intact limb was applied, the primates resorted back to the use of the affected limb to perform essential activities such as grooming and feeding. These findings provided the foundation for the constraint-induced therapy (CIT) approach, also referred to in literature as the *CIMT* or *forced use therapy* approaches. The original focus of CIT was to foster motor return in clients experiencing chronic upper limb paralysis. Recently, several modified forms CIT (mCIT) have evolved in an attempt to expand the content and intensity of CIT. In 2012, Nijland et al. published their review of CIT literature from which they designed a treatment protocol that extends CIT from chronic to acute stages of stroke, as early as in the first 5 weeks of onset.

The original CIT approach for clients with chronic stroke required the use of a constraint device, such as a mitt or sling, applied to the unaffected extremity of a client with hemiparesis, 14 hours per day for 2 weeks (Page, Sisto, Levine, Johnston, & Hughes, 2001, p. 584) while promoting active engagement in daily routines. Though evidence-supported functional improvement in the coordinated use of the affected extremity, particularly in clients with chronic cardiovascular accidents, several barriers to the successful integration of the approach in intervention were identified. The chief barrier highlighted was the investment of time required by the client (and therapist) over the 2-week interval. This duration of 14 hours per day can quickly lead to frustration and poor compliance and therefore negative results. As a result, Page, Sisto, and Johnston modified the CIT approach in 2000, decreasing intensity to 5 hours per day, 5 days per week, for a duration of 10 weeks. To date, recommendations can vary from 0.5 to 6 hours per day, 3 to 5 times per week, for 2 to 10 weeks (Lin, Wu, Liu, Chen, & Hsu, 2009). "Numerous studies of stroke patients have shown that CIT and its derivatives significantly improve motor ability and functional use of the affected limb . . . ." (Lin et al., 2009).

Given the evidence in support of it, the CIT/CIMT approach will continue to gain visibility; however, this method is not suitable for all clientele, and the exact method with the best outcomes is still under debate (Reiss, Wolf, Hammel, McLeod, & Williams, 2012). Attention must also be paid to the potential safety risk posed by constraining the unaffected extremity of a client who has sustained a neurological injury.

The Neurodevelopmental Theory: A Review of NDT, PNF, Rood, and Brunnstrom Approaches

Per the neurodevelopmental theory, the four most traditional and commonly implemented approaches for coordination are the Bobath or NDT approach, Kabat's proprioceptive neuromuscular facilitation (PNF) approach, the Rood approach (Stroup & Snodgrass, 2005), and the Brunnstrom approach. As mentioned earlier, each of these approaches share in the principles of neural plasticity further enhanced by the promotion of repetition. However, these approaches differ in that they also harbor a shared belief that it is through eliciting reflexive movements along the developmental continuum that coordinated movement will be restored. Given the complexity of this belief, the use of these approaches often warrants continuing education on behalf of the therapist. Additional information regarding continuing education opportunities in these areas may be found in Appendix A.

The NDT (Bobath) approach, developed by Dr. Karel and Berta Bobath, a 1940s husband-and-wife team (one a neurologist and the other a physical therapist), places emphasis on the accurate interpretation of sensory input to produce refined motor output (Luke, Dodd, & Brock, 2003). Dysfunction in coordination is a result of abnormal sensation and, specifically, abnormal sensations of the upright posture. Without postural control in the core musculature, a client is unable to

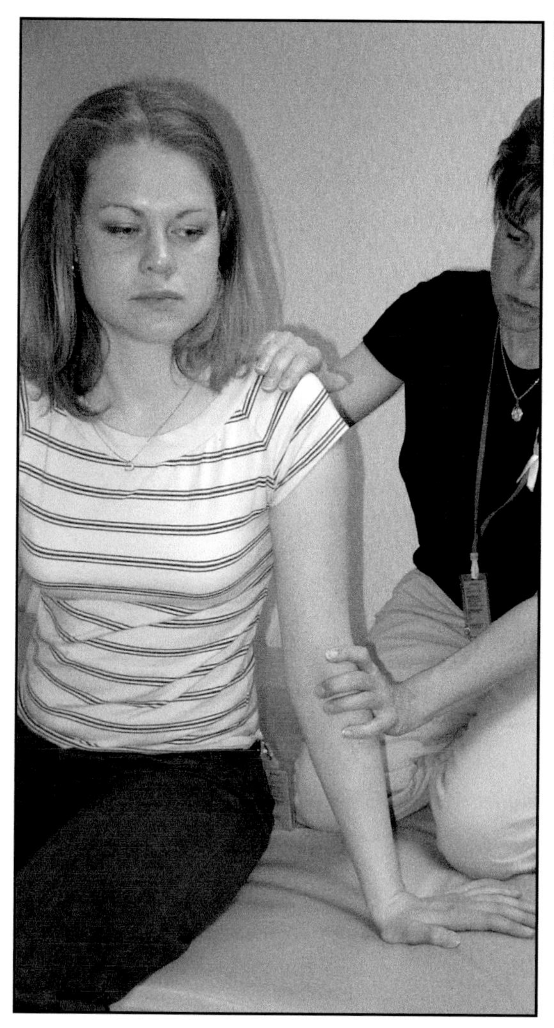

Figure 2-15. Demonstration of a typical weight-bearing position throughout the upper extremity. Support and stability is provided by the therapist at the elbow and shoulder joint structures as the client leans toward the positioned extremity to bear body weight through shoulder, elbow, and wrist joints of the upper extremity.

produce coordinated motion in the distal extremities. Therefore, much of the approach emphasizes the establishment of postural stability and alignment by employing techniques of weight-bearing and weight shifting (Raine, 2009). Here, the occupational therapist is fostering exaggerated sensory input by means of bearing weight directly through affected extremities to improve both interpretation via feedback and resulting motor output (Figure 2-15). With regard to weight shift, the occupational therapist promotes reaching, either in a functional capacity or with the use of a therapeutic ball, out of the base of support to introduce graded opportunities for challenging the core stability or underlying postural control. Figure 2-16 is an illustration of this technique. These restorative methods, guided by specific handling techniques designed to inhibit reflexive movement (key points of control), secondarily improve distal mobility or coordination of the extremities. Of note, though NDT is a historically popular restorative approach in rehabilitation, "to date, researchers have not found evidence that NDT is more effective than any other approach" (Krug & McCormack, 2009) when compared and contrasted with other methods of intervention.

Herman Kabat, a neurophysiologist, developed the PNF approach in the 1940s that again focuses on the developmental sequence of motor performance, yet with a strategic focus on agonist and antagonist muscle relationships (Schultz-Krohn, Pope-Davis, Jourdan, & McLaughlin-Gray, 2013).

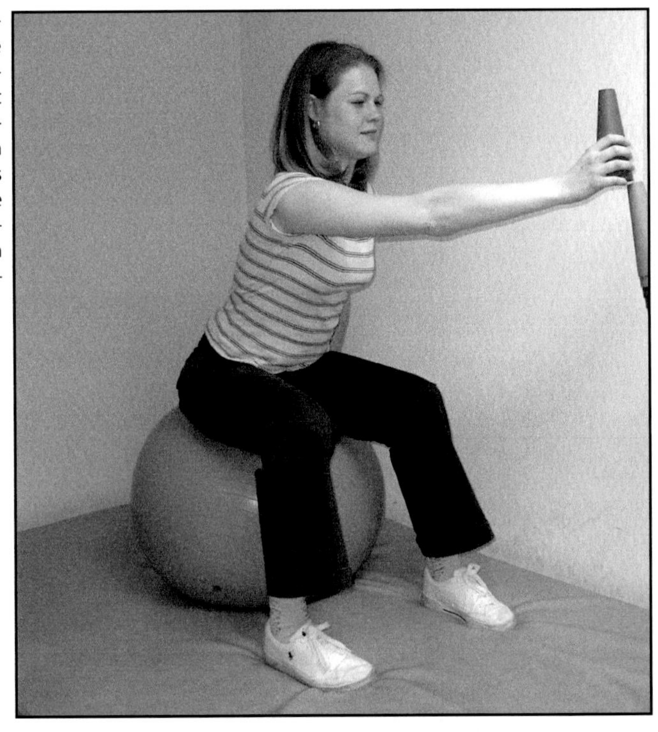

Figure 2-16. An example of how weight-bearing can be promoted throughout the trunk and lower extremity while also challenging postural control by reaching out of the base of support. Though an occupational therapist's primary focus is on engagement in functional activity, at times the use of cones is adopted. This procedure minimizes distraction, redirecting attention to the challenge demanded by both balancing and weight shifting in the presence of compromised proximal stability.

The foundation of this approach is found in the belief that human motion occurs in a curvilinear plane and requires the entire system to execute accurately. Function is a result of the fine orchestration by the central nervous system among antagonist and agonist muscle contractions. Restorative techniques of PNF foster gross motor motions in diagonal or curvilinear (Figure 2-17) patterns to best simulate functional motion and progress as dictated by typical motor development. Emphasis is placed heavily on repetition as the manner of retraining the motor control centers to specific sensory input and facilitated by way of verbal or tactile cuing. Upon regaining a cooperative relationship among the muscular system as a whole, coordination is therefore improved. Research on the efficacy of this approach is limited (Shimura & Kasai, 2001). In support, Westwater-Wood, Adams, and Kerry (2010) found in a critical review of evidence that current research demonstrates trends toward the effectiveness of PNF as an approach to rehabilitation in a variety of patient populations. Conversely, Kraft, Fitts, and Hammond (1992) found PNF to be the least effective method of intervention when compared to techniques of electrical stimulation in clients who had experienced a chronic stroke.

Margaret Rood, who was versed in both occupational and physical therapy professions, developed the Rood approach in the 1950s (Schultz-Krohn et al., 2013). This approach addresses coordination deficits secondarily by prioritizing restorative techniques used to normalize muscle tone. Tone will be specifically addressed in a later subsection, while coordination remains the focus here; thus, only a portion of the Rood Approach is directly applicable. As do the NDT and PNF approaches, Rood emphasizes the developmental nature of motor control and the importance of postural alignment or stability. As in PNF, these techniques foster unison between agonistic and antagonist musculature, and as in both PNF and NDT, repetition of normally coordinated movement patterns fosters restoration.

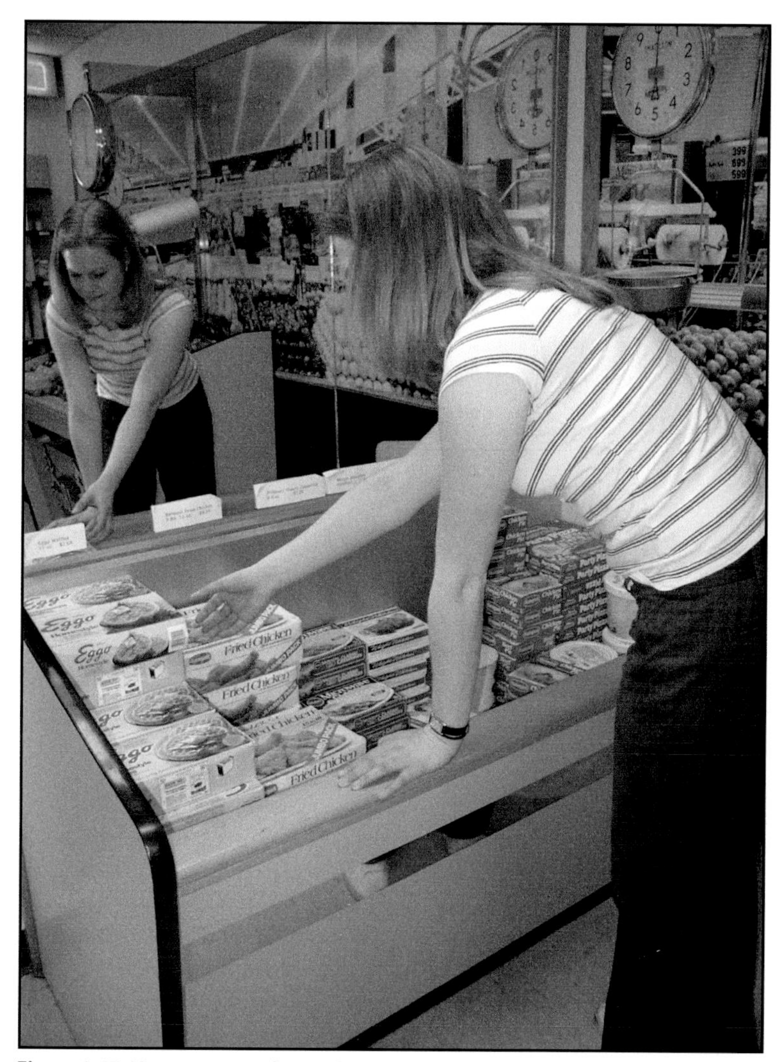

Figure 2-17. Movement in a diagonal or curvilinear pattern integrated into the execution of a functional activity.

With the Rood approach, clients are placed in positions reflective of typical development, referred to as *ontogenic positions*. These include prone on elbows and/or quadruped, which require the subconscious co-contraction of heavy-work or large proximal and stabilizing musculature. Clients are then requested to engage in meaningful activity using consciously controlled light-work or distal mobilizing musculature while maintaining the ontogenic position. Figure 2-18 is an illustration of this technique. There is a lack of literature identifying the efficacy of the Rood approach. However, Stroup and Snodgrass (2005) have stated that although "her work is of interest, it is not as widely accepted as NDT or PNF" (p. 49). In addition, other authors have stated: "Subsequent understanding of motor recovery in adults with acquired brain injuries has negated the value of using a developmental model. In fact, today, the emphasis is on providing movement practice to patients in natural context" (Sabari, Capasso, & Geld-Glazman, 2014).

The Brunnstrom approach, developed by Signe Brunnstrom in 1970, is not as commonly seen as NDT or PNF treatment approaches. Per Bertoti (2004), "the actual approach to intervention is considered outdated and inappropriate today, [although] Brunnstrom is credited with two main

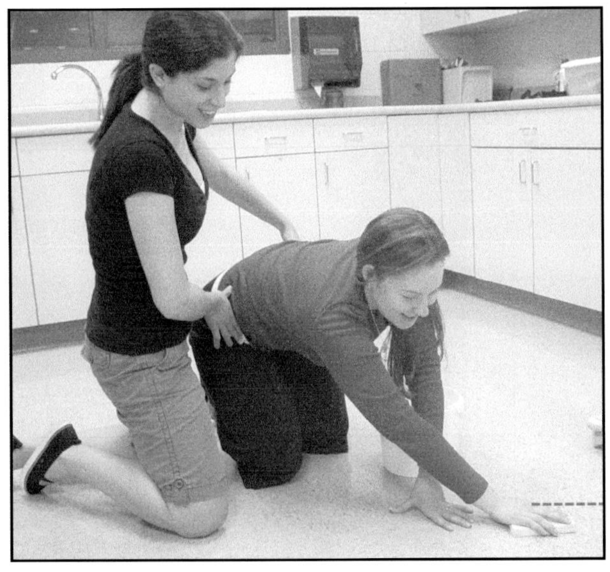

Figure 2-18. This demonstration illustrates the use of ontogenic positioning as a technique of weight-bearing in the restoration of coordinated movement. Here, challenge is provided along the developmental sequence, specifically, the quadruped position. To increase meaningfulness, cones can be replaced with cleaning the floor once the client has established improvement in coordinated movement.

contributions which are still valuable: a description of the stereotypical synergy patterns and recovery stages of . . . [clients] seen following a cerebrovascular accident (CVA)" (p. 189). It is therefore only these two concepts that will be discussed further in this chapter.

Brunnstrom, after observing "thousands of stroke survivors" (Bertoti, 2004), documented the similarities in movement patterns and commonly seen phases of recovery. The patterning of the upper and lower extremity were characterized by dominating flexion or extension positions in the affected limbs, typically flexion of the upper and extension of the lower. Brunnstrom found that these synergistic patterns, occurring along a recognizable pattern of recovery, could be recruited to produce normal movement experiences for clients by way of associated reactions or brainstem reflexes (Katz, Alexander, & Klein, 1998). Because synergies are the result of tonal abnormalities, they are only introduced here and will be discussed in further detail within the Restorative Techniques for Tone section of this chapter. In brief, tonal abnormalities directly affect coordination.

According to Brunnstrom, the goal of occupational therapy intervention lies within managing the characteristics at each stage of recovery and by facilitating techniques that progress the client to the next stage. Techniques progress from postural or proximal trunk control to distal hand and wrist control by first using reflexive movements, which are also known as associated reactions. Progress is made to the point of using only verbal cuing to promote voluntary motor control of the affected limb. Again, Brunnstrom's findings are of most clinical significance in the descriptions provided by the patterning and stages of recovery and the approach continues to hold meaning as a tool of restoration in common day practice (Katz et al., 1998).

Finally, some occupational therapists may use the simple principle of exaggerated sensory input to directly modify motor output when addressing issues of coordination. This technique is illustrated by the use of weighted everyday items such as utensils (Figure 2-19) to amplify typical sensory input and therefore refine motor output. This is a common technique in the presence of tremors such as is seen in Parkinson's disease, for example. These types of weighted items are readily available for purchase through the manufacturers listed in Appendix A. In addition, the use of weighted cuffs placed on extremities during engagement in personally meaningful and functional activity produces similar effects. Efficacy studies of this modified technique are limited, and it requires further exploration.

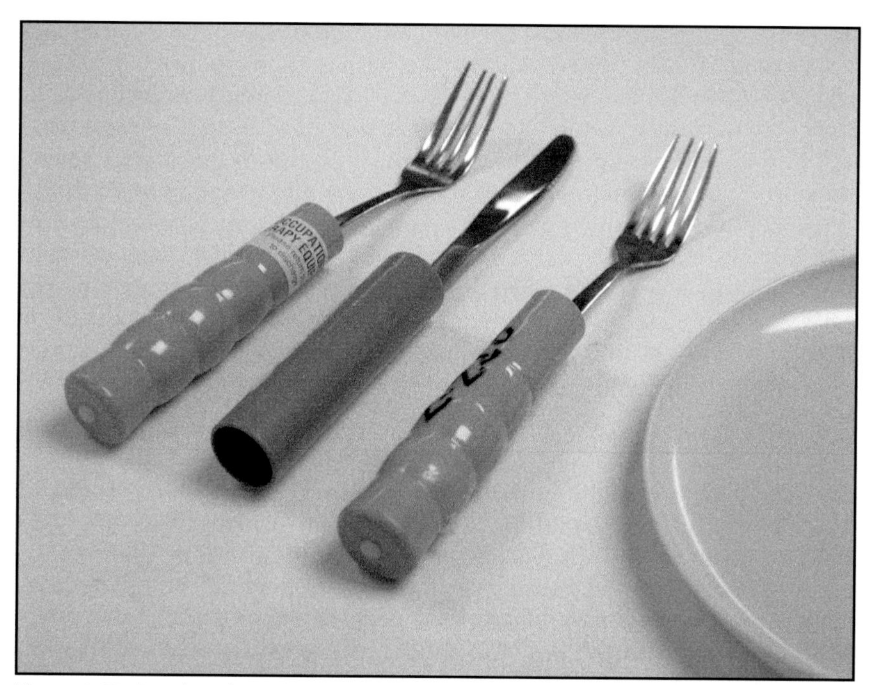

Figure 2-19. Samples of weighted utensils employed to exaggerate sensory input and refine motor output in the task of feeding.

It should be noted the most promising type of intervention is providing task-oriented training within the context of the client's natural activity. This shift away from strict neuromuscular techniques, such as Rood and NDT, to task-oriented intervention was referred to as a "paradigm shift" (Rao, 2011, p. 124), which began in the 1960s but has taken a stronger place in intervention as the occupational therapy community increased the emphasis on function/occupation within practice (2011).

Special Considerations

The foremost consideration that must be made on behalf of clients with issues of coordination is personal safety. A lack of coordination increases the incidence of both orthopedic and various soft-tissue injuries, including sprains and strains. The likelihood for falls, cuts (such as with a knife or shaver), and even burns as a result of involuntary movements is significant and must be addressed with proactive educational measures provided by the occupational therapist as they relate to everyday routines. Low-tech adaptive equipment may also be recommended to ensure client safety. These techniques will be further explored in Chapters 3 and 4.

It is also important to reiterate the nature of the underlying cause of coordination deficits, whether injury or illness to the brain or CNS. With this in mind, the occupational therapist must evaluate the client's cognitive status to appropriately adjust the restorative methods selected to address coordination. For example, a client with limited attention may not be able to participate in a structured activity for greater than 5 minutes. However, as a retired farmer, the same client is able to attend to the task of simple tabletop gardening for up to 20 minutes. Selecting appropriate methods for clients with cognitive issues will greatly increase the likelihood of successful restoration and will be discussed further later in this chapter.

Shumway-Cook and Woollacott (2012) note the significance of time in methods related to recovery versus compensation. The authors note that in the past, it was believed that the CNS was more rigid and less alterable over time (2012). More current investigation highlights the incredible capacity of the CNS to regenerate and reorganize over time. Time is an important factor for the therapist to consider as it relates to the specific injury or illness underlying the limitation in coordination. For example, Parkinson's disease and MS are progressively degenerative, yet over a lengthier period of time than Huntington's or Creutzfeldt-Jakob diseases. Some diseases, such as peripheral neuropathy, are caused by a loss in sensory input, while others result in loss of strength (e.g., myasthenia gravis or ALS). Again still, some are chronic and progressive in nature while others are not. These are all critical considerations the occupational therapist must attend to while developing an individualized intervention plan with a client and specifically as to whether they would benefit most from restorative or compensatory strategies to address issues of coordination.

Maintenance Programs

As with previously reviewed foundational skills, maintenance programs for coordination issues should also emphasize the infusion of the skills of everyday living. The occupational therapist should encourage those activities and tasks the client identifies as daily routine and naturally infuse concepts of motor learning, such as repetition and postural stability. Tying shoes, buttoning a shirt, applying toothpaste to a toothbrush, using the telephone or a television remote, typing on a computer keyboard, or having a game of bridge or bingo all require motor coordination and represent excellent tools for the occupational therapist to enforce as part of the individualized maintenance program. Emphasis should be placed not on the activity itself, but rather repeated practice over time to facilitate improved coordination overall.

Restorative Techniques for Tone

Definitional Analysis

Tone is defined by the Framework (AOTA, 2014) as a client factor relative to neuromusculoskeletal and movement-related functions. More specifically, it is categorized as a function of muscles. However, it is important to note that tone also directly affects the functions of joints and therefore movement in general. This concept is less obvious in the categorizations and definitions provided by the Framework document.

Again, additional definitions from other sources are included here to better illustrate the functional significance of tone as a foundational skill for engagement in meaningful occupation. Muscle tone specifically is defined as "the state of slight contraction usually present in muscles which contribute to posture and coordination" (Venes, 2009, p. 2332). Shumway-Cook and Woollacott (2012) elaborate that a "certain level of tone is present in a conscious and relaxed person" (p. 168), which is not apparent using electromyography (EMG) or a record of muscle activity. Therefore, electrical impulses of the skeletal muscle are not required to maintain an individual's level of tone; or quite simply, tone is not a function of consciousness (Shumway-Cook & Woollacott, 2012).

Notoriously, tone harbors ambiguity when presented by definition alone. Further discussion is required to gain more insight as to how a change in tone can be responsible for such an array of biomechanical limitations within the client's experience. For purposes of illustration, it is plausible to liken tone to the "electricity" that runs through the human body, just as electricity runs through the walls of a house. When electricity in a house is either lowered or increased, an effect is produced on each and every item plugged into the wall sockets. Recall conditions of periodic "brownouts" during hot summer days when many residents of the neighborhood were using their air conditioners. The demand for electricity exceeds the supply and the appliances are no longer producing their expected functions or desired effects. This case is the same when speaking of tone as the "electricity" running through the human body.

Tone is, in essence, the "electricity" that continuously runs through the body at a relatively static rate. Tone, therefore, allows a client to produce movement on demand just as plugging a lamp into a socket would allow for light on demand. Yet, similar to the "brownout" analogy, the level of tone within the human body may not always allow for optimal movement. Too little tone, or hypotonia, would then produce slowed, uncoordinated movement with hyperflexibility noted at the joint structures; too little tension or resistance to movement is produced by the muscles (Bertoti, 2004). The extreme of this is characterized as flaccidity or a condition in which tone is completely absent (Bertoti, 2004). Conversely, high tone, also referred to as *hypertonia*, may produce fast, jerky, equally uncoordinated movement with limited flexibility noted at the joint structures and too much tension or resistance to movement produced in the muscles (Bertoti, 2004). The extremes of hypertonia can be further categorized as either spasticity, an increase in tone dependent upon the reaction of the stretch reflex to movement (Trompetto et al., 2014), or rigidity, an increase in tone not directly related to the velocity of movement, and typically can involve agonist/antagonist (Sanger et al., 2003). Various other categorizations of tonal abnormalities exist, yet with these most prevalent examples we are better able to visualize the functional implications that changes in muscle tone may have for the successful engagement in occupation.

In concluding the definitional analysis of tone, it is also important to note that an individual's level of tone may vary from moment to moment or day to day. Common illustrations of this phenomenon include walking outside on a brisk winter day, as compared to a warm summer's one, or even having an unexpected visitor enter a room and startle its occupants. These situations cause a temporary increase in your body's level of tone or readiness to respond (Bertoti, 2004). Significantly, the spike in tone is temporary. Occupational therapy intervention becomes necessary when the fluctuations in tone are long-standing and, therefore, impede functional performance as is seen in a variety of neurologically based health conditions.

Modes of Injury or Illness

Muscle tone is a function of neuromusculoskeletal and movement-related functions as outlined by the Framework (AOTA, 2014) and therefore is directly affected by illness or injury to the CNS. An array of health conditions may cause fluctuations in tone that in turn cause an individual to experience dysfunction. Many of these conditions lie in the categorizations of acquired brain injuries and spinal cord injuries. Either a result of external force inflicted on the central nervous system itself, as seen in traumatic brain injury and traumatic spinal cord injury, or internal mechanisms, as seen in degenerative diseases, vascular abnormalities, and infections, each can cause disruptions or alterations in the nerve impulses to the area of the brain responsible for the production of smooth, voluntary movement.

Hematomas, or tumors of blood, are commonly seen in both traumatic and nontraumatic injury (Beers et al., 2006). Whether formed as a result of external trauma or internal bleeding from a vascular hemorrhage, they also present an example of injury that may result in tonal abnormalities. Arteriovenous malformations, characterized by an abnormality in the junction between arteries and veins within the brain (Beers et al., 2006), tumors of the brain itself, or even ischemic circumstances, may also disrupt tonal impulses and potentially impede volitional movement.

Tonal abnormalities are also associated with a variety of degenerative disease processes. Clients with Parkinson's disease may exhibit rigidity or an increase in muscle tone of the agonist and antagonist muscles simultaneously (Schultz-Krohn, Foti, & Glogoski, 2013). In MS, spasticity may be present in one case yet absent in another. Furthermore, with Huntington's disease, chorea-type tonal patterns may be observed as involuntary, irregular movements of the extremities that are exacerbated by stress, absent during sleep, and spastic in cases of early onset (Schultz-Krohn et al., 2013).

The previous examples represent only a few of the conditions that commonly disturb muscle tone within the body. Just as tone is challenging to define, it also presents a challenge in identifying all possible modes of injury or illness. Some clients with acquired brain injury may present with hypertonia, while others present with spasticity, clonus, chorea, or may be spared tonal abnormalities altogether. Additionally, clients commonly still experience fluctuations from hypotonia to hypertonia over the period of recovery from illness or injury. In all, any approaches the occupational therapist may choose to address tone must be client- and case-specific, changing in focus along with the healing process and sensitive to the prognosis of the injury or illness causing the disturbance itself.

Restorative Techniques: Motor Control, Motor and Biomechanical Frames of Reference

Foremost, prior to discussing the restoration of tone specifically, it is important to reemphasize the symbiotic relationship that exists between tone and coordination. Each skill relies heavily on the other to successfully produce the functional movement that is necessary to engage in personally meaningful activity. As a result, various techniques for the restoration of coordination will appropriately overlap with those used to address tonal abnormalities. In illustration of this point, tone immediately follows coordination in sequence of this chapter.

Per the Framework (AOTA, 2014), which classifies muscle tone as a neuromusculoskeletal function, the restoration of tone has historically been grounded in the traditional neurodevelopmental theories. These techniques have also been criticized for lacking in evidence and based within an outdated understanding of how the nervous system recovers after insult or injury (Galea, 2012). Conventional rehabilitative practice has also incorporated the use of PAMs under the biomechanical theory to address issues of muscle tone. With the most recent evolution of the motor control and motor learning frames over the last 15 years, there is increasing evidence in support of task-oriented approaches that guide and inform techniques implemented to normalize tone. This theory has also embraced the more contemporary technologies available today, including robot-assisted therapy and the SaeboFlex (Saebo Incorporated) device. This area of techniques is only beginning to emerge, and further studies are necessary to generalize the task-specific practice to occupational performance (Fasoli, 2011).

There are several strategies used to restore abnormalities in tone by the occupational therapist. Those guided by the theory of motor control and motor learning serve to address this function on a general level, not specific to a particular quality of muscle tone. Strategies of the neurodevelopmental and biomechanical theories are targeted to either decrease excessive tone (techniques of inhibition) or increase conditions of low tone (techniques of facilitation). Restoring muscle tone with the goal of functional and fluid movement within and among one's environment is often a challenge for therapists. As such, issues of tone are thought to be managed rather than remedied by a comprehensive team of rehabilitation specialists working together to preserve function and prevent deformity. Overall, additional studies are needed to decipher which of the traditional approaches, or combination thereof, hold the most promise for the effective management of tonal abnormalities over time.

Contemporary Approaches: Robot-Assisted Therapies and the SaeboFlex

Advancements in rehabilitative technologies have undoubtedly changed the practice of occupational therapy and will continue to shape the future of the profession. As Fasoli notes in her review of rehabilitative technology, "[They] are not expected to replace occupational or physical therapists, but they will become part of their treatment arsenal to optimize functional performance after a disabling event" (2011, p. 281). Robot-assisted devices are designed to produce repetitive movement patterns in a task-specific manner that retrains the nervous system and motor control centers. The devices currently available are fairly expensive but are also felt to be cost-effective by providing high-intensity, quantifiable intervention with minimal supervision by the therapist in a health care environment in which time is ever more valuable (Fasoli, 2011). The number of different upper extremity (UE) devices is rapidly increasing, particularly as evidence shows great promise with regard to their therapeutic value. Fasoli (2011) highlights the MIT-MANUS and InMotion2 (Interactive Motion Technologies), the Mirror Image Motion Enabler (MIME)/PUMA 560 (Staubli Unimation Inc), the Reo Therapy System (Motorika Ltd), and the ARMeo (Hocoma) among several others, including those targeted specifically to hand function, and notes the need for training in order to select the appropriate device to achieve desired outcomes. Refer to Appendix A for additional resources on robot-assisted devices.

Developed by brothers John Farrell, OTR/L, and Henry Hoffman, MS, OTR/L, the SaeboFlex is a custom-fit, dynamic orthotic device that allows a client with moderate tonal abnormalities resulting from neurological injury to produce functional grasp and release patterns of the wrist and hand (Northwest Hospital & Medical Center, 2005). Refer to Appendix A for additional resources on the SaeboFlex. The device places the wrist and fingers into extension. It is from this position that the client actively grasps, while the dynamic, spring-loaded outriggers assist in the extension required for release. These patterns are repeated in 45-minute sessions, three times per week over 4 weeks with a trained occupational therapist (see Appendix A for additional information on training opportunities) and are supplemented by a home-based program designed to foster greater use of the device over time (Northwest Hospital & Medical Center, 2005). Over the years, Saebo has added several new devices to their product line, including the SaeboReach dynamic orthotic and the SaeboStretch dynamic resting hand splint, all of which are demonstrating positive results in clinical trials focusing on improvements in the functional range of hemiparetic upper extremities (Hoffman & Blakey, 2011).

In 2007, Farrell, Hoffman, Snyder, Giuliani, and Bohannon published the results of a pilot study concluding that the SaeboFlex device and its training can yield improved wrist extension and decrease in muscle tone for the effective treatment of post-stroke hemiparesis. A more recent study yielded similar results (Stuck, Marshall, & Sivakumar, 2014)

Traditional Approaches of Inhibition

Electrical Modalities

Surface electromyographic biofeedback (sEMG) is a technique employed by the occupational therapist with advanced training (see Appendix A) for the re-education and relaxation of muscular tone. With this modality, a recording of muscle activity is transcribed into visible data along a computer screen by way of electrodes that have been placed strategically along the affected musculature. The therapist manually sets an audible alert at a predetermined level of resting muscle activity. The client is then instructed to attempt to relax, and once the preset level of resting muscle activity is achieved, an alert provides auditory or visual feedback. This serves to reinforce the client of the volitional strategies taken that have effectively decreased muscle tone. Research has demonstrated that the sEMG biofeedback method has demonstrated statistically significant results in the effectiveness of decreasing hypertonia following cases of CVA specifically (Rao, 2011).

TENS has also been suggested as an inhibitory technique by Watanabe (2004). The theory behind the use of TENS directly relates to the function it holds as an effective modality in the management of chronic pain. Wantanabe (2004) suggests that "pain can increase reflex-afferent activity, so a modality which inhibits this input could [also] decrease spasticity" (p. 48).

NMES has also been employed more recently as a means to inhibit conditions of excessive tone. Stowe et al. reported in 2013 that although evidence in support of this prior to 2008 was limited, more recent investigations have shown improved performance following the use of NMES on spastic muscle tissue in both post-acute and chronic stroke survivors. Evidence is also emerging in the use of FES for the reeducation and retraining of motor impairment during task-specific activity engagement (Bellew, 2012). Technologies are emerging at rapid rates that combine the use of electrical stimulation to normalize tone and movement patterns. An example is found in the NESS H200 (Bioness Inc), where studies have shown promising results in treating spasticity of the UE. In all, the skilled and trained use of electrical modalities to restore functional use of the UE is an option that occupational therapists should consider as an effective intervention strategy given continuing education and competency.

Positioning Techniques

Gillen (2011) describes the method of proper positioning as an effective means to maintain the normal tension and length of soft tissue following insult or injury to the nervous system. In review of the many different positioning strategies employed by occupational therapists, Gillen found there was no particular consensus on a specific technique but rather much variability among protocols (2011). The efficacy of positioning as a treatment method lies in preventing further disability or contractures rather than remediating the underlying spasticity. To prevent further disability or contractures, the therapist will promote positions of bilateral symmetry among joints to provide both stretch to involved musculature and the appropriate length tension to uninvolved musculature throughout the day, in both supine or seated positions (Barnes, 1998). This can be supported by the application of positioning items such as foam wedges, strapping, or pillows to achieve the most optimal posture for a client with spasticity, while also minimizing the potential for permanent muscle fiber shortening or contracture formation.

Serial casting is a relatively common, aggressive technique employed by occupational therapists as a tool for the treatment of spasticity. With this approach, one therapist passively places the affected extremity in a position of maximal stretch, often only possible through applying direct pressure to the tendon insertion of the affected muscle. Direct pressure at a tendonous insertion point mechanically causes that muscle to be inhibited (Rust, 2014), thereby allowing for maximal passive range to be achieved. At this point a second therapist applies a protective barrier on the skin, additional padding at bony prominences of the limb to minimize pressure areas, and finally the casting material. Plaster is often used due to its conformability and strength. Once dry, the cast is then cut longitudinally using a cast cutter along both the medial and lateral aspects to create a "bivalve." The bivalve construction allows for maximal ease in application of the cast. An individualized wear schedule is devised according to tolerance and with close monitoring to prevent skin breakdown at areas of increased pressure (e.g., the styloid processes or olecranon process of the UE). As a complement to the wear schedule, the client is also prescribed a PROM program designed to promote the appropriate length-tension relationship among involved musculature, minimize disuse, and prevent contractures or adhesions of the soft tissue. With noted improvement in the passive range at the affected joint, the casting process is repeated at the newly achieved length of prolonged stretch and the wear schedule modified accordingly.

Although this approach is widely used, it is "labor-intensive and relatively expensive" when compared with implementing a prefabricated, low-load, prolonged stretch device designed to achieve the same desired effect (Vandyck & Mukand, 2004, p. 13). Refer to Appendix A for manufacturers of low-load, prolonged stretch devices. Efficacy studies yield positive correlations among the PROM available at affected joints after implementation of serial casting. However, Gillen (2011) highlights studies that contradict this conclusion. These studies found that prolonged immobility, such as is fostered through serial casting, likely achieves its intended results through promoting muscle atrophy versus directly influencing muscle tone. Evidence such as this should be considered when crafting the individualized treatment plan.

Thermal Modality Techniques

Cameron (2009) describes using cold pack application (cryotherapy) at the temperature of 10°C as an effective means of inhibiting tone achieved by "first, a decrease in gamma motor neuron activity and later, a decrease in afferent spindle and Golgi tendon organ (GTO) activity" (p. 137). To achieve this effect, the cold application must be provided for a duration of 10 to 30 minutes, paying careful attention to indications and precautions outlined for the use of this physical agent modality (see Table 2-21). Price, Lehmann, Boswell-Bessette, Burleigh, and deLateur (1993) studied the efficacy of cryotherapy on hypertonicity and concluded that statistically significant reduction can be measured up to 1 hour after application. Therefore, this technique produces relatively short-term effects in reducing muscle spasticity.

Neurodevelopmental/Sensorimotor Techniques

The neurodevelopmental techniques (also referred to as sensorimotor techniques) of NDT, PNF, and Rood all ascribe to be methods of addressing hypertonia. This area of techniques harbor little evidence to support the claim and are in need of further study to validate efficacy. However, traditionally, occupational therapists have implemented these techniques in the clinic to address conditions of hypertonia, and therefore they are included in this discussion.

The NDT (Bobath), PNF, and Rood approaches mutually share a foundation in techniques that are slow in speed as tools to foster the inhibition of tone. Slow stroking as outlined by Rood, promoting slow controlled movement patterns outlined by NDT, and using the slow relaxation methods outlined by PNF all emphasize the speed of implementation to provide necessary sensory and vestibular input that then relaxes the system and decreases the heightened level of muscle tone (Schultz-Krohn et al.,2013).

With NDT specifically, upright positioning of the body, or the facilitation of postural control, holds significant importance in normalizing tone. Per NDT, dysfunction is housed in the abnormality of core posture and is commonly seen following neurological insult. For example, as a result of sensory loss, a client may avoid weight-bearing on the affected side due to a fear of falling. "Muscle tone also tends to increase with other threats, registered as stress" (Cameron, 2009, p. 99). Hence, restoration must begin by re-establishing security for the client in core stability, which is a precursor to distal mobility. Therefore, the techniques of NDT are executed to facilitate postural control and promote normal weight-bearing experiences. This then secondarily addresses the tonal abnormality by minimizing the emotion of fear.

The NDT approach also specifies the use of trunk rotation, scapular retraction, and a forward pelvic position (or, in general, the proper positioning and length of proximal musculature) as cornerstones to promote the normalization of tone (Levit, 2014). Emphasis is placed on deep pressure applied by the therapist and at proximal key points of control (as described earlier in restoration of coordination) to elicit the necessary lengthening of affected musculature (Chae, Sheffler, & Knutson, 2008) and/or achieved by techniques of weight-bearing through the affected extremity. Whether by promoting through engagement in functional activity (Figure 2-20) or in isolation, the NDT weight-bearing technique promotes a prolonged stretch to affected muscles and presents another tool of inhibition for the occupational therapist to consider.

Margaret Rood also describes position-specific techniques to address muscle spasticity. With this approach, emphasis is placed on positions of the traditional developmental sequence, or ontogenic positions, described earlier with coordination.

With the PNF approach, muscle contraction and hold patterns are outlined as effective means for normalizing spasticity. Schultz-Krohn et al. (2013) report that facilitating these rhythmic

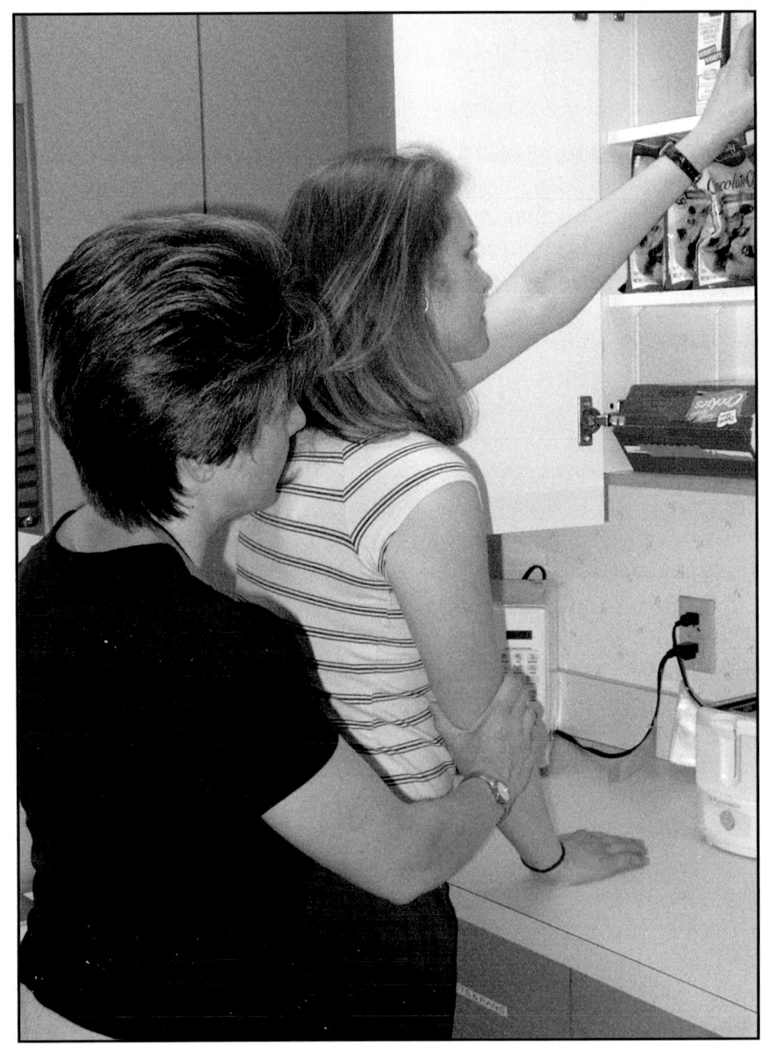

Figure 2-20. Weight-bearing through the upper extremity, promoted by functional reaching during the engagement of meaningful occupation.

rotational movements is effective in decreasing spasticity and increasing range of motion. Other theorists have outlined the use of the same technique for inhibition of tone, generally termed *repeated contractions* in the PNF approach as techniques of reciprocal innervation (Ivanhoe & Reistetter, 2004).

Pharmaceutical Techniques

It is significant to note the growing evidence in support for using medically prescribed pharmacological agents as the primary effective method in managing conditions of hypertonia. Gillen (2011) reports baclofen, diazepam, dantrolene sodium, and tizanidine, as the most common sampling of medications used to treat issues of increased muscle tone in a post-stroke population specifically. Other pharmacological agents implemented in cases of more persistent spasticity include Botox (botulinum) injections, phenol blocks, and implantable pumps that provide continuous interthecal administration. However, Gillen notes that these approaches remain experimental and

Table 2-20
Remedial Techniques for Tonal Abnormalities

Inhibition Techniques	Shared Techniques	Facilitation Techniques
• Relaxation techniques • Neutral warmth • Slow rocking • Light joint compression • Serial casting • Tendon pressure • Prolonged cooling • TENS	• Weight-bearing • Positioning • Biofeedback	• Heavy joint compression • Quick stretch • Tapping • Brushing • Vestibular stimulation • Icing • Associated reactions • NMES

require additional investigation to validate their longer-term efficacy in the management of this motor disorder (2011).

Traditional Approaches of Facilitation

Electrical Modalities

Electrical stimulation has been clearly demonstrated to be "a valuable facilitation tool for . . . [clients] with primary movement disorders" (Bertoti, 2004). Bertoti (2004) goes on to report that with augmentation of muscle activity via NMES, the degree of hypotonia is temporarily found to normalize. Chae, Sheffler, and Knutson (2008) further support this conclusion in their examination of electrical stimulation to decrease the incidence of shoulder subluxation, a common complication of excessively low UE tone, or flaccidity. As a PAM, continuing education is required to implement this technique both safely and effectively. Refer to Appendix A for additional information and resources on the use of PAMs by an occupational therapist and Table 2-24 for an outline of indications and contraindications for the use of NMES. Additional benefits have also been found in the use of EMG biofeedback as a modality to facilitate increased muscle tone (Gillen, 2011), similar to that described earlier as a technique for inhibition. For facilitation, the client's attention is directed to effective measures taken in efforts to increase hypotonic muscle activity.

Neurodevelopmental/Sensorimotor Techniques

As depicted in Table 2-20, the same sensorimotor approaches outlined earlier as techniques of inhibition also prescribe strategies for the facilitation of low tone.

As mentioned earlier in this segment, NDT outlines techniques used in general to normalize tone, whether hyperactive or hypoactive, as they present in typical or synergistic patterns. Therefore, the methods presented by NDT are the same in cases of both inhibition and facilitation. Trunk rotation, scapular retraction, and forward pelvic position are promoted to normalize low tone in the proximal musculature and through the use of handling techniques at identified key points of control. Weight bearing is intended to assist in regulating overall abnormalities in tone throughout the body, as was discussed in the inhibitory section. Recent evidence is lacking on the use of the NDT approach after neurological insult. In an extensive review of current literature designed to measure the efficacy of the NDT approach, Kollen et al. (2009) indicated that "there was no evidence of superiority of Bobath [NDT] on sensorimotor control of upper and lower limb, dexterity, mobility, activities of daily living, health-related quality of life, and cost-effectiveness (p. e89).

The authors go on to recommend that therapists should rely upon evidence-based guidelines as a framework from which the most effective treatment should be derived.

Various other facilitatory techniques are outlined by the Rood approach, including quick stretch, brushing, vestibular stimulation, vibration, light touch, and icing (cryotherapy) as tools in normalizing low tone. A quick stretch to the affected muscle fibers, followed by rapid and repetitive tapping along the same muscle belly during an attempted movement, is believed to both inhibit the antagonistic muscle and activate the reflexive stretch response of the agonistic, or affected muscle (Rood, 1962). Quick, vestibular stimulation in an anterior-posterior or medial-lateral plane has been reported in this treatment to elicit protective reflexes and therefore assist in promoting an increase in tone. Quick icing or quickly swiping the skin surface with ice similarly was completed to produce a protective withdrawal reflex, again acting as a technique to temporarily increase the level of tone. These techniques have been replaced in recent intervention with functional electrical stimulation, relaxation strategies, and medications for spasticity relaxation, etc. (Sabari, Capasso, & Feld-Glazman, 2014).

The Brunnstrom approach describes specific patterns of recovery, each characterized by alterations in tone, which occur following CVA. Brunnstrom emphasizes that recovery follows a developmental sequence: proximal to distal musculature, flaccid to spastic tonal patterns, and followed by the return of normal movement patterns. Intervention is focused on facilitating and managing the underlying patterns of tone, also known as synergies, which present in varying degrees along each stage of the recovery process. Brunnstrom recruits the use of associated reactions, otherwise described as brainstem reflexes (e.g., asymmetrical tonic neck reflex [ATNR]), to evoke movement where it was otherwise nonexistent due to the lack of sufficient muscle tone (Trombly Latham, 2014). Hence, resistance to movement in the unaffected extremity will elicit a synergistic pattern of heightened tone in the affected extremity and potentially allow for the production of movement. For example, resisted grasp in the unaffected hand will cause a grasping pattern of movement in the affected hand allowing for potentially functional use (Trombly Latham, 2014). This movement is then physically experienced by the client and practiced readily in order to achieve normal movement patterns. The Brunnstrom approach also outlines the use of repetitive tapping, quick stretch, and brisk stimulation or brushing to facilitate tone, similar to the Rood approach described previously.

Special Considerations

Clients presenting with tonal abnormalities are also susceptible to an array of secondarily harmful conditions that warrant the attention of the occupational therapist. As a normal level of tone within the musculature allows for optimal movement, too little or too much tone hinders movement and may also cause further disability. This principle can be best illustrated in situations of joint subluxation and contracture formations.

In the absence of tone, the joint structures and the capsule specifically become laxed or stretched due to the overpowering, unopposed force of gravity on extremities in the upright position. This allows the humeral head to fall or sublux from the glenoid fossa and is commonly observed in clients who have experienced CVAs. Shoulder subluxations are not only painful for clients, but also potentially harmful due to the excessive stretch on nerves and blood vessels that can secondarily lead to complicating conditions including complex regional pain syndrome (CRPS) or adhesive capsulitis. It is the responsibility of the occupational therapist to be attentive to joint laxity to minimize the likelihood of complications. Intervention strategies include proper positioning and support against gravity that can be achieved by adding a hemi-tray (Figure 2-21), arm trough, lap tray, or, though controversial for fostering further disuse, a shoulder sling. It should be noted that a lap tray is considered a restraint unless the client can remove it independently. Regardless of which equipment is being incorporated, the therapist must attend to a careful wear schedule that

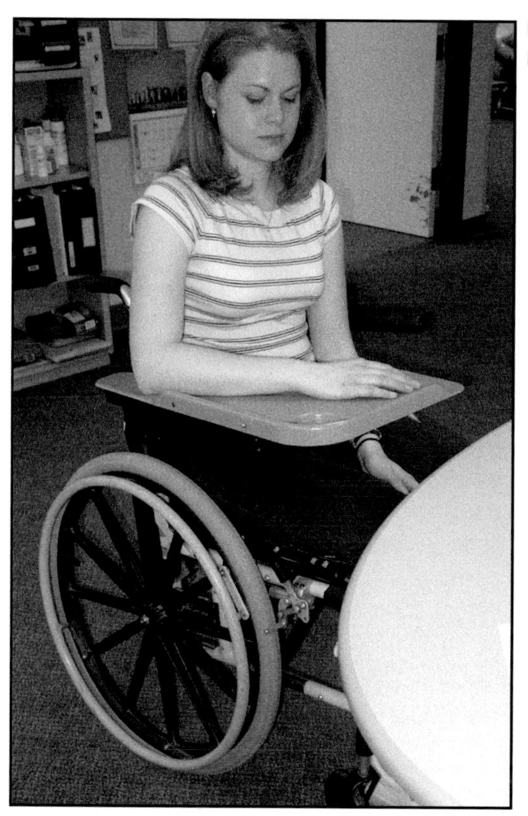

Figure 2-21. Demonstration of the use of a hemi-tray to provide proper positioning of the upper extremity.

minimizes disuse while also providing necessary protection from excessive joint distraction or severity of subluxation (Gilmore, Spaulding, & Vandervoort, 2004).

In cases of spasticity, sustained contraction of the muscle tissue can produce damaging contractures within muscle fibers themselves. The prevention of contractures, or permanent shortening of muscle fibers, is routinely a focus of intervention that employs such aggressive measures as serial casting and low-load, prolonged stretch devices, both described earlier in this subsection.

It is also important to note the significance of the scapulohumeral rhythm (Neumann, 2010) when remediating tonal issues of the UE. The occupational therapist must attend to the collaborative relationship between the scapula and the humerus (scapulohumeral rhythm)to foster a return of normal movement patterns throughout the entire UE. In cases of low tone, the scapula may become malaligned in its orientation to the thorax, commonly referred to as *scapular winging.* Likewise, in cases of high tone, the scapula may become fixed relative to the thorax. Each condition directly impedes the scapulothoracic joint and, therefore, biomechanically prevents full shoulder movement in the upper ranges of motion.

When addressing tone, the underlying significance of an individual's preferences and his or her aversions or fears are of added importance to the occupational therapist. A proven and strong correlation exists between a client's emotional status and their level of muscle tone. For example, a client who is particularly averse to cold will not find prolonged icing or cryotherapy to be an effective technique of inhibition. Similarly, a client who is particularly fearful of anticipated pain with movement will be less likely to benefit from the technique of prolonged stretch. It is critical that the occupational therapist openly communicate with the client and establish trusting, therapeutic rapport to ascertain which options may present as most effective in managing individual tonal issues.

As a final note, consideration should also be paid to the therapeutic benefits of aquatic therapy interventions to address issues of tone. For example, supported floating using assistive floatation devices in a warm water pool may be found particularly relaxing for a client and therefore an effective technique of tonal inhibition. In a study conducted by Kesiktas et al. (2004) entitled "The Use of Hydrotherapy for the Management of Spasticity," water-based intervention programs were found to be "helpful in decreasing the amount of medication required" (p. 273) for conditions of spasticity, and "when compared to the control group, the use of hydrotherapy produced a significant decrease in [muscle] spasm severity" (p. 272). Alternately, exercise in a cool water environment may have a facilitatory effect on muscle tone. A specialized aquatic technique, watsu or water shiatsu uses slow rocking movements provided passively by the therapist with the goal of inducing a deep state of relaxation. The primary purpose of this relaxed state is to allow for natural, rotational movements of the limbs and trunk with the goal of equalizing the body's meridians or pathways of energy as described in Eastern medical philosophies (Chon, Oh, & Shim, 2009). This deepened state of relaxation also promotes a reduction of spasticity. As a precaution, clients who are fearful of water would not benefit from aquatic intervention strategies because emotion directly affects degree of muscle tone. Additional training is recommended for aquatic intervention, particularly in the use of watsu techniques. Refer to Appendix A for more information on aquatic rehabilitation.

Techniques at a Glance

See Table 2-20 for an outline of the most commonly employed techniques for the inhibition of tone, the facilitation of tone, and those that are effective in either case of tonal abnormality.

Maintenance Programs

Due to their specialized nature, restoration techniques for tone are not traditionally carried over into client-facilitated maintenance programs. Rather, these techniques are an integral component of the clinic-based therapy sessions themselves. This is not to say that with demonstrated safety and independence in the use of weight-bearing, for example, a client and his or her caregivers would not be supported in the desire to continue the use of techniques outside the therapy session. In fact, techniques including NMES are being found to be most effective at higher frequency and are feasible for clients' home-based use with training (Doucet, 2012).

Techniques of proper positioning, including casting and splinting applications, are traditionally seen as maintenance approaches for affected extremities. The goal for such methods is to maintain the ideal length of the connective tissues that underlie the production of movement. For example, a wrist cock-up splint would provide the ideal length of stretch for finger flexors in the absence of active wrist extension. Again, as is always the case with positioning tools, a client-specific wear schedule must be created to minimize the disuse of the area affected and prevent complications including decubiti formation, muscle atrophy, or contractures. For illustration, this may include only nighttime application followed by an early morning AROM program designed to restretch the immobilized soft tissues. Independence with application of all required positioning devices must also be established prior to execution as part of a maintenance program.

Restoration of the Primary Functional Skills at a Glance

The restorative techniques discussed in this chapter are summarized in Table 2-21 (pain and edema), Table 2-22 (sensation: hyposensitivity and hypersensitivity), Table 2-23 (range of motion), and Table 2-24 (strength).

Restorative Techniques for Cognition and Perception

Definitional Analysis

Per the Framework (AOTA, 2014), both perception and cognition are categorized as specific mental functions embedded within client factors and body functions. This is a broad categorization for these skill areas, each considered comprehensive and influential in the execution of performance and active engagement in meaningful activity. Mental functions in general are then further subdivided into categories of global mental functions and specific mental functions.

Mental functions provide a general overview of those subskills that collectively allow for effective and meaningful interaction within the environment and among other individuals from day to day. Specific mental functions include attention, memory, perception, thought, and emotion, while global mental functions include consciousness, orientation, temperament, personality, and energy or drive. These categories are deeply interdependent. Collectively, they allow an individual to demonstrate ability through engaging in occupation. Hence, both cognition and perception are also described as performance/process skills within the Framework document (AOTA, 2014). In this context, examples of cognitive and perceptual skills include attending, choosing, initiating, sequencing, searching, organizing, and adjusting in order to complete a given task successfully.

Specific mental functions elaborate on skills commonly associated with cognition and emphasize the relationship among one's perceptual functions and the thinking process. These include attention, memory, thought, judgment, and emotional regulation (AOTA, 2014). The significance of perception and its impact on cognition is further illustrated by including functions of the interpretation of sensory input from tactile, visual, auditory, olfactory, and gustatory senses. The complexity of these processes is also captured in the performance skill of emotional regulation, highlighting the need for one to cope, control, persist, and respond appropriately to a given situation in order to successfully display ability. More so, all are also directly affected by the contextual and performance patterns inherent to the individual performing the task. As the body of knowledge regarding the intricacy of these functions and skills continues to grow and expand rapidly, so too must the rehabilitative strategies occupational therapists use in an attempt to restore cognitive perceptual impairments.

"Traditionally, rehabilitation efforts have been aimed at restoring or compensating for basic cognitive deficits such as attention or memory, whereas higher-level cognitive processes have not always been taken into consideration" (Katz & Maeir, 2011, p. 13). Katz and Maeir (2011) describe the concept of higher-level cognitive functioning further by integrating the foundational skills of cognition with those of perception and emotional regulation that combined to allow for awareness and control of one's problem solving and learning during goal-directed tasks. Developmental psychologists refer to this set of skills as *metacognition*, whereas neurorehabilitation models prefer the term *executive functioning* (Katz & Maeir, 2011). Both highlight the importance of adaptation and accommodation, or flexibility of mind, in the refined execution of collective cognitive perceptual skills. The restorative strategies implemented after neurological injury or illness in the areas of cognition and perception must also embrace this refined integration as the ultimate goal to maximize independent participation in everyday occupational tasks.

Table 2-21
Remedial Techniques for Pain and Edema

Pain and Edema Modality or Intervention Techniques	Cold pack	Ice bath (Gillen & Burkhardt, 2004)	Contrast bath (Cochrane, 2004)	Vapocoolant spray
Rationale/Indications for Use	Desensitize pain receptors and decrease pain Typically, 24 to 48 hours after injury to address edema, pain exacerbations of arthritis, acute bursitis or tendonitis, spasticity, acute or chronic pain secondary to muscle spasm	Desensitize pain receptors as well as quick vasomotor restriction	Desensitize pain receptors as well as create rapid vasoconstriction and vasodilation	Decrease muscle spasms and trigger point discomfort for a short period of time (10 to 15 min) (Bracciano, 2000)
Average Length of Time per Session	10 to 20 minutes	3 to 5 seconds and repeated 2 to 3 times	6 to 10 seconds repeated 2 to 3 times	2 to 3 sprays (Micholovitz, 1990)
Process	• One layer of towel between the client and the cold pack • Cold pack is placed over or around the area of pain/edema	• Ice bucket is placed on the floor • Arm is placed in the ice water for 3 to 5 seconds and then removed • Repeat 2 to 3 times	• Ice and warm water buckets are placed on the floor • Arm is placed in the ice water for 3 to 5 seconds • Arm is placed in the warm water for 3 to 5 seconds	• Position client with identified muscle on passive stretch • Spray bottle is inverted at 30 degree angle, about 45 cm from skin • Muscle or trigger point sprayed in unidirectional sweeping motion 2 to 3 times
Precautions (With all physical agent modalities, always monitor and protect underlying skin)	Avoid use with clients having significantly impaired circulation or hypersensitivity to cold; avoid application over wounds, prolonged placement over superficial nerves, compromised cognitive status Vapocoolant spray cannot be used if client or therapist is pregnant			

(continued)

Table 2-21 (continued)

Remedial Techniques for Pain and Edema

Pain and Edema Modality or Intervention Techniques	Moist heat pack	Paraffin wax	Fluidotherapy thermal mode
Rationale/ Indications for Use	Stiff joints, subcutaneous adhesions, contractures, chronic arthritis, subacute or chronic cumulative trauma, neuromas, spasms	Circumferential heating for stiff joints, subcutaneous adhesions, contractures, chronic arthritis, subacute or chronic cumulative trauma	Programmable and adjustable heat, adjustable fan for stiff joints, subcutaneous adhesions, contractures, chronic arthritis, subacute or chronic cumulative trauma, neuromas, spasms
Average Length of Time per Session	15 to 20 minutes	15 to 20 minutes	15 to 20 minutes
Process	• Six to eight layers of towels between the client and the moist heat pack • Moist heat pack is placed over or around the area of pain/edema	Hand is dipped into paraffin five times, wrapped in plastic, and then wrapped in a towel	Machine is preheated Extremity is placed into the heated corn husks and the "sleeve" is wrapped around the client's extremity
Precautions (With all physical agent modalities, always monitor and protect underlying skin)	Acute injury, diminished sensation, decreased circulation, compromised cognitive status, tumors or cancers, acute edema, deep vein thrombosis, pregnancy, bleeding abnormalities, infection, advanced cardiac disease, underlying skin, some case of rheumatoid arthritis where client may experience exacerbation following heat (Shankar & Randall, 2002)		

(continued)

Table 2-21 (continued)

Remedial Techniques for Pain and Edema

Pain and Edema Modality or Intervention Techniques	Iontophoresis (see Figure 2-1)	Transcutaneous Electrical Nerve Stimulation (TENS)
Rationale/ Indications for Use	Promotes healing and decreases pain and edema through using electric currents to deliver transcutaneous prescription medications such as corticosteroids and analgesics	Interrupts the pain cycle at the spinal level (Cameron, 2003)
Average Length of Time per Session	Typically 20 to 30 minutes depending upon client tolerance (Bracciano, 2000)	Time can vary from 15 to 45 minutes depending upon the condition and other chosen parameters (Bracciano, 2000)
Process	• Medication is injected into the iontophoresis pad • Medication pad is placed over the area of pain/ edema • Dispersive pad is placed on the same side of the body at any location (typically low back, shoulder, or thigh) • Parameters should be set at a low current density to prevent irritation such as 05 mA/cm^2	• Stimulation sites selected based upon the condition and client goals • 3 areas to facilitate current flow are motor, trigger, and acupuncture points (Bracciano, 2000) • Further training is required to become competent in the different protocols utilized with TENS
Precautions (With all physical agent modalities, always monitor and protect underlying skin)	Pregnancy, skin lesions or sensitivity, allergy to medications used, cardiac pacemaker or arrhythmias, placement over the carotid sinus, blood clots, impaired sensation, malignant tumor	Presence of cardiac pacemakers, pregnancy, tumors/malignancy, epilepsy, over the ocular orbits or carotid sinus, active infection, peripheral vascular disease, cardiac disease, mucosal surfaces, compromised cognitive status Caution must be used in clients experiencing acute pain symptoms or undiagnosed pain (Shankar, 2002)

(continued)

Table 2-21 (continued)

Remedial Techniques for Pain and Edema

Pain and Edema Modality or Intervention Techniques	Compression
Rationale/Indications for Use	Decreases edema through facilitation of the return of edematous fluids to the heart for efficient removal from the system (Cameron, 2003)
Average Length of Time per Session	Time varies with form of intervention and the degree of edema
Process	• Positioning of an affected area in elevation above the heart allows for gravitational forces to engage in removing excess fluids • Aquatic rehabilitation techniques recruit the principles of hydrostatic pressure to circumferentially compress affected areas (Salzman, 1998) • Wrappings, garments such as Isotoner (Totes Isotoner Corp) gloves (see Figure 2-3) • Electric pumps which provide timed, intermittent compression via filling a sleeve surrounding the area with air
Precautions (With all physical agent modalities, always monitor and protect underlying skin)	Extensive/overly prolonged compression that can cause further circulation problems, decreased sensation, presence/risk of blood clots, open wounds/infections/cellulitis, systemic febrile illness malignancy, fragile skin, acute cardiac disease, pregnancy (Shankar & Randall, 2002) *(continued)*

Table 2-21 (continued)

Remedial Techniques for Pain and Edema

Pain and Edema Modality or Intervention Techniques	Massage • Retrograde massage through manual compression (subacute) • Manual lymph drainage (chronic conditions)
Rationale/Indications for Use	• Retrograde massage: Decreases edema through providing compression to the affected tissues • Manual lymph drainage: Decreases edema through use of specialized techniques to elicit a release of "trapped" lymph within the circulatory system (Cameron, 2003)
Average Length of Time per Session	• Retrograde massage: 10 to 20 minutes • Manual lymph drainage gradual increase from 20 minutes to a maximum of 60 minutes
Process	Retrograde massage: 1. Place the client in a position which is respectful of comfort, yet also considerate to elevation above the heart Pillows, etc should be used to maximize client's level of comfort 2. Clarify with the client any possible allergies to skin lotions or creams 3. Ideally, a lanolin-based or vitamin E cream is applied to all surfaces of the skin in the area where massage will be applied to decrease friction produced by massaging technique 4. Therapist begins to provide pressure sensitive to the client's discomfort and moving in a direction toward the heart Pressure should be circumferential, or provided to all surfaces of the skin simultaneously (see Figure 2-4) 5. This "mechanical pumping", in the distal to proximal direction and using the lanolin-based cream to decrease friction between surfaces, is a frequently used remedial technique in addressing subacute edema for 3 to 5 minutes at the intensity of 4 to 6 times per day (Prosser & Conolly, 2003) Manual lymph drainage: Lymphedema is a specialty area within occupational therapy and requires additional training for proficiency
Precautions (With all physical agent modalities, always monitor and protect underlying skin)	*See Compression

(continued)

Table 2-21 (continued)

Remedial Techniques for Pain and Edema

Pain and Edema Modality or Intervention Techniques	ROM • AROM • AAROM • PROM	Manual therapies (therapeutic touch) • Crainiosacral • Myofascial release • Strain counter strain (subacute or chronic)
Rationale/ Indications for Use	Promotes movement to limit the accumulation of fluids and the pain/adhesions associated with guarding or misuse of an extremity (Cameron, 2003)	Though each has its own unique approach, collectively, these techniques are founded on the belief dysfunction arises from tensions occurring throughout the body and techniques implemented are intended to restore uniformity throughout the system
Average Length of Time per Session	Time varies with particular technique	Time varies with particular technique
Process	Example of AROM exercise for edema/pain: • Tendon gliding (see Figure 2-4) completed five repetitions twice daily until edema is effectively diminished (Prosser & Conolly, 2003)	Due to the specialized nature of these techniques, continuing education is required to ensure safe and successful implementation Refer to Appendix A for additional information and resources on these specialized technique options
Precautions (With all physical agent modalities, always monitor and protect underlying skin)	See Table 2-24	Due to the fact that these are specialized areas, precautions are dependent and individualized for each technique

Table 2-22

Remedial Techniques for Sensation: Hyposensitivity and Hypersensitivity

Sensation: Hyposensitivity Modality or Intervention Techniques	Sensory retraining: Direct sensory input • Buckets • Wands • Textures	Sensory retraining: Functional activities
Rational/Indications for Use (For complete descriptions see narrative information)	Direct sensory input applied to re-educate the client of these sensations	"therapy aimed at enabling a person to regain contact with his or her environment; (via sensory input and) includes body awareness exercises and sensory activities utilizing objects" (Jacobs & Jacobs, 2004, p 213)
Average Length of Time per Session	Time varies	Time varies
Process	Intervention is initiated by having the client organize the sensory stimulation bins or dowels in a sequence of least to most abrasive, then begin with stimulation via the texture which is tolerated, applied directly to the affected area (Waylett-Rendall, 2002) Graded progression to less abrasive textures is then guided by the therapist with particular attention to the client's ability to feel the texture Vibration can also be added post intervention with dowels/textures	• Provide clients with an array of opportunities that provide engagement in familiar sensory experiences of all kinds • Retraining activities may include an array of activities such as a fine motor task in identifying coins to those of a gross motor nature such as moving the arm above the head so as to successfully brush hair • Emphasis is not so much placed on the type of item or movement, but rather to recruit other perceptions, such as vision, in retraining the "sense" the item or movement provides
Precautions	Do not allow client to begin with a texture that is abrasive and can cause undetected irritation to the skin Avoid any sharp objects	See direct sensory input

(continued)

Table 2-22 (continued)

Remedial Techniques for Sensation: Hyposensitivity and Hypersensitivity

Sensation: Hyposensitivity Modality or Intervention Techniques	Desensitization: Direct sensory input • Buckets • Wands • Textures • Vibration	Fluidotherapy: Nonthermal or thermal effect depending on client's tolerance and preference
Rational/Indications for Use (For complete descriptions see narrative information)	Desensitization of sensory receptors	Corn husk contact can be graded by fan control allowing progressive input Temperature can also be graded
Average Length of Time per Session	10 minutes, 3 to 4 times per day	15 to 20 minutes
Process	Intervention is initiated by having the client organize the sensory stimulation bins or dowels in a sequence of least to most abrasive, then begin with stimulation via the texture which is tolerated, applied directly to the affected area (Weylatt-Rendall, 2002) Graded progression to increasing more abrasive textures is then guided by the therapist with particular attention to the client's level of comfort Vibration can also be added post intervention with dowels/textures	• If thermal, machine is preheated • Client's extremity is placed in the fluidotherapy machine and the "sleeve" is wrapped around the client's extremity • Fan setting begins low and is increased as tolerated • Heat setting begins low and is increased as tolerated within therapeutic range of 38° C to 506° C • If open wound/skin lesions/infections, cover prior to placing hand into machine
Precautions	*Do not over stimulate as this may result in pain	If thermal, please see precautions under Pain and Edema table; if nonthermal, no further precautions

Table 2-23
Remedial Techniques for Range of Motion

Sensation: Hyposensitivity Modality or Intervention Techniques	PROM • Completed by caregiver • Pendulum exercises (Codman) • Self ROM	AROM/AAROM • Pulleys • Shoulder wheel • Arm ergometer • ROM arch • Wall ladder • Work hardening equipment, such as BTE (see Figure 2-9)
Rational/Indications for Use (For complete descriptions see narrative information)	Maintain ROM, prevent contractures, adhesions, and joint deformities (Pedretti, 1990)	Increase ROM, prevent contractures, adhesions, and joint deformities (Pedretti, 1990)
Average Length of Time per Session	Completion requires approximately 15 minutes, 3 times per day	Completion requires approximately 15 minutes, 3 times per day
Process	• Caregiver: move extremity through entire range of joint • Pendulum: Client bends forward at the waist using the unaffected arm as support on a stable surface • All the affected arm to hang down to the floor • The body is moved so that the momentum of the body causes the arm to move in a straight line for ward/back and side to side, as well as clockwise/counter-clockwise in a circle (www.Draubreysmith.com) • Self-ROM: See Figures 2-6 and 2-7	See Figure 2-8 for a sample AROM program
Precautions	Dislocation of a joint, myositis ossificans, infection or inflammatory conditions within the joint, recent surgical procedure, unhealed fracture, marked osteoporosis, carcinoma of the bone or any fragile bone condition, significant hypermobility, significant pain, hemophilia, hematoma in the joint	See PROM

(continued)

Table 2-23 (continued)

Remedial Techniques for Range of Motion

Sensation: Hyposensitivity Modality or Intervention Techniques	Moist heat packs	Fluidotherapy thermal mode	Ultrasound (continuous setting: thermal) (see Figure 2-2)
Rational/Indications for Use (For complete descriptions see narrative information)	To promote tissue elasticity in preparation for the stretch associated with range exercises as well as to minimize the perception of pain at the session start.	To promote tissue elasticity in preparation for the stretch associated with range exercises as well as to minimize the perception of pain at the session start.	Promotes tissue healing and removal of waste products generated by the healing process.
Average Length of Time per Session	15 to 20 minutes	15 to 20 minutes	15 to 20 minutes, 3x/week, alternating days, approx. 10 treatments.
Process	• Six to eight layers of towels between the client and the moist heat pack • Moist heat pack is placed over or around the area of pain/ edema	Machine is pre-heated. Extremity is placed into the heated corn husks and the "sleeve" is wrapped around the client's extremity. Heat setting within therapeutic range of 38° C to 50.6° C. If open wound/skin lesions/infections, cover prior to placing hand into machine.	• Parameters vary from: 1.0 to 2.0 W/cm^2 for 5 to 8 mins, 1 or 3 MHz • Ultrasound coupling gel is placed on the site of injury. • Wand is moved slowly and without stopping (Bracciano, 2000)
Precautions	• See fluidotherapy and thermal ultrasound	Acute injury, diminished sensation, decreased circulation, compromised cognitive status, tumors or cancers, acute edema, deep vein thrombosis, pregnancy, bleeding abnormalities, infection, advanced cardiac disease, some case of rheumatoid arthritis where client may experience exacerbation following heat.	

Table 2-24
Remedial Techniques for Strength

Strength: Modality or Intervention Techniques	Strength training • Hand grippers • TheraPutty/TheraBand • Free weights/wrist weights • BTE	Isometric exercises
Rationale/Indications for Use (For complete descriptions see narrative information)	Given that strength is a remedial skill for successful engagement in functional activity, occupational therapy practitioners commonly must address strength specifically in order to assist the client in regaining independence in desired occupations	Static strengthening in which muscular contraction/tension occurs without shortening or lengthening of the muscle. Typically used after injury rehabilitation or surgical procedures as the first stage of strengthening. (Robergs & Roberts, 2000)
Average Length of Time per Session	Used as a precursor to functional activity, therefore no more than 15 minutes	Hold each attempt for 5-10 seconds, 10 times, 1-2 times per day, daily. pending level of tolerance and progress. (Caution: Do not hold breath! Contraindicated for clients with cardiac and hypertension as isometrics can increase blood pressure.)
Process	TheraBand, TheraPutty, or hand grippers are generally color-coded by the manufacturer to illustrate for the therapist and client alike, the idea of graded resistance (see Figures 2-10, 2-11, and 1-12)	Exercises may be performed lying, sitting, or standing depending upon client's abilities and body part being strengthened. The client tightens and holds the contraction or may hold the body part against a resistance such as a wall or table. Example: Tightening the quadriceps muscle in a sitting position or holding the wrist into extension against the side of a table. (Caution: Do not hold breath! Contraindicated for clients with cardiac and hypertension as isometrics can increase blood pressure)
Precautions	*See isometric/isokinetic exercises	Inflammation, significant pain, recent fracture, bone carcinoma or any fragile bone condition, significant spasticity, cardiovascular conditions, hypertension, chronic obstructive pulmonary disease, any condition where fatigue might exacerbate the condition, and arthritis

(continued)

Table 2-24 (continued)

Remedial Techniques for Strength

Strength: Modality or Intervention Techniques	Isokinetic exercise	Isotonic exercises • Concentric • Eccentric
Rationale/Indications for Use (For complete descriptions see narrative information)	Achieved through the use of exercise machines designed to strengthen muscles while working at a regulated speed and resistance (Robergs & Roberts, 2000)	Strengthening exercises which involve a shortening and lengthening contraction of the involved muscle against a constant load or resistance. Typically used in the subacute stages of healing (Robergs & Roberts, 2000)
Average Length of Time per Session	Repetitions can vary from 8 to 20 times depending on client goals. Sets will vary from 1 to 3, depending upon client tolerance and progress. Typically performed on alternating days	Repetitions can vary from 8 to 20 times depending on client goals. Sets will vary from 1 to 3, depending upon client tolerance and progress. Typically performed on alternating days
Process	Exercise machines are used in therapy clinics to achieve the desired resistance and velocity. Examples include: • Cybex • BTE PrimusRS • Biodex • Lido • KinCom • Isocom	Exercises may include calisthenics, weight training with free weights or machines or progressive resistance exercise (PREs). This involves the use of gradually increasing resistance over time and progress
Precautions	Inflammation, significant pain, recent fracture, bone carcinoma or any fragile bone condition, significant spasticity, cardiovascular conditions, hypertension, chronic obstructive pulmonary disease, any condition where fatigue might exacerbate the condition, and arthritis	*See isometric/isokinetic exercises

(continued)

Table 2-24 (continued)

Remedial Techniques for Strength

Strength: Modality or Intervention Techniques	Progressive resistive exercises (PREs)	Work simulator • BTE • ERGOS
Rationale/Indications for Use (For complete descriptions see narrative information)	Uses a specific method based on outlined parameters to strengthen	This equipment option offers greater control in grading the resistance provided to muscle tissue as well as the unique capacity to simulate of planes of motion related to functional activity
Average Length of Time per Session	Time is dependent on number of repetitions/sets completed, however a recommended frequency is to complete each of the above 1 time per day over 4 to 5 days per week	Movements or activities are simulated through the use of tool/equipment choices and body positioning. Repetitions can vary from 8 to 20 times depending on client goals. Sets will vary from 1 to 3, depending upon client tolerance and progress. Typically performed on alternating days
Process	1. Assess the client's overall maximal strength level within the defined area (i.e., right upper extremity) or the maximal weight through which the client is able to complete a full ROM with coordinated movement. 2. Foster 10 repetitions of muscle contraction within the defined area using weights equal to 50% of the determined maximal capacity 3. Follow with 10 repetitions of muscle contraction within the defined area using weights equal to 75% of the determined maximal capacity 4. Complete with 10 repetitions of muscle contraction within the defined area using weights equal to 100% of the determined maximal capacity	For example, with the BTE Work Simulator, available attachments for are designed to simulate particular aspects of a given functional activity such as driving, golfing, or opening a jar. Resistance is increased, or decreased, via the simple, and even fractional, adjustment in the software programming
Precautions	See isometric/isokinetic exercises	Same as strengthening precautions listed earlier in this table

(continued)

Table 2-24 (continued)

Remedial Techniques for Strength

Strength: Modality or Intervention Techniques	Neuromuscular electrical stimulation (NMES) or functional electrical stimulation (FES)
Rationale/Indications for Use (For complete descriptions see narrative information)	"The efficacy of electrical stimulation for the purposes of strengthening has been exclusively studied and is well established" (Bertoti, 2004) Used to externally elicit active muscle contraction, and therefore, secondarily addresses issues of strength
Average Length of Time per Session	Time varies with chosen protocols and the tolerance of the clients
Process	Electrical stimulation is provided via electrode placement over given motor points located along a weakened muscle's length. The electrical impulses then elicit contraction of the designated musculature and produce an active concentric contraction. Depending on the client, a variety of wave amplitudes, duty cycles, and frequencies will be appropriate. Further training in electrical stimulation is required
Precautions	Presence of cardiac pacemakers, pregnancy, tumors/malignancy, epilepsy, over the ocular orbits, carotid sinus, or heart areas, blood pressure abnormalities, obesity, active infection, peripheral vascular disease, cardiac disease, mucosal surfaces, skin conditions such as eczema, impaired sensation, compromised cognitive status. Caution should be taken in case of compromised circulation due to clotting or thrombus, in cases of prosthetic implants, and in the presence of degenerative disease processes. Caution must be used in clients experiencing acute pain symptoms or undiagnosed pain

barrier to active engagement in meaningful occupation via the incomplete representation of one's surrounding environment.

Visual fixation describes the ability to sustain focus on an object within the environment. It is important to note that difficulty in this subskill can be either primary in nature or secondary to other issues, such as a cognitive inability to attend.

Oculomotor control involves various subskills that together allow for fluent movement of the eyes. These include aspects of visual fixation as well as saccadic eye movements (scanning) and smooth eye pursuits. In essence, in order to visually attend to one object within the visual field, a client must be able to fix (fixation) their vision on the object, make necessary fractional adjustments in eye position to maintain the object within the line of sight (saccades), and follow the object, while sustaining focus, as it moves through space (smooth eye pursuits). These skills collaborate to enable observation of movement through all visual fields and without the need to reposition the head. Deficits within this area can prevent a client from reading.

Visual spatial inattention is most commonly the result of a CNS lesion that disrupts the ability to visually attend to each and all visual fields spontaneously. In most circumstances, the impairment is seen with right-brain lesions resulting in a disruption of visual attention to items in the left visual hemisphere. Clients presenting with inattention may present with a rightward gaze preference that is often further complicated by concurrent visual field cuts, discussed previously, or body neglect, to be discussed later in this subsection. In isolated visual inattention, a client will respond to cues of redirection; however, this is not the case when field cuts and/or body neglect are additionally present. Again, the ability to accurately view the surrounding environment impedes successful engagement in an array of functional tasks ranging from activities of daily living to leisure and social pursuits.

Praxis

Praxis is a component of motor planning and refers to one's ability to create and execute a motor response to effectively interact within his or her environment. Apraxia (literally without praxis) further describes the inability to create or execute a motor plan in the absence of any other underlying sensory, strength, or coordination deficit. Apraxia is further categorized into two separate types based upon the manifestation of the actual deficit: ideomotor apraxia and ideational apraxia (Jacobs & Simon, 2015).

Ideomotor apraxia is "the inability to translate an idea into motion" (Jacobs & Simon, 2015, p. 141). Conversely, ideational apraxia describes the inability to conceptualize the sequence of a motor plan, thereby affecting the execution of a purposeful motor task (Jacobs & Simon, 2015). The functional implication of the latter type manifests with greater severity when compared to that of an ideomotor origin due to the absence of the client's ability to understand the concept of movement itself. For example, a client with ideomotor apraxia may not be able to mimic the task of brushing teeth regardless of verbal prompts provided, yet is observed doing so successfully on his or her own during the regular morning routine. With ideational apraxia, the client may attempt to comb his or her hair when presented with the toothbrush, demonstrating a deficit in the conceptualization of the use for this tool.

Additionally, the term *constructional apraxia* may also be categorized here, but "*constructional disorder* is now favored over the previously used term . . . since the deficit does not clearly fall within the definition of apraxia" (Phipps, 2013, p. 642). Zoltan (2007) describes clients as having difficulty replicating or creating two- to three-dimensional designs, via copying or drawing, either spontaneously or upon command. She outlines research studies that link this specific disorder directly with a client's ability to either prepare meals or dress accurately.

Body Scheme Disorders

Body scheme is a general categorization of skills required to spatially orient one's own body parts. Deficits within this area include somatognosia, unilateral body neglect, anosognosia, and issues of distinguishing right from left, or right-left discrimination. As a group, these deficits present significant functional impairment.

Somatotopagnosia describes deficits in which a client may have difficulty recognizing his or her own body parts and/or is unable to differentiate between the body parts of others versus his or her own (Jacobs & Simon, 2015). The client may be unable to follow a request to point to his or her nose or leg regardless of whether the request is made verbally or by imitation. Asking the client to draw a person on a sheet of paper may yield an arm in place of a leg, two arms and no representation of legs, or even extremities in the absence of a trunk.

Unilateral body neglect is a condition in which the client lacks the integration of sensory input on one half of the body, resulting in a lack of awareness of the existence of that side of the body. For example, a client may only draw one half of the body when asked to draw a person, may only dress one half of their body during the morning routine, or comb only one half of the hair on his or her head. Typically, neglect of the left half of the body is again, indicative of right-brain involvement and may or may not be accompanied by visual field cuts or visual inattention of the same side. Anosognosia represents an extreme form of unilateral body neglect characterized by a lack of acceptance or even denial of paralysis experienced within the body (Jacobs & Simon, 2015). Confusion and confabulation may also accompany this disorder as illustrated by the client who claims his or her paralyzed limb has simply "always had a mind of its own" or who falls from the bed when attempting to stand, stating, "It's just asleep." This deficit is commonly associated with a concurrent cognitive impairment, although not always (Zoltan, 2007).

Deficits resulting in impairment of right-left discrimination are characterized by a client's inability to follow therapist commands such as "Point to your left knee" or "Raise your right hand." Impaired right-left discrimination is "considered by some to be a rare but striking disorder" (Zoltan, 2007, p. 143).

Finger agnosia is a body scheme disorder causing difficulty in naming fingers or identifying the finger touched and a decreased ability to imitate gestures. Clients often present with bilateral involvement, resulting in poor manipulation skills involving coordination of the fingers. Because the hand and fingers represent the cornerstone of function, finger agnosia can pose significant limitations in one's ability to perform functional, everyday tasks (Zoltan, 2007).

Agnosias

Agnosias related to perceptual deficits (but not specifically to body scheme disorders mentioned previously) include visual agnosia, visual object agnosia, prosopagnosia, simultagnosia, visual-spatial agnosia, tactile agnosia, auditory agnosia, and apractognosia. These types of agnosias result in the lack of recognition of familiar items or people due to the perceptual misinterpretation of input from visual, tactile, proprioceptive, and auditory systems alone (Zoltan, 2007). Because these occur infrequently and because intervention is similar as for body scheme disorders, intervention for these particular disorders will not be specifically addressed.

Visual Discrimination Skills

Visual discrimination refers to the ability to distinguish characteristics among items viewed. Visual discrimination is further classified into five subtypes: form discrimination, depth perception, figure ground, spatial relations, and topographical orientation (Zoltan, 2007).

Form discrimination involves visual recognition of objects, shapes, color, and edges regardless of the context in which they are presented. When form discrimination is affected by injury or illness, clients may not be able to recognize subtle changes in form and properly adjust the motor response. Zoltan (2007) cites the classic example of a client attempting to use a water pitcher as a urinal.

Depth perception, or stereopsis, involves the ability to judge distance within the environment such as is needed for reaching to grasp a container of milk in the refrigerator. It is a skill that demands accurate visual input to produce accurate motor output. Deficits in this area may present as "undershooting" or "overshooting" when attempting to retrieve common everyday items needed to engage in daily occupations (Zoltan, 2007).

Figure ground involves the ability to perceive the foreground from the background. Though similar to depth perception and form discrimination, this skill specifically requires the ability to distinguish items that are closest to or furthest from oneself based on variations in color, texture, shape, and/or shadow. For example, a deficit in figure ground may hinder a client's ability to locate a white shirt placed on the white bedspread or, for that matter, the white buttons on a white shirt, thereby impairing the overall level of independence with the task of dressing (Zoltan, 2007).

Spatial relations refers to the ability to judge the relationship of items to oneself and each other. This includes the subconscious interpretation of what is seen, such as the control knobs of a water faucet located to each side of the water spout itself. For instance, to use the water faucet, one must be able to gauge the distance between oneself and the faucet as well as the components of the faucet, including the orientation of right versus left (hot/cold), above versus below (faucet/basin), and on versus off. A client experiencing deficits with spatial relations would have difficulty following requests such as, "Can you hand me the dish towel hanging next to the refrigerator?" (Zoltan, 2007).

The final subskill of visual discrimination is topographical orientation, which refers to one's ability to navigate the environment, both immediately and on a more global scope (Jacobs & Simon, 2015). This skill results from the ability to recognize familiar settings and conceptualize the relationship of one place to another. A deficit in this skill area, or topographical disorientation, may prevent a client from locating the bathroom adjoining his or her room or identifying the route necessary to get from one point in the community to another. As outlined by Zoltan (2007), remedial techniques are not generally attempted in this subskill area, with preference given to strategies of compensation or adaptation.

Common Frames of Reference for Perceptual Intervention

In general, the prevailing frame of reference that guides restorative intervention methods implemented by the occupational therapist is Toglia's dynamic interactional approach (Cole & Tufano, 2008). Per Cole and Tufano (2008), the dynamic interactional approach (DIA) views dysfunction in part as an inability to "select and use processing strategies to organize and structure incoming information." Refer to Chapter 3 for a brief analysis of this frame of reference. DIA is based on the concept that the brain has the capability of both healing and adapting for dysfunction or neural plasticity, a principle that is described with more detail within the coordination subsection of this chapter. Methods prescribed here foster the repetition of sensorimotor experiences that in turn foster overall relearning for the system. Many of the methods implemented are also based in concepts of teaching/learning integrated into routine, everyday task performance.

Restorative Techniques for Perception

The occupational therapist must implement several underlying techniques as preparatory methods to promote the restoration of perceptual skills. The most commonly employed techniques are summarized below and presented in Tables 2-25 through 2-28, which outline specific methods as they relate to the terminology previously reviewed.

The use of cuing and chaining (forward and backward) are frequently implemented as both restorative and compensatory approaches employed by the occupational therapist when addressing

Table 2-25

Remedial Techniques for Visual Processing

Visual Processing Skill Area	Remedial Strategies
Ocular alignment	Use of eye patches with attention to a wear schedule that fosters strengthening of the affected eye while avoiding weakening of the non-affected eye; table top worksheet tasks that promote ocular alignment such as reading or following moving targets.
Visual fields	Use of anchoring techniques (Figure 2-22) are common where the occupational therapist will place a yellow (for example) border to the affected side and then use graded tactile and verbal cues reminding the client until they are able to see the yellow anchor. This provides the client with an environmental cue indicating that they are seeing the full visual field. Frequently combined with acts of function, such as eating a meal, in table top worksheet tasks, or with computer generated tasks which foster improved attention to the affected side. If anchoring continues, it becomes an adaptive/compensation or maintenance technique, as seen in Chapters 3 and 4.
Visual fixation	Due to the nature of the close relationship among scanning and fixation, the most commonly implemented remedial technique used here is reading. Therapist will grade these tasks from letter identification to reading a paragraph (Zoltan, 1996).
Oculomotor control and scanning	Fostering functional engagement in tasks requiring the skill of scanning, saccades, and smooth eye pursuits (Figure 2-23). The client may be asked to locate various items within their room, home, or hospital environment; identify the price of grocery items by locating price tags; and locate various items within a newspaper. Table-top worksheets or computer generated programs that foster scanning, or even participation in crossword puzzles pending level of interest.
Visual spatial inattention	Most commonly, techniques described above in the visual field section are repeated here so many times that they occur simultaneously. The occupational therapist may also use external stimulus, such as bright colors and/or lights in the affected area along with graded cuing statements to promote attention to that side during any functional tasks. Table top worksheets, such as bisecting lines, as well as a computer generated program specific to inattention are also commonly used tools.

perceptual deficits. Cuing is provided as a form of graded assistance during the performance of functional activities. Cuing is graded not only by the quantity of cues offered by the therapist but also the manner in which they are provided. For example, a client may be offered tactile, verbal, and kinesthetic cues. When the client's performance improves, the occupational therapist will then grade to using only verbal or visual cues, fostering increased independence with performance demands. For example, a client who has a visual field cut may be reminded to attend to the affected side during the morning routine by having the therapist rub the affected extremity in addition to verbal reminders to look to that side during task execution. The occupational therapist may then grade the cues provided by eliminating the tactile cues and using only verbal (or even written) cues to remind the client to attend to the affected side, thereby promoting increased independent participation in the grooming task.

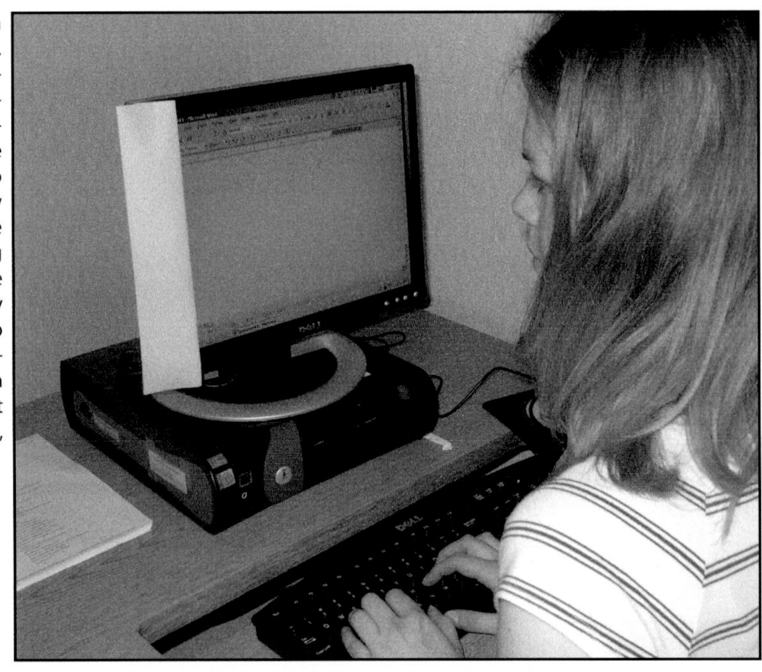

Figure 2-22. Demonstration of an anchoring technique. While engaging in the functional task working at a computer, the occupational therapist will provide cues to guide the client's visual attention to the left side by placing a yellow strip along the left edge of the computer screen. Repeating this technique enables the individual to independently use the brightly colored strip as a cue that he or she is seeing all of what is placed in front of him or her whether it is a computer screen, a book, or a newspaper.

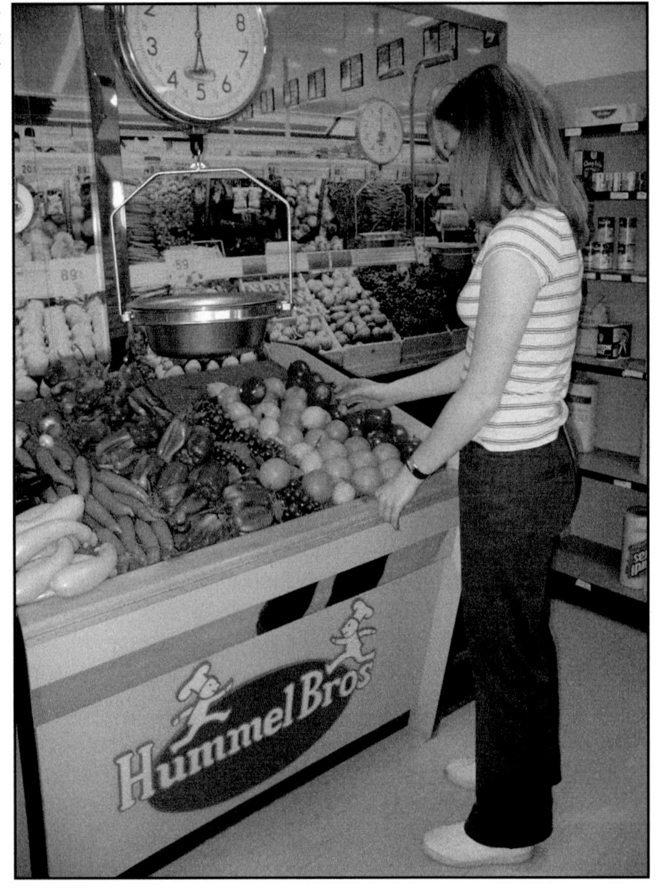

Figure 2-23. Sample of a functional environment where the occupational therapist is able to employ the restoration of oculomotor control and scanning.

Table 2-26 Remedial Techniques for Ideational and Ideomotor Apraxias
Use of hand-over-hand techniques (tactile, proprioceptive and kinesthetic cuing) depicted in Figure 2-24 are most commonly implemented within the context of functional task engagement (such as dressing or washing) where the OT will physically move the affected body part for the client. Repetition is then promoted in the patterns of functional movement and frequently follow a developmental sequence. The OT may also use graded verbal cues as performance improves yet is seen mostly as a frustration to clients in the initial stages of recovery. Chaining is also implemented so as to ensure client successes.

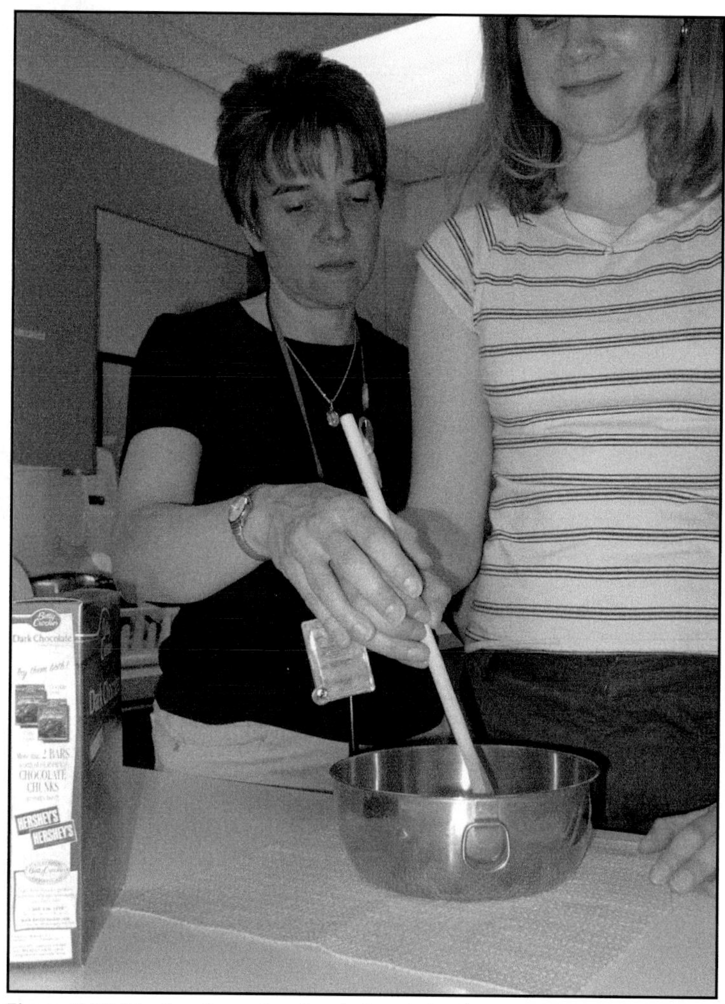

Figure 2-24. The hand-over-hand technique is implemented by the therapist to specifically provide exaggerated proprioceptive, kinesthetic, and tactile input as normal movement patterns in the presence of apraxia.

Finally, it is important to note that the therapist must allow for ample processing and response time in the performance of functional activity for a client with perceptual deficits. Adjusting time constraints for the completion of a given task also becomes a potential method for restoration.

TABLE 2-27

REMEDIAL TECHNIQUES FOR BODY SCHEME

Body Scheme Skill Area	Remedial Strategies
Somatognosia	Use graded tactile, verbal, and visual cues to increase awareness of body parts within the context of engaging in a functional task. In addition, the OT will frequently provide these cues in association with choices for the client and then grade this level of assistance (e.g., "Is this your hand or your foot?" while gently stroking the hand). Methods also include participation in body puzzles or computer generated programs fostering improved body orientation.
Finger agnosia	Fostering improved performance in functional tasks via repeated attempts, chaining, and cuing. The OT may provide nonadversive tactile stimulation (refer to sensation section) to isolated digits regularly requesting identification of the specific digit given added sensory input. A developmental progression is generally followed moving from gross grasp patterns to more precise movement of the fingers demanded in the engagement of functional activity
Unilateral body neglect/ anosognosia	Use of hand over hand techniques to physically guide the client's attention to the affected extremity using the unaffected extremity. Fostering added sensory input to the affected extremity via rubbing with appropriate textures prior to engagement in functional tasks. Occasionally, aspects of the NDT, such as weight-bearing through the affected extremity, may also be implemented just prior to functional task participation to again, provide added sensory stimulation. Therapist cuing and chaining are regularly graded during these activities.
Right-left discrimination	Most commonly, the OT will initiate visual cuing techniques to foster success with functional tasks. This may include the use of a wrist weight on the dominant hand during functional activities and be graded to simply a colored wrist band as performance and accuracy improves. Again, common to see cuing, chaining techniques as well as the provision of choice to enable success.

In addition, the therapist must be aware that the return to function begins at the lowest skill level, subsequently building upon those foundations to promote the overall restoration of the perceptual skill. For example, a client must have good attention skills in order to have short-term memory. Subsequently, good short-term memory skills are needed to have intact topographical orientation. This again illustrates the complex interrelationship between cognitive and perceptual skill execution.

Cognition

REVIEW OF COGNITIVE TERMINOLOGY

In order to best outline restorative techniques for cognitive deficits, a prioritized overview of the coinciding subskills and related terminology is provided again below.

Table 2-28

Remedial Techniques for Visual Discrimination

Visual Discrimination Skill	Remedial Strategies
Form discrimination	Use of graded verbal, visual cues and the use of vision to foster improved performance are commonly implemented. Clients may be requested to repeat various functional tasks which require form discrimination such as sorting items, for example, a bag of bolts or a drawer of utensils (Zoltan, 1996).
Depth perception	Functional activity engagement requiring of reach and grasp (Figure 2-25), table top worksheets, and computer generated programs designed for remediation of this skill are frequently implemented. Heavy emphasis may also be placed on verbal guidance, or cues, through the act of reach so as to retrain the sense of depth during functional movement patterns.
Figure ground perception	Scattering of everyday common objects and requesting the client point to the requested item (Zoltan, 1996). Use of cuing and grading of size and degree of subtle qualities inherent of the objects provided and requested are common.
Spatial relations	Repetitive use of graded verbal techniques as well as provided choices to promote success. For example, "Your shirt is on the shelf above your socks" or "The toothpaste is in the drawer beneath the sink." Hand-over-hand techniques may also be of assistance in guiding the client through the excursion of the required movement.

Orientation

Orientation is most commonly described in three facets: one's ability to recognize self, place, and time (Jacobs & Simon, 2015). A client experiencing disorientation may be unable to recall his or her name, birth date, family members (orientation to self), or location (orientation to place) and/or unable to state the present time, day, month, year, or season (orientation to time). Commonly, a state of disorientation will cause clients to become easily lost or frustrated due to repetitive prompting for what was once customary information, such as, "Where are we now?" or "How old are you?" Clients may also be observed asking the same questions repetitively, lacking the recall to realize they had already been asked previously.

Attention

Commonly, arousal is considered a component of attention because they are interrelated. One is unable to attend without first being aroused or alert. Zoltan (2007) describes alerting as the degree to which one is prepared to mobilize attention and notes that this level may fluctuate depending on the state of one's CNS. The ability to mobilize or focus one's attention on a given task is considered a building block for an array of higher level mental functions including memory and problem solving. Therefore, attention (and alerting) must be addressed with priority by the occupational therapist in a bottom-up approach with the goal of remediating overall cognitive functions.

Memory

Memory is defined as one's ability to successfully encode, store, and retrieve information as required to engage and re-engage successfully in purposeful activity (Zoltan, 2007). This area is

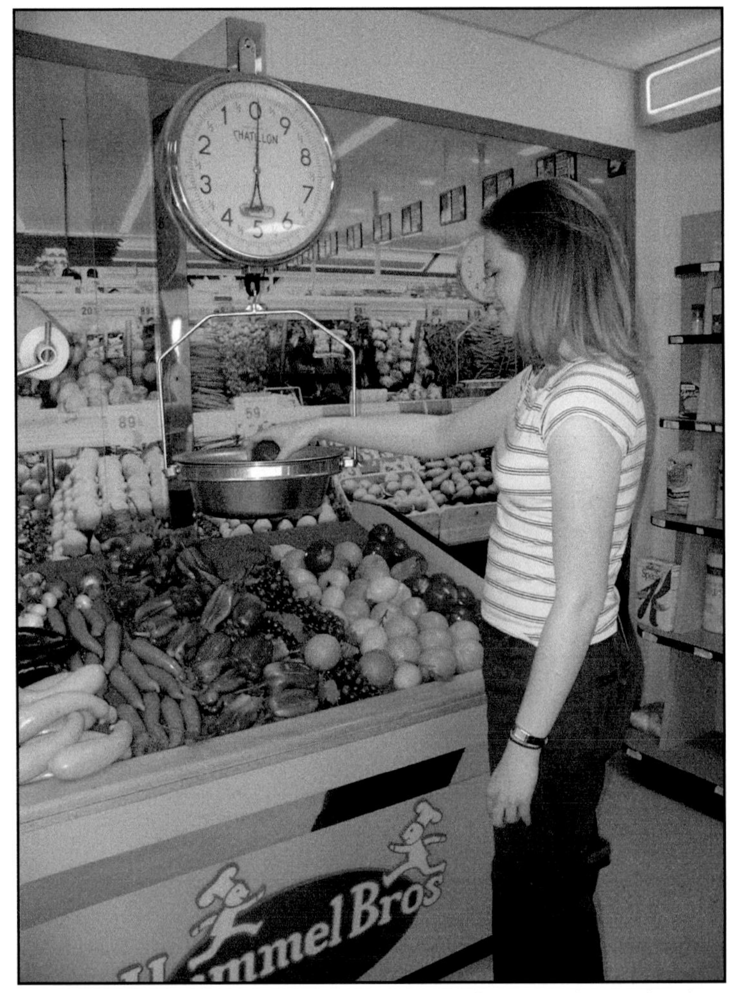

Figure 2-25. Again using the grocery store as an illustration, having the client place items within the scale is a functional example requiring the integration of depth perception in addition to several other perceptual skills.

contingent on attention and perception. For example, without the ability to attend to a task, the client may be unable to create memory about an experience. Similarly, without having the ability to recognize various situations accurately, as is seen with perceptual disturbances, it becomes increasingly difficult to form the accurate memory of a given experience for future reference. In addition, varying types of memory exist, and one type may present a barrier for a client while another a strength. Most frequently, memory is classified as short-term or long-term, reflective of the extent to which the information is stored within the brain.

Short-term memory describes storing information for the purpose of immediate recall, either within seconds, minutes, or hours. Long-term memory characterizes processing events to be recalled after a period of days and years after the initial event. Limitations in either category can significantly impede a client's ability to function safely and independently within the environment.

Executive Functions

The term *executive functions* is used to describe a variety of higher-level, multistep cognitive skills combined. As noted earlier in this subsection, this term is often used interchangeably with *higher-level cognitive* or *metacognitive functions* (Katz & Maeier, 2011). These skills include initiation, self-awareness and insight, planning and organization, problem solving, and mental flexibility. Impairments in this area of cognition is often coined *dysexecutive syndrome* (Zoltan, 2007).

Initiation describes the ability one has to begin engagement in a given task without overreliance on prompts (Gillen, 2009). A client with decreased initiation may have great difficulty starting tasks, regardless of any comorbid cognitive deficit. The client simply is unable to get started despite having no issues with completing the task to its entirety once the activity has been initiated. The converse of initiation is the skill of termination; a client with decreased termination is unable to cease engagement in the activity or task regardless of the fact it has been already been completed. This is also referred to as *perseveration* (Jacobs & Simon, 2015).

Self-awareness and *insight* are terms used to describe the degree to which clients are aware of their deficits. Compromise in this area presents the occupational therapist with a great challenge because the client is unaware of deficits, causing significant concern for the client's safety and well-being. This lack of deficit awareness may be so intense in some cases that attempts to foster insight into disability will yield aggressive rebuttal or uncharacteristic hostility toward the therapist.

Planning and organization are skills that enable one to formulate goals or objectives and a coinciding plan that allows for the achievement of those goals. It is arguable that all task participation on a daily basis is a result of planning and organizing. For example, one must rise in the morning, decide what needs to be completed that day, apply priorities, assess time constraints, develop a plan, identify potential barriers to success, and then execute the plan. Not only does this process call upon planning and organizing as executive functions, but it also requires memory, orientation, attention, and mental flexibility (Zoltan, 2007).

Problem solving, as indicated previously, is critical to carry out functional tasks successfully throughout the day. As was the situation with planning and organization, problem solving is also a skill that is dependent on others, such as insight, impulse control, reasoning, and mental flexibility (Zoltan, 2007). For example, the client may have planned a visit to the local grocery store to obtain supplies necessary to prepare a meal. In executing this plan, the client discovers that he or she has missed the bus that would provide transportation to the grocery store or that the supplies required to prepare the meal are out of stock. The client must first identify the problem and then consider alternate plans that will continue to allow for success in achieving the ultimate goal. These alternate plans may include calling a cab, waiting for the next bus, or substituting ingredients required to prepare the planned meal. Each of these options will require additional consideration of time constraints, feasibility, cost, and overall foresight. This illustrates a classic example of the capacity to problem solve.

Mental Flexibility

Mental flexibility provides one with the ability to "initiate, stop, and switch actions depending upon feedback from the environment and related actions" (Zoltan, 2007, p. 269). Clients who demonstrate impairment with mental flexibility may appear very literal or concrete in their thought process or contributions to conversation. They may be unable to shift their thinking from one topic to the next and back again (often referred to as multitasking) or are commonly observed to be perseverative (consumed by one thought) on superficial experiences in the immediate environment or those offering ease in association. As with most cognitive skills, mental flexibility is dependent on other skills including memory, attention, and problem solving; hence, deficits in any one or more of these areas may also manifest themselves in terms of mental flexibility.

Acalculia

Acalculia is a term used to describe difficulty with calculations. It is often taken for granted how frequently one uses their ability to perform calculations on a daily basis: to manage funds, complete simple money transactions, maintain a suitable budget, identify the costs of items necessary to purchase, use the telephone, or even to address mailing envelopes (Zoltan, 2007). Acalculia is a specific disorder in the processing of any numeric information. The deficit can result from perceptual or processing impairments, as illustrated by a client who may see a 6 as a 9 (perceptual) versus one who may not comprehend the concept behind the symbol + versus — or ×. These types of deficits may present concurrently or in isolation.

Theory of Cognitive Intervention

Toglia's dynamic interactional approach (DIA) is predominately used to guide intervention when working with clients experiencing cognitive deficits. Originally based on learning theory and now updated by Toglia to include metacognition (insight into own capabilities), this theory emphasizes the retraining of cognition in a hierarchical manner while embracing the principle of neural plasticity. It addresses orientation, attention, visual processing, motor planning, cognition, occupational behaviors, and effort (Cole & Tufano, 2008).

Restorative Techniques for Cognition

Prior to outlining the specific approaches employed by the occupational therapist, it is paramount to discuss key concepts in maximizing success when working with clients experiencing issues with cognitive ability. The most commonly implemented techniques are summarized within Table 2-29, outlining specific methods as they relate to the terminology reviewed earlier.

Foremost, the therapist must always consider the benefits of a nondistracting environment to further enable success for a client with cognitive issues. Aspects most easily modified include the lighting, smells, and sounds typical of the area where intervention is planned to occur. A less stimulating environment may enhance results for a client who is distractible, whereas the opposite would be preferred when attempting to promote increased arousal.

Techniques of restoration should regularly coincide with the execution of everyday routines and habits. This is achieved by aggressively infusing a client's premorbid routines as inherently motivating methods for reestablishing independence. For example, a client who has just awoken may wander around his or her unfamiliar hospital room, seemingly anxious, irritable, and unable to self-engage in any task. Yet, when the client is verbally prompted to take his or her typical morning shower, he or she is then able to locate all necessary items and complete the task with supervision only as a means of ensuring safety.

As with addressing perception, the occupational therapist addressing cognition will benefit from the use of repetitive and frequent verbal, tactile, and visual cuing; methods of chaining; and overall skills in gradation to facilitate the successful completion occupational tasks. Also of note is the occupational therapist who will, at specific times avoid providing cues altogether to offer the client an opportunity to plan, organize, and problem-solve with as little assistance as possible. This technique is commonly employed to assist a client in developing awareness or insight into their areas of weakness. For example, the occupational therapist may ask the client to make a simple meal, such as his or her usual breakfast choice, and provide supervision only for the purpose of ensuring safety. The client may forget to plug in the toaster or place the coffee grinds in the coffee maker as a result of his or her inability to accurately sequence. When the bread is not toasted or the coffee remains merely water, an exaggerated opportunity has been provided for the client to identify a problem and find a solution, while also concretely illustrating that skills once executed with ease might now require more attention after the incidence of injury or illness.

Finally, it is important to reiterate that cognitive skills are hierarchical in nature, a concept embraced by the cognitive rehabilitation theory. Fundamental cognitive skills represent the foundation for restoration to re-establish execution of higher-level, executive skills. For example, without being cognitively alert, attention to task is not possible. Furthermore, without attention,

TABLE 2-29

REMEDIAL TECHNIQUES FOR COGNITIVE RETRAINING

Cognitive Skill	Remediation Strategies
Orientation	Regularly requesting client orientation responses that foster the use of graded cues for accuracy such as looking out windows for signs of season; adoption of a daily planner outlining important personal information with the use of regular prompting to promote automatic use.
Attention	Foster the active engagement in activities of premorbid interest such as playing a game of cards, knitting, or drawing for example, gradually increasing time constraints; use of computer generated programs designed to improve attention skills; implement reward system such as engagement in a preferred task for 5 minutes followed by 2 minutes of therapist-selected tasks; include activities that require physical activity as this often assists in promoting attention.
Memory	Provide verbal cuing via choice of two in prompting responses; implement regular structure into the daily routine; table top memory drills or games, where deemed age appropriate.
Initiation	Foster engagement in activities of premorbid interest and routine; provide incentives and client-specific rewards for goal attainment; provide multisensory environment with colors, light, and the use of graded verbal, tactile, and visual cuing.
Self-awareness/ insight	Videotaping, role playing, photo collages of premorbid activity engagement, self reflective questioning, engagement in activities of everyday living while allowing for feedback through self reflection, active participation of family members, and/or significant others within intervention so as to provide "nonthreatening" feedback regarding deficit areas.
Planning and organization	Techniques of preplanning and organizing through developing specific daily schedules; table top worksheet activities, and computer generated programs which require preplanning and organization; participation in a supervised community outing planned by the client.
Problem solving	Allow the client to engage in a functional activity such as a simple cooking task; use graded cuing and provide choices to assist in identifying errors and support in finding solutions for those errors.
Mental flexibility	Fostering engagement in an activity that requires both visual and auditory interpretation (e.g., participation in a group-based exercise program); implement the use of computer generated programs designed to foster improved mental flexibility skills.
Generalization	Provision of experiences that require generalization such as reading directional signs in the clinic as well as out in the community as a means of navigation or locating items in one pharmacy as compared to another.
Acalculia and calculations	Computer generated programs and/or table top worksheet tasks, assist the client in paying simple bills or placing a phone call.

completion of a task may not be possible. The therapist must then follow a bottom-up approach that prioritizes those fundamental skills in order to realistically plan methods of intervention.

Special Considerations for Cognitive Perceptual Intervention

There are many special considerations for selecting occupational therapy intervention strategies for clients who have cognitive, perceptual, or cognitive and perceptual deficits. The most important are summarized in the following paragraphs.

Foremost, it is important that the occupational therapist engage the family, significant others, and potential caregivers in the carry-over of techniques very early on to foster the optimal intensity and repetition required to regain these skills. Training should be provided early on and modified as necessary so that they are also able to foster recall and independence with cuing. As many clients with cognitive or perceptual issues are hospitalized for the initial rehabilitation phase, families are often requested to adorn the hospital room with familiar items including typical items of their morning routine (e.g., hair brush), personal items, and photographs of loved ones. This also allows the therapist to infuse these familiar items into treatment sessions as an opportunity to promote success for the client.

The occupational therapist must also be considerate of the client's available support systems and their significance during the healing process. Working with clients who have sustained cognitive and/or perceptual deficits often requires educating those significant others wishing to provide this much-needed support. Education is frequently provided by request when questions arise stemming from the observation of uncharacteristic behaviors demonstrated by the client. The therapist must always use caution, as the explicit sharing of client-specific information is restricted by federal legislation. The Health Insurance Portability and Accountability Act (HIPAA) of 1996 (PL 104-191) was enacted, in part, to preserve the privacy of a client's health information.

Client safety is also of paramount importance when working with those who have impaired cognition and/or perception. As discussed previously, some clients with cognitive issues may experience bouts of hostility and frustration. This is a recognized level of the recovery process, outlined by the Rancho Los Amigo (RLA) scale, as the RLA IV level. The RLA scale is a measurement tool devised at the Rancho Los Amigo Hospital in Downey, California, that defines eight distinct levels through which individuals generally progress during the healing process and in the case of brain injury specifically. Each level is characterized by a set of observable behaviors. For example, RLA level I is characterized by complete nonresponsiveness, and level VIII is defined by a return to a purposeful and appropriate level of cognitive functioning (Tipton-Burton, McLaughlin, & Englander, 2013). Refer to Figure 2-26 for a brief summary of the Ranchos Los Amigo scale levels of cognitive functioning. In cases of RLA level IV, client safety as well as that of the treatment team are important, while always recalling that hostility is a symptom of the injury in a given phase of recovery and not necessarily the client's cognitive intent.

Maintenance Programs

With regard to maintenance programs for clients with cognitive and/or perceptual deficits, it must be emphasized that recovery can vary greatly from client to client. Some improve at a faster rate yielding discharge directly to the home with continued outpatient services, while others require discharge to a more structured transitional living program prior to returning home. Often, it is this proposed discharge environment that will direct not only efforts of restoration but also the specific maintenance program recommended for the client.

The maintenance program will typically emphasize the specific carry-over of any and all techniques found to be successful for fostering maximal independence during treatment sessions. Careful consideration should also be paid to the societal acceptance of recommended techniques to enhance the probability of carry- over. For example, a client with memory issues would be more

RANCHOS LOS AMIGOS SCALE OF COGNITIVE FUNCTIONING

RLA I: No Response
Client is nonarousable; no response to stimlus of any type.

RLA II: Generalized Response
Client can initiate gross reactions to stimuli in some manner.

RLA III: Localized Response
Client begins to respond with more appropriate gestures such as turning head to the sound of a familiar family member. May also respond to simple commands such as "squeeze my hand."

RLA IV: Confused-Agitated
Client gains alertness in state of confusion displaying heightened reactions to simple requests, such as aggressive outbursts or emotional lability. Behavior is often characterized as inappropriate and internally driven with respect to societal norms or expectations.

RLA V: Confused – Inappropriate – Nonagitated
Client is able to consistently respond to simple commands, requires prompting and structure in all tasks, incongruent, inappropriate, emotional responses may continue yet are less aggressive in nature.

RLA VI: Confused – Appropriate
Client is gaining ability to engage in goal oriented and purposeful behavior. Attention is improving along with the ability to follow commands with less structure provided. Remains confused, though appropriate in reaction to events leading up to injury and the characteristics of the injury (insight).

RLA VII: Automatic – Appropriate
Client is able to function in a structured daily routine without assistance though continues to require supervision for safety in multi-stepped tasks or in those lacking in definite structure. Behavior is considered automatic and rote in nature.

RLA VIII: Purposeful – Appropriate
Client is aware of remaining limitation as well as all events leading to injury. He/she is able to perform in all areas of occupation, however, may continue to require supports for higher level executive functioning skills such as work or money management, for example.

Figure 2-26. Original scale, levels of cognitive functioning, 1980. (Reprinted with permission of Ranchos Los Amigos Medical Center, Downey, California, Adult Brain Injury Service.)

likely to actively adopt the use of a handheld organizer in assisting with the recall of daily routines over a cumbersome notebook filled with check lists.

Finally, the importance of local community-based resources should be formally identified and provided to clients and their caregivers. This may include a variety of support services including support groups, vocational rehabilitation programs, driving rehabilitation programs as applicable, or contact information regarding accessible housing, local means of transportation, or market places for assistive technology needs. This individualized, comprehensive, and proactive approach often leads to a maximal level of independence for clients who have experienced cognitive perceptual impairments.

Summary Questions

1. Define *restoration* and discuss the "bottom-up" approach to intervention.
2. List and describe restorative techniques for pain management, sensation, ROM, and strength.
3. Discuss precautions and contraindications related to techniques described in each subsection of this chapter.
4. Discuss the potential limitations to occupational therapy practice in terms of the use of PAMs.
5. Discuss the impact of modes of injury on foundational skill areas.

Acknowledgments

A special thanks to Anne Walczak, OTR\L, Supervisor of SCINO and Medical Rehabilitation Programs at Gaylord Hospital, Wallingford, Connecticut, and to Carolyn Matrian, who at the time of original publication was a fieldwork level II student from Ithaca College, New York, on affiliation at Gaylord Hospital, for their demonstrations illustrated within this chapter's photographs.

Additional thanks are extended to the editors of this text, Catherine Meriano, JD, MHS, OTR/L, and Donna Latella, EdD, OTR/L, for their enduring vision, resourcefulness, contributions, and patience throughout the lengthy process of completing this chapter.

Strengthening		
Acute strengthening post CVA	Bartolo, M., De Nunzio, A. M., Sebastiano, F., Spicciato, F., Tortola, P., Nilsson, J., & Pierelli, F. (2014). Arm weight support training improves functional motor outcome and movement smoothness after stroke. *Functional Neurology, 29*(1), 15-21.	Spring loaded arm exercise device improved strength greater than traditional therapy.
Long-term strengthening post CVA	Signal, N. E. J. (2014) Strength training after stroke: Rationale, evidence and potential implementation barriers for physiotherapists. *New Zealand Journal of Physiotherapy, 42*(2) 101-107.	Discusses barriers and potential outcomes for strength training post CVA
Interventions for individuals with motor impairments post CVA	Nilsen, S. M., Gillen, G., Geller, D., Hreha, K., Osei, E., & Saleem, G. T. (2015) Effectiveness of interventions to improve occupational performance of people with motor impairments after stroke: An evidence-based review. *American Journal of Occupational Therapy, 69*(1), 6901180030p1-9.	Literature review with findings for a variety of topics, including strengthening/ROM interventions.
Intervention approaches for the shoulder	Cavanaugh, J. T., & Rodeo, S. A. (2014) Nonoperative rehabilitation for shoulder instability. *Techniques in Shoulder & Elbow Surgery, 15*(1), 18-24.	Review of a variety of causes of instability as well as the interventions best suited for positive outcomes.
Table compiled by Pam Hewitt, MS, OTR/L, AAFC and Catherine Meriano, JD, MHS, OTR/L.		

Sensation	
Sensation and completion of activities	Hill, V. A., Fisher, T., Schmid, A. A., Cabtree, J., & Page, S. J. (2014). Relationship between touch sensation of the affected hand and performance of valued activities in individuals with chronic stroke. *Topics in Stroke Rehabilitation, 21*(4), 339-346
Assessment/treatment for sensation post CVA	Borstad, A. L., & Nichols-Larsen, D. S. (2014) Assessing and treating higher level somatosensory impairments post stroke. *Topics in Stroke Rehabilitation, 21*(4), 290-295.
Learning-based sensory intervention post CVA	Byl, N. N., Pitsch, E. A., & Abrams, G. M. (2008) Learning-based sensorimotor training for patients stable after stroke. *Neurorehabilitation and Neural Repair, 22*(5), 494-504.
Sensory retraining with discrimination versus stimuli training	Carey, L., Macdonell, R., & Matyas, T. (2011) SENSe: Study of the Effectiveness of Neurorehabilitation on Sensation: A randomized controlled study. *Neurorehabilitation and Neural Repair 24*(4), 304-313.
Impact of sensation from the client perspective	Doyle, S. D., Bennett, S., & Dudgeon, B. (2014) Upper limb post-stroke sensory impairments: the survivor's experience. *Disability and Rehabilitation, 36*(12), 993-1000.
Table compiled by Pam Hewitt, MS, OTR/L, AAFC and Catherine Meriano, JD, MHS, OTR/L.	

REFERENCES

Almhdawi, K., Mathiowetz, V., & Bass, J. (2014). Assessing abilities and capacities: Motor planning and performance. In M. V. Radomski & C. A. Trombly Latham (Eds.), *Occupational therapy for physical dysfunction* (7th ed., pp. 242-275). Philadelphia, PA: Lippincott Williams & Wilkins.

Aquatic Exercise Association. (2010). *Aquatic fitness professional manual* (6th ed.). Champaign, IL: Human Kinetics.

American Occupational Therapy Association. (2014). Occupational therapy practice framework: Domain & process (3rd ed.). *American Journal of Occupational Therapy, 68*(Suppl. 1), S1-S48.

Artzberger, S. M., & White, J. (2011). Edema control. In G. Gillen, *Stroke rehabilitation: A function-based approach* (3rd ed., pp. 307-325). St Louis, MO: Mosby.

Barber, L. (1990). Desensitization of the traumatized hand. In J. Hunter, L. Schneider, E. Mackin, & A. Callahan (Eds.), *Rehabilitation of the hand* (3rd ed., pp. 721-730). St Louis, MO: Mosby.

Barnes, M. P. (1998). Management of spasticity. *Age and Aging, 27*(2), 238-245.

Beers, M. H., Porter, R. S., Jones, T. V., Kaplan, J. L., & Berkwits, M. (Eds.). (2006). *The Merck manual of diagnosis and therapy* (18th ed.). Whitehouse Station, NJ: Merck Research Laboratories.

Bellew, J. W. (2012). Clinical electrical stimulation: Application and techniques. In S. L. Michlovitz, J. W. Bellew, & T. P. Nolan (Eds.), *Modalities for therapeutic intervention* (5th ed., pp. 241-277). Philadelphia, PA: F.A. Davis.

Bertoti, D. B. (2004). *Functional neurorehabilitation through the life span.* Philadelphia, PA: F.A. Davis.

Bottomley, J. (2009). T'ai Chi: Choreography of mind and body. In C. Davis (Ed.), *Complementary therapies in rehabilitation* (3rd ed.). (pp. 137-158). Thorofare, NJ: SLACK Incorporated.

Breines, E. B. (2013). Therapeutic occupations and modalities. In H.M. Pendleton & W. Schultz-Krohn (Eds.), *Pedretti's occupational therapy: Practice skills for physical dysfunction* (17th ed., pp. 729-754). St Louis, MO: Elsevier.

Cameron, M. H. (2003). *Physical agents in rehabilitation: From research to practice* (2nd ed.). Philadelphia, PA: Saunders.

Cameron, M. H. (2009). *Physical agents in rehabilitation: From research to practice* (3rd ed.). Philadelphia, PA: Saunders.

Chae, J., Sheffler, L., & Knutson, J. (2008) Neuromuscular electrical stimulation for motor restoration in hemiplegia. *Topics in Stroke Rehabilitation, 15*(5), 412-426.

Chon, S. C., Oh, D. W., & Shim, J. H. (2009). Watsu approach for improving spasticity and ambulatory function in hemiparetic patients with stroke. *Physiotherapy Research International, 14* (2): 128-136.

Cole, M. B., & Tufano, R. (2008). *Applied theories in occupational therapy: A practical approach.* Thorofare, NJ: SLACK Incorporated.

Doucet, B. M. (2012). Neurorehabilitation: Are we doing all that we can? *American Journal of Occupational Therapy, 66*(4), 488-493.

Dutton, M. (2012). *Orthopedics for the physical therapy assistant.* Sudbury, MA: Jones & Bartlett Learning.

Falvo, D. (2009). *Medical and psychosocial aspects of chronic illness and disability* (4th ed.). Sudbury, MA: Jones and Bartlett Publishers.

Farrell, J. F., Hoffman, H. B., Snyder, J. L., Giuliani, C. A., & Bohannon, R. W. (2007). Orthotic aided training of the paretic upper limb in chronic stroke: Results of a phase 1 trial. *NeuroRehabilitation, 22*(2), 99-103.

Fasoli, S. E. (2011). Rehabilitation technologies to promote upper limb recovery after stroke. In G. Gillen (Ed.), *Stroke rehabilitation: A function-based approach* (3rd ed., pp. 280-306). St Louis, MO: Mosby.

Galea, M. P. (2012). Physical modalities in the treatment of neurological dysfunction. *Clinical Neurology and Neurosurgery, 114*(5), 483-488.

Gillen, G. (2009). *Cognitive and perceptual rehabilitation: Optimizing function.* St Louis, MO: Mosby.

Gillen, G. (2011). Upper extremity function and management. In G. Gillen, *Stroke rehabilitation: A function-based approach* (3rd ed., pp. 218-279). St Louis, MO: Mosby.

Gillen, G., & Burkhardt, A. (2004). *Stroke rehabilitation: A function-based approach* (2nd ed.) St. Louis, MO: Mosby.

Gillen, G., & Rubio, B. (2011). Treatment of cognitive-perceptual deficits: A function-based approach. In G. Gillen, *Stroke rehabilitation: A function-based approach* (3rd ed., pp. 501-533). St Louis, MO: Mosby.

Gilmore, P. E., Spaulding, S. J., & Vandervoort, A. A. (2004). Hemiplegic shoulder pain: Implications for occupational therapy treatment. *Canadian Journal of Occupational Therapy, 71*(1), 36-47.

Hoffman, H. B., & Blakey, G. L. (2011). New design of dynamic orthoses for neurological conditions. *NeuroRehabilitation, 28*, 55-61.

Horak, F. B. (1991). Assumptions underlying motor control for neurologic rehabilitation. In M. J. Lister (Ed.), *Contemporary management of motor control problems: Proceeding of the II STEP Conference* (pp. 11-27). Alexandria, VA: Foundation for Physical Therapy.

Houglum, P. A. (2010). *Therapeutic exercise for musculoskeletal injuries* (3rd ed.) Champaign, IL: Human Kinetics.

Huntley, N. (2008). Cardiac and pulmonary diseases. In M. V. Radomski and C. A. Trombly Latham (Eds.), *Occupational therapy for physical dysfunction* (6th ed.) (p. 1302). Philadelphia, PA: Lippincott Williams & Wilkins.

Ivanhoe, C. B., & Reistetter, T. A. (2004). Spasticity: The misunderstood part of the upper motor neuron syndrome. *American Journal of Physical Medicine and Rehabilitation, 83*(10 Suppl.), S3-S9.

Ivey, J., & Mew, M. (2010). Theoretical basis. In J. Edman (Ed.), *Occupational therapy and stroke*. Malden, MA: Wiley-Blackwell.

Jacobs, K., & Simon, L. (2015). *Quick reference dictionary for occupational therapy* (6th ed.). Thorofare, NJ: SLACK Incorporated.

Katz, D. I., Alexander, M. P., & Klein, R. B. (1998). Recovery of arm function in patients with paresis after traumatic brain injury. *Archives of Physical Medicine, 79*, 488-493.

Katz, N., & Maeir, A. (2011). Higher-level cognitive functions enabling participation: Awareness, and executive functions. In N. Katz (Ed.), *Cognition, occupation, and participation across the life span* (3rd ed., pp. 13-40). Bethesda, MD: AOTA Press.

Kesiktas, N., Paker, N, Erdogan, N., Gulsen, G., Bicki, D., & Yilmaz, H. (2004). The use of hydrotherapy for the management of spasticity. *Neurorehabilitation and Neural Repair, 18*(4), 268-73.

Kollen, B. J., Lennon, S., Lyons, B., Wheatley-Smith, L., Scheper, M., Buurke, J. H., . . . Kwakkel, G. (2009). The effectiveness of the Bobath concept in stroke rehabilitation: What is the evidence? *Stroke, 40*(4), e89-e97.

Kraft, G. H., Fitts, S. S., & Hammond, M. C. (1992). Techniques to improve function of the arm and hand in chronic hemiplegia. *Archives of Physical Medicine and Rehabilitation, 73*, 220-227.

Krug, G., & McCormack, G. (2009). Occupational therapy: Evidence-based interventions for stroke. *Missouri Medicine, 106*(2), 145-149.

Langenbahn, D. M., Ashman, T., Cantor, J., & Trott, C. (2013). An evidence-based review of cognitive rehabilitation in medical conditions affecting cognitive function. *Archives of Physical Medicine and Rehabilitation, 94*(2), 271-286.

Langhammer, B., & Stanghelle, J. K. (2000). Bobath or Motor Relearning Programme? A comparison of two different approaches of physiotherapy in stroke rehabilitation: a randomized controlled study. *Clinical Rehabilitation, 14*(4), 361-369.

Langhammer, B., & Stanghelle, J. K. (2010). Can physiotherapy after stroke based on the Bobath concept result in improved quality of movement compared to the Motor Relearning Programme. *Physiotherapy Research International, 16*(2), 69-80.

Levit, K. (2014). Optimizing motor behavior using the Bobath approach. In M. V. Radomski & C. A. Trombly Latham (Eds.), *Occupational therapy for physical dysfunction* (7th ed.). (pp.675-676). Philadelphia, PA: Lippincott Williams & Wilkins.

Lin, K., Wu, C., Liu, J., Chen, Y., & Hsu, C. (2009). Constraint-induced therapy versus dose-matched control intervention to improve motor ability, basic/extended daily functions, and quality of life in stroke. *Neurorehabilitation and Neural Repair, 23*(2), 160-165.

Luke, C., Dodd, K. J., & Brock, K. (2003). Outcomes of the Bobath concept on upper limb recovery following stroke. *Clinical Rehabilitation, 18*, 888-898.

Mathiowetz, V., & Bass-Haugen, J. (1994). Motor behavior research: Implications for therapeutic approaches to central nervous system dysfunction. *American Journal of Occupational Therapy, 48*, 733-745.

Neumann, D. A. (2010). *Kinesiology of the musculoskeletal system: Foundations for physical rehabilitation* (2nd ed.). St. Louis, MO: Mosby.

Nijland, R., van Wegen, E., van der Krogt, H., Bakker, C., Buma, F., Klomp, A., . . . van Kordelaar, J. (2012). Characterizing the protocol for early modified constraint-induced movement therapy in the EXPLICIT-Stroke trial. *Physiotherapy Research International, 18*(1), 1-15.

Northwest Hospital & Medical Center. (2005, June/July). What's new in rehab? Retrieved June 10, 2006, from http://www.saebo.com/customers/104072910252887/filemanager/NewsletterJune_July2005.pdf

O'Toole, M. T. (Ed). (2003). *Miller-Keane encyclopedia and dictionary of medicine, nursing, and allied health.* Philadelphia, PA: Saunders.

Page, S. J., Sisto, S. A., & Johnston, M. V. (2000). Modified constraint-induced therapy in stroke: a case study. *Archives of Physical Medicine, 81*(12), 1620.

Page, S. J., Sisto, S. A., Levine, P., Johnston, M. V., & Hughes, M. (2001). Modified constraint-induced therapy: a randomized feasibility and efficacy study. *Journal of Rehabilitation Research and Development, 38*(5), 583-590.

Phipps, S. (2013). Assessment and intervention of perceptual dysfunction. In H. M. Pendleton & W. Schultz-Krohn (Eds.), *Pedretti's occupational therapy: Practice skills for physical dysfunction* (17th ed., pp.631-647). St Louis, MO: Elsevier.

Price R., Lehmann, J. F., Boswell-Bessette, S., Burleigh, A., & deLateur, B. J. (1993). Influence of cryotherapy on spasticity of the human ankle. *Archives of Physical Medicine and Rehabilitation, 74*(3), 300-304.

Prosser, R., & Conolly, W. B. (Eds.). (2003). *Rehabilitation of the hand & upper limb.* Edinburgh, Scotland: Butterworth-Heinemann.

Raine, S. (2009). The Bobath concept: Developments and current theoretical underpinning. In S. Raine, L. Meadows, & M. Lynch-Ellerington, (Eds.), *Bobath concept: Theory and clinical practice in neurological rehab* (Chapter 1). Ames, IA: Blackwell Publishing.

Rao, A. K. (2011). Approaches to motor control dysfunction: An evidence-based review. In G. Gillen, *Stroke rehabilitation: A function-based approach* (3rd ed., pp.117-155). St. Louis, MO: Mosby.

Reiss, A. P., Wold, S. L., Hammel, E. A., McLeod, E. L., & Williams, E. A. (2012). Constraint-induced movement therapy (CIMT): Current perspectives and future directions. *Stroke Research and Treatment, 2*, 159391.

Robergs, R. A., & Roberts, S. (2000). *Fundamental principles of exercise physiology: For fitness, performance, and health.* Boston, MA: McGraw-Hill.

Robinson, K., Kennedy, N., & Harmon, D. (2011). Is occupational therapy adequately meeting the needs of people with chronic pain? *American Journal of Occupational Therapy, 65*(1), 106-113.

Rood, M. S. (1962). The use of sensory receptors to activate, facilitate, and inhibit motor response, autonomic and somatic, in developmental sequence. In C. Sattely (Ed.), *Approaches to the treatment of patients with neuromuscular dysfunction* (Study Course VI, 3rd International Congress WFOT, pp.26-37). Dubuque, IA: W. C. Brown.

Rust, K. (2014). Managing deficit of first-level motor control capacities using rood and proprioceptive neuromuscular facilitation techniques. In M. V. Radomski & C. A. Trombly Latham (Eds.), *Occupational therapy for physical dysfunction* (7th ed., pp. 679-680). Philadelphia, PA: Lippincott Williams & Wilkins.

Sanger, T. D., Delgado, M. R., Gaebler-Spira, D., Hallett, M., Mink, J. W., Task Force on Childhood Motor Disorders. (2003). Classification and definition of disorders causing hypertonia in children. *Pediatrics, 111*(1), e89-e97.

Schatman, M. E. (2009). Interdisciplinary chronic pain management: Perspectives on history, current status, and future viability. In S. M. Fishman, J. C. Ballantyne, & J. P. Rathmell (Eds.), *Bonica's management of pain* (4th ed., pp. 1523-1532). Baltimore, MD: Lippincott Williams & Wilkins.

Schrepfer, R. (2007). Aquatic exercise. C. Kisner & L. A. Colby (Eds.). *Therapeutic exercise: Foundations and techniques* (5th ed., pp.273-293). Philadelphia, PA: F. A. Davis Co.

Schultz-Krohn, W., Pope-Davis, S. A., Jourdan, J. M., & McLaughlin-Gray, J. (2013). Traditional sensorimotor approaches to intervention. In H. M. Pendleton & W. Schultz-Krohn (Eds.), *Pedretti's occupational therapy: Practice skills for physical dysfunction* (17th ed., pp. 796-830). St Louis, MO: Elsevier.

Schultz-Krohn, W., Foti, D., & Glogoski, C. (2013). Degenerative diseases of the central nervous system. In H. M. Pendleton & W. Schultz-Krohn (Eds.), *Pedretti's occupational therapy: Practice skills for physical dysfunction* (17th ed.). (pp 916-953). St Louis, MO: Elsevier.

Sebastin, S. J., (2011). Complex regional pain syndrome. *Indian Journal of Plastic Surgery, 44*(2), 298-307

Shankar, K., & Randall, K. D. (2002). *Therapeutic physical modalities.* Philadelphia, PA: Hanley & Belfus.

Shimura, K., & Kasai, T. (2001). Effects of proprioceptive neuromuscular facilitation on the initiation of voluntary movement and motor evoked potentials in upper limb muscles. *Human Movement Science, 21*(1), 101-113.

Shumway-Cook, A., & Woollacott, M. H. (2001). *Motor control: Theory and practical applications* (2nd ed.). Baltimore, MD: Lippincott Williams & Wilkins.

Shumway-Cook, A., & Woollacott, M. H. (2012). *Motor control: Translating research into clinical practice* (4th ed.). Baltimore, MD: Lippincott Williams & Wilkins.

Sinclair, M. (2008). *Modern hydrotherapy for the massage therapist.* Baltimore, MD: Lippincott Williams & Wilkins.

Singh, V. K., Prem, V., Karvanan, H. (2014). Integrated neuromuscular inhibition technique reduces pain intensity on upper trapezius myofascial trigger point. *Physiotherapy and Occupational Therapy Journal, 7*(1), 11-19.

Smith, A. (2005). Codman's exercises, otherwise known as pendulum or tic-toc exercises. Retrieved July 15, 2007, from http://www.draubreysmith.com/codman.htm.

Starkey, C. (2013). *Therapeutic modalities* (4th ed). Philadelphia, PA: F.A. Davis.

Stoney, C. M., Wallerstedt, D., Stagl, J. M., & Mansky, P. (2009). The use of complementary and alternative medicine for pain. In R. J. Moore (Ed.), *Biobehavioral approaches to pain* (pp. 381-408). New York, NY: Springer Science+Business Media.

Spicher, C., Kohut, G., & Miauton, J. (1999). At which stage of sensory recovery can a tingling sign be expected? *Journal of Hand Therapy, 12*(4), 305.

Stowe, A. M., Hughes-Zahner, L., Barnes, V. K., Herbelin, L. L., Schindler-Ivens, S. M., & Quaney, B. M. (2013) A pilot study to measure upper extremity H-reflexes following neuromuscular electrical stimulation therapy after stroke. *Neuroscience Letters, 535*, 1-6.

Stroup, E. L., & Snodgrass, J. (2005). The motor control model: Treatment applications and research considerations. *Advance for Occupational Therapy Practitioners, 21*(3), 48-49.

Stuck, R. A., Marshall, L. M., & Sivakumar, R. (2014). Feasibility of SaeboFlex upper-limb training in acute stroke rehabilitation: A clinical case series. *Occupational Therapy International, 21*, 108-114.

Taub, E., Uswatte, G., & Pidikiti, R. (1999). Constraint-induced movement therapy: A new family of techniques with broad application to physical rehabilitation—A clinical review. *Journal of Rehabilitation Research and Development, 36*(3), 237-251.

Thomas, H. (2012). *Occupation-based activity analysis.* Thorofare, NJ: SLACK Incorporated.

Tipton-Burton, M., Mclaughlin, R., & Englander, J. (2013). Traumatic brain injury. In H. M. Pendleton & W. Schultz-Krohn (Eds.), *Pedretti's occupational therapy: Practice skills for physical dysfunction* (17th ed., pp. 887-915). St Louis, MO: Elsevier.

Trombly Latham, C. A. (2014). Optimizing motor behavior using the brunnstrom movement therapy approach. In M. V. Radomski and C. A. Trombly Latham (Eds.), *Occupational therapy for physical dysfunction* (7th ed.) (p. 667-678). Philadelphia, PA: Lippincott Williams & Wilkins.

Trompetto, C., Marinelli, L., Mori, L., Pelosin, E., Curra, A., Molfetta, L., & Abbruzzesel, G. (2014). Pathophysiology of spasticity; Implications for neurorehabilitation. *BioMed Research International*, 2014, 354906.

Vance, C. G. T., Dailey, D. L., Rakel, B. A., Sluka, K. A. (2014). Using TENS for pain control: the state of the evidence. *Pain Management, 4*(3), 197-209.

Vandyck, W., & Mukand, J. (2004). Reducing contractures after TBI. *OT Practice, 9*(19), 11-15.

Venes, D. (Ed.). (2009). *Taber's cyclopedic medical dictionary* (21st ed.). Philadelphia, PA: F.A. Davis.

Watanabe, T. (2004). The role of therapy in spasticity management. *American Journal of Physical Medicine and Rehabilitation, 83*(10 Suppl), S45-S49.

Waylett-Rendall, J. (2002) Desensitization of the traumatized hand. In E. J. Mackin, A. D. Callahan, A. L. Osterman, T. M. Skirven, L. H. Schneider, & R. R. Hunter (Eds), *Hunter, Mackin and Callahan's rehabilitation of the hand* (5th ed., pp. 693-700). St. Louis, MO: Mosby.

Westwater-Wood, S., Adams, N., & Kerry, R. (2010). Narrative review: The use of proprioceptive neuromuscular facilitation in physiotherapy practice. *Physical Therapy Reviewers, 15*(1), 23-28.

Wietlisbach, C. M., & Branham, F. D. B. (2014). Physical agent modalities and biofeedback. In M. V. Radomski & C. A. Trombly Latham (Eds.), *Occupational therapy for physical dysfunction* (7th ed.) (p. 558-588). Philadelphia, PA: Lippincott Williams & Wilkins.

Woodson, A. M. (2014). Stroke. In M. V. Radomski & C. A. Trombly Latham (Eds.), *Occupational therapy for physical dysfunction* (7th ed., pp. 999-1041). Philadelphia, PA: Lippincott Williams & Wilkins.

Zoltan, B. (2007). *Vision, perception, and cognition: A manual for the evaluation and treatment of the neurologically impaired adult* (4th ed.). Thorofare, NJ: SLACK Incorporated.

3 Activities of Daily Living

Catherine Meriano, JD, MHS, OTR/L
Donna Latella, EdD, OTR/L

Chapter Objectives

By the end of this chapter, the student will be able to do the following:

- Define activities of daily living (ADLs) as pertains to the Occupational Therapy Practice Framework (the Framework).
- Describe specific models/frames of reference as related to ADLs.
- Comprehend safety issues as related to ADLs.
- Delineate between the role of the occupational therapist and the occupational therapy assistant as they pertain to the occupation of ADLs.
- Comprehend and identify social participation implications as related to decreased independence in ADLs.
- Describe the impact of contextual and environmental factors on ADLs.
- Identify appropriate ADL intervention strategies based on various performance skills and client factors.
- Identify specific ADL compensation/adaptation strategies.
- Identify general ADL remediation strategies.
- Identify ADL compensation/adaptation intervention strategies related to vision, perception, and cognition.
- Identify general ADL maintenance strategies.

Introduction

ADLs are defined by the American Occupational Therapy Association (AOTA) as "activities which are oriented toward caring for one's own body (adapted from Rogers & Holm, 1994, pp. 181-202)—also called basic activities of daily living (BADL) or personal activities of daily living (PADL)" (AOTA, 2014, p. S19). This chapter will first discuss general aspects of all ADLs. These will include methods and frames of reference for intervention, safety, psychological issues, the role of

Meriano C, Latella D.
Occupational Therapy Interventions: Function and Occupations, Second Edition (pp 137-247).

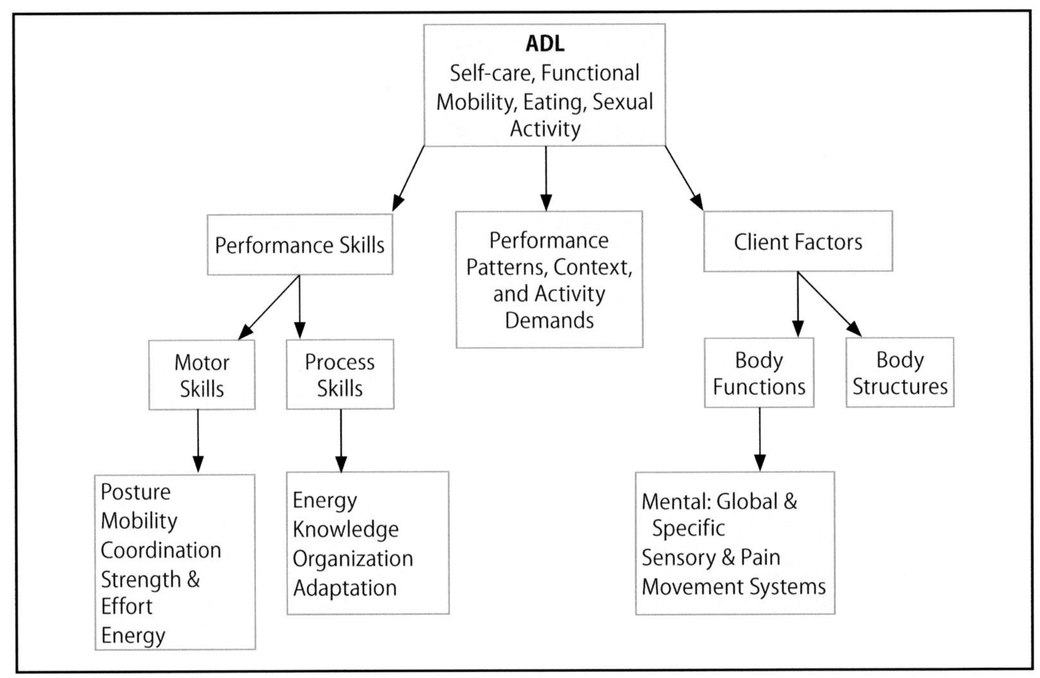

Figure 3-1. Components of ADLs. (Adapted from American Occupational Therapy Association. (2014). Occupational therapy practice framework: Domain and process (3rd ed.). *American Journal of Occupational Therapy, 68*(Suppl. 1), S1-S48.)

the occupational therapy assistant, as well as the Framework definitions of context and environment, performance patterns, and activity demands. Following these topics, interventions for ADLs are discussed in the categories of self-care (e.g., bathing, hygiene, dressing, feeding, and toileting skills), functional mobility, eating/dysphagia, and sexual activity. In each of these categories, different intervention approaches as described in Chapter 1 will be discussed. These approaches are remediation, compensation/adaptation, and maintenance. In addition, compensation and adaptation interventions will be broken down further based on whether the compensation is "changing the task" or "changing the tools." Figure 3-1 depicts the areas of the AOTA Framework that will be addressed in this chapter. Similar charts are placed throughout the chapter in reference to the information within each area covered.

Because ADLs are often addressed in conjunction with other interventions and because occupational therapy intervention is a continuum of client care, references will be made to other sections of the book throughout this chapter. Information regarding the AOTA Framework document from Chapter 1 and the client factors, motor skills, and performance skills discussed in Chapter 2 and later chapters will be referenced as appropriate.

Method of Intervention: Bottom Up vs Top Down

As stated in Chapter 1, intervention for ADLs can follow one of two approaches. The first approach, according to Zoltan (2007) is called the bottom-up approach. If using the bottom-up approach, the occupational therapist would decide to provide intervention for foundational activities that impact ADLs. For example, if after the completion of a task analysis, the occupational therapist determines that the client has limited ADLs as a result of fine motor coordination deficits, the intervention would be provided for the remediation of fine motor coordination deficits, as described in Chapter 2. The reasoning behind this approach is based on the idea that if fine motor coordination skills are remediated, then ADL skills will also improve.

The negative aspect of this approach is that carry-over or generalization to ADLs is not guaranteed by the fact that foundational skills are present in isolation. As discussed in Chapter 1, carry-over includes completing the same task in a similar setting. Generalization is the ability to complete a similar task in a variety of settings. While some researchers have found that individuals completing exercises on one upper extremity (UE) demonstrate improved performance of the same exercise on the contralateral extremity (Nagel & Rice, 2001), this does not necessarily guarantee carry-over to ADLs. One reason may be because rote exercise does not hold meaning to the individual as would a purposeful activity. Fasoli, Trombly, Tickle-Degnen, and Verfaellie (2002) found that "motor actions during material-based occupation appeared to be strongly influenced by the added purpose and meaning derived from the use of tools and objects" (2002, p. 126). More recently this finding was again established using games with children after they experienced burn injuries. (Omar, Hegazy, & Mokashi, 2012). While this study was completed with children, games or other meaningful activities would yield the same results in adults, because "the patient interest is aroused and provides an incentive for this active participation in the therapeutic program" (Omar et al., 2012, p. 266). It is also interesting to note the reverse carry-over from ADLs to foundational skills may be found. Nelson, Konosky, Fleharty, Webb, Newer, and Hazboun (1996) found that despite the same amount of tone present in clients who had a cerebral vascular accident, those who completed functional tasks were found to have greater return of supination than those who completed rote exercise.

Because carry-over to ADLs as well as foundational skills can be found when using functional activities, the second approach, referred to as *top-down* by Zoltan and *the occupational therapy intervention process model* (OTIPM) by Fisher, is generally preferred (Fisher, 2002; Zoltan, 2007). Using this approach, the occupational therapist would perform ADL skills incorporating remediation for functional activity deficits into the session. Using the same fine motor coordination skills as the deficit, the occupational therapist would be sure to include buttoning, opening of a small container such as for toothpaste, and other fine motor tasks into the ADL session. Providing opportunities to perform these tasks in different situations is critical to generalization (Zoltan, 2007).

While the top-down approach is preferred, both of these approaches have merit. The therapist must use clinical judgment to determine which approach works best for each individual client and each clinical setting. If a client is in an acute care hospital and clothes are not available, then the top-down approach is not realistic. On the other hand, if a client has significant cognitive deficits along with the fine motor deficits, the top-down approach will offer better carry-over to ADLs. This section of the book will discuss primarily top-down approaches, as the bottom-up approaches were already addressed in Chapter 2.

Frames of Reference for ADL Intervention

There are a variety of frames of reference that can be utilized when working on ADLs. Chapter 1 discussed the client-centered models such as the person-environment-occupation-performance (PEOP) model, and the person-environment-occupation (PEO) model, as well as systems models such as the model of human occupation (MOHO) and the ecology of human performance.

In addition to these, therapists using the top-down approach may also use frames of reference based on clients' specific situations. For a client who is aging, a developmental frame of reference such as Jung's spiritual stages, Erickson's psychosocial stages, or Levinson's life transitions may be utilized (Cole, 2012).

For a client who has experienced a traumatic brain injury or a cerebral vascular accident in whom behavior changes are apparent, a behaviorist theory such as behavior modification may be employed. Behavior modification is based on environmental reinforcers in order to shape behavior (Cole, 2012). This same client may have cognitive deficits and will require a cognitive frame of reference such as Toglia's multicontextual approach, which includes metacognition and self-awareness. This frame of reference emphasizes retraining cognition that occurs through hierarchical intervention and brain plasticity (Cole, 2012).

Because behavior modification is based on environmental feedback, better carry-over should be demonstrated again with the use of functional activities rather than rote exercise. This is also true of cognitive rehabilitation. According to Cole, "cognitive strategies are always taught in the context of an activity" (2012, p. 168).

Safety During ADL Interventions

One of the primary concerns during any type of ADL is client safety. Because ADLs include hot water, sharp objects, and other safety hazards, it is vital that therapists monitor these safety hazards and provide client and caregiver education. Safety concerns will be addressed throughout this section with specific tasks as examples.

Implications for Psychological Impact on ADLs

The occupational therapy practitioner must not concentrate so heavily on the functional aspects of recovery that the psychological aspects are overlooked. Because ADLs are typically very personal experiences, there can be a significant psychological impact on a client when there are limited ADL skills. The roles of the individual and the impact of decreased ADLs on the family or work context can be significant. For example, when the family breadwinner is suddenly not only unable to support his family but cannot even feed himself, his self-esteem and family interactions can be significantly changed. In addition, most clients are going to be uncomfortable or embarrassed when unable to perform personal tasks such as washing or cleaning themselves after using the toilet.

In general, the psychological issues that arise can be dealt with during the ADL sessions. There are times however, when these issues become too overwhelming for the client. For example, if a client is showing signs of significant depression and this is impacting his or her motivational level for ADLs, more time needs to be devoted to addressing the depression. Typically, even in settings where the main focus is on physical rehabilitation rather than psychological, these psychological interventions are reimbursable as long as these interventions relate back to the functional status of the client.

Context And Environment of ADLs

Therapists often have thought of the context as the environment where ADLs take place. The importance of this context was underscored with the work of Gibson and Schkade (1997). Their study found that occupational therapy intervention that was focused on the roles and contexts identified as important by the clients resulted in higher levels of independence and less restrictive discharge environments (1997). In addition, studies have indicated the benefits of client-centered occupational therapy interventions (Guidetti et al., 2012; Kristensen et al., 2011). Client-centered

Table 3-1 Context and Impact on Activities of Daily Living	
Context	**ADL Example**
Cultural	Cultural and societal beliefs regarding frequency of bathing
Physical (relates to space demands)	Accessibility to bathroom or bedroom layout
Social	Expectations of spouse to assist with ADLs even if the client has the skills
Personal	Socioeconomic status impacting ability to change the physical environment of ADL space
Temporal	Time of day when client prefers to complete certain ADLs

intervention often include the environment with the most meaning for the client. According to the AOTA Framework, context and environment go beyond just the physical space. Environment "refers to the external and social environments that surround the client," and contexts "include cultural, personal, temporal, and virtual" (AOTA, 2014, p. S28). These general definitions were explained in Chapter 1, but Table 3-1 describes examples of how some of these contexts can be related to ADLs. In order to work with clients in a holistic manner, the context and environment must be considered and incorporated into the intervention plan of the individual client.

Performance Patterns Related to ADLs

Along with context, the performance patterns of the client's ADLs must also be considered when formulating an intervention plan. As discussed in Chapter 1, performance patterns include habits, routines, rituals, and roles according to the AOTA Framework (2014). When establishing an intervention plan, it is essential to determine the client's habits and routines regarding ADLs. For example, some clients prefer to sponge-bathe, others to shower, and still others to soak in the tub. Each of these routines will change the type of interventions provided.

A client's role(s) within the family unit as well as society may also impact ADLs. For example, if the role of the client is the caregiver, it may be difficult for others to step in to care for this client because they have never had to experience that role within the family. Another example would be if the expectation within a society is for the spouse, rather than health care professionals, to care for the ill family member. These societal and family roles are often interdependent within the cultural context as described above.

Activity Demands of ADLs

The activity demands of ADLs include the required tools, space, time, foundational skills, and social skills to complete different ADL tasks (AOTA, 2014). As with performance patterns, aspects of activity demands are also related to the client's context. Table 3-2 provides examples of activity demands and ADLs.

Table 3-2

Activity Demands and the Relationship to ADLs

Activity Demands According to AOTA Framework (2014)	Examples Related to ADLs
Objects	ADL supplies or equipment
Space demands (relates to physical context)	Bathroom space available for ADLs
Social demands	Expectations of the individual to perform ADLs independently
Sequence and timing	Steps and sequencing required to complete ADLs properly
Required actions	Foundational skills required to complete ADLs
Body functions and structure	ROM and anatomical parts (hands) required for ADL completion

The Role of the Registered Occupational Therapist/ Occupational Therapy Assistant

Intervention for ADLs can be completed by occupational therapists or occupational therapy assistants. Both have adequate training and knowledge regarding most ADL tasks. As stated in the introduction chapter of this text, the occupational therapist and occupational therapy assistant create a team effort for providing intervention to each client. In this chapter, the term *occupational therapist* represents both of these professionals.

The information provided regarding ADLs is primarily entry-level information for both occupational therapists and occupational therapy assistants. If further training is required beyond entry-level skills, this will be indicated with particular areas of intervention, such as dysphagia.

Self-Care: Bathing, Hygiene, Dressing, Feeding, and Toileting

The definitions of these self-care activities according to the AOTA Framework (2014) are as follows:

- "Bathing, showering: Obtaining and using supplies; soaping, rinsing, and drying body parts; maintaining bathing position; and transferring to and from bathing positions" (p. S19).
- "Personal hygiene and grooming: Obtaining and using supplies; removing body hair (use of razors, tweezers, lotions, etc.); applying and removing cosmetics; washing, drying combing, styling, brushing and trimming hair; caring for nails (hand and feet); caring for skin, ears, eyes, and nose; applying deodorant; cleaning mouth; brushing and flossing teeth; or removing, cleaning, and reinserting dental orthotics and prosthetics" (p. S19).
- "Dressing: Selecting clothing and accessories appropriate to time of day, weather, and occasion; obtaining clothing from storage area; dressing and undressing in a sequential fashion; fastening and adjusting clothing and shoes; and applying and removing personal devices, prosthesis, or orthoses" (p. S19).

- Feeding: "The process of (setting up, arranging, and) bringing food (fluids) from the plate or cup to the mouth" (AOTA, 2000a, p. S19; O'Sullivan, 1995, p. 191).
- Toileting and toilet hygiene: "Obtaining and using supplies; clothing management; maintaining toilet position; transferring to and from toileting position; cleaning body; and caring for menstrual and continence needs (including catheters, colostomies, and suppository management)" (p. S19).

It should be noted that the AOTA Framework document also includes personal device care as a separate self-care activity. The definition is provided below; however, this category will be incorporated into toileting, bathing, hygiene, and dressing because it is typically incorporated into these interventions rather than completed in isolation.

The definitions of these ADLs according to the AOTA Framework (2014) are as follows:

- "Personal device care: Using, cleaning, and maintaining personal care items, such as hearing aids, contact lenses, glasses, orthotics, prosthetics, adaptive equipment, and contraceptive and sexual devices (p. S19).

Evaluation of ADLs

While the focus of this text is intervention, evaluations will be discussed briefly because they are an important component of the intervention plan. The first step of any evaluation is the completion of an interview or an occupational profile with the client. This allows the therapist to gather information regarding the client's motivating factors, goals, discharge needs, etc. One tool that can quickly and easily be administered to assist in this process is the Canadian Occupational Performance Measure (COPM). This tool allows the client to identify areas of occupation in which he or she would like to improve (Law, Baptiste, Carswell, McColl, Polatajko, & Pollock, 1998). Using a functional approach, the therapist would then begin to evaluate specific ADLs that the client desires to work on and that are required for discharge planning. The COPM is available for purchase through AOTA. While there are many evaluations available, a few examples of formal evaluations include the performance assessment of self-care skills (PASS), the assessment of motor and process skills (AMPS), the Arnadottir OT-ADL neurobehavioral evaluation (A-ONE), and the functional independence measure: guide for the uniform data set for medical rehabilitation (FIM). These evaluations have been chosen because they all begin with function. This text is emphasizing the top-down approach, and these tools fit well with this approach. In addition, the AMPs and the A-ONE assess cognition and perception along with ADLs, allowing for a more holistic evaluation of the client.

The performance assessment of self-care skills (PASS), developed by Rogers and Holm (1989), includes 26 activities that can be evaluated as a whole or individually. Eight of the 26 items are related to ADLs as defined by AOTA, and the client is scored based on independence in completing a task, safety during the task, as well as the appropriate completion or outcome of the task. This evaluation has two versions, clinic and home; therefore, it can be used in multiple settings. The tasks are the same for the two versions but the materials are different, so this evaluation can be utilized in the home even if it has previously been used in the clinic. Training is required prior to using the PASS, but after training the tool is available to the clinician for use.

The AMPS, developed by Fisher (2001), evaluates both motor and process skills through the use of ADLs. The clients are scored based on their "effort, safety, efficiency, and independence" (www.ampsintl.com). This tool has excellent validity and reliability as well as cultural sensitivity (a significant number of international subjects were included in the research of this tool). Unlike with the PASS, the client is not asked to perform a task as he or she normally would, but rather is given a specific set of instructions. In general, however, therapists will be able to locate tasks that are appropriate for clients due to the large number of tasks available in the evaluation tool. Documentation of this tool is completed on the computer, and training is required. Information regarding training can be found at www.ampsintl.com and in Appendix A.

The A-ONE, developed by Arnadottir (1990), evaluates ADLs and correlates them to neurobehavioral deficits, such as apraxia, agnosias, and neglect. ADL tasks, when using this tool, are completed by the client without specific directions to complete the task in a particular way. Scoring is based on the client's independence as well as any neurobehavioral impairments noted during the ADL task. Training is required for use of this tool. Information regarding this evaluation tool can be found in Arnadottir (1990).

While based on function, the functional independence measure (FIM) is the most limited of the evaluation tools listed; however, it is one that is frequently used by rehabilitation facilities. One reason for the frequent use of this tool is the fact that training is cost-effective and completed fairly quickly compared to that of the other tools above. A second reason is that the FIM is often used in an interdisciplinary format with speech therapy, occupational therapy, physical therapy, and nursing filling out different sections. The FIM evaluates self-care, continence, mobility/locomotion, communication, and social cognition. The scores are simply 1 to 7 and there is no opportunity to explain why the level is below the 7 or independent score. One client may have perceptual deficits and another cognitive, but both could have the same score. Administrators like the FIM because the standardized results can be sent to the Uniform Data Systems for a fee, and the facility will receive "benchmark" outcome data comparing like facilities (www.udsmr.org).

In addition to standardized and formal evaluations, informal evaluations are also created by individual facilities. The advantage of these is the low cost; however, the reliability and validity of these tools is not tested. Examples of informal evaluations include self-care evaluations; home evaluations to address the context, safety, and function of the client in whatever environment is planned for after discharge; and table-top cognitive/perceptual evaluations. Because table-top activities are not generally directly related to function and often not of value to the client, these are discouraged in favor of more functional assessments. For more information regarding specific evaluation tools, see Appendix B.

Remediation of Self-Care

Remediation of self-care skills using the "top-down" approach will typically include completion of an ADL session. By completing this session, the therapist can incorporate performance skill issues, such as decreased fine motor skills or decreased cognitive skills; however, the focus is on practicing the actual skills that the client will utilize on a daily basis. Remediation by definition is improving the skills, not adapting them; therefore, practice and training are the cornerstones of this approach. In addition, context, activity demands, performance patterns, and safety must be considered as discussed earlier in this chapter. For remediation to be most successful, the environment and activity demands must be as close as possible to the performance of this task in the client's actual environment.

One technique used for remediation is *backward chaining*. This technique, as described in Chapter 1, allows the client to finish the task rather than start it and stop once he or she has "failed." By using this technique, the client gains confidence in his or her skills, and a stronger rapport is established with the therapist. As the therapist decreases the assistance given, the client continues to gain skill and confidence, eventually becoming independent. If the therapist is unable to decrease assistance, then remediation is no longer an appropriate approach.

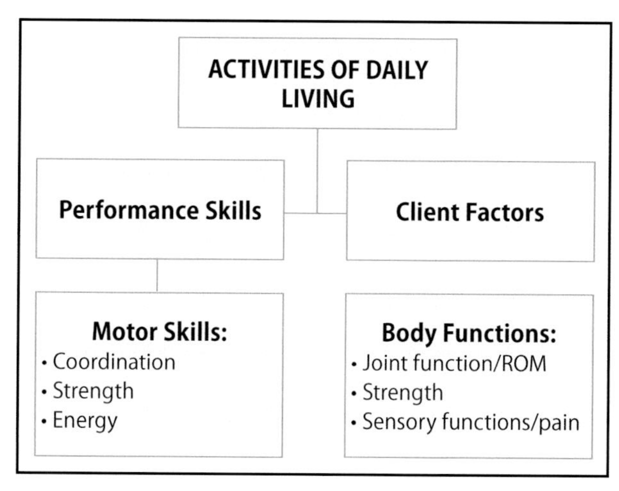

Figure 3-2. Components of performance skills /client factors related to ADLs. (Adapted from American Occupational Therapy Association. (2014). Occupational therapy practice framework: Domain and process (3rd ed.). *American Journal of Occupational Therapy, 68*(Suppl. 1), S1-S48.)

Compensation/Adaptation of Self-Care Deficits for Clients With Physical Limitations: Performance Skills/Client Factors

As stated in Chapter 1, the AOTA Framework uses the term *modify* as well as *compensation* and *adaptation*. Other resources will distinguish between adaptation and compensation by stating that adaptation occurs when the environment is changed and compensation occurs when the task or environment is changed (Zoltan, 2007). In practice, many therapists use these terms interchangeably. For these reasons, the compensation and adaptation sections are broken down into "change of task" and "change of tools" for maximum clarity.

Both compensation and adaptation can be used to achieve short- or long-term goals with clients. If a client will be quickly discharged from a facility, a therapist may use compensation/adaptation to allow the client to regain independence until further remedial therapy can improve the self-care skills. For other clients, remediation is not appropriate due to the underlying pathology; therefore, compensation/adaptation will be the best choice of intervention for a longer period of time. Once these compensations and adaptations become a permanent part of the self-care routine, they are considered "maintenance" according to the AOTA Framework (2014) (Figure 3-2). Maintenance will be discussed later in this chapter.

Because the form of compensation/adaptation depends largely on the underlying pathology or symptoms of the pathology, the intervention strategies discussed below have been broken down into sections based on a grouping of symptoms. For self-care, these groupings are clients with motor skill deficits and clients with processing skill deficits.

Interventions for these groupings are not exclusive, and overlap may exist. For example, a client may demonstrate hemiparesis, cognitive deficits, and perceptual deficits at the same time. In this situation, a therapist must utilize clinical judgment as to which combination of approaches will be appropriate for this particular client.

Other factors that will determine the form of compensation/adaptation include the context of the client upon discharge from therapy, the performance patterns of the client, the activity demands of the task, and the individual preferences of the client.

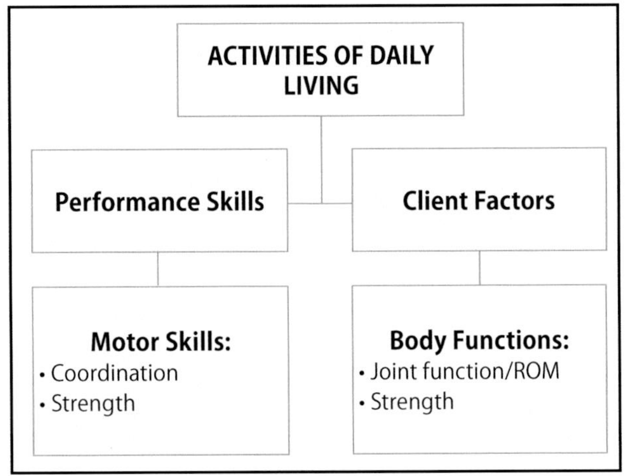

Figure 3-3. Relationship of ROM, strength, and coordination to ADLs. (Adapted from American Occupational Therapy Association. (2014). Occupational therapy practice framework: Domain and process (3rd ed.). *American Journal of Occupational Therapy, 68*(Suppl. 1), S1-S48.)

Compensation/Adaptation Interventions of Self-Care for Range of Motion, Strength, and Coordination Deficits

Range of motion (ROM), strength, and coordination are found in the AOTA Framework document under motor skills and body functions (2014) (Figure 3-3). Definitions of these can be found in Chapter 2.

While modes of injury were discussed in Chapter 1, those related to ROM, strength, and coordination specifically will be reviewed again. The most common neurological pathologies leading to deficits in these three areas are cerebral vascular accident (CVA) and head injury; however, clients with a variety of neurological pathologies could demonstrate deficits. In addition, many clients with orthopedic or traumatic injuries, burns, arthritis, or other joint dysfunction will demonstrate deficits in these areas. While some clients will experience bilateral deficits, it is more common for there to be unilateral injury. For this reason, the self-care section will more often refer to an "affected" versus "unaffected" extremity. In addition, the range of function within these categories is tremendous. One client could have mild weakness, allowing a great deal of function, while another client could have hemiplegia, with no function or tone noted in the arm. Certainly, the intervention for these clients is markedly different. It is vital to understand the basic concepts of intervention for populations of clients but tailor each intervention plan to the unique characteristics, interests, and environment of the client sitting before the therapist.

For clients with motor deficits, many self-care tasks are generally impacted. It is best to first attempt to change the task, rather than add adaptive equipment, because there is less of a financial burden and often less to confuse an individual client. In addition, if the adaptive equipment is for some reason unavailable, the client's skills are significantly impacted.

However, there are times when tools such as adaptive equipment and durable medical equipment (DME) will offer greater opportunities for the client. One approach to providing compensation/adaptation for the client with limited or no use of one side of the body is to provide tools that are available for the general population. Today a large number of self-care products are available in a pump dispenser for bathing and hygiene. These products can easily be used with one hand, and their availability makes them easy to replace for the client when necessary. If liquid products are not desirable to the client, "soap on a rope" or a suctioned holder such as the Little Octopus (Patterson Medical Holdings) can be used. Other tools available to the general public are elastic pants to increase the ease of donning pants, shoes with hook/loop fasteners instead of laces, and button extenders created for shirt collars that can be used for shirt cuffs.

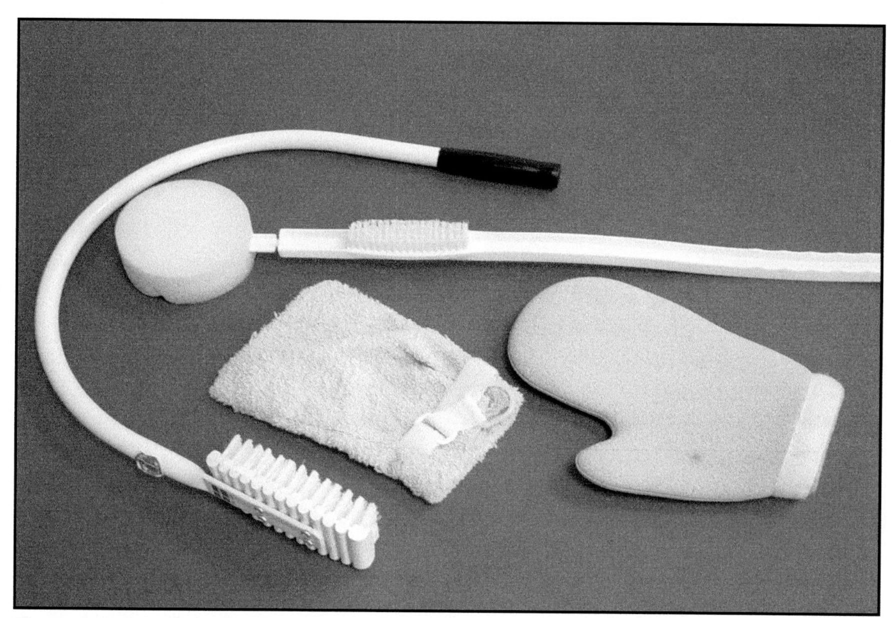

Figure 3-4. Sample bathing equipment: wash mitts, long-handled back brush, and long-handled sponge.

In addition to these commonplace tools, adaptive equipment is also available. Examples of these tools include long-handled sponges, wash mitts, and adapted bath brushes (Figure 3-4). As discussed in Chapter 1, there are considerations that must be addressed prior to providing training with adaptive equipment. These considerations include cost, client preferences, and insurance coverage.

Another alternative to adaptive equipment is to change the environment, thus altering the task. Moving items within easy reach in cabinets, closets, and drawers will provide greater independence to the client without the need for reachers or other adaptive equipment.

Bathing

Changing the Task to Achieve Independence

During self-care, the client who does not have functional use of one UE needs to learn to function with the remaining extremity. For bathing, the clients are typically able to use the unaffected extremity to complete these tasks, particularly if the dominant arm is the unaffected arm. There may be some difficulty with washing related to standing to wash, but this will be discussed later under toileting.

Changing the Tools to Achieve Independence

Clients with motor deficits can use adaptive equipment throughout self-care activities. For example, during bathing, a client can be given a wash mitt that allows for the soap to be placed in the mitt. With this tool, a client will no longer drop the soap while trying to wash. (An alternative to this tool is for the client to buy any type of bath sponge and use pump soap to apply onto the sponge.) For clients with limited lower extremity (LE) ROM, a long-handled sponge will allow them to wash the LEs without leaning forward. After washing, a towel can be wrapped around the sponge to dry the LEs as well.

For information regarding bathroom equipment such as raised toilet seats and shower seats, please refer to the section on functional mobility later in this chapter.

Grooming/Hygiene

Changing the Task to Achieve Independence

The majority of hygiene tasks can also be completed utilizing the unaffected extremity. Some bilateral tasks such as drying or styling hair, painting nails on the unaffected hand, and flossing teeth will be more difficult. In addition, "personal care devices" (AOTA, 2014) often require bilateral use. It is difficult to put in a hearing aid battery or contact lenses with only one extremity. Some clients will eliminate these difficulties by changing the task completely—choosing to change to a hairstyle that requires no styling, eliminating nail polish, or wearing glasses instead of contact lenses. While it is not generally recommended for the therapist to encourage clients to limit activities they enjoyed prior to an injury or illness, these activities may not hold a great deal of value to certain clients, and still other clients may prefer the limitations over the frustration of attempting the activities. Of course, adaptive equipment, as discussed below, is another option.

Changing the Tools to Achieve Independence

A variety of tools are available to assist clients who demonstrate motor deficits. For the client with limited use of one extremity, there are hygiene tools that suction to the sink such as denture brushes, nail brushes, or nail clippers. Again, mainstream items such as pump toothpaste or pump shampoo will also assist as well. There are even stands available to the general public that hold a hair dryer for individuals with limited arm strength or ROM. Other tools have extended handles and will hold toothbrushes, combs, brushes, etc., allowing for function even with limited motor skills.

Feeding

Changing the Task to Achieve Independence

Clients with limited motor skills will generally have difficulty holding utensils and cups to feed themselves. One way to change the task is to choose foods that allow greater independence. A sandwich or other finger foods may be easier for the clients to bring to their mouths than soup or peas on a spoon. This choice takes a great deal of coordination with the client, the family, and the dietary department. It is typically not a permanent solution because it would be too limiting to the client, but it provides greater independence until the client regains functional skills for other foods.

Changing the Tools to Achieve Independence

As stated earlier, many clients with motor deficits will be fairly independent in feeding if the unaffected side is also the dominant side. The tasks that will cause difficulty for even this client are the tasks requiring two hands such as cutting food and opening containers. For clients who have use of the dominant arm, as well as those who do not, there are multiple pieces of adaptive equipment. Again, we first look for tools available to the general public. Cardboard milk and juice containers with screw-top openings rather than the traditional openings are one example. Once these possibilities have been examined, appropriate adaptive equipment is reviewed. Examples of equipment for feeding are rocker knives for one-handed cutting, swivel spoons to avoid spilling with tremors, adapted handled utensils for clients with limited grip, scoop dishes, nonslip mats to avoid plate slippage, and covered cups to avoid spilling. Examples of adaptive equipment for feeding are shown in Figure 3-5.

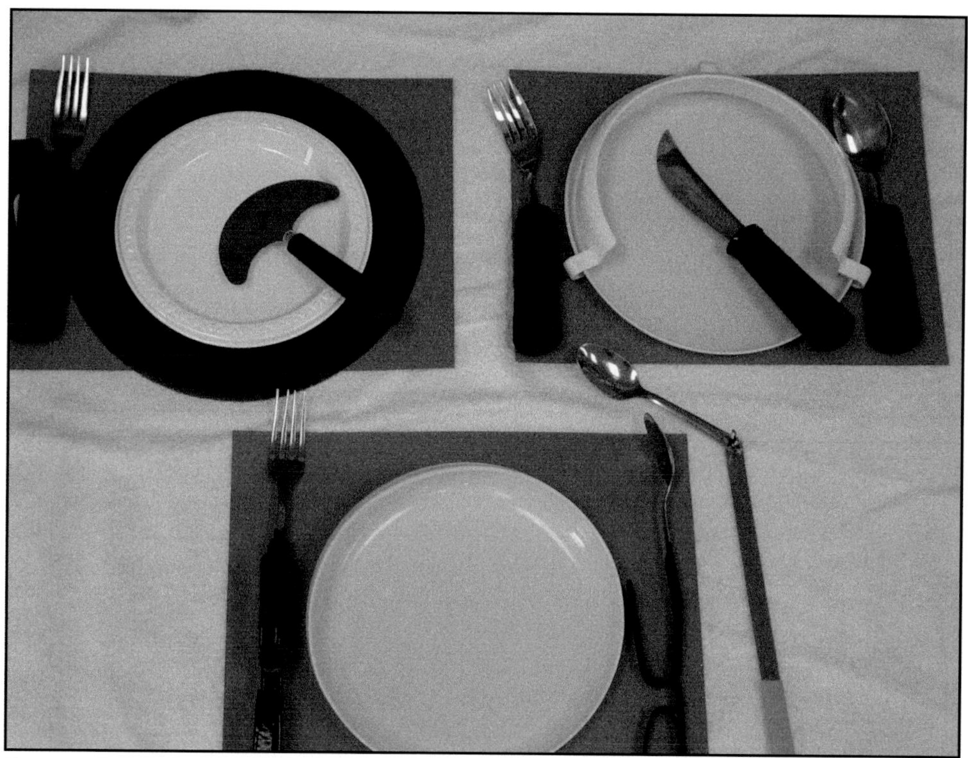

Figure 3-5. Sample feeding equipment: adapted utensils/dishes and dycem.

Dressing

Changing the Task to Achieve Independence

Dressing is the most difficult task for the majority of individuals with motor deficits. One-handed dressing techniques do allow for independence; however, practice is required as these techniques are new to clients. In general, the client should dress the affected extremity first, and undress the affected extremity last. As stated earlier, there is a large range of function among individuals with motor deficits. This text will describe the methods that should be used for clients with the most severe deficits: hemiparesis or hemiplegia. If the client has some function of the affected side, he or she should always be encouraged to use it during dressing tasks. This may alter the methods described below, but these methods are only general guidelines that should be tailored to fit each individual client.

For dressing the upper half of the body, the client should be sitting either in a chair or at the edge of the bed, depending on sitting balance skills. If there is any concern regarding a client's sitting balance, a chair must be utilized for the safety of the client. In addition, the chair should have armrests to allow for greater support of the client, as well as a firm surface to assist in standing.

Generally, the first step in dressing for women is to put on a bra. There are a few methods available to change this task. The first is to hook the bra ahead of time and then put it on over the head as if it were a pullover shirt. The method for a pullover shirt is discussed below. This works well with women of smaller build. The second method is to use the unaffected arm to push the hook of the bra behind the body, followed by reaching across the front of the body to bring the bra hook to the front midline. The bra can then be hooked in front with the unaffected arm and rotated around the body until the cups are in the front. The bra strap is placed on the affected arm and pulled up

Table 3-3 Steps to Don a Bra
1. Keep bra hooked and put on as pullover shirt.
2a. Using unaffected arm, push hook behind the back.
2b. Using unaffected arm, reach across the body and bring hook to front.
2c. Using unaffected arm, hook bra in front and rotate bra around body until cups are in front.
2d. Bring strap onto affected arm and then unaffected arm.
3a. Using unaffected arm, front-hook bra or adapted bra is hooked in front.
3b. Bring strap onto affected arm and then unaffected arm.

the arm as far as possible. The unaffected arm is then place into the other bra strap and pulled up in place. Front closure bras or adapted bras can also be used; however, these will be discussed below as "changing the tools." Table 3-3 summarizes the different steps to putting on a bra.

Some women will chose to wear an undershirt rather than a bra, and many men will also wear undershirts. The undershirt, as well as any other types of shirts, sweaters, or sweatshirts that go on over the head, are put on using the "pullover" method. Again, the client dresses the affected arm first. This is often the most difficult part, particularly for clients with little to no function of the affected UE. Short-sleeved shirts are easier to begin with because there is less length to pull onto the affected extremity. The first step is to gather the shirt sleeve of the affected arm using the unaffected arm. This gathered sleeve is placed on the lap in front of the affected arm so the unaffected arm can be used to place the affected arm into the gathered sleeve (Figure 3-6). The sleeve is then pulled up the affected arm as far as possible, at least over the elbow. If the shirt is pushed over the shoulder, this will allow greater ease when the shirt is brought over the head. Once the affected arm is in the sleeve, the client puts the unaffected arm into the other sleeve and brings the shirt over his or her head, or brings the shirt over the head first, and then places the unaffected arm into the sleeve (Figure 3-7). This will depend on client preference. Lastly, the client reaches behind the back to straighten out the shirt. It is often necessary to push the shirt over the affected shoulder with the unaffected arm as the shirt gets caught on the front of the shoulder. Table 3-4 summarizes the methods for donning a pullover-type shirt.

Clients with severe motor impairments may have difficulty with this method because the weakened wrist and hand may flex as the shirt sleeve is being pulled up and can result in the shirt sleeve getting stuck. Some clients prefer to use an alternate method in order to get the affected extremity into the sleeve. These clients use the unaffected arm to enter the end of the sleeve of the affected arm. They reach through this sleeve and grab the affected hand. The sleeve is then pulled over the affected hand by either pushing against the lap or pulling with the teeth. Once the hand is out of the sleeve, the unaffected arm can be used to pull the sleeve up the affected arm. The remainder of the process is the same.

For clients who choose to wear a button-down shirt, the method is slightly different. The same methods described above are used to get the affected arm into the sleeve. Once the affected arm is in the sleeve, the client reaches across the body and holds the label of the collar or the end of the collar, depending on comfort, with the unaffected arm. The client then brings the collar around the back and places the unaffected arm into the sleeve. Once straightened with the unaffected arm, the client then buttons the shirt with the unaffected arm (Figure 3-8). If there are buttons at the cuffs, the client can button the cuff of the affected arm using the unaffected arm. For the affected arm, the client can either keep the cuff buttoned or add elastic buttons (which will be discussed later). In

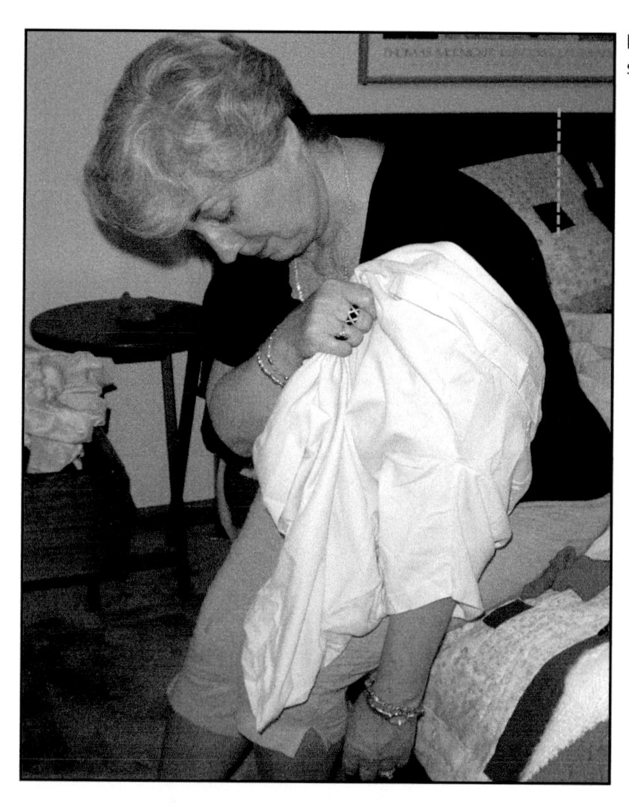

Figure 3-6. Client places affected arm into sleeve.

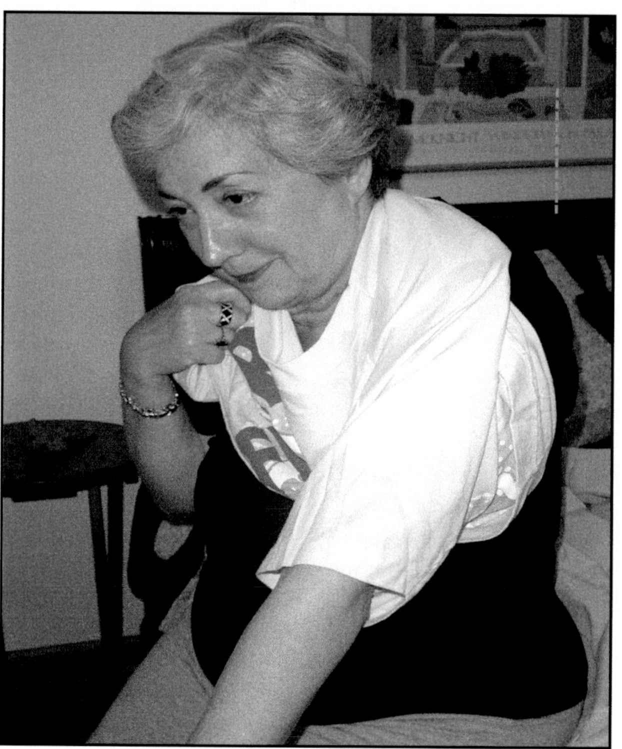

Figure 3-7. Client dons shirt over head.

Table 3-4 Steps to Don a Pullover Shirt
1. Gather the shirt sleeve and place on the lap.
2. Use the unaffected arm to place the affected arm into the sleeve of the shirt.
3. Pull the sleeve up the affected arm as far as possible: at least over the elbow, preferably over the affected shoulder.
4. Place the unaffected arm into the sleeve.
5. Pull the head opening over the head.
6. Reach behind the back to straighten the shirt.

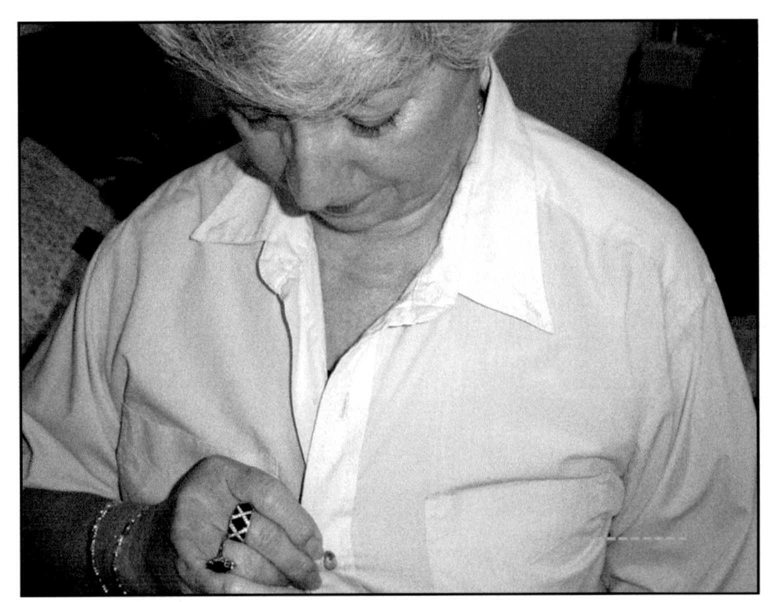

Figure 3-8. Client buttons shirt with unaffected arm.

addition, a client can also choose to keep all buttons closed and put on a button-down shirt using the pullover shirt method. This works best with clients with smaller frames. Table 3-5 summarizes the method to don a button-down-type shirt.

LE dressing includes shoes, socks, underwear, protective garments (as needed), and pants. Underwear and pants are put on in the same manner. The affected leg is placed in the pant leg first, followed by the unaffected leg. There are different methods to get the affected leg into the pants based on the client's sitting balance skills as well as the function of the LE. If the client is able to safely bend forward and place the pants or underpants on the floor, he or she can then use the unaffected arm or leg to lift the affected leg into the pants/underwear. The client can then lean forward and pull the pants/underwear up onto the affected leg. This method works best if the client has enough strength in the affected leg to lift the heel off of the floor. If the affected leg has no function, the pants/underwear can be difficult to pull up. In addition, some clients prefer to put the affected leg onto a small foot stool (Figure 3-9). This provides a shorter distance to reach as well as a better angle to pull once the pants/underwear are being pulled up.

If a client does not have the ability to reach forward, the affected leg can be lifted with the unaffected arm and crossed over the unaffected leg. Once in this position, the client can use the

Table 3-5
Steps to Don a Button-Down Shirt
1. Gather the shirt sleeve and place on the lap.
2. Use the unaffected arm to place the affected arm into the sleeve of the shirt.
3. Pull the sleeve up the affected arm as far as possible, at least over the elbow and preferably over the affected shoulder.
4. With the unaffected arm, reach across the body and hold the label or the end of the collar.
5. Bring the collar around the back to the unaffected side.
6. Place the unaffected arm into the sleeve.
7. Straighten the shirt and button.

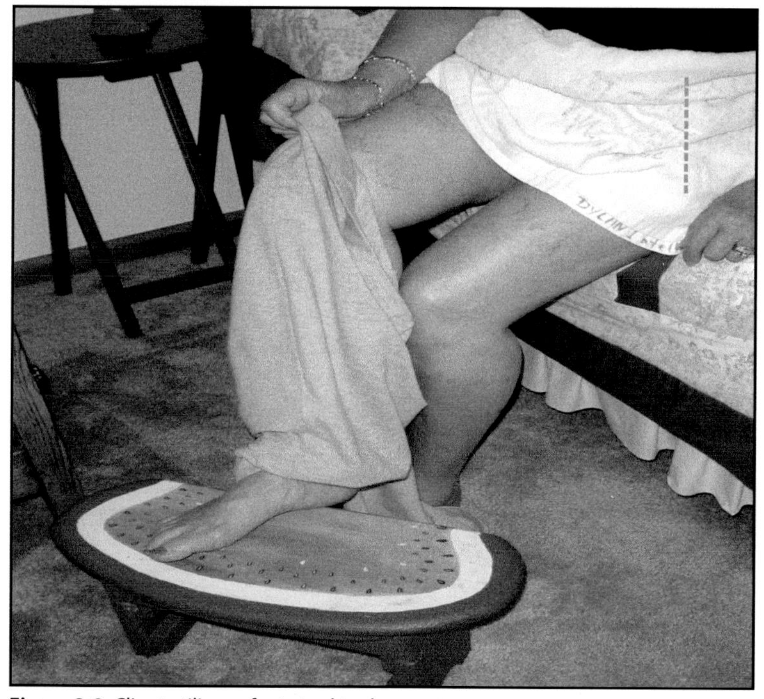

Figure 3-9. Client utilizes a foot stool to don pants.

unaffected arm to take hold of the affected ankle and pull the ankle/foot up so the affected foot is placed onto the unaffected thigh (Figure 3-10). With the affected foot now close to the client, it is not necessary to lean forward. The client can place the pants/underwear over the foot with the unaffected arm and then hold the pants while guiding the affected leg off of the unaffected leg. As the affected leg is lowered, it will automatically enter the pant leg or go through the leg hole of the underwear. At this point, the unaffected leg can be placed in the other pant/underwear leg. It should be noted that clients who have severe hemiparesis might have difficulty keeping the affected leg on the unaffected leg because it will fall forward too quickly. If this happens, the client and therapist need to determine how best to keep the foot in place long enough to get the pant leg on. If able, some clients pull the affected leg higher up the unaffected thigh, others place the unaffected leg on a foot stool to utilize the forces of gravity, and still other clients simply learn to move quickly

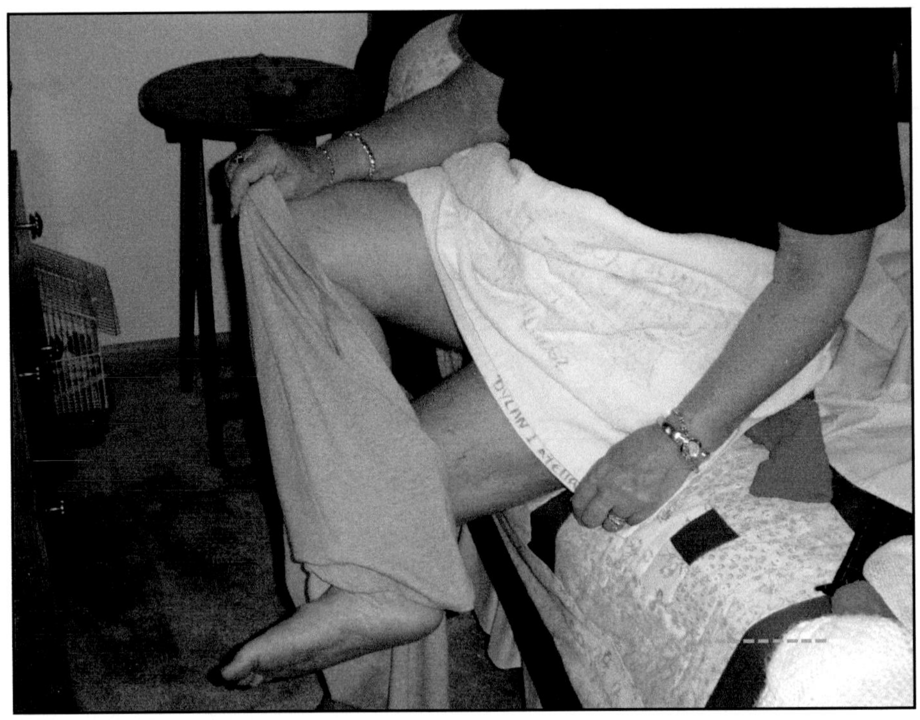

Figure 3-10. Client dons pants on the affected side.

to apply the pant leg. If these methods are unsuccessful or causing greater frustration to the client, then adaptive equipment may be a better choice.

Prior to standing, clients should check to see if the pants are still under either foot. If this has occurred, the client should pull up the pants so he or she is not stepping on them when standing and hiking the pants. If mobility is an issue, it is best to complete the above steps for both the under- wear and the pants so the client will only be required to stand once to hike up both garments. If mobility is not an issue, then the client can be asked to stand each time a garment is put on. While standing, the client uses the unaffected arm to pull up both sides of the pants/underwear. Many clients also prefer to complete any closures while standing. This is beneficial for a few reasons. First, most of us complete this task while standing, so this will simulate a more traditional and ingrained method for clients. Second, closures are more likely to bunch up or become misaligned when sitting. Other clients prefer pants with an elastic waist so closures are not an issue. Note that if the client did not use this type of pants prior to the injury, this may be considered "changing the tools" of the task as discussed later. Table 3-6 summarizes the steps to don pants. If a client requires a smaller protective garment in his or her underwear, this can be applied prior to standing up. These usually are pressed into the underwear with adhesive that can be used once strips of paper are removed from the protective garment. Larger garments, such as adult diapers, may be worn with or without underwear. Some of these protective garments are put on like underwear, and the methods described above can be used. Others are put on like a traditional diaper, which is a more difficult process for clients with hemiparesis. One method to don these adult diapers is to lightly fasten the side so they can be put on like underwear and then tightened once standing. This will only work if the fasteners can be readjusted after the first use. Some fasteners will rip the adult diaper if refastening is attempted. Another method is to partially place the adult diaper inside underwear. The underwear acts as a cradle to the adult diaper affording the client the opportunity to straighten and fasten the adult diaper using the affected arm without the diaper

Table 3-6

Steps to Don Pants

1a.	Place garments on the floor and use the unaffected leg/arm to place the affected leg into the hole of the garments.
1b.	Place the affected leg onto a foot stool and reach forward to put the garment over the foot.
1c.	Cross the affected leg over the unaffected leg using the unaffected arm. Pull the affected foot onto the unaffected thigh and place the garment over the foot.
2.	Once the affected leg is placed into the garment, place the unaffected leg into the other hole.
3.	Pull up the pants until all material is free of the feet.
4.	Stand and hike up the pants using the unaffected side.
5.	Close fasteners.

falling to his or her knees. This method is not well received at some facilities because it creates an extra step when the soiled adult diaper needs to be changed. Lastly, clients with better LE mobility are able to stand long enough to place the adult diaper between the legs. Once in place, these clients can hold the adult diaper between the legs long enough to fasten the diaper on the sides with the unaffected extremity. Ideally, clients will become continent again after an illness and will be able to function without adult diapers; however, for some clients, these will remain a necessity.

The last two items to be donned are shoes and socks. Some clients prefer to put on socks before pants, others after pants. In either case, the methods for donning socks are similar to putting on pants. Depending on the sitting balance skills of the client, he or she can either lean forward to put the sock over the affected foot or bring the affected foot up to the lap, as explained earlier, in order to put on the sock. The most difficult part of putting on socks is usually getting the socks over all the toes with one hand. Some clients prefer to hook the sock on one side of the foot and pull it over the other using the unaffected arm. Others prefer to place the unaffected hand into the top of the sock and then abduct all of the fingers (Figure 3-11). This causes the top of the sock to open wide enough for the client to then slip the top of the sock over all the toes at once. With the toes in the sock, the client can then use the unaffected arm to pull up the sock. Again, if the client is using the "lap" method, as the leg is lowered it will enter into the sock. Once the affected leg is completed, the same methods can be used for the unaffected foot in order to don the sock.

The last item is the shoes. For safety, it is best if clients wear shoes with rubber soles and good support. This often means wearing sneakers or another form of tie shoes. While donning shoes can be difficult, tying is often the hardest part. The method chosen to don the shoes will once again depend on the client's safety while leaning forward. If a client has good sitting balance, the shoe is placed on the floor with the tongue of the shoe pulled back as far as possible. The client then places the foot of the affected leg into the shoe using the unaffected arm. Once the foot is placed, the client will need to pull the back and/or the tongue of the shoe to get the foot properly placed in the shoe.

If the client does not have sufficient sitting balance to use this method, the affected leg should be placed on the unaffected thigh, as done earlier for pants and socks, and then the shoe is placed over the foot. In this position, the client can push the shoe on by holding the bottom of the shoe or by pulling the back of the shoe.

If the client is able to get the shoes on with the shoes tied, this simplifies the method as it avoids the need to tie shoes. Certainly each new pair will need to be tied initially, but once tied in a double knot, the shoes can stay tied. If the shoes need to be tied each time, the client will need to learn

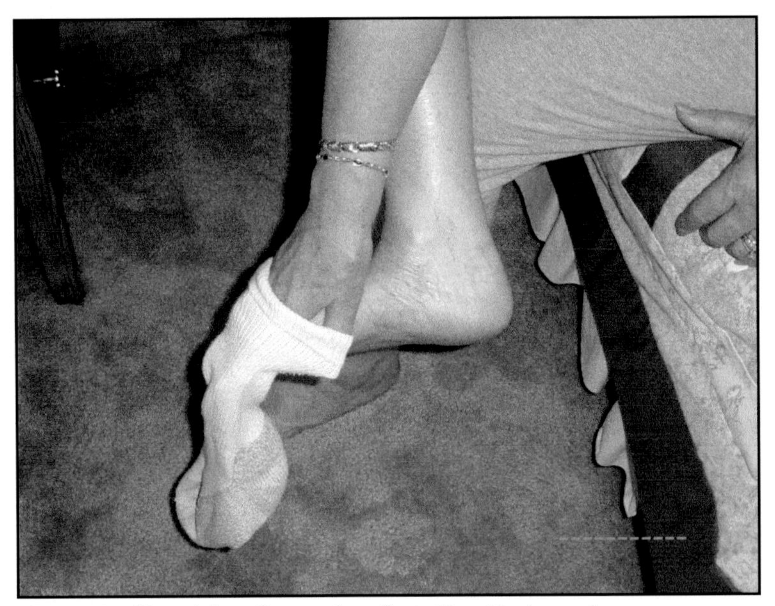

Figure 3-11. Client abducts fingers of unaffected hand to don socks.

to tie with one hand or use adaptive equipment such as elastic laces. (Using elastic laces would constitute "changing the tool.")

To tie a shoe with one hand, the laces must be removed from the shoe and a knot is tied in one end. The lace is then put through the shoes from side to side. This allows a traditional look to the lace, but only one lace is left at the end. The client leaves the lace hanging to the side and forms a small loop by pulling up the lace between the last two lace holes. The client then reaches through this loop with the index finger and thumb grabbing the hanging lace closest to the last lace hole (Figure 3-12A). A second small loop is formed with this piece of lace, as the first loop is pulled tight around this new loop. This process is completed again with the client reaching through the second loop to pull the lace closest to the loops. This time the client pulls the third loop larger and tighter so the shoe will not untie (Figure 3-12B). If there is a great deal of lace left, this can be tucked into the side of the shoe. To untie the shoe, the client simply pulls the end of the lace and all of the loops will untie.

The above methods are sufficient for most individuals with limited motor skills; however, one particular population requires different instructions. The clients who have had a total hip replacement cannot lean forward or cross the legs because of the "total hip precautions" after surgery. For these clients, changing the task is not a possibility, but changing the tools is required and will be discussed on the following page.

Changing the Tools to Achieve Independence

During dressing, a client can utilize a variety of adaptive equipment such as button hooks for one-handed buttoning, elastic laces for the shoes, sock aids to put on socks, reachers for donning and doffing pants/underpants, and long-handled shoe horns to limit leaning forward while donning shoes. Figure 3-13 depicts examples of dressing and hygiene tools.

For the clients with a diagnosis of total hip replacement, these pieces of adaptive equipment will be vital. The typical equipment provided consists of a reacher and/or a dressing stick, elastic shoelaces, and a long-handled shoehorn. These are shown in Figures 3-13 and 3-14. As stated earlier, total hip precautions will significantly limit the client's ability to dress the affected leg. These

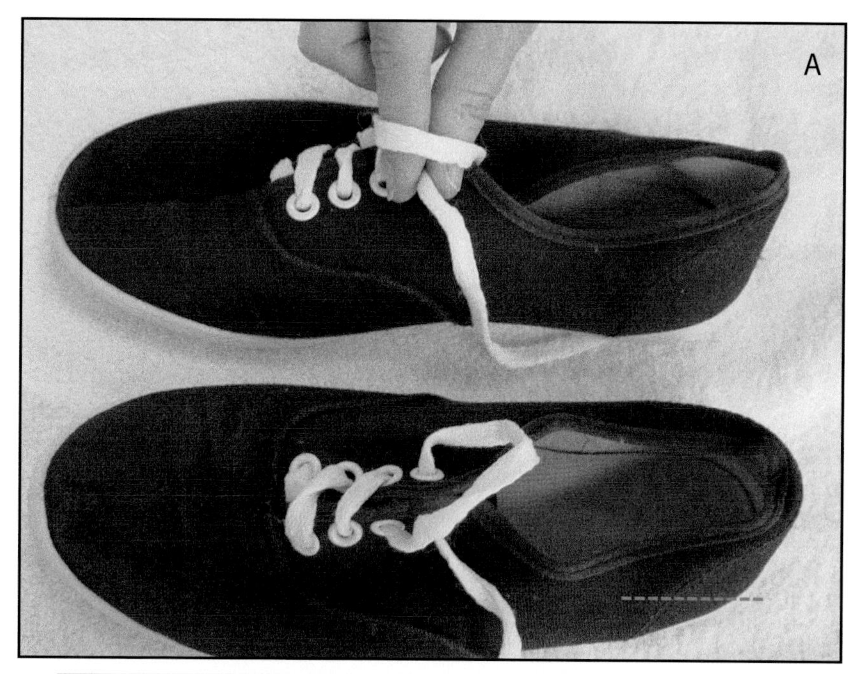

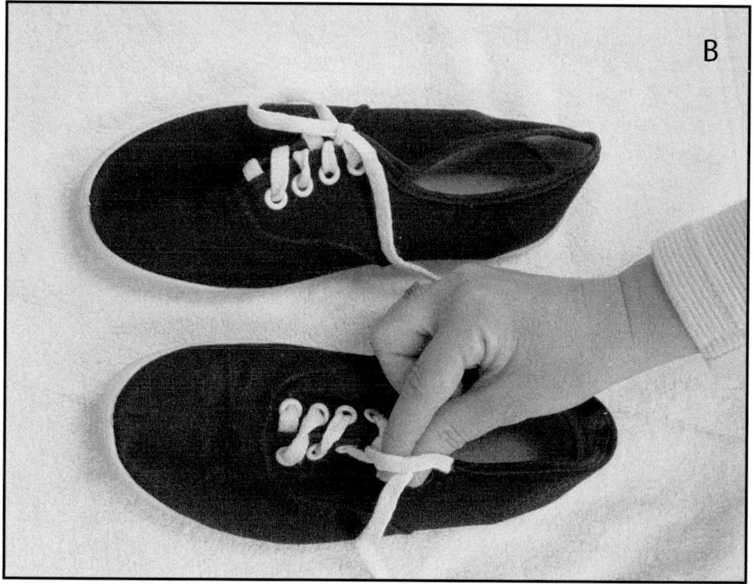

Figure 3-12. (A) One-handed shoe tying: steps 1 and 2. (B) One-handed shoe tying: steps 3 and 4.

precautions depend on the anterior or posterior surgical intervention, but in general clients should not flex the hip past 90 degrees, adduct the hip past neutral, or internally/externally rotate the hip until cleared by the physician to do so (Fairchild, 2013). This clearance may not occur for several weeks to months, depending on the healing progress of the client. These clients will require a dressing stick or reacher to put on pants/underwear, a sock aid, and elastic laces. Some clients will also require a long-handled shoehorn. In addition, a raised toilet seat is typically required. This will be discussed later in this chapter.

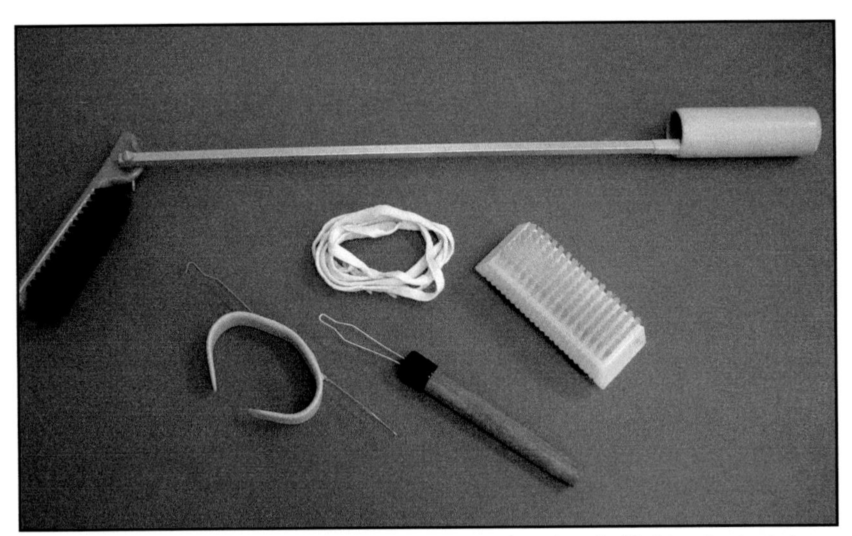

Figure 3-13. Sample dressing and hygiene equipment: long-handled hairbrush, elastic laces, button hooks, and suction nail brush.

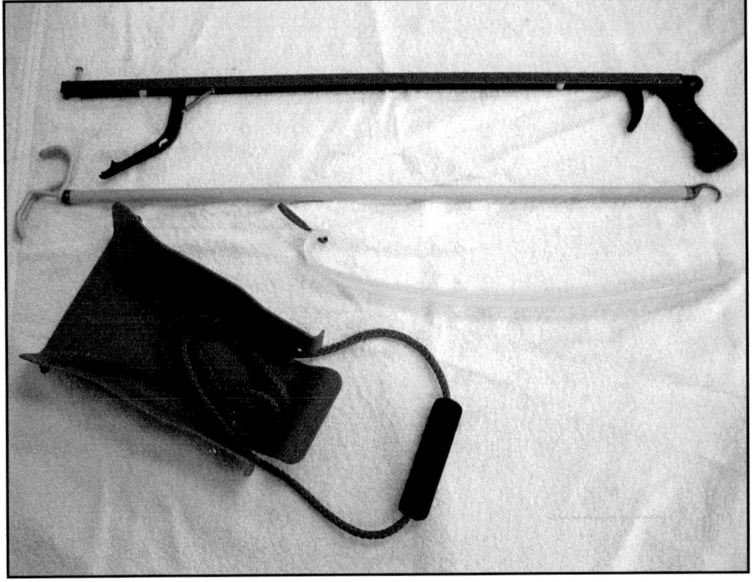

Figure 3-14. Equipment for LE dressing: reacher, dressing stick, long-handled shoehorn, sock aid.

Toileting

Changing the Task to Achieve Independence

The aspects of toileting that cause the most difficulty for clients with motor deficits are the transfers on/off the toilet and clothing management. Other issues can also cause problems such as use of toilet paper and menstrual and bowel/bladder management tools.

Transfer skills will be addressed under "functional mobility" later in this section. The task of clothing management can be improved by having the client prepare prior to the transfer. If

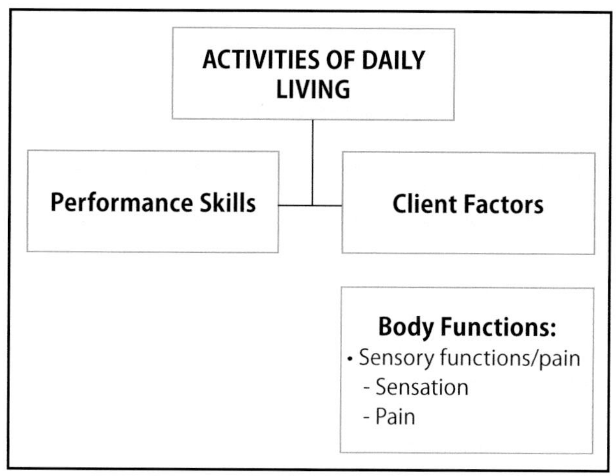

Figure 3-15. Relationship of sensation/pain to ADLs. (Adapted from American Occupational Therapy Association. (2014). Occupational therapy practice framework: Domain and process (3rd ed.). *American Journal of Occupational Therapy, 68*(Suppl. 1), S1-S48.)

possible, the client should undo the belt and top button of the pants if present. This will allow the client to release the pant zipper once at the toilet and quickly lower the pants. Underwear can be pulled down with the unaffected extremity. It is important not to allow the pants to fall to the floor prior to the completion of the transfer. This may cause a hazard while transferring if the clothing becomes entangled in the client's feet.

To increase independence with cleaning and the use of menstrual and bowel/bladder management tools, it is important to place all necessary items in a location where the client can reach them with the unaffected extremity. This may require relocation of the toilet paper dispenser and the use of baskets near the toilet for supplies.

Changing the Tools to Achieve Independence

Adapted tools may be required if the client is unable to properly maintain personal care due to limited motor skills. Tools that can be provided include flushable wipes instead of toilet paper, lengthened suppository inserters to increase ease, and adapted catheter or colostomy bags to allow for emptying without full bilateral hand use. Some of these adaptations are available commercially, but some are created for the particular client by the therapist. An example of this would be removing the elastic bands typically provided with a catheter leg bag and replacing these with hook-and-loop fastener straps if the client is unable to fasten the elastic bands.

Compensation/Adaptation Interventions of Self-Care for Clients With Decreased Performance Skills/Client Factors: Sensation and Pain

Sensation and pain can be found in the AOTA Framework document under client factors (AOTA, 2014; Figure 3-15). While this area of the document covers all sensory issues, only sensation changes and pain will be addressed in this section. Changes in sensation can be a result of central nervous system damage, such as CVA or head injury, or peripheral nervous system damage, such as nerve lacerations. These forms of injury typically cause hyposensitivity, or a decrease in sensation (Jacobs & Simon, 2015).

Sensation changes can also lead to hypersensitivity, an increase in sensation (Jacobs & Simon, 2015). Some clients can interpret hypersensitivity as pain. Typically, hypersensitivity occurs with trauma, such as an amputation, or surgical repair, such as carpal tunnel surgery, but some clients with central nervous system and peripheral nervous system injuries also experience hypersensitivity, such as clients with chronic regional pain syndrome (previously referred to as *reflex sympathetic dystrophy*). For additional information regarding modes of injury, refer to Chapter 1.

While it is important to understand a client's diagnosis and prognosis, this section will discuss only the hypersensitivity and hyposensitivity symptoms resulting from these varied diagnoses. Because these two areas of sensation are opposites by definition, they are also treated differently. Pain management will be addressed briefly in this section but more in-depth in the maintenance section.

Hypersensitivity

Clients experiencing hypersensitivity, will often be fearful of interventions because they may experience pain. It is vital to provide only as much sensory input as the individual client can tolerate. While remediation may center on decreasing the hypersensitivity through input, compensation/adaptation interventions will attempt to keep the client independent while the hypersensitivity is still present. Remediation is preferred over compensation/adaptation because it encourages use of the affected extremity; therefore, the techniques below should generally not be employed as long-term strategies.

Changing the Task to Achieve Independence

The primary way to change the task when hypersensitivity is present is to utilize the unaffected extremity to "check" situations first, such as water temperature. This will allow the client to use both extremities without overstimulating the hypersensitive extremity.

- Bathing example: Water should always be checked with the unaffected hand to ensure proper temperature. Water pressure on showers may need to be lowered to offer less stimulation. Some showers allow this adjustment at the shower controls or showerhead.
- Grooming/hygiene example: Electric razors or toothbrushes may provide too much stimuli to the affected extremity; therefore, the client may need to hold the grooming tool with only the unaffected extremity until increased stimulation is tolerated.
- Feeding example: The pressure required to cut certain harder food items may aggravate the client's affected extremity. The client can either reverse hands, which many find difficult, or use repeated lighter cuts with a knife rather than apply heavy pressure.
- Dressing example: For some, simply pulling clothes over the affected extremity is too much stimulation. Sleeves should be left unbuttoned and preferably should be without a taper on the end. This will allow the extremity to be placed through the sleeve with minimal contact.
- Toileting example: Generally, there will be little impact on toileting; however, if the affected extremity is the dominant side, the client may need to learn to clean him or herself with the nondominant hand. Women will also need to learn to apply feminine products with the nondominant hand.

Changing the Tools to Achieve Independence

The majority of tools provided in all areas of ADLs are intended to protect the hypersensitive area of the extremity, typically the hand.

- Bathing example: A glove can be worn during bathing if the temperature of the water aggravates the affected extremity. Often, warm water is soothing; however, certain clients may find this aggravating to the injury. If water pressure adjustments are required, as mentioned above, and controls are not adjustable, a new showerhead or a hand-held shower may be required.

- Grooming/hygiene example: As stated earlier, electric razors and toothbrushes may cause overstimulation; therefore, regular razors and toothbrushes may be required until the client can tolerate the vibration of the electric tool. If grasping any grooming/hygiene tools is painful, handles can be built up to allow larger grasp.
- Feeding example: If the pressure of cutting is not tolerable to clients, they can utilize rocker knives to spread out the pressure, or utilize one-handed cutting boards with the unaffected extremity. If grasping utensils is painful, handles can be built up to allow a larger grasp.
- Dressing example: Shirts with elastic at the sleeves should not be worn and gloves can be purchased one size larger in order to allow less stimulation when donning and doffing.
- Toileting example: As stated earlier, generally toileting is not impacted by hypersensitivity to the extent that introduction of tools is required.

Hyposensitivity

As discussed previously, remediation is preferred to compensation/adaptation because this encourages use of the extremity; however, most strategies listed below are employed to allow greater safety until sensation returns. For clients with permanent sensory loss, these strategies may become maintenance techniques.

Changing the Task to Achieve Independence

- Bathing example: Clients should always check the temperature of water with the unaffected extremity to avoid any scalding.
- Grooming/hygiene example: Clients should look into any drawers prior to reaching in with the affected extremity. This will avoid cuts from sharp objects such as tweezers or razors. Clients may also choose to reach in with the unaffected extremity, but cuts to this extremity remains less safe than avoiding any cuts by looking first.
- Feeding example: When cutting food, the clients should always observe to avoid cutting the affected extremity.
- Dressing example: The client should check elastic sleeves to ensure they are not too tight on the affected extremity.
- Toileting example: If the affected extremity is the dominant side, the client may need to learn to clean him or herself with the nondominant hand. Women will also need to learn to apply feminine products with the nondominant hand.

Changing the Tools to Achieve Independence

- Bathing example: A thermostat can be installed on a single shower/bath or the hot water heater's thermostat can be adjusted to limit the temperature of water to avoid scalding.
- Grooming/hygiene example: If the hyposensitivity has occurred on the face as well as an extremity, electric razors are preferred to avoid any cuts.
- Feeding example: If holding food to cut it is unsafe, a one-handed cutting board can be utilized to avoid cutting the affected extremity.
- Dressing example: Clothing with elastic at the end of the sleeves should be avoided. This can cause pressure unbeknownst to the client. This is true of outerwear and gloves as well.
- Toileting example: Generally, toileting is not impacted by hyposensitivity to the extent that introduction of tools is required.

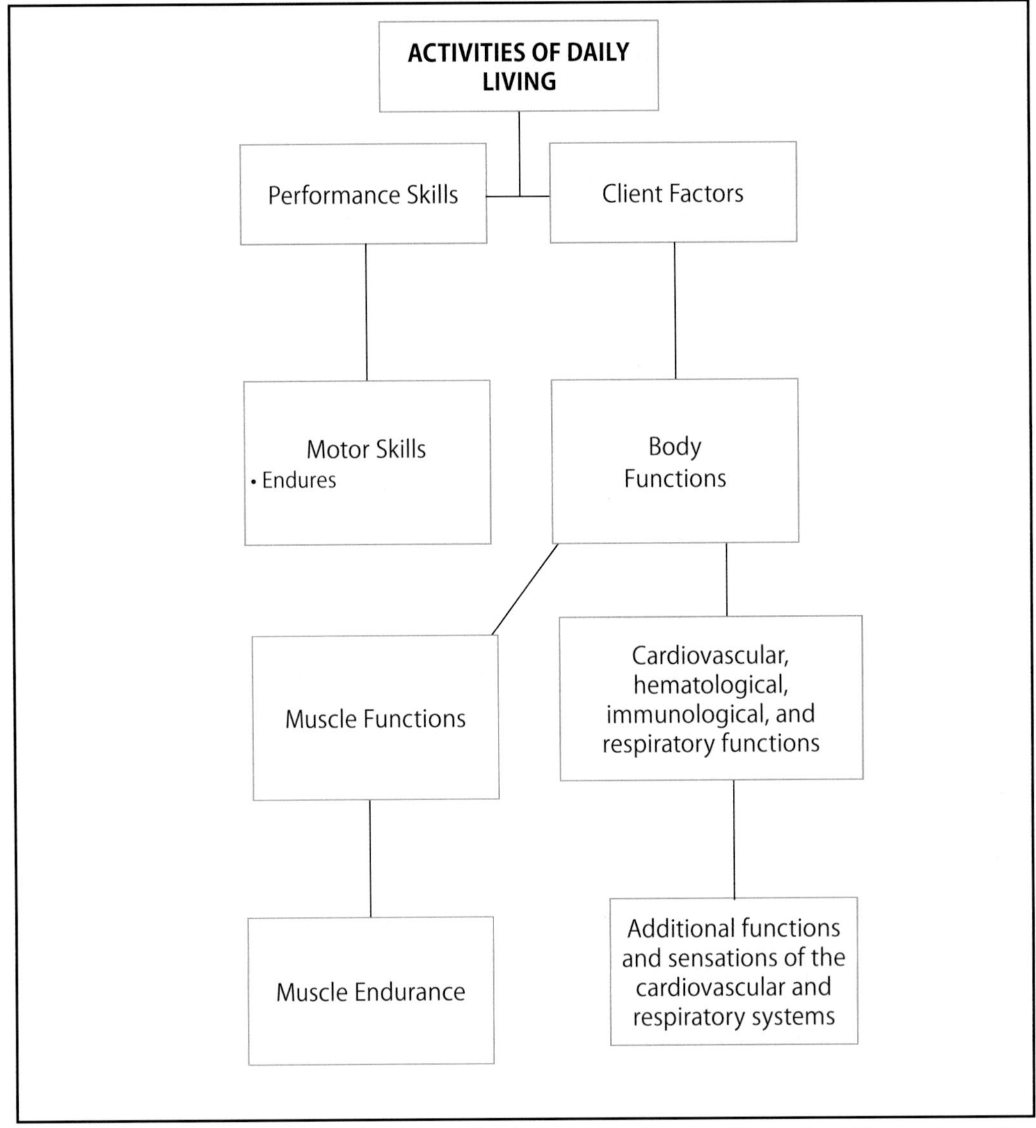

Figure 3-16. Relationship of energy/endurance to ADLs. (Adapted from American Occupational Therapy Association. (2014). Occupational therapy practice framework: Domain and process (3rd ed.). *American Journal of Occupational Therapy, 68*(Suppl. 1), S1-S48.)

Compensation/Adaptation Interventions of Self-Care for Clients With Decreased Client Factors-Body Functions: Endurance/Energy

Energy is located in the AOTA Framework (2014) under global mental functions as well as neuromusculoskeletal and movement-related functions, but the definition is the same; therefore, it will be addressed as one area (Figure 3-16).

Decreased energy or endurance can be caused by a large number of pathologies. Most obvious is when a client has cardiac or pulmonary deficits that directly impact the ability to get oxygen to the muscles. Other clients will have decreased endurance due to immobility after a hospitalization or injury. Others have slowly limited activity over a longer period of time, leading eventually to decreased endurance for activities.

The most common intervention methods used to increase endurance are two-fold. The first intervention is to build up the client's endurance by completing tasks. As stated earlier, this can be done using a bottom-up approach such as repetitive exercises with no or light weights. Examples of these include pulley exercises or arm ergometers. These interventions are considered "remedial," and more information regarding them can be found in Chapter 2. A top-down approach will utilize graded functional activities to increase endurance.

The second aspect of increasing the client's functional skills is referred to as energy conservation. This is a compensatory/adaptive strategy because the education provided to the client is aimed at teaching the client to change behaviors, thus allowing the client to be less tired. Most of these principles have a similar theme: plan activities to limit exertion. Examples of these are listed below for each self-care activity.

Changing the Task to Achieve Independence

- Bathing example: Have all supplies required for bathing in one convenient location. Also, clients can complete showers or baths on a day when little else is planned and when energy is not typically drained (e.g., the end of the day is usually more tiring).
- Grooming/hygiene example: Have all supplies required for grooming/hygiene in one convenient location. Plan trips to nail salons for the midmorning and limit other plans that day.
- Feeding example: Eat meals in a relaxed environment with sufficient time allowed. Rushing through meals increases tension and can cause fatigue. If eating at a restaurant, limit plans for the remainder of that day. If eating a regular meal is too tiring, clients may choose to eat smaller meals throughout the day.
- Dressing example: Sit, rather than stand, while dressing. Put clothes away in outfits for ease of use each morning. Arrange clothes and drawers to allow easy access to clothes most often used. Rotate this with the seasons, if necessary.
- Toileting example: Straining while on the toilet can not only be dangerous for the heart but can utilize a great deal of energy. Attempt to utilize the toilet for bowel movements when ample time is available. This will avoid significant straining in order to rush.

Changing the Tools to Achieve Independence

Many of the tools discussed previously will also assist the client with decreased endurance. It is important for the tools chosen to be lightweight so they are not contributing to fatigue. Larger equipment, such as seats, should be placed in a permanent location in order for the client to further conserve energy by not moving them.

- Bathing example: Use a shower seat to conserve energy when seated. Use a long-handled sponge to wash LEs, decreasing the need to bend/reach.
- Grooming/hygiene example: While standing at the sink, use a small foot stool to rest on one leg while applying makeup or drying hair to limit fatigue. Lightweight blow-dryers or blow-dryer stands are available that can limit fatigue.
- Feeding example: Generally, no feeding tools are required.
- Dressing example: Adaptive equipment such as long-handled shoe horns, elastic laces, sock aids, and reachers can decrease the need to bend/reach. As stated earlier, the weight of these tools should be considered. If too heavy, they may increase fatigue rather than decrease it.

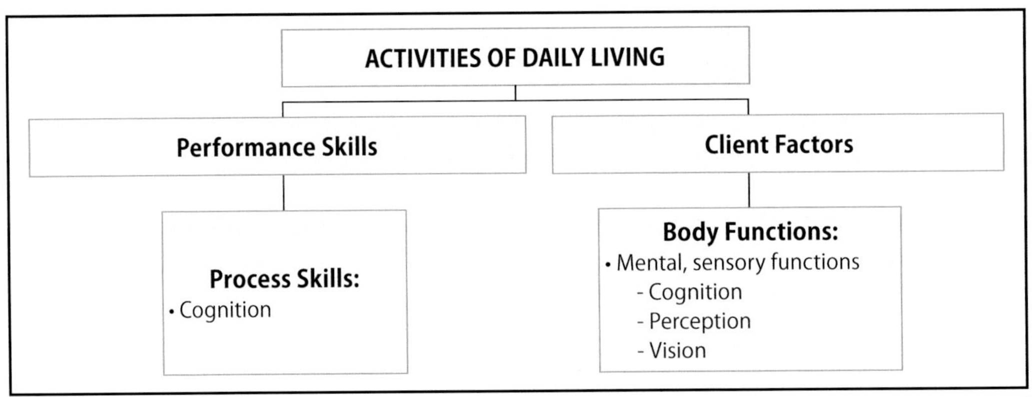

Figure 3-17. Components of performance skills/client factors related to ADLs. (Adapted from American Occupational Therapy Association. (2014). Occupational therapy practice framework: Domain and process (3rd ed.). *American Journal of Occupational Therapy, 68*(Suppl. 1), S1-S48.)

- Toileting example: Utilization of laxatives, stool softeners, or fiber products, under the supervision of a physician, can reduce straining while on the toilet.

Compensations/Adaptations of Self-Care Deficits for Clients With Cognitive, Perceptual, or Visual Limitations: Performance Skills/Client Factors

This section will focus on the impact of cognitive, perceptual, and visual deficits upon ADL performance (Figure 3-17). Many conditions may lead to these deficits, primarily those of a neurological origin. As an example, Dodge, Kadowski, Hayakawa, and Yamakawa (2005) found that cognitive impairment increases the risk of eventual decline in ADL/IADL skills with clients who have sustained a CVA. Depending on the amount of cognitive impairment, subjects who had baseline independence in ADL/IADL skills lost a significant portion of function within a short period of time, particularly in the older-adult group. AOTA has published a position statement regarding cognition and cognitive rehabilitation stating, "Cognition is integral to effective performance across the broad range of daily occupations" (2013, p. S9). In addition, a recent study regarding Parkinson's disease dementia (PDD) stated, "A detailed ADL evaluation that detects relevant impairment is thus the most important part of the [differential] diagnosis of PDD" (Liepelt-Scarfone et al., 2013, p. e82902). This statement further highlights the important link between cognition and ADLs.

In general, cuing, as described in Chapter 1, is considered to be a useful tool for remediation as well as compensation/adaptation. For this reason, it will be addressed throughout the section. It is also important to note that the functions discussed in the following section begin at the lowest skill level and are reliant upon the skill before. For example: A client must have good attention skills in order to have short-term memory, and must have short-term memory to have topographical orientation.

The AOTA Framework (2014) presents perceptual and cognitive deficits within two sections of the document. The first section, Client Factors-Body Functions, addresses basic mental functions such as cognitive and perceptual skills. The Framework (2014) defines these basic cognitive skills as necessary to complete, manage, and modify ADL tasks.

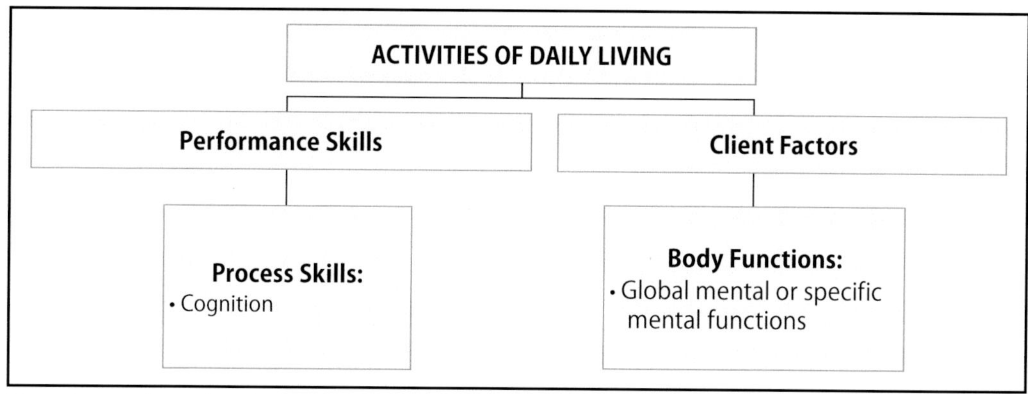

Figure 3-18. Relationship of cognition to ADLs. (Adapted from American Occupational Therapy Association. (2014). Occupational therapy practice framework: Domain and process (3rd ed.). *American Journal of Occupational Therapy, 68*(Suppl. 1), S1-S48.)

A second section of the AOTA Framework (2014) also addresses cognitive as well as perceptual deficits. The deficits are discussed under a subsection of Client Factors, Body Function Categories. These body function categories are the affective, perceptual, and additional cognitive skills required to complete ADL tasks.

Body function categories are divided into the following global mental functions and specific mental functions:

- Global mental functions: These include consciousness functions (arousal level, level of consciousness) and orientation.
- Specific mental functions: Attention, memory, perception (visual-spatial), thought functions (e.g., recognition, categorization, generalization), higher-level cognitive functions (e.g., judgment, concept formation, time management, problem solving, decision making), and mental functioning (e.g., motor planning, specifically dressing apraxia) (AOTA, 2014).

The format of this section of the text is a brief introduction to the topic and examples of compensation/adaptation interventions. Examples of appropriate activities will be listed. Some ADL examples will not be listed because these tasks may be inappropriate or not possible for a client with the deficits presented. For specific definitions, please refer to Chapter 2.

Compensation/Adaptation of Self-Care for Clients With Decreased Performance Skills/Client Factors: Cognitive Deficits

See Figure 3-18.

Performance-Process Skills

Table 3-7 briefly presents the subcategories of performance skills because these skills are typically addressed in a less formal manner within most ADL intervention plans.

Client Factors: Body Functions—Global Mental Functions

As stated earlier, global mental functions include consciousness and orientation. Consciousness is further divided into arousal level and level of consciousness (AOTA, 2014). Examples of appropriate activities will be listed below, although may not be possible to attempt ADLs with clients who have significantly decreased arousal levels.

Table 3-7

Process Skills and ADL Examples of Each

Process Skill Subcategories	Examples of ADL Compensation/Adaptation Interventions
Energy	
Paces	Provide client with a clock and chart with estimated amount of time required for each category of ADL tasks
Attends	Refer to Specific Mental Functions category
Knowledge	
Chooses	Offer two or more options and play out scenario of choices with client. For example, allow client to choose the red shirt or the white shirt to match the purple pants
Uses	Provide checklist of ADL items and brief description of what they are used for, such as a razor or step stool
Handles	Demonstrate to client use of tools or materials. Observe for carry-over at next session. For example, demonstrate how to hang pants neatly in closet
Heeds	Provide daily checklist to document each time ADL task is completed
Inquires	Provide written directions for ADL tasks. Request that client ask one or more questions regarding safety in ADLs/session
Temporal Organization	
Initiation	Use external cues during intervention such as a bell or alarm clock to begin washing/dressing, for example. Address strategies to develop internal initiation cues
Sequencing	Provide client with ADL board containing the written steps of bathing, dressing, etc
Organizing Space and Objects	
Searches/Locates	Provide external cuing such as labels or signs to assist with locating ADL objects or tools
Gathers	Provide checklist of items needed for bathing, dressing, or hygiene to assist client in gathering needed materials
Organizes	Provide client with daily reminders, lists, or calendars. Assist client in organizing closet, drawers, and shelves, as needed
Restores	Label shelves, drawers, and closets to assist in putting items away
Navigates	Use contrasting colors in physical contexts. Instruct client to use tactile cuing when navigating in bathroom and bedroom environments
Adaptation	
Notices/Responds	Grade environmental, nonverbal, or perceptual cues in bathroom and bedroom, as appropriate
Accommodates/Adjusts	Problem-solve alternative actions or scenarios with client. For example, client should attempt toileting skills in bathrooms with different layouts
Benefits	Assist client/family in problem-solving various ADL issues that may occur upon discharge home and plan for adaptations

Consciousness or Arousal Level

Zoltan (2007) describes arousal level as "alerting" or a level of alertness that fluctuates depending on the state of one's CNS and prepares for mobilization to attention.

The occupational therapy intervention at this level is very limited in terms of functional performance. Initially, the client's level of alertness may be very limited, not allowing for even the simplest of ADL training. Of particular concern with a low arousal level is the task of eating. This task will be addressed in the eating/dysphagia section later in this chapter.

Changing the Task to Achieve Independence

The client's level of arousal or ability to participate in the task will dictate the need or readiness to change the method. The therapist may need to see the client for several short sessions per day. Depending on the client's response, the physical context may need to be changed. For example, a less distractible environment may allow the client to better attend, or more likely a moderate amount of sensory stimulation such as noise/sound may improve the client's level of alertness (e.g., upbeat music).

The client may benefit from simple verbal instructions and potentially tactile cuing. Instructions and verbal communication may be upgraded as the client's level of alertness increases.

- Bathing and hygiene example: As levels of alertness increase and the client is able to sit upright in bed, the therapist may begin addressing simple ADL skills, which are continuously graded, as necessary. The basic intervention may involve asking the client to brush hair, brush teeth, or wash face and/or hands. In addition, as levels of alertness and attention improve, the therapist may encourage the client to begin using ADL strategies to improve memory. (Refer to the memory section of this chapter for further details on memory.)
- Feeding example: Prior to feeding, arousal levels can be improved by providing a stimulating environment (bright and colorful) and positioning the client upright. (Refer to the positioning section of this chapter if adaptations are required to achieve an upright posture.) The texture and temperature of the food may also alert the client. For example, cold foods may increase alertness. Finger foods may also increase alertness.
- Dressing example: Dressing may not be appropriate until the level of alertness improves to the point that the client can interact. The client may be able to participate in a simple task such as putting on a "johnny coat."
- Toileting example: Depending on the level of alertness, attempting to toilet out of the bed may keep the client more alert to complete the task. If toileting in bed, a task such as bridging may cause the client to become more alert. (Refer to the functional mobility section of this chapter for more information on bridging.)

Changing the Tools to Achieve Independence

Any tools used with clients who have a decreased level of alertness should be kept very simple with items added gradually, as the client tolerates. One tool should be introduced at a time, while ensuring safety.

- Bathing example: Begin with a familiar tool such as a washcloth that may be a very bright, alerting color and texture. Use the warm water and touch of the washcloth as an alerting tool.
- Hygiene example: Adapt oral care by assisting the client to cleanse his or her mouth with a disposable oral swab. This adaptation is important because the client's level of alertness and/or oral motor status may not be ready for the amount of liquid created with using toothpaste. As levels of alertness improve, the activity may be graded to using a toothbrush and toothpaste.

- Feeding example: Brightly colored plates or placemats under the food may increase alertness. Providing foods of particular interest to a client, such as a favorite food, may also be alerting.

Orientation

Orientation is an individual's awareness of time, person, and/or place. Deficits in orientation may typically present with memory loss and problems with new learning. Because the strategies for improving orientation must be reinforced with all skills throughout the day by the entire rehabilitation team and family, the interventions below are presented in general terms. In addition, much of orientation interventions are centered on visual/verbal cuing and consistency.

Changing the Task to Achieve Independence

- General ADL examples: The session may informally involve orientation training as well. It is important to remember that carry-over with orientation is very much dependent on memory skills. The client's daily patterns, such as routines, should be consistent and structured as much as possible, particularly as arousal levels improve. The client's physical context should be consistent, well-organized, and if possible simulate the client's natural environment for self-care tasks. For example, if feeding can occur in a small dining room rather than in the client's room, the client will be better oriented to mealtime.

The therapist may see the client either during or after breakfast, providing verbal orientation to the time of day as related to the ADL task. The method may be changed by asking the client basic orientation questions during the ADL task. This should occur throughout the day with the assistance of staff and family.

Changing the Tools to Achieve Independence

- General ADL examples: Basic orientation tools may begin with only a simple calendar or sign of the day and date. As the level of arousal improves, the method may be changed by introducing additional orientation boards. The boards may incorporate ADL information such as mealtimes and bathing, dressing, and therapy schedules.

As the client's participation in therapy improves, familiar ADL items should be brought from home such as clothes, grooming items, and a watch.

Client Factors: Body Functions—Specific Mental Functions and Global Mental Functions

Specific mental functions include attention, memory, perception, thought functions, and mental functions of sequencing complex movement, emotions, self, and time. Global mental functions include consciousness, orientation, temperament and personality, energy and drive, and sleep (AOTA, 2014).

Attention

Zoltan (2007) discusses the impact of attention deficits on the client's ability to learn and focus on ADL skills. Attention is a building block for higher-level specific mental functions such as memory and problem solving and therefore must be addressed first.

Changing the Task to Achieve Independence

Clients who have conditions that affect attention skills must begin ADL training with the simplest of tasks, in a short intervention time that is adapted with improvement. It is important for caregivers to speak simply and slowly and allow for processing time (Zoltan, 2007). In addition, distraction should be kept at a minimum, although gradually introduced as the client is ready. The physical context should remain the same until the client demonstrates he or she is ready for generalization and/or gradation.

- Bathing and hygiene example: Intervention may begin at the bedside and progress to the bathroom sink by encouraging the client to brush hair, brush teeth, or wash face. ADL intervention may be adapted by asking the client to wash the upper half of the body and progressing in the next session to the entire body, as able. The task may be further adapted by progressing to the shower. The environment should be without distractions at first, with appropriate distractions added as the client improves.
- Feeding example: Prior to attempting feeding, the environmental distractions should be eliminated. Food items of particular interest to the client or with varied textures and colors can also increase attention to feeding. In order to decrease distractions, smaller meals should be presented to the client. Verbal or visual cuing to stay on task may be required but should be graded.
- Dressing example: Provide only the required clothes with each step and gradually provide more clothing. The environment should be without distractions at first, with appropriate distractions added as the client improves. Backward chaining where the occupational therapist initiates the task and asks the client to complete it or forward chaining where the client is required to complete only a small portion of a task and then the occupational therapist finishes the task may be attempted. Chaining should be graded as improvement is noted.
- Toileting example: With a compensation/adaptive approach, Zoltan (2007) recommends that the client vocalize the task in a step-by-step manner. For toileting, the client should vocalize each step of what to do from the time he or she experiences the urge to void to entering the bathroom, attending to perianal care, attending to clothing, and finally washing hands at the sink.

Changing the Tools to Achieve Independence

In general, for all ADLs, the environment should be without distractions at first, with appropriate distractions added as the client improves. Tools utilized for the ADLs should be limited until the client has demonstrated improvement. Additional examples are provided for feeding and dressing regarding tools.

- Feeding example: To decrease distractions, limited utensils should be provided. Colorful plates may increase attention but can also be distracting depending on the individual client.
- Dressing example: If a client is having difficulty donning pants, socks, and shoes, a step stool in front of the bedside chair may assist the client in reaching his or her feet with all three tasks. Additional tools may be added as appropriate and as the client's attention improves.

Memory

Although there are many types of memory and memory deficits, this section will focus on intervention strategies related to ADLs with an adaptive/compensation approach.

Changing the Task to Achieve Independence

Intervention strategies during ADLs, in general, may be adapted by providing the client with an ADL schedule. For individuals who have limited carry-over, involve him or her in developing the schedule. The same strategy may be implemented for creating lists of items needed for bathing, dressing, hygiene, and toileting, as well as basic instructions for carrying out ADLs.

Chunking and grouping (Zoltan, 2007) is a method used to organize categories, objects, and function of items to be recalled. These methods can be utilized in general for all ADLs. The client is asked to group like items together (all items for brushing teeth) and repeat the steps verbally to increase retention of information. Additional specific examples are provided for feeding and dressing.

- Feeding example: Regularly scheduled meals with consistent routines will benefit memory skills.
- Dressing example: This "story method" (Zoltan, 2007. p. 223) is a strategy whereby a client is encouraged to create a story about what is to be recalled. The client will create a story regarding the steps involved, items needed, and physical context involved with getting dressed.

Changing the Tools to Achieve Independence

For all ADLs, cuing tools may be used as a strategy to increase memory through the use of alarm clocks or timers, memory notebooks, or labeling of ADL items and storage areas. The clocks and timers are utilized to remind the clients of a task or a portion of a task that requires completion. These are often used for IADLs such as cooking and medications but can also be utilized for tasks such as toileting and bathing. A memory notebook will provide visual cues for completion of tasks. Another type of memory notebook, suggested by Zoltan (2007), is the utilization of audiotapes that provide step-by-step instructions for tasks. Visual cues can be used to label items as to their use or label storage for easy retrieval of items.

In addition, when memory is impacted, some cuing may be required to increase compliance. One study found that using videotapes of family members asking the client to complete a task increased compliance (O'Connor, Smith, Nott, Lorang, & Mathews, 2011).

The specific mental functions, which are addressed less formally and/or less frequently, within intervention plans, are presented in Table 3-8.

Compensation/Adaptation Interventions of Self-Care for Clients With Decreased Performance Skills/Client Factors: Perceptual Deficits

As depicted in Figure 3-19, the Framework (2014) addresses perceptual functions under client factors, but particular perceptual topics are not listed. The topics chosen for discussion below have been determined from the authors' clinical practice as well as current references that will be discussed throughout.

General compensatory or adaptive strategies that apply to clients diagnosed with perceptual deficits center around safety and environmental context. These general strategies include:

- Maximize safety in all situations by removing unsafe objects as necessary.
- Educate client and all caregivers regarding functional limitations.
- Practice in a variety of physical contexts.

Visual Fixation/Scanning

Visual fixation involves the voluntary ability to sustain gaze while visually attending to a task or an object in the environment. Scanning allows the eye to follow an object without simultaneous head movement. While saccadic eye movement is typically symmetrical (e.g., reading), scanning during functional activities involves less predictable patterns that are more complicated (Zoltan, 2007).

Table 3-8

Specific Mental Functions and Examples of ADL Compensation/Adaptation Strategies

Specific Mental Function Subcategories	Compensation/Adaptation Intervention Strategies
Thought Functions	
Recognition	During ADL session, ask client to identify typical ADL items, familiar individuals, or objects in the room. Label drawers and shelves
Categorization	Educate client/family regarding organizing ADL items into categories such as shirts on one side of closet and pants on another or bathing items on one shelf of the bathroom and grooming on another
Generalization	Address ADLs in a variety of possible situations, such as bathing at the sink and shower, and dressing in the bathroom and bedroom
Higher-Level Cognitive Functions	
Judgment	Teach client to ask for help when unsure of safety. Ask client open-ended questions in order to think out loud before acting
Concept formation	Have client keep an ADL journal or log with daily schedule, progress, goals, and achievements
Time management	Provide ADL schedule. Use clock or timer, as needed
Problem solving	Alter environment to improve skills such as with external cues and written instructions. Explore possible strategies with client
Decision making	Provide client with two or more options for safe and appropriate decision making, before acting. Allow client to think out loud

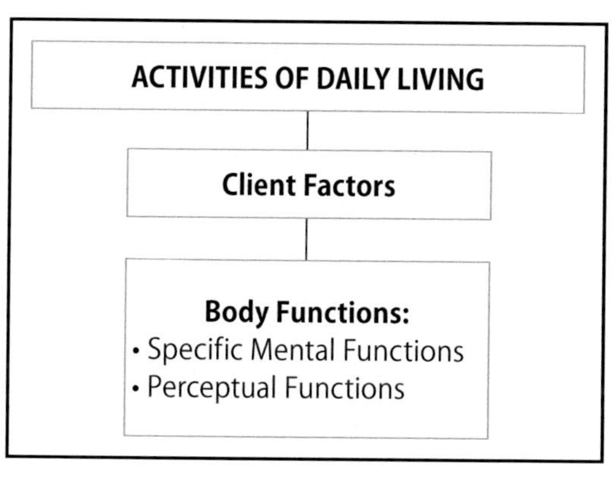

Figure 3-19. Relationship of perception to ADLs. (Adapted from American Occupational Therapy Association. (2014). Occupational therapy practice framework: Domain and process (3rd ed.). *American Journal of Occupational Therapy, 68*(Suppl. 1), S1-S48.)

Changing the Task to Achieve Independence

Provide cuing as needed. Cuing can be verbal or tactile when guiding the client to anchor the initiation of scanning (from left to right) and when controlling the speed of scanning.

- Bathing example: The client should place his or her hands to the left/right of the labels on bottles to anchor reading. Bathing items should be routinely placed in certain locations to limit the scanning required to find needed items.

- Grooming/hygiene example: The client may experience difficulty in finding the toothbrush on the right side of the sink. The therapist may cue or anchor the client to the middle of the visual field at the water spout. The therapist may then verbally cue the client to scan to the right of the spout. If verbal cuing is unsuccessful, the therapist may use tactile cuing by having the client touch the spout with the right hand and scan his or her eyes to the right, as the hand moves toward the toothbrush.
- Feeding example: Cuing may be required at first to find all items on the plate or table.
- Dressing example: When retrieving clothes from the closet, the client may be cued to anchor using touch as well as vision. Anchoring would begin on the left side of the closet with the client gradually scanning to the right. With this method, the client would then retrieve all clothing needed, including cuing to scan toward the floor for his or her shoes.
- Toileting example: Cuing may be required at first in order to scan to find sanitary products or toilet paper.

Changing the Tools to Achieve Independence

- Bathing example: Brighten tools in shower/tub in order to increase ability to fixate on the object.
- Grooming/hygiene example: Brighten tools placed in a predictable pattern at the sink, tray table, or bureau.
- Feeding example: Brighten placemats or sides of tray table.
- Toileting example: A brightly-colored sticker may be placed to the left of the toilet tissue holder, in order for the client to anchor upon it and scan to the right in order to locate the paper.

Visual Inattention/Visual Neglect

The impact of unilateral neglect on ADLs is significant. In reviewing various intervention approaches to unilateral neglect, Lin states, "unilateral neglect has been associated with poor recovery in everyday life functioning," and one conclusion of this research was that retraining to improve daily skills should include functional tasks (Lin, 1996). In addition, awareness of the inattention may play a role. Tham, Ginsburg, Fisher, and Tegner (2001) found that clients who were educated regarding the disability and became more aware of the disability demonstrated greater improvement in ADL skills even when specific ADL intervention was not provided.

For those clients who are unable to become aware of the inattention, the therapist will need to modify and simplify the physical context as much as possible. Gradual grading of activities will also be required. For example, begin by providing all objects within the client's intact visual field and incorporate visual scanning through head as well as eye movements during functional activities.

It should also be noted that analysis of the literature has found limited evidence to support intervention for neglect. These analyses appear to review remedial interventions, which would lead therapists to rely on adaptations/compensations as discussed here (Bowen & Lincoln, 2007; Kerkhoffa & Schenkb, 2012). A recent review completed for the Cochrane database concluded cognitive remediation interventions were not sufficiently proven to be effective for neglect (Bowen, Hazelton, Pollock, & Lincoln, 2013). This is further evidence that intervention completed in the context of function may have better results than traditional cognitive interventions.

Changing the Task to Achieve Independence

In general for all ADLs, placing the items required for the task within the available visual field will increase performance. As stated above, cuing the client to compensate by turning the head

Table 3-9

Body Scheme Disorders and Examples of ADL Compensation/Adaptation Strategies

Body Scheme Disorder	Compensation/Adaptation Strategies: Task and/or Tools Changed
Autotopagnosia	During ADLs use verbal cues to increase awareness of body parts with a functional approach. For example: Ask client to pick up the part of the body that goes inside the shoe (Zoltan, 1996)
Finger agnosia	Adapt ADL environment to increase safety and finger dexterity
Unilateral body neglect	Adapt ADLs by using reminders or daily activity list to complete entire task(s) to compensate for neglect
Right–left discrimination	Provide adaptations to instructions during ADL instruction. For example, when dressing, provide tactile cuing to locate items, or state that the "shirt is next to the pants"

along with moving the eyes may also increase performance. Additional examples are provided below for hygiene and dressing.

- Hygiene example: While brushing hair, if client neglects affected side of the head, guide his or her hand to that side and verbally cue to attend.
- Dressing example: Use tactile and/or verbal cuing to encourage awareness of affected side.

For example, as the client is donning a shirt, touch the client's affected UE while verbally cuing to attend to that side.

Changing the Tools to Achieve Independence

- Bathing example: Avoid a handheld shower to ensure the water washes over the entire body.
- Grooming/hygiene and dressing example: Utilize a mirror during tasks to encourage visualization of the entire body/face.
- Feeding example: Provide client with an adapted dish that has two to three dividers. Instruct client to turn dish clockwise into intact visual field each time a divider is emptied.
- Toileting example: Position toilet tissue within client's field of vision. After toileting, position client in front of bathroom mirror in order to fully hike pants and tuck in both sides of shirt.

Body Scheme

Body scheme is a foundation skill that uses sensory or internal awareness of the body and the spatial relationship of the body parts to one another (Jacobs & Simon, 2015; Zoltan, 2007). Because there are multiple forms of body scheme disorders, each one cannot be reviewed individually. For this reason, Table 3-9 identifies the most common forms of body scheme disorders as well as examples of compensatory or adaptive interventions for these.

Visual Discrimination

Visual discrimination involves the ability to distinguish between various objects or forms in relation to the environment (Zoltan, 2007). Because there are multiple forms of visual discrimination disorders, each one cannot be reviewed individually. For this reason, Table 3-10 identifies the

Table 3-10

Visual Discrimination and Examples of ADL Compensation/Adaptation Strategies

Visual Discrimination Disorder	Compensation/Adaptation Strategies: Task and/or Tools Changed
Form discrimination	Adapt environment by placing all hygiene items upright. Label item and store items in habitual pattern
Depth perception	Teach client to compensate by using other sensory skills such as tactile. For example, client should use touch to locate the toothbrush when reaching for it
Figure ground perception	Adapt ADL environment to increase cognitive awareness by carefully organizing items in a non-cluttered area. For example, put only a few items on shelf in bathroom
Spatial relations	Label all ADL storage areas and replace items to consistent areas
Topographical orientation	Adapt ADL environment through the use of simple pictures. For example, hang a picture of a dress on the clothes closet

most common forms of visual discrimination disorders as well as examples of compensatory or adaptive interventions for these.

Motor Planning

Motor planning involves the individual's ability to organize and perform movements in order to carry out purposeful activity (Jacobs & Simon, 2015). Apraxia is a category of motor planning deficits whereby impairments of purposeful movement or skills do not involve coordination, sensory deficits, visual/perceptual issues, language deficits, or cognitive deficits alone (Jacobs & Simon, 2015).

Dressing apraxia is a specific motor planning deficit related to perceptual and cognitive skills. Zoltan (2007) describes dressing apraxia as a disorder in body scheme or spatial relations rather than a motor or physical dysfunction. Clients demonstrate difficulty in proper orientation of clothing. For example, a client may put an arm in a pant leg, a sock on a hand, or a shirt on upside down. While dressing apraxia is a common motor planning deficit, other self-care examples are also provided below.

Changing the Task to Achieve Independence

- Bathing, hygiene and toileting example: Provide brief, one-step verbal cues or directions, such as, "Wash your face."
- Feeding example: Finger foods or foods easily placed on utensils (soup versus mashed potatoes) may decrease motor planning difficulties.
- Dressing example: The therapist should attempt the dressing task in several ways in order to assure success. First, various setups should be tried, such as dressing at the edge of the bed, in front of a mirror, or in a bedside chair. The therapist should consider presenting one piece of clothing to the client at a time or lay out all items at once.

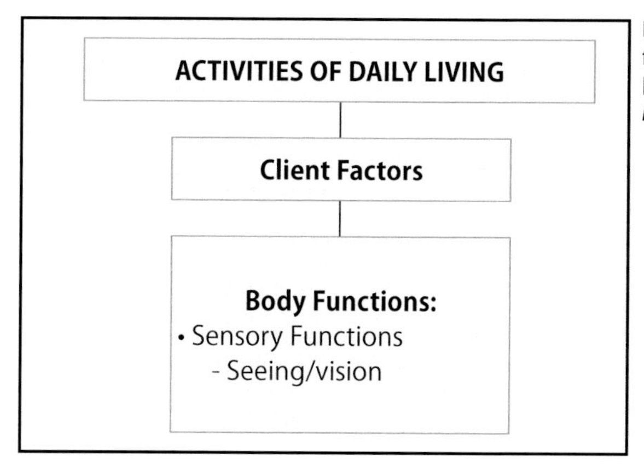

Figure 3-20. Relationship of vision to ADLs. (Adapted from American Occupational Therapy Association. [2002a]. *Occupational therapy practice framework: Domain and process.* Bethesda, MD: AOTA.)

Changing the Tools to Achieve Independence

In general for all ADLs, limit the use of tools because these may increase motor planning deficits. If tools are required, introduce them one at a time. For dressing, tools may include adaptation of clothing as described below.

- Dressing example: Adaptations may be made to the client's clothing such as labeling or color-coding the inside, top, right, or left. Buttoning a shirt may also be a very difficult task for a client with dressing apraxia. Strategies for success include having the client use tactile and visual input, as well as color-coding the button with the buttonhole. Instructions to button from the bottom up or top down may also work for a client with this deficit. Typically, the use of adaptive equipment may further confuse a client with dressing apraxia, particularly if ideational apraxia, which affects the ability to use tools, is also present.

Compensation/Adaptation Interventions of Self-Care for Clients With Decreased Performance Skills/Client Factors: Vision

See Figure 3-20.

Low Vision

When addressing low vision (visual acuity) with a compensation/adaptive approach, the focus is primarily on changing the task within the client's environment or physical contexts. Typically, individuals with low vision are able to independently perform basic ADL skills with or without simple task modifications. Higher-level ADL skills that involve safety issues (distinguishing hot from cold or identifying sharp objects) or require vision (such as reading directions) are usually a challenge.

There are many general issues to consider before providing ADL intervention with clients who have low vision. While specific examples will be described for each self-care task, the general strategies listed here should be utilized in conjunction with the specifics listed later in this section.

- Ensure client's glasses are available and fitted correctly.
- Provide any directions in simple, large print.
- Decrease clutter in environment.
- Use automatic, motion-controlled lighting.

- Control the amount of natural light in environment in order to decrease glare.
- Use Braille labels as appropriate.
- Use assistive technology, as described in Chapter 5, which provides auditory or tactile feedback.
- Use contrast whenever possible.
- Organize belongings in a systematic, predictable routine in order to locate easily on a daily basis.
- To prevent slippage, remove bath mat when not in use.
- Install grab bars in tub/shower.

Changing the Task to Achieve Independence

- Bathing example: Organize items within reach, in a systematic location. For example: always place similar-looking shampoo and conditioner in designated locations to avoid confusion.
- Grooming/hygiene example: Organize items within reach, in a systematic location. For example, always place sharp razors in the same location to avoid cuts. Use fingers as a guide when applying makeup and purchase makeup that has been chosen in the past or have a friend evaluate a new color.
- Feeding example: Place food items in a consistent location, using a system such as the clock method. For example, place the juice at 12 o'clock and the coffee at 3 o'clock.
- Dressing example: Do not place light clothes upon white bed sheets or blankets. When dressing, encourage client to use a systematic approach to organizing clothes by colors, styles, and appropriate weather (Cohen, 2001).
- Toileting example: If items are similar in shape or size, always place them in particular locations so they do not get mixed up (e.g., tampons that are "plus size" versus "slim").

Changing the Tools to Achieve Independence

- Bathing example: When bathing, provide soap that is a different color than the sink and a bath mat, towel, slippers, and robe that are brightly colored.
- Grooming/hygiene example: Increase contrast using bright labels and large print. Braille can also be put on items if the client is taught how to use this. Another alternative is to place distinct textures on certain items that look similar, such as deodorant and hairspray. Use a magnifying mirror for makeup and shaving.
- Feeding example: Use brightly colored placemats, contrasting the color of the dining table and the tableware. If food items appear similar in color, place them on different color plates to distinguish.
- Dressing example: During dressing activities, encourage use of touch and texture to identify matching clothing (Cohen, 2001). Provide bright, solid-colored clothes, as able.
- Toileting example: Color-code baskets with bright colors to distinguish different feminine hygiene products (e.g., panty shield versus maxi-pads) and other similar-looking products.

Visual Fields

Visual fields are the areas of vision that are seen without movement of the eyes or head (Jacob & Simon, 2015). Deficits may present on one side of the visual field in one or both eyes.

Changing the Task to Achieve Independence

- Bathing example: Provide client and caregivers with strategies for cuing into affected visual fields in order to locate all bathing supplies in the shower or tub. Place items in reach within intact visual field.
- Grooming/hygiene example: Provide client and caregivers with strategies for cuing into affected visual fields in order to locate all grooming and hygiene supplies. Place items in reach within intact visual field, particularly any items that can be sharp, such as a razor or tweezers.
- Feeding example: Provide client and caregivers with strategies for cuing into affected visual fields in order to locate all food and drink on the table. Seat client where items may be in reach of intact visual field.
- Dressing example: Provide client and caregivers with strategies for cuing into affected visual fields in order to locate all clothes in the closet or drawers. If clothes are picked out for a client, place items in reach within intact visual field.

Changing the Tools to Achieve Independence

For all self-care tasks, most adaptive equipment or tools will not provide assistance. Reminder cards can be placed within the client's visual field to remind the client to scan for other self-care items. Depending on the task, a large red strip can be placed on the affected side of the self-care tools and the client can be trained to scan until the strip is visualized. This will allow the client to view all items. In general, changing the task, as described above, will provide better compensation and adaptation by the client.

Maintenance of Self-Care Skills

For clients who are not suited for remediation and have plateaued with adaptation and compensation attempts—either due to prognosis, diagnosis, or their personal choices—maintenance will be the ultimate approach. For clients who are able to participate in remedial interventions, there will be a period of time when remediation is still being attempted and it is unclear when maintenance begins. It is difficult to determine when adaptation and compensation become maintenance; however, once it is determined that a change in task or a change in tool is to be utilized long term, maintenance has certainly begun. Maintenance is more likely to occur for clients with chronic illnesses such as arthritis or degenerative illnesses such as Parkinson's disease. A particular symptom of any disease may become chronic, such as pain, causing maintenance to be appropriate.

It is important to note that the maintenance approach can still be a reimbursable service. While this is not the focus of this book, coverage is typically available for maintenance as long as skilled services are still required. Many clients, however, will not require skilled occupational therapy services once the above strategies are taught or the tools are mastered. If a diagnosis is progressive in nature, further evaluation of these strategies and tools may be required to maximize function throughout the progression of the disease.

Functional Mobility

This section will focus on the impact of functional mobility upon ADLs. The Occupational Therapy Framework (AOTA, 2014) categorizes functional mobility as a subsection of ADLs, which is an area of occupation. The Framework defines functional mobility as "moving from one position or place to another (during the performance of everyday activities) such as in-bed mobility, wheelchair mobility, and transfers" (AOTA, 2014, p. S19). Transfers include surfaces such as bed, bedside chair, wheelchair, toilet, tub/shower, floor, and car. In addition, functional mobility includes ambulation related to functional activities and transporting items. Fairchild (2013) discusses trunk control, positioning, and bed mobility as components of functional mobility. These functional mobility categories must be addressed in a hierarchical nature (Radomski & Latham, 2014). For example, adequate trunk stability and control must be achieved before trunk mobility. Furthermore, bed mobility should be addressed before chair transfers, and toilet transfers before tub transfers. More specifically, Fairchild (2013) discusses how in order to achieve independence in functional mobility skills, important positioning/bed mobility activities are required, which include moving upward/downward, side to side, rolling, turning over, and from supine to sitting. These activities typically preclude attempts at actual transfers. In addition, functional mobility should be addressed in as many environmental contexts as possible in order to assure generalization and transfer of learning.

Necessary equipment for possible independence and safety in functional mobility will also be addressed. Functional mobility equipment generally includes devices for positioning, bed mobility, transfers, wheelchair mobility, ambulation, and overall safety.

Because mobility training is a top-down approach, it is discussed in this chapter. In addition, within the topic of mobility, it is important to note that the remedial and compensatory approaches to intervention often blend. Refer to Chapter 2 for a discussion of mobility issues as related to ROM, strength, coordination, etc.

Remediation techniques for functional mobility include daily practice of skills through repetition, chaining (forward and backward), cuing, and incorporating preparatory methods into intervention sessions (refer to Chapter 1). There are several foundational skills necessary for progression to independent transfers and functional mobility. These skills include sufficient joint ROM and flexibility, adequate muscle strength, endurance to tolerate the activity, and adequate visual-perceptual and cognitive skills for safety. Specifically, sufficient UE strength is required for most transfers and functional mobility using an assistive device. A remediation example is as follows: Prior to transferring out of bed, the occupational therapist may supervise the client in an exercise program at bed level, which includes ROM, Thera-Band (Hygenic Corp), and/or the use of handheld weights to increase UE strength. Next, the therapist may practice previously learned techniques such as rolling, supine-to-sit, and sit-to-stand at the edge of the bed using above remediation techniques, as applicable.

Compensation/Adaptation of Functional Mobility Deficits for Clients With Physical Limitations

When addressing functional mobility issues during ADL tasks, several performance skills and client factors must be considered (see Figure 3-2). These have been previously defined in Chapters 1 and 2 and will follow the same format as discussed previously.

Performance Skills: Motor Skills

Motor and praxis skills during functional activities involve moving and interacting with the environment, tasks, and objects (AOTA, 2014). These skills include bending and reaching, positioning, pacing, coordinating, maintaining balance, posture, and manipulating mobility, which are defined as follows:

- Positioning involves putting self in an appropriate distance in order to complete the task successfully.
- Pacing involves the tempo of movements to complete a task.

Table 3-11

Activity Demands and Examples of Impact on Functional Mobility

Activity Demands According to AOTA Framework (2002a)	Examples Related to Functional Mobility
Objects	Assistive devices such as a wheelchair, walker, or cane.
Space demands (relates to physical context)	Space available to maneuver assistive devices.
Social demands	Expectations of the individual to perform functional mobility independently.
Sequence and timing	Steps and proper sequencing required to complete functional mobility with or without an assistive device.
Required actions	Foundational skills required to complete functional mobility.
Body functions and structure	ROM and anatomical parts (hands/legs) required for functional mobility skills.

- Coordinating involves using body parts to interact with BADL objects in order to complete a functional performance activity. Coordination includes manipulation and the flow of movement to complete activity.
- Manipulating involves using objects to complete a task.

Performance Patterns Related to Functional Mobility

When establishing an intervention plan, it is essential to determine the client's habits and routines regarding functional mobility. For example, a client may have habitually transferred out of bed on the same side for many years. After sustaining a CVA, the client may because of hemiplegia need to get out of bed on the opposite side, particularly for safety reasons. Therefore, while being sensitive to previous habits, the therapist must educate the client and family on the need to create a new habit.

A client's role(s) within the family may also be impacted by changes in functional mobility. A client who is now wheelchair-bound may not be able to partake in a habitual family hike or take the family pet out every morning. It is the occupational therapist's job to work with the client and family to compensate or adapt the previous roles to the new disability.

Activity Demands of Functional Mobility

The activity demands of functional mobility include the required tools, space, time, foundational skills, and social skills to complete applicable tasks (AOTA, 2014). Similar to performance patterns, aspects of activity demands are also related to the client's context. Table 3-11 provides examples of activity demands and functional mobility.

Table 3-12

Levels of Assistance

Dependent transfer	Client is unable to participate in transfer
Maximum-assist transfer	Client performs 25% of transfer
Moderate-assist transfer	Client performs 50% of transfer
Minimum-assist transfer	Client performs 75% of transfer
Contact guard transfer	Client requires hands-on for guidance or possible loss of balance
Supervision transfer	Client does not require physical assist, although may need verbal cues for safety/performance
Distant supervision transfer	Client is approaching independence, although may need occasional reminders
Independent transfer (with or without an assistive device)	No assistance, cuing, or reminders needed for safety or performance

Client Factors: Body Functions—Neuromusculoskeletal and Movement-Related Functions

- Functions of joints and bones including mobility and stability of joint and bone functions (e.g., PROM, postural alignment, and joint mobility)
- Muscle power (strength), tone, and endurance
- Motor reflexes, involuntary movement reactions/functions, motor control, and gait pattern functions

There are many specific types of transfers that will be addressed in detail later in this section. Transfers are further designated by the level of assistance required. These levels are described in Table 3-12. Depending on the physical abilities of the client, mental status, and safety abilities, an additional therapist or health care professional may be needed during transfers, at least initially. The therapist should always ask for assistance before beginning the transfer if the need for a second individual is possible.

It is very important to accurately assess the client according to these levels in order to accurately document baseline status and client progress. Accurate documentation of functional transfers/mobility is also vital for similar communication between health care professionals. Specific documentation includes the cross-discipline knowledge of transfer levels of assistance as depicted in Table 3-12. In addition, caregivers may also be provided with accurate training and education regarding the client's status.

Precautions and General Information for Functional Mobility

There are many precautions that must be considered and anticipated during all levels of assistance and types of transfers. General transfer precautions and safety techniques are listed in Table 3-13. The client's safety during transfers is a primary concern, and the therapist is ultimately responsible for safe transfers. The therapist must have a baseline assessment of the client's mental and physical status in order to predetermine the type of transfer to attempt as well as the potential level of assistance needed.

Table 3-13
General Transfer Precautions and Safety Techniques

1. Client should wear proper shoes. If shoes are not available, then slipper socks should be worn
2. Assess client's perceptual and cognitive status prior to performing transfers
3. Assess client's physical capabilities prior to performing transfers
4. Ensure all lines attached to client are protected
5. Stabilize or lock all surfaces
6. Adjust surfaces for safety and ease of transfer
7. All unneeded equipment and furniture should not obstruct the transfer
8. Preplan the steps and setup of the transfer (selection and position of equipment)
9. Use a safety/transfer belt
10. Anticipate possible safety issues that may occur
11. Position the client properly before beginning the transfer
12. Instruct client regarding safety issues and steps of the transfer and demonstrate, as able
13. Be knowledgeable of and use good body mechanics at all times. Instruct caregivers as well
14. Know your own limitations and ask for assistance, preferably before the transfer, if needed
15. Instruct client not to hold onto the therapist when transferring. Do not grasp client's upper extremities during transfers
16. Do not leave the client alone after transferring, particularly on an unfamiliar or less stable surface, such as a tub bench
17. After the transfer is completed, ensure proper positioning and safety (e.g., lock wheelchair brakes, return side rails of bed)
18. Be aware of any special conditions which may be exacerbated during the transfer, such as a shoulder subluxation or total hip replacement

Prior to the transfer, the therapist must determine the best position for him or herself and the client in order to prevent injury. It is typically safest for the therapist to be in front of and slightly to one side of the client (often the weaker side).

General Transfer Tools

Table 3-14 lists many tools that may be used for transfers from any surface, including bed level, standing, toileting, and showering during functional mobility. The tools will be referred to during the remainder of this section.

Compensation/Adaptation for Trunk Control

Trunk Control: Stability Before Mobility

Conditions that affect the client's central nervous system, such as stroke and spinal cord injuries, may impair trunk control. Individuals will not be able to engage in tasks that involve trunk mobility until adequate trunk control and strength have been achieved. Decreased trunk control will impact many areas of function including functional mobility, safe eating, independence in

Table 3-14

Functional Mobility Tools

Slide board	Made of wood or plastic, this device is placed under the client's buttocks to act as a bridge when transferring between one surface and another. This is typically used with clients who have paraplegia, amputation(s), severe LE weakness, or are unable to weight-bear
Bed rails	May be permanently part of a hospital bed or portable to fit most typical bed mattresses
Tub/toilet rails	Rails may be portable or installed permanently in the tub. Toilet rails are typically permanent. Placement is important for accessibility
Commode	A seat with a cut-out opening that holds a bucket. Used for toileting when necessary at the bedside or when the bathroom is inaccessible
Walker basket	Typically a lightweight metal or plastic device that attaches to the front of the walker in order to transport small items safely
Leg-lifter	A soft device with a large loop on one end in which the client places the foot or thigh of the affected LE. A loop on the opposite end is held in order for the UEs to move the limb in bed or to the edge of the bed
Trapeze	A triangular metal device secured on a frame above the client's bed. The client uses the trapeze for leverage when performing bed mobility tasks such as supine to long-sitting and to the edge of the bed
Rope ladder	An actual ladder device in which one end is attached to the foot of the bed and the others held by the client in order to pull to a sitting position in bed
Transfer belt	A sturdy belt used during transfers, which gives the therapist something to hold onto (other than the client) while guiding/assisting the client. The belt serves as an additional safety method
Draw sheet/pad	An additional sheet or thin pad placed directly under the client. It is used by health professionals/caregivers to hold onto while assisting the client with bed mobility

ADLs, interaction with the environment, and safety. Therefore, trunk or postural control must be a priority in order to achieve the simplest of functional outcomes.

Clients with decreased trunk control typically have the following postural weaknesses: posterior pelvic tilt, unequal weight-bearing through ischial tuberosities, lumbar spine flexion, kyphosis, lateral flexion of the spine, and head/neck malalignments (Gillen, 2011). Trunk control interventions should then begin with proper positioning of the client in order to address these postural issues.

Trunk Control: Mobility

Before beginning techniques to improve trunk mobility, the client must begin in a proper seated position. The therapist may use techniques throughout attempts at improving trunk mobility such as cuing, demonstration, hands-on techniques to "feel" the movement, or the use of a mirror. The overall goals are to improve trunk strength, balance, symmetry, and control during functional activities (Gillen, 2011).

- Examples of bed-level ADL tasks that may require trunk control movements: bathing and dressing, weight shifting while toileting, reaching at the sink for grooming items, and sitting at the kitchen table at mealtime.

Changing the Task to Achieve Independence

The therapist may provide handling techniques during ADL tasks. Handling includes providing external support to the trunk or allowing the client to feel the desired movement under the direction of the therapist. This handling may be graded according to the needs of the client (Gillen, 2011). For example, the therapist may provide support to the client's lumbar area as he or she is leaning forward over feet to don pants. In addition, the therapist may encourage increased trunk motion during this task, through handling techniques, as the client is ready.

Reaching tasks may challenge and encourage improved trunk control by the placement of objects in various reaching distances from the client's position (Gillen, 2011). For example, while the client is seated in front of the sink for brushing teeth, the therapist may place the wheelchair slightly farther from the sink than typical, the toothbrush on the counter, and the toothpaste on a shelf slightly higher than the counter.

Changing the Tools to Achieve Independence

As extremities are being incorporated into ADL tasks that involve weak trunk musculature, tasks will become increasingly more challenging. Therefore, trunk supports may be utilized to free the extremities for function. These aids include pillows, cushions, lap trays, and lumbar or lateral supports.

The client may not be ready to be challenged by increasing reach activities. In this case, the environment may be adapted by placing items at a closer distance. Adaptive equipment to enhance independence while improving trunk control and strength may be introduced such as a long-handled sponge and shoe horn, reacher, and sock aid. The client may also need a commode or shower seat with a high back for increased trunk support when toileting and showering.

The client's home may require additional modifications as the trunk improves. Modifications may include high-back chairs with arms instead of sitting on a very soft, low couch or using a chair with arms at the kitchen table. If trunk mobility is significantly decreased, the client may benefit from a hospital bed with electronic controls and bed rails until strength improves.

Trunk control activities typically begin on a stable surface such as a chair or mat. As the client improves, an unstable or movable surface may be introduced (Gillen, 2011). Unstable surfaces include the use of therapy balls, rocker boards, or bolsters. Basic trunk control exercises may be used as preparatory methods to ADLs, including reaching, catching, and throwing activities, for example, as the client is ready. Actual ADLs may be encouraged on an unstable surface such as a bolster, beginning with a very simple task, such as buttoning a shirt. Activities must be graded very carefully in order to encourage success, safety, and security.

Compensation/Adaptation for Bed Mobility

Bed mobility activities include rolling from supine to side-lying, side-lying to supine, supine to prone, prone to supine, supine to sitting at edge of bed or long-sitting, bridging, moving upward/downward, and from side to side. Equipment for bed mobility may include bed rails, trapeze, draw sheet, leg-lifter, ladder rope, and special mattresses.

Bed mobility training is not only a precursor to transfer training and independence, but also vitally important for preventing decubiti and/or contractures, which result from lack of movement and position changing. In addition, rolling side to side and sitting upright in bed are necessary skills for building independence in ADLs (Radomski & Latham, 2014). The client should be encouraged to assist the therapist as much as possible, whether it is with head movements, UE positioning, and/or LE movements. The amount of assistance given by the therapist should be graded and gradually decreased, as able (see Table 3-12). For example, as the client rolls from supine to side-lying, the therapist may initially offer moderate assistance at the knees and shoulder

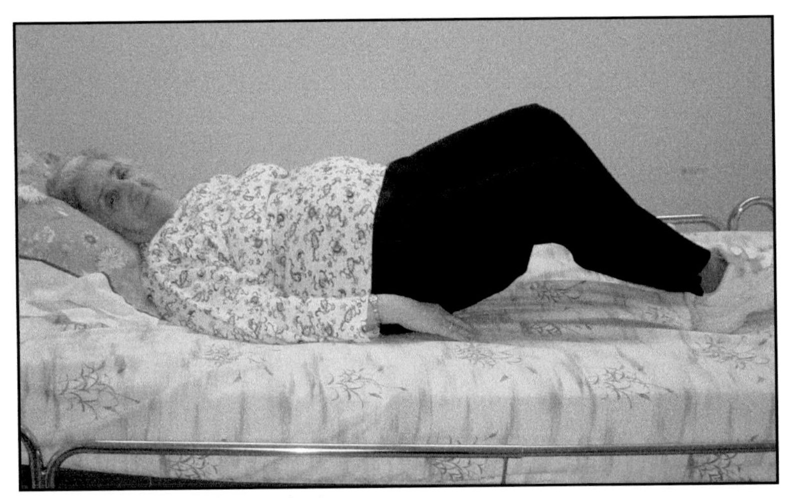

Figure 3-21. Client bridging in bed.

to complete the task. As the client improves, the movement may be graded by offering only minimal assistance at the knees and shoulder, or grading may be completed by only offering moderate assistance at one body part versus two.

The first issue with bed mobility should be reducing the friction between the client and the surface of the bed or mat. For example, using a draw sheet under the client will help to decrease friction. Whenever possible, reduce the effects of gravity and/or use gravity to assist the activity. For example, by lowering the head of the hospital bed, the client may use gravity to assist when attempting to "scoot" back in bed. Proper body mechanics are also a priority for the safety of the client as well as the therapist and will be addressed later in this section as each movement and transfer is described.

Moving Side to Side

The client should be encouraged to assist with bed mobility as much as he or she is able. When moving side to side while supine, the client should be instructed to flex at the hips and knees with feet flat on the mattress. One UE should be beside the trunk and the other abducted. The client is instructed to push both feet, elbows, and head into the mattress while lifting the pelvis upward. This technique is commonly referred to as bridging (Figure 3-21). The pelvis should then move toward the abducted UE. Then, the client repositions the extremities in order to move again, if needed. The client should be instructed to move both to the right and left. Initially, the movement may be performed by the therapist offering assistance for bridging, and then the activity is graded by decreasing the amount of hands-on assistance offered.

Moving Upward/Downward

When moving upward while supine, the client should be instructed to flex at the hips and knees with feet flat on the mattress and heels close to the buttocks. The elbows should be flexed and placed close to the trunk while the shoulders are pulled up toward the ears. The client is asked to bridge (as described earlier) and move upward by pushing with the LEs and depressing the scapula. The client will reposition to move upward again, if necessary.

When moving downward while supine, the client will partially flex the hips and knees with feet flat on the bed. The elbows are flexed next to the trunk and the shoulders depressed. The client is instructed to bridge while pushing into the bed with the elbows, head, and heels. The client moves

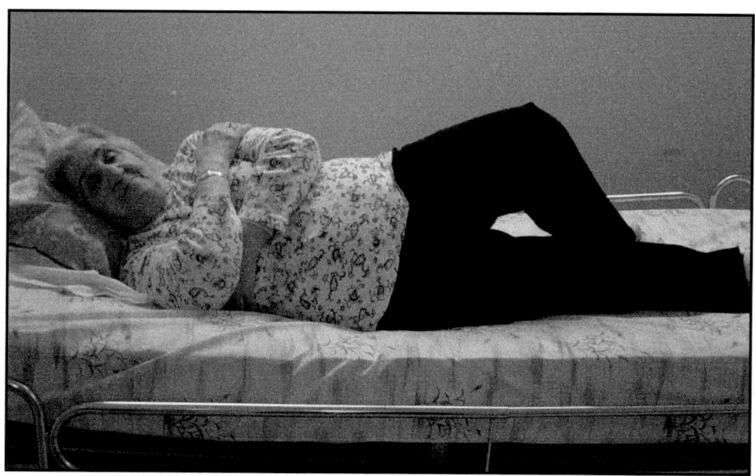

Figure 3-22. Client rolling to the right.

downward by pulling the LEs, pushing upward with the shoulders, and pushing downward with the elbows and forearms. The client is requested to reposition to repeat above, if needed.

Again, these movements may be graded by the therapist after initially offering hands-on assistance.

- Examples of bed-level ADL tasks that may require these movements: For a client on bed rest, the caregiver may rely on the client to perform/assist with these movements in order to make or change the bed. Clients tend to slip downward in the bed, and not only are they uncomfortable, but it is difficult to assist them to an upright position for safe eating. Therefore, the technique of moving upward is very important. Also, bridging is important when hiking pants in bed, placing a bed pan, and donning protective garments.

Changing the Task to Achieve Independence

The method may be changed by adjusting the levels of assistance. For example, the therapist may need to assist the client in flexing the hip and knees. The client may also need assistance in maintaining this position. The therapist may also assist with bridging, if needed. Instead of this strategy, the client may attempt the activity independently without flexing the hip/knees and only pushing down with the head and heels, with lower extremities extended (Fairchild, 2013).

Changing the Tools to Achieve Independence

The use of bed rails or a trapeze may assist the client with bed mobility as needed. The therapist may assist the client with actually moving to the side by using a draw sheet, as needed.

Moving From Supine to Side-Lying

The client is initially requested to move to one side of the bed (see section on moving side-to-side). When rolling to the right, the client is instructed to reach across the midline with the left UE while lifting the flexed left LE over the right LE (Figure 3-22). The client flexes the neck and uses abdominal muscles in order to roll. Side-lying may be maintained by placing the right hand on the bed and flexing both LEs. The client may need to slightly lean the shoulders toward the left side to further maintain the position, but not too far as the client will fall into a prone position. The same technique may be used for the left side.

- Examples of bed-level ADL tasks that may require these movements: Moving to side-lying is important for placing a bed pan, cleansing the perianal area, hiking pants in bed, donning protective garments, and inspecting a client's back and buttocks for possible pressure areas or decubiti.

Changing the Task to Achieve Independence

As needed, the therapist may assist the client by facilitating movement at the hip, knee, shoulder, head, or UE. The therapist ascertains which areas may need the most assistance. As the client strengthens, less assistance is provided.

Changing the Tools to Achieve Independence

The use of bed rails or a trapeze may assist the client with bed mobility as needed. The therapist may assist the client with actually moving to the side by using a draw sheet, as needed.

Moving From Supine to Prone

The client is initially requested to move to one side of the bed. The client is then asked to roll as previously described, except the UE is placed under the side of the body or the shoulder is flexed close to the right ear. The client is then instructed to roll into a prone position (staying away from the edge of the bed).

Changing the Task and Tools to Achieve Independence

These strategies are described previously under moving side to side and moving supine to side-lying.

Moving From Prone to Supine

While in a prone position, the client is instructed to move to one side of the bed. In order to roll to the right side, the client should position the right UE under the right side of the body or flex the right shoulder and place it by the right ear. The left hand is placed flat on the bed near the left shoulder. The left hip and knee are either slightly flexed or extended. The client is instructed to push with the left UE, lift the LE over the right LE, and roll to side-lying (staying away from the edge of the bed).

- Examples of bed-level ADL tasks that may require these movements: Most clients have difficulty moving out of a prone position or are not comfortable in it. If prone is comfortable, skin may be inspected in this position and pressure taken off the heels. Most ADLs do not require this position for completion of tasks. Therefore, lying or moving into a prone position is not typically of high priority.

Changing the Task to Achieve Independence

As needed, the therapist may assist the client by facilitating movement at the LE, head, or UE. The therapist ascertains which areas may need the most assistance. As the client strengthens, less assistance is provided.

Changing the Tools to Achieve Independence

A draw sheet may be used to assist the client with this movement.

Moving From Supine to Long-Sitting

While the client is supine, instruct the client to prop on both elbows. The client must use abdominal muscles and gradually push up with alternating UEs in order to weight-bear on both hands.

- Examples of bed-level ADL tasks that may require this position: In a long-sitting position, the client may eat at bed level, perform hygiene tasks, bathe UE, and/or don a bra, shirt, or hospital gown.

Changing the Task to Achieve Independence

As an alternative method, the client may roll into side-lying and gradually push with UEs into long-sitting.

Changing the Tools to Achieve Independence

If the client is in a hospital bed and is unable to prop on elbows, he or she may use the electronic controls to elevate the head of the bed and position automatically into long-sitting. With the above alternative method, the client may use the bed rails for rolling into side-lying and pushing with UEs. A rope ladder or trapeze may assist with either method above.

Moving From Supine to Sitting at the Edge of the Bed

Instruct client to bridge slightly to the edge of the bed (see Figure 3-21), leaving enough room to roll into side-lying. Follow above procedures for rolling into side-lying. Position client with hips and knees flexed while maintaining side-lying (see Figure 3-22). Once in this position, the client pushes the lower extremity over the edge of the bed. Instruct the client to push with the UEs, head, and trunk following. The LEs gradually pivot in order to dangle over the edge of the bed.

- Examples of ADL tasks at the edge of the bed: As long as sitting balance is intact, the client may perform many ADL tasks at the edge of the bed such as feeding, hygiene, bathing and dressing the UEs, bathing the front of the LE, and donning socks and shoes. LE tasks may be more difficult as they require excellent sitting balance. Various mattresses such as those filled with air may not allow for safe sitting balance and activities at the edge of the bed.

Changing the Task to Achieve Independence

The therapist will offer assistance as necessary with each step of the task. The therapist may need to offer assistance with sitting balance at the edge of the bed.

Changing the Tools to Achieve Independence

The client may use the bed rails, trapeze, or rope ladder for assistance with pivoting to a sitting position. The bed rail may assist in maintaining a sitting position. Long-handled adaptive equipment such a long-handled sponge may assist the client with ADLs at the edge of the bed.

Special Considerations for the Client With Neurological Symptoms

Typically, it is easier for a client with hemiparesis to roll toward the affected side as the unaffected side is able to actually perform the activity. Before rolling, the affected UE is positioned close to the body. Rolling toward the unaffected side requires more effort of the affected extremities, as able. The client reaches for and holds onto the wrist of the affected extremity while hooking the unaffected foot under the ankle of the affected LE. The client then uses the unaffected extremities to assist with rolling to the unaffected side. The therapist will provide levels of assistance as necessary (see Table 3-12).

Clients who have neurological weakness or paraplegia of the LEs will rely on UE function and strength for bed mobility. In particular, the client will use shoulder and scapula muscles for rolling and triceps, as well, for propping on elbows to long-sitting. The client will also use the UEs to move and position the LEs. Precautions must be taken to protect an unstable glenohumeral joint, which may be at risk for subluxation.

Changing the Task to Achieve Independence

The therapist or caregiver may assist with LEs and/or affected UE, as needed.

Changing the Tools to Achieve Independence

Assistive devices such as a trapeze, rope ladder, leg-lifter, or bed rails may also assist with independence.

Special Considerations for the Client With Orthopedic Injuries

Clients who have had a total hip replacement will require specific precautions with bed mobility depending upon the surgical procedure. Clients who have had both an anterolateral approach and posterolateral approach are typically recommended to initially lie supine with a wedge between both LEs in order to ensure hip precautions. It is not typically recommended for a client to sleep on or roll to the affected side. Clients with hip replacements may benefit from a trapeze above the bed (Fairchild, 2013).

Clients who have an LE amputation are instructed to use the unaffected side for eventual independent bed mobility. This is achieved through flexing the hip and knee while pushing the foot of the unaffected LE into the mattress (Fairchild, 2013).

Changing the Task to Achieve Independence

The client should compensate by using the UEs for assistance with mobility whenever possible. The therapist or caregiver will offer assistance, as needed.

Changing the Tools to Achieve Independence

Bed rails and/or a trapeze may assist with bed mobility.

Adaptation/Compensation for Transfers

The most important concept to remember with transfer training is that each client will be unique in his or her own assistance needs, limitations, safety issues, and frustration tolerance (refer to Table 3-13). Adaptations must be made for each situation and physical context as well, while keeping generalization of skills in mind. New therapists should never hesitate to ask for assistance when a transfer may be too difficult to perform alone, as safety is the priority. In addition, the therapist must be aware of the client's status at the time of the intervention session, as skill levels may change rapidly toward the positive or negative. The therapist not only needs to check the most recent documentation but also inquire with nursing and/or other available team members prior to initiating the session. The proper steps of a transfer are listed below.

1. Always use a transfer belt during functional ambulation.
2. Maintain a wide stance closely behind or on the affected side of the client.
3. With one hand, hold the transfer belt and with the other, guide the client's anterior shoulder across the chest or the trunk, as needed. Do not hold onto clothes or client's UE.
4. Position feet anterior-posterior: The outside foot should be in front of the other foot as well as between the client's foot and the assistive device. The inside foot should be positioned behind the outside foot as the client moves forward.

Table 3-15
Weight-Bearing Abbreviations and Definitions

- *Non-Weight-Bearing (NWB)*: The client is not to place any weight on the affected extremity.
- *Toe-Touch Weight-Bearing (TTWB)*: The client may rest the affected extremity on the floor, but no weight is to be applied to the foot.
- *Partial Weight-Bearing (PWB)*: The client can place some weight onto the affected extremity, but not full pressure.
- *Weight-Bearing as Tolerated (WBAT)*: This generally indicates that there are no medical restrictions, but pain may limit the client's ability to bear weight on the affected extremity.
- *Full Weight-Bearing (FWB)*: There are no medical restrictions, allowing the client to place all body weight on the affected extremity.

5. Move forward in the same direction as the client without crossing feet.
6. If the client loses balance backward, position behind the client in order for him or her to lean back, while assisting the client to re-gain balance.
7. If the client loses balance to the side toward the therapist, allow the client to lean into the therapist while using the transfer belt to assist in regaining balance.
8. Whenever it is too difficult to assist the client in regaining balance, the therapist or caregiver should quickly consider carefully assisting the client to the floor.

This section will cover all levels and types of transfers including sit-to-stand, stand-pivot, toilet, tub, car, and lift transfers. Performance of ADL skills will be incorporated where applicable.

Prior to asking a client to stand, the occupational therapist must be aware of the weight-bearing status of the client. The weight-bearing status is determined by the physician. The generally accepted abbreviations and definitions of weight-bearing are listed in Table 3-15.

Sit-to-Stand Activities

When performing sit-to-stand activities from any surface, it is important for the client to have supportive footwear. The therapist will use a transfer belt and review procedures with the client. Before beginning, both transfer surfaces must be stable, which includes locking wheelchair and hospital bed brakes. The therapist positions him or herself in front of the client (and slightly to the weak side if necessary) offering LE stabilization, as needed with his or her own knee or foot (Figure 3-23). The client is requested to "scoot" to the edge of the surface (bed, wheelchair, chair, mat, etc.) as much as safely possible, using one or both hands flat on the surface to push off. The client may also push off with the bed rail or armrest on one side, but not an assistive device such as a walker, as it will be unstable. Feet should be placed flat on the floor about 6 to 10 inches apart and slightly behind the knees (Fairchild, 2013). The client is requested to lean forward with the shoulders above the knees. The therapist holds onto the transfer belt (and is using good body mechanics), while the client pushes off with the UEs and gradually straightens LEs into standing (Figure 3-24). At this time, the client may hold onto an assistive device such as a walker or quad cane in order to safely balance.

- Examples of ADL tasks that use sit-to-stand activities: Functional standing activities may be included in this area. Examples of functional sit-to-stand activities are toileting, bathing perianal area, hiking pants, and retrieving clothes from closet or bureau.

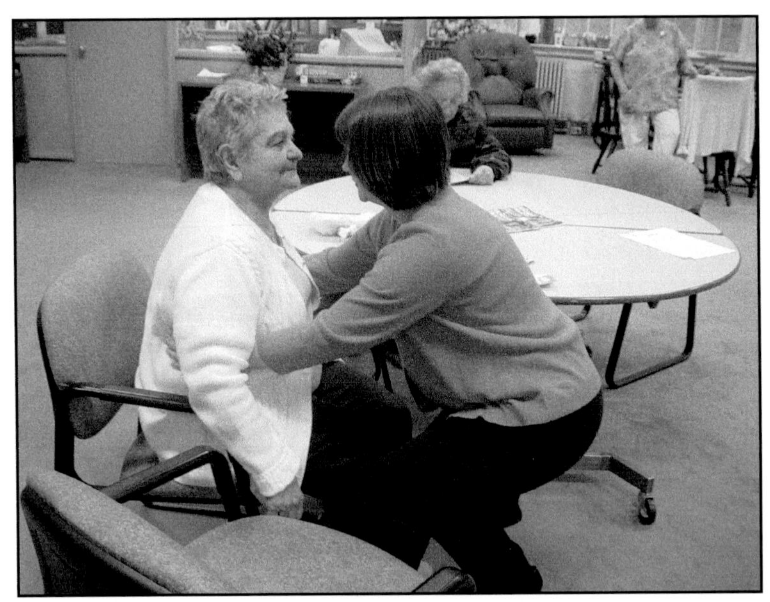

Figure 3-23. Start position for sit-to-stand.

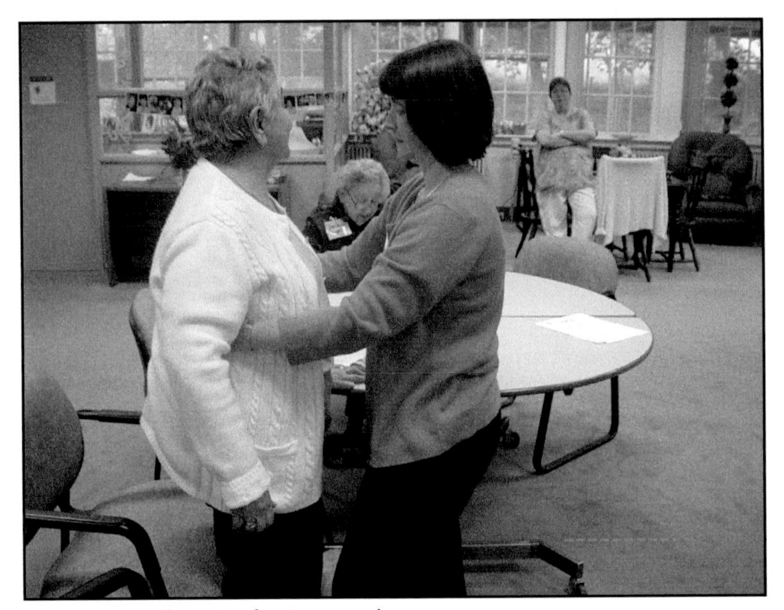

Figure 3-24. End position for sit-to-stand.

Changing the Task to Achieve Independence

If no rails or armrests are available, the client may push off of thighs or use both edges of the sitting surface.

Changing the Tools to Achieve Independence

Clients can use well-installed grab bars to pull up into standing, rather than pushing off of the chair. Raised seat surfaces will generally allow greater ease of standing. For the bathroom, raised toilet seats are available. For other chairs, the legs can be made longer. There are rare instances when the therapist may allow the client to use one extremity held on the walker to stand with the other on the sitting surface. The therapist must supervise the client closely and provide instructions for safety.

Stand-Pivot Transfers

Stand-pivot transfers are used with clients who are unable to take at least a few steps to or from the transfer surface. This transfer is initiated in the same manner as a sit-to-stand activity, although the client will not have an assistive device ready for maintaining balance. As the client stands, the therapist stays close to assist with stability and balance. Once the client is in a full standing position, the client and therapist pivot simultaneously. The client is then gradually guided into sitting as he or she reaches back for the sitting surface (rail, armrest, cushion, etc.).

- Examples of ADL tasks that use stand-pivot activities: See toilet transfers.

Changing the Task to Achieve Independence

It is advisable to perform this transfer to the affected side as well, in the event a nonpredictable environment is not set up for a transfer to the unaffected side. If a client requires assistance from two individuals, a second may stand to the side or in back of the client, also using the transfer belt. The method may need to be changed completely if two or more professionals are unable to pivot the client. Alternative methods may include a manual "lift" by two or more professionals or a mechanical lift (refer to manual/mechanical lift information later in this section).

Changing the Tools to Achieve Independence

Refer to the information regarding intervention with the client who has a neurological injury or illness below.

Issues for the Client With Neurologic Deficits

- Client typically will stand-pivot to unaffected side and pivot on unaffected LE or foot.
- If one UE is hemiparetic, only one UE may be able to assist with the task.
- If client has a subluxation, a sling may be used for transfers and functional mobility only. The use of the sling will help to protect the subluxation during the transfer. It should be removed when client is sitting or lying because extended use of the sling or shoulder immobility may encourage adhesive capsulitis.

Issues for the Client With Orthopedic Deficits

- Client typically will stand-pivot to unaffected side and pivot on unaffected LE or foot.
- Total hip replacement (THR) precautions must be followed for clients who have sustained certain hip replacements (refer to section on THR precautions).

Transfers to Surfaces With an Assistive Device

Transfers using an assistive device are appropriate for a client able to take at least a few steps to or from the transfer surface. Again, ensure all surfaces are stable and locked. This transfer is initiated in the same way as a sit-to-stand activity with the device ready for maintaining balance upon standing (Figure 3-25). Once standing balance and stability have been achieved, the therapist may either assist or supervise the client to the transfer surface. When the client is ready to sit, if he or she is using a walker, the device should be placed directly in front of him or her, but not be held while sitting. Instead, the client should reach back for the transferring surface with one or both UEs, as able (Figure 3-26). If the client is using a hemi-walker, quad cane, or cane, the device will

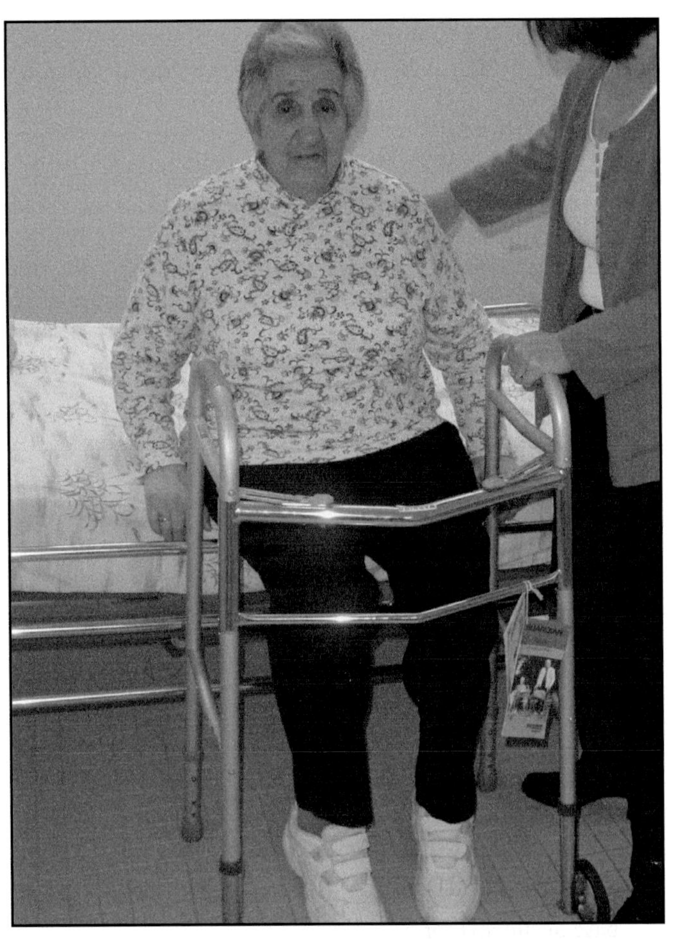

Figure 3-25. Sit-to-stand with adaptive ambulation device.

remain on the side on which the client ambulates with it; but again, it is not held while sitting. Once sitting, the client should "scoot" fully back on the surface.

- Examples of ADL tasks that use transfers with an assistive device: The client transferring with an assistive device may be carrying bath or clothing items from one surface to another in the bedroom or bathroom. Also see toilet transfers.

Changing the Task to Achieve Independence

As the client progresses, the transfer surfaces may be placed farther away from each other.

Changing the Tools to Achieve Independence

After consulting with the rehabilitation team, the client may be ready to progress to the next level of an assistive device or take a few steps to transfer without a device, if safe. The client who uses a walker may benefit from a walker basket.

Issues for the Client With Neurologic Deficits

- There is a possible need for a sling in clients with UE subluxation, although a sling for the affected extremity should be used with extreme caution and only during transfers/functional mobility in order to protect the shoulder from subluxation (or further injury).

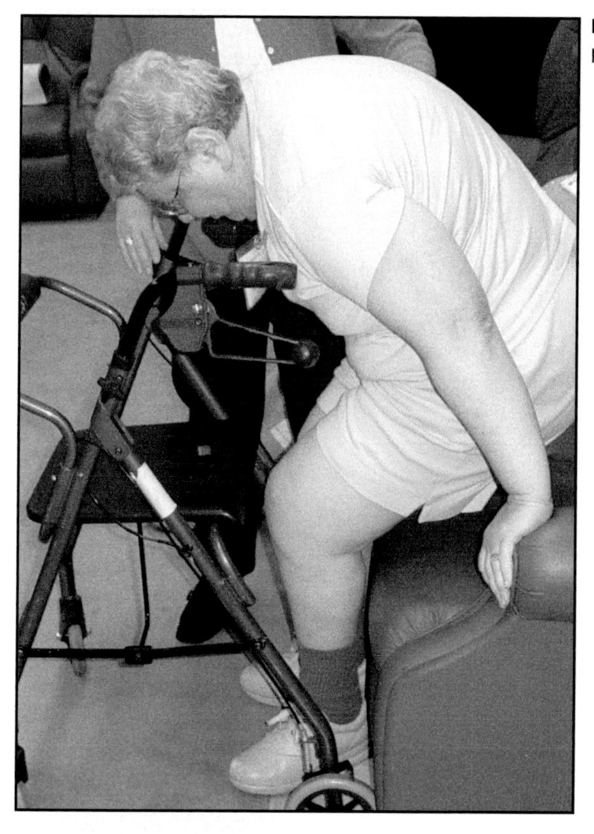

Figure 3-26. Client safely reaches back for chair prior to sitting.

- Client with hemiparesis will most likely need a hemi-walker initially, as it provides a wider base of support for balance.

Issues for the Client With Orthopedic Deficits

- Client may need platform crutches or platform walker with UE injuries if weight-bearing is contraindicated on the wrist joints.

Slide Board Transfers

Slide board transfers are appropriate for clients who have paraplegia of the LEs, bilateral amputations, severe LE weakness, or are unable to weight-bear on both LEs. The slide board is used as a bridge to transfer from one surface to another. The client must have adequate ROM and strength of both UEs, good sitting balance, and trunk mobility. The therapist applies the transfer belt. The transfer begins by equalizing the surfaces, as able. For example, when transferring from a hospital bed to a wheelchair, the bed should be positioned at a close level to the wheelchair. Both transferring surfaces must be stable and locked. Typically, a wheelchair is positioned at up to a 90-degree angle to the transferring surface (Figure 3-27). The client (with therapist's assistance as necessary) places the slide board under the buttocks by weight-bearing on the opposite extremity and elongating the trunk to the side. The client/therapist ensures the board is secured properly under the buttocks and on the transferring surface. The client leans forward slightly and weight-bears on both UEs, which should lift his or her body up slightly with each attempt. As this occurs, the client also moves across the board toward the transferring surface. The therapist positions in front of the client and may need to guide the LEs during the transfer.

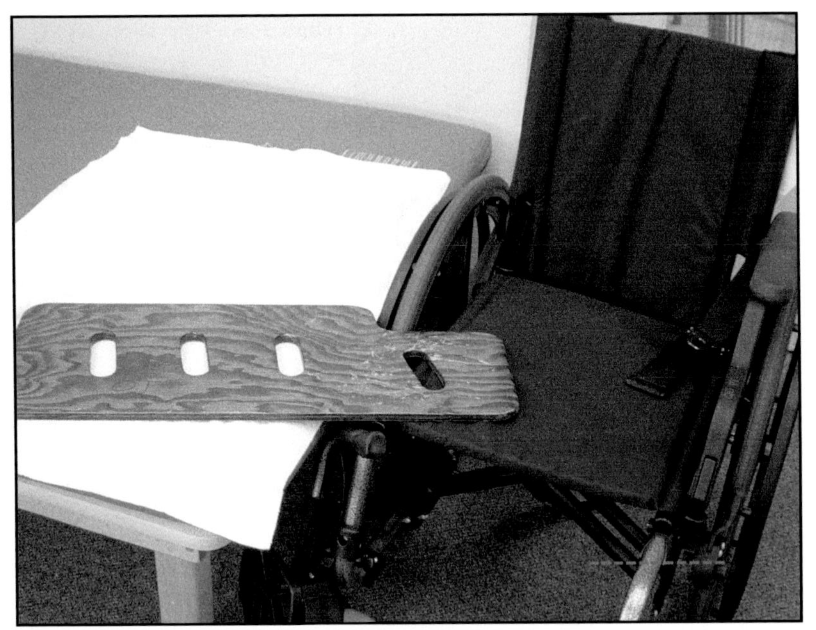

Figure 3-27. Slide board and wheelchair positioned.

- Examples of ADL tasks that use slide board activities: Slide board transfers are generally used to transfer to many surfaces during ADLs, including toilet and tub bench transfers.

Changing the Task to Achieve Independence

Typically, the therapist assists/supervises while positioned in front of the client. This positioning may vary depending on the setup of the transferring environment. For example, in a small bathroom, the therapist may not fit in front of the client and may have to position behind or beside the toilet or tub bench during the transfer. Car transfers may also need an alternative method.

Changing the Tools to Achieve Independence

A pillow case, a towel, or powder may be put on the board to decrease friction and increase ease of transfer. If the client is unable to handle or place the slide board successfully, the transfer may be performed as a bump-over without the slide board. With this technique, there cannot be any armrests on chairs. Also, the transfer surfaces must be of equal height and as close together as possible. The therapist must first ensure client safety and cognitive skills.

Issues for the Client With Neurologic Deficits

- Client may need assistance secondary to poor sitting balance.
- Transfer toward strong side, if possible.
- Clients with paraplegia of both LEs may become independent with slide board transfers.
- Client with UE hemiparesis may not have sufficient UE strength/function to perform transfer.

Issues for the Client With Orthopedic Deficits

- Clients who have sustained bilateral amputations without prosthetic devices may require the use of slide board transfers.

- Clients who have a non-weight-bearing status of both LEs may require slide board transfers. This is typically a temporary situation.

Toilet Transfers

Toilet transfers may use any of the above transfer techniques depending on the size and setup of the bathroom(s) the client uses. The limitations of space within most bathrooms as well as safety procedures are the primary considerations when planning for eventual independence with transfer training. Often, a standard wheelchair will not fit into the client's bathroom, requiring alternative plans for toileting. For example, with a client who is unable to ambulate and the wheelchair does not fit in the bathroom, the best option would be to use a commode at the bedside. Aside from modifying techniques for limitations in space within most bathrooms, the above procedures for the many types of transfers remain the same.

- Examples of ADL tasks that use toilet transfer activities: Before the actual transfer, the therapist and client need to plan how LE clothing will be pulled down and hiked. Often, it is helpful to loosen belts and closures before transferring (being careful clothes do not fall to the floor during the transfer). Before toileting, the client will need to maintain standing balance to further loosen and pull down garments and then to cleanse and hike after toileting.

Changing the Task to Achieve Independence

The positioning of the wheelchair by the toilet may have to be modified due to the size and setup of the bathroom. The position of the therapist may also need to be modified. The client may not be able to transfer to the unaffected or stronger side. An alternative method for slide board or bump-over methods may be a forward/backward toilet transfer. For example, the wheelchair is placed directly in front of the toilet and the client slides on and off the toilet in a forward/backward manner, facing the back of the toilet.

Changing the Tools to Achieve Independence

The client may benefit from a raised toilet seat and rails. If there is a counter within reach on one side of the toilet, it may be used to push off. A commode may be placed over the toilet with the bucket taken out, as an alternative tool. This commode may also be placed by the bedside at night.

Issues for the Client With Neurologic Deficits

- Whenever possible, the client should transfer to/from the strong side.
- The client may benefit from a raised toilet seat or commode over the toilet.

Issues for the Client With Orthopedic Deficits

- Clients who have had back surgery, hip replacement, or knee replacement(s) may require a raised toilet seat for a successful transfer.
- Clients may also benefit from the use of rails.

Tub/Shower Transfers

Safety issues are of a higher concern with tub/shower transfers. It is recommended to have rails, a handheld shower, and a skid-proof bath mat outside and inside of the tub/shower stall; occasionally it is also recommended to remove shower doors. Often tub benches cannot fit when shower doors are present. At least initially, clients are not recommended to transfer directly to the floor of the bathtub. Instead, a transfer tub bench or shower seat is recommended (Figure 3-28). Transferring to a transfer tub bench requires similar techniques to those presented above. The

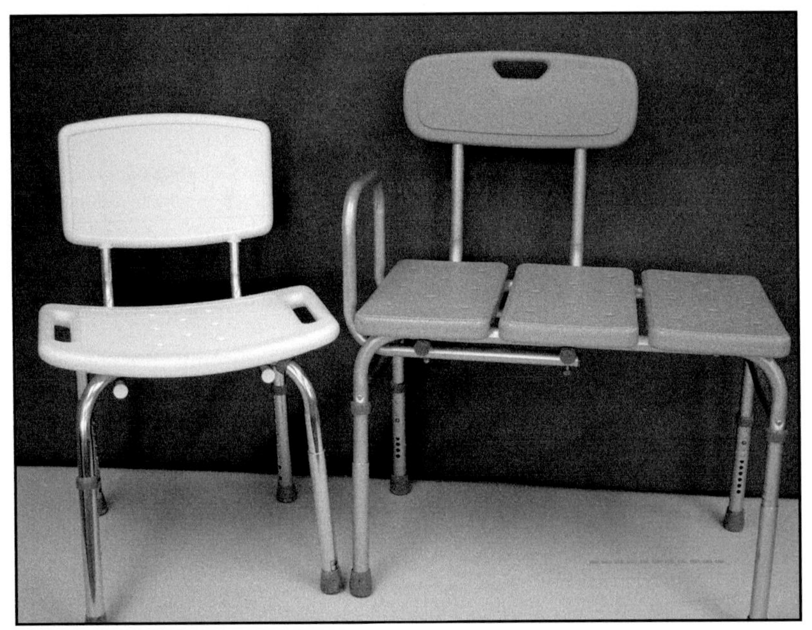

Figure 3-28. Tub bench and shower seat.

therapist may need to provide additional assistance with lifting LEs over the height of the tub. If no rails are present, the therapist may need to offer further assistance for safety, balance, and stability.

Transferring over the height of the tub or ledge of a shower stall will require additional explanation as well as strength, balance, and mobility on the client's part. The therapist applies the transfer belt, and the client either ambulates to the tub/shower or stands from the wheelchair with procedures presented above. For example, the shower head may be to the right when the client is facing the tub/shower. When standing beside the tub or shower, the client stands at an angle slightly facing and to the side of the tub or shower. If the client is able to hold the assistive device in the left hand, he or she may continue to do so. If it is held in the right, the client will need to let go of the device and grab onto a handrail, which should be placed at the front of the tub/shower. If there is no rail, the client may hold the therapist's hand. The client will then step into the tub with the stronger LE while slightly facing the tub/shower and follow with the other extremity. The client may either grab onto a rail on the inner wall of the tub/shower with the left hand or reach for the shower seat. The client will then face the showerhead, feel the seat behind his or her knees, continue to hold the rails, then reach back for the shower seat with one hand and sit.

- Examples of ADL tasks that use tub/shower activities: While simulating the transfer and sitting on a shower chair/bench, the client's trunk stability must be assessed. As applicable, one-handed shower techniques may be initiated, with or without use of a handheld shower. Adaptive equipment may be used for one-handed bathing. The therapist must plan with the client how the perianal area will be bathed, particularly if there is no cut-out in the seat. If a sit-to-stand is required for this task, the client and therapist should simulate the skill prior to the actual shower.

Changing the Task to Achieve Independence

Instead of slightly facing the tub, the client may side-step into the tub. This method is preferable if the stronger LE is able to step in first. This method may be necessary due to lack of space. When the client is ready, transfers to sitting on the floor of the tub may be attempted with great caution, supervision, and good judgment.

Changing the Tools to Achieve Independence

The client may not be able to use a tub transfer bench due to lack of space or the expense of the tool. Often, a sturdy plastic lawn chair may fit in the tub as a shower seat and be much more affordable. Many prefabricated tub/showers have built-in shower seats, as well. The safety of these seats must be evaluated before use.

Issues for the Client With Neurologic Deficits

- Safety concerns in clients who, for example, are impulsive, are experiencing neglect, or have significantly decreased balance include a greater risk of falling when the floor or bath is wet or slippery.

Issues for the Client With Orthopedic Deficits

- Secondary to possible THR precautions, casts, open wounds, staples, etc., the client may not be able to take a shower and will need to sponge-bathe.

Manual or Two-Person Lift Transfers

For clients who are fully dependent in transfers, two individuals may be needed to lift the client to a bed, mat, wheelchair, or commode. The techniques depend on the surface transferring to and from, as well as the size of the client. The client will be positioned with the head and trunk flexed and UEs folded in front of the body (Fairchild, 2013). One therapist will position behind the client using a wide base of support. The therapist reaches under the client's axilla and around the chest to grasp the client's forearms. The second therapist faces the side of the client's LEs and grasps them by holding one arm under the client's upper thighs and the other under the lower legs. (Alternative LE lift: the second therapist faces the client's LE in order to lift both LEs at the knees.) The therapists will count, "One, two, three, lift." As the lift begins, they both must lift the client high enough to clear the height of the wheelchair while moving the client sideways toward the transferring surface. Proper body mechanics on the part of the therapists is vital.

- Examples of ADL tasks that use manual lift activities: Because this transfer is being dependent in nature, there are no ADL tasks directly related.

Changing the Task to Achieve Independence

See previous section. A third individual may either be needed to stand by or assist at the axilla or with the LEs. An alternative two-person method involves the therapists positioned on each side of the client distributing the client's weight more evenly. A negative aspect of the lift is that it often requires the client to be carried farther than the first method. Each therapist uses a forearm to cradle the client's thigh, and the other crosses the client's posterior upper trunk to grasp the other therapist's forearm. The client's UEs are placed over the therapist's shoulders (Fairchild, 2013).

Changing the Tools to Achieve Independence

If the client may be too heavy or his or her safety is an issue, a mechanical lift should be used.

Issues for the Client With Neurologic Deficits

- The client may be especially fearful of the transfer if visual/perceptual and/or cognitive issues are present.

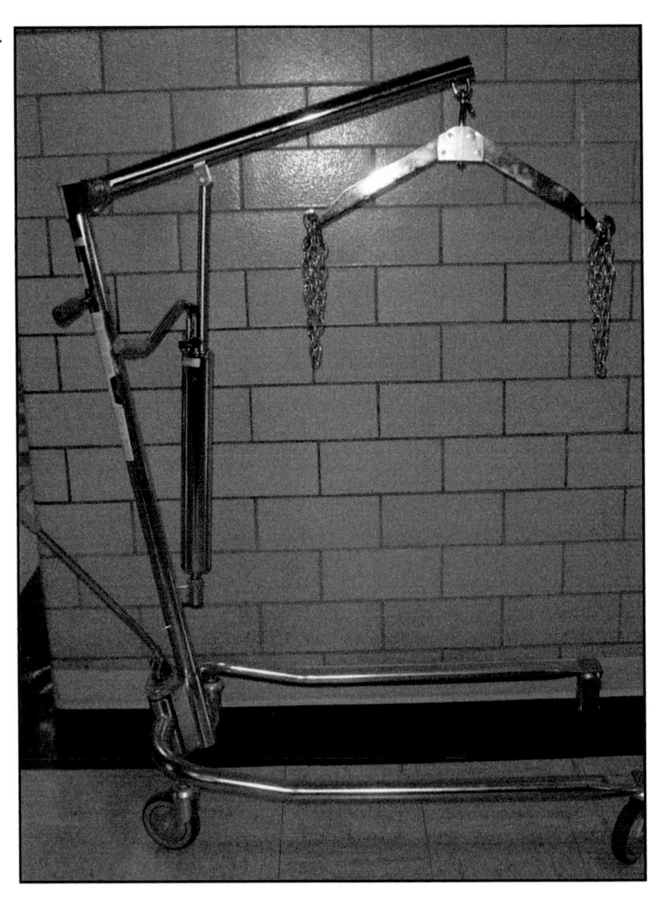

Figure 3-29. Mechanical lift.

- If a client is at level IV of the Ranchos Los Amigos scale, for example, an agitated state may decrease the safety of the transfer.

Issues for the Client With Orthopedic Deficits

- Be aware of possible decubiti when rolling the client and placing a transfer pad. The client may be at risk for a decubiti secondary to friction from being manually transferred.

Mechanical Lift Transfers

Mechanical lift transfers are categorized as dependent in nature, as are manual lifts. A hydraulic lifting device, such as the Hoyer patient lifter may be used for clients who are either too heavy and/or require extensive lifting and assistance (Figure 3-29). Caregivers need to be educated in the use of the mechanical lift, as with other transfers. Clients may be transferred to most surfaces, including the toilet and commode. Caution is necessary however, if the client's mental status or sitting balance may necessitate supervision or assistance when arriving at the transfer surface.

The mechanical lift transfer also involves explaining the steps of the activity to the client before beginning. The steps are as follows:

1. While at bed level, the sling component of the lift must be positioned under the upper trunk, buttocks, and upper thigh of the client by rolling him or her from one side to the other (see bed mobility techniques).

2. The lift should be positioned perpendicular to the bed and as close as possible with the spreader bar over the client's chest.
3. The chains or straps of the sling are attached to the spreader bar.
4. The control valve then is partially opened in order to gradually lower the spreader bar until the chains/straps can be attached to the sling.
5. Then the valve is closed to prevent the spreader valve from lowering further.
6. The chains or straps are attached to the sling, directing the S hooks away from the body.
7. Make adjustments and check all attachments as needed.
8. Ask the client to fold his or her UEs over the chest.
9. Elevate the client by pumping the handle until he or she is elevated off the bed.
10. Slowly move the lift from the bed, with a second person guiding the client's LEs.
11. Guide the client to the transferring surface with his or her buttocks positioned directly over the seat/surface.
12. Gradually open the control valve, which will slowly lower the client to the surface.
13. Guide the client's body toward the surface and close the valve.
14. Remove the chains or straps from the sling, leaving the sling in place for the transfer back to the bed or another surface.

- Examples of ADL tasks that use mechanical lift activities: As stated, clients may be transferred via the mechanical lift to the toilet or commode. Adapted raised toilet seats, transfer pads with cut-outs, and rails are typically necessary for safety, hygiene, and sitting balance.

Changing the Task to Achieve Independence

As the client's ability to participate improves, the mechanical lift may not be needed.

Changing the Tools to Achieve Independence

A sling with an opening at the perianal area may be used for clients who are lifted to a commode/toilet. A client may need to have multiple slings, with one at the upper body and one at the buttock area.

Getting Up From the Floor

Getting up from the floor is an important segment of rehabilitation for independence. If a client falls or needs to get up from the floor, the ideal position to begin with is prone. The client will then push him or herself to a quadruped position and then to kneeling, half-kneeling, and then standing.

- Examples of ADL tasks that involve getting up from the floor: This transfer may also be used when getting out of the floor of the tub.

Changing the Task to Achieve Independence

If the client is unable to get into a prone position, he or she may logroll to side-lying, push to side-sitting, and then move to a quadruped position.

Changing the Tools to Achieve Independence

The client may also hold onto a nearby stable object for assistance.

Car Transfers

Car transfers may be initiated with any of the various techniques above, as appropriate. For example, the therapist may perform a stand-pivot transfer with the client to the car seat. Slide board transfers or transfers using a walker or any other assistive device may also be attempted. The difference in a car transfer is with the approach to the car seat. With any of the types of transfers, the client will typically need to take a backward approach to the car seat. The client needs to back into the car seat and feel it behind the LEs before sitting. The client will need to reach back for the side of the car and/or dashboard when sitting. The open car door may be an obstacle for assistive devices as well as the therapist. Therefore, careful step-by-step planning of this transfer is necessary.

After the client sits, he or she may need assistance in pivoting in order to sit straight in the seat and lift both LEs over the edge of the car.

Changing the Task to Achieve Independence

The transfer approach may be easier for the client if he or she sits in the back seat of the car. Transferring into a van or SUV will be much more of a challenge. Clients will have difficulty because of the height of the vehicles and may either need to be lifted or use a ramp or step stool.

Changing the Tools to Achieve Independence

As noted above, a ramp or step stool may be needed. Step stools may only be used with clients who have good mobility and strength. Because of the lack of stability with a step stool, the client must be closely assisted or supervised. Also, the client may not be able to access the car seat with his or her walker or wheelchair; therefore, for this transfer only, he or she may need to have handheld assistance from the therapist, as appropriate. In addition, an adaptive device called the HandyBar (Avenue Innovations & Avin) is a tool designed to provide assistance with car transfers. The HandyBar fits in the striker plate of the car door to allow for a secure hand hold when standing or entering the car.

Functional Ambulation for Clients With Physical Limitations

Basic foundation skills for functional ambulation include sufficient weight-bearing on the LEs, good LE ROM and strength, dynamic balance, and an adaptability to temporal and physical contexts.

Functional ambulation involves a repetition of movements called the gait cycle. The gait cycle involves two phases, the stance phase and the swing phase. The stance phase is when the heel contacts the ground and begins to bear weight until the foot is fully on the ground. Next, the heel lifts off the ground to make the mid-stance phase and then the push-off, which involves weight-shift forward onto the toes. Then, the foot is ready to leave the ground.

The swing phase involves the leg swinging forward with the foot clearing the ground. This is called liftoff or the early swing phase. The late swing phase is when the leg decelerates and gets ready for heel contact.

It is important for occupational therapists to have a basic understanding and working knowledge of the gait cycle in order to properly use observations and evaluate, plan, and execute interventions related to functional mobility and specific to the client's needs and related condition. Also, a good understanding of functional ambulation will allow for effective communication with physical therapy as well as other team members. For example, the occupational therapist may need to communicate to the physical therapist and/or other team members any changes in status or specific needs regarding a client during functional mobility. Through this team process, making recommendations and decisions requires basic knowledge of other health care practitioners' skills and roles.

Table 3-16

Functional Mobility Assistive Devices

Device	Description
Wheelchair: manual, electric	Client with upper extremity function will typically use a manual chair.
Scooter	
Walker: standard, rolling, platform, 3-wheeled walker	Platform walker is used for clients who have sustained a UE injury and have weight-bearing restriction. Rolling walker is used with clients who do not have the strength to lift a standard walker. A three-wheeled walker offers more stability and has brakes.
Hemi-walker	One-handed walker with four legs to offer a wide base. It is held in the unaffected UE and is made for individuals with hemiparesis/hemiplegia.
Quad-cane: large and small-based	A smaller base of support than a hemi-walker, but larger than a straight cane. Also has four legs. Base comes in two sizes.
Straight cane	Smallest base of support. May be used by client with neurological, orthopedic, or general balance conditions.
Crutches: axillary, platform, and Lofstrand	Platform crutches are also used for clients who have sustained a UE injury and have restrictions. Lofstrand crutches are used when less stability/support is needed than with axillary crutches (Pierson, 1996).

Changing the Task to Achieve Independence

Compensation during functional mobility may require a change in the weight-bearing status of the client (see Table 3-15).

Changing the Tools to Achieve Independence

Functional ambulation is an important aspect in achieving independence in ADLs. In order to achieve as much independence as possible as well as ensure safety, stability, balance, and support, clients may require an assistive mobility device. Table 3-16 lists the many devices available, ranging from those offering the most assistance/stability (wheelchairs and walkers) to those offering the least (straight cane). See Figure 3-30 for sample assistive devices. The choice of assistive device also involves the client's ability to use one or both of the UEs.

Refer to the section on wheelchair mobility for descriptions of the power and manual wheelchairs. Clients who may only be able to ambulate short distances, such as from the bedroom to the bathroom, may need a manual wheelchair or a scooter for longer distances, such as community mobility. In addition, the use of a wheelchair or scooter during ADLs may allow the client to sit and rest when needed and free up the UEs, particularly when both hands are needed for a task.

In general, walkers offer maximal bilateral stability, balance, and support for individuals who have the use of both UEs. Types of walkers include standard, rolling, three-wheeled, and platform walkers. A standard walker must be slightly lifted off the ground with each step during ambulation. When negotiating corners, the standard walker must also be carried or lifted during the turn. The rolling walker is often helpful for individuals who cannot lift the walker or have an ataxic gait. For these individuals, it is usually easier to push the walker with each step, although turning corners may be more difficult. Also, clients who move too quickly or have difficulty stopping may not be safe with a rolling walker. These walkers may offer a folding option for fitting in a car, closet, or smaller space. A walker basket may fit in the front of most walkers in order to carry light items.

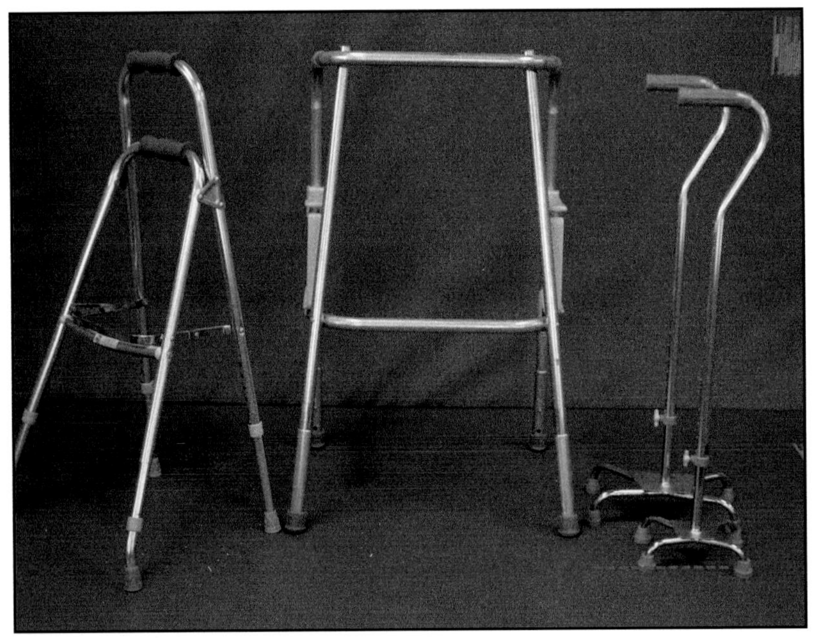

Figure 3-30. Sample ambulation devices.

A three-wheeled walker that has larger, pneumatic wheels and hand brakes offers more stability and safety. Often, the three-wheeled walker will have a fold-down seat, offering rest periods for individuals with decreased endurance. This walker is capable of carrying heavier objects, although it is not indicated for clients who lean on the walker for support. The width and turning radius is larger and it is more difficult to store, particularly in a car.

Platform walkers may be of the standard or rolling type and are fitted with either a single or double platform for the UE(s) to rest on. These are typically used for clients who require a walker for ambulation but have either UE weight-bearing restrictions or significant deformities of wrists/hands that make grasping the walker too difficult. For example, a client with bilateral Colles' fractures may need this type of walker because of weight-bearing restrictions and bilateral cast restrictions/immobility.

The hemi-walker is a one-handed walker typically used with individuals with hemiplegia who have limited to no use of the affected extremity. The hemi-walker offers a wide base of support and stability to be used on the unaffected side of the body.

Quad canes are four-pronged and provide less support and stability than the hemi-walker but more than a straight cane. Quad canes are offered in two sizes: large-based and small-based. Quad canes may be used for clients with neurological conditions who have progressed from a hemi-walker or for any individual who needs more support and stability than that offered by a straight cane but does not need a walker.

Straight canes offer the smallest base of support and are used for individuals with mild balance and stability issues. Canes tend to be easier to use on stairs and narrow areas and are easily stored.

Axillary crutches are used for individuals needing less stability and support than a walker provides and allow for increased speed of ambulation. Crutches require good standing balance and UE strength. They are easily used on stairs, stored, and transported. Lofstrand crutches allow the client to place the forearm in a cuff attached to the crutch versus positioning the device under the axillary area, decreasing injury to the axillary area and making them easier to use on stairs. They are used when less stability/support is needed than with axillary crutches. Platform crutches use a similar attachment as the platform walker for individuals with weight-bearing or UE issues that limit gripping of handles.

Changing the Tools to Achieve Independence

The tools in Table 3-16 may be adapted depending upon the client's strength, ROM, balance, safety/cognition, and levels of assistance needed.

Changing the Task to Achieve Independence

The tasks of functional mobility may be adapted by changing the weight-bearing status of the client, as applicable.

- Examples of ADL tasks that use functional mobility activities: ADL tasks involving the above tools include ambulating to the bathroom, toilet transfers, shower transfers, and ambulating to the closet to retrieve clothes.

Compensation/Adaptation for Wheelchair Mobility

A manual wheelchair is typically used by clients who have sufficient UE ROM and strength of one or both limbs for propulsion of the chair. One or both LEs may also assist with propulsion. A powered wheelchair or motorized scooter are appropriate for clients with limited or no UE function or who have significantly decreased endurance. Typically, in order for a client to use a scooter, he or she will need to be independent with transfers and have good trunk control. When evaluating for the type of chair needed, the client's home, work, community, and transportation issues must be considered. The client must be instructed on mobility in all of the physical contexts of their lifestyle. Training is required and is best if tailored to the client's specific context (Reid, Laliberte-Rudman, & Hebert, 2002; Sakakibara, Miller, Souza, Nikolova, & Best, 2013). Through regular practice, intervention has been shown to increase wheelchair speed, endurance, and handgrip strength, particularly when a functional approach is taken, such as with propelling to meals and social events. In addition, nursing home residents have reported that wheelchair use increased feelings of independence, physical well-being, and emotional well-being (Simmons, Rahman, & Dietz, 1996; Sakakibara et al., 2013). Increased wheelchair mobility will, furthermore, improve involvement in occupation, social participation, work, and roles, thereby increasing quality of life and overall satisfaction.

Wheelchair mobility training typically begins in the rehabilitation clinic using a smooth surface in an uncluttered environment. The client must also be instructed in using the parts of the chair such as brakes and removable leg/armrests. Outside wheelchair mobility training must address propulsion on uneven surfaces/terrain, negotiating crowds and obstacles, narrow spaces, and accessibility in general.

- Examples of ADL tasks that use wheelchair mobility activities: Wheelchair mobility involves many functional activities such as transfers into and out of an adapted shower stall, retrieving clothes from the closet/bureau, and general accessibility to the bathroom.

Basic Wheelchair Propulsion

- Bilateral UE Propulsion: The client grasps the top of the wheelchair hand rims and pushes forward or pulls backward equally. When turning right or left, the client holds one hand rim still while pulling/pushing the other hand rim in the desired direction.
- Propulsion With One UE and One LE: Typically, such as with hemiplegia, the functional UE and LE to be used are on the same side, although the technique may be adapted for contralateral sides. The client grasps the hand rim on one side and pushes/pulls in the desired direction, while the LE works in the same direction. The foot may assist with turning as well.

- Bilateral LE Propulsion: The client uses the heels and soles of the feet to propel the chair in the desired direction, including turning the chair (Fairchild, 2013).

Changing The Task To Achieve Independence

The caregiver may offer assistance as needed with propulsion. The task may be broken down into small steps initially, such as with attempting turns or using both the UEs and LEs simultaneously.

Changing the Tools to Achieve Independence

The hand rims may be adapted for ease of propulsion. The chair may also be lowered for clients using the LE(s) for propulsion. The client may need to wear leather gloves in order to increase grip on the hand rims as well as for comfort.

Wheelchair Mobility on Ramps

Using a ramp for wheelchair mobility allows the client accessibility when stairs or the entrance to a van/bus or doorway are too high. The Americans with Disability Act ([ADA]28 CFR 36, §4) has specified regulations for the length, slope, and texture of a ramp. For every inch of rise, there must be 12 inches of ramp length; if the step is 4 inches high, the ramp must be 48 inches long.

Techniques for ascending (forward facing) a ramp involve leaning forward from the trunk and pushing on the hand rims with a smooth forward motion. Moving the center of gravity forward is essential to avoid tipping backward. Descending (forward facing) a ramp involves positioning the hips to the back of the chair and sitting upright from the trunk (Fairchild, 2013) or leaning backward slightly. The client should place the palms of the hands on the hand rims, keeping the fingers extended for safety. While applying even pressure on the hand rims, the client controls or slows down the forward motion of the chair during the descent (Fairchild, 2013). It is not recommended to use the hand brakes to slow the movement down the ramp.

Changing the Task to Achieve Independence

If a forward-facing approach is not successful, the client may attempt a backward-facing approach with ascending/descending. The client may require assistance for this task.

Changing the Tools to Achieve Independence

Wheelchairs may be adapted for specific needs, such as with a hemiplegic arm trough (Figure 3-31), anti-tip devices, high/low backrests, and desk arms.

Wheelchair Wheelies

Wheelchair wheelies are an advanced skill that allows the client to elevate the caster wheels in order to manage curbs and sidewalks or to clear heights on the ground or floor. The therapist must first evaluate the client for safety, judgment, good UE strength, coordination, and balance while in the chair. The therapist must also prepare for possible falls backward in the chair before the client fully acquires the skills necessary to perform this technique (Radomski & Latham, 2014).

Initiating the wheelie involves the client grasping onto the anterior hand rim and quickly pulling back on the hand rims with both hands. After this motion is completed, the hands are then moved posterior on the wheel rims. In this position, the chair frame is then rotated backward with a quick forward push on the wheel rims and a quick stop. This causes the caster wheels to elevate and the wheelchair to balance only on the back wheels (Radomski & Latham, 2014).

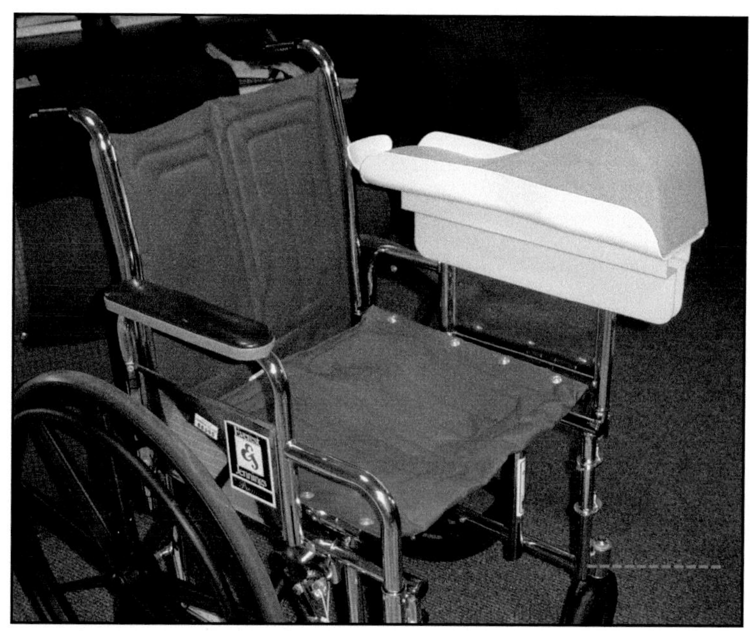

Figure 3-31. Arm trough on a wheelchair.

Wheelchair Mobility With Curbs and Steps

Although the need to negotiate curbs or steps in the community is becoming less and less frequent secondary to the ADA laws, there are still many circumstances in which the client will need to know how to ascend/descend a curb or step. Clients who are deemed capable of performing a wheelie in a manual wheelchair may become independent with this skill. Ascending and descending a curb or steps using a powered chair or a scooter is not feasible, except for specialized chairs made for this purpose.

Ascending a curb or step is initiated by the client performing the wheelie with the casters positioned on the curb. Then, the client leans forward, gives a strong push on the hand rims with the UEs, and propels the rear wheels onto the curb or step.

Descending uses a backward approach with the client leaning forward in the chair, pushing the hand rims backward, causing the back wheels to roll down the curb or step. The client may also use a forward-facing approach by using the wheelie position and pushing the back wheels off the curb/step.

In many instances, the client will need assistance with this task, particularly with decreased UE strength, decreased balance, and safety issues. For example, the client may be assisted with the wheelie component of the task or after the chair is in the wheelie position.

Descending more than one or two steps is a much more challenging and dangerous task, while ascending is not a feasible independent task. Two individuals should provide dependent mobility when ascending/descending several steps. When ascending, one individual stands behind the chair, which is positioned against the steps, while the second individual is in front. While tipping the chair backward, the individual in the back holds the handles and pulls the chair up each step. The individual in the front holds and balances the chair by the leg rests or frame. Descending involves the individual in the front guiding and holding onto the chair to control the speed, while the individual in the back assumes the same position, pushing the chair down each step. Proper body mechanics for both individuals providing the dependent mobility are essential (Radomski & Latham, 2014).

Changing the Task to Achieve Independence

As above, the client may need the assistance of one or two individuals in order to complete the task. Forward-facing and backward-facing approaches may be attempted. In case of emergency, the appropriate client may be educated in ascending/descending stairs while sitting on the buttocks, using the UEs to bump up or down the stairs.

Changing the Tools to Achieve Independence

The wheelchair may be adapted with anti-tip devices. The weight of the wheelchair may also be a consideration.

Opening Doors While Propelling a Wheelchair

Propelling a wheelchair using a "self-closing" device to open/close doors involves client education in regard to safety techniques as well as working against resistance from the door (Fairchild, 2013). When propelling through a door that opens away from the client, he or she must position the wheelchair at an angle facing the door latch. As this is done, the client reaches for the doorknob or latch with a quick, strong push. The client may need to stabilize the wheelchair by holding onto one hand rim in order to prevent the chair from rolling backward. Then, the chair is quickly propelled through the doorway. The client may need to simultaneously hold the door open with one hand.

When propelling through a door that opens toward the client, the chair should be positioned at an angle facing the door hinges. The client reaches for the doorknob or latch with a quick, strong pull. Again, the client may need to hold the door open with one hand to prevent rolling backward. Several small pulls may be needed to open the door far enough.

Changing the Task to Achieve Independence

Moving through the door at an angle decreases the width needed to open the door and pass through, although if the chair does not fit at an angle, the approach should be facing the door. Because of the weight/resistance of a self-closing door, the client may require assistance.

Changing the Tools to Achieve Independence

Propelling the wheelchair without a self-closing device involves positioning the chair facing the door at an angle that is either facing the door latch or the hinges. The client will need to open the door only wide enough for the chair to fit through and follow the above procedures for opening the door, although less force is needed. The client will then turn the chair in order to close the door once through. When propelling the wheelchair through automatic doors, the client must first position him or herself far enough away for the doors to open safely without getting hit. The client may also benefit from an adapted doorknob turner or handle.

Getting On/Off an Elevator While Propelling a Wheelchair

The client may use a forward or backward approach when entering and exiting an elevator. Safety issues include uneven surfaces or a space between the floor of the elevator and the floor of the landing, causing wheels to stop rolling or dropping into the space and/or the chair to tip forward; inability to reach the elevator buttons; or the doors attempting to close before the client is fully in or out of the elevator.

Changing the Task to Achieve Independence

The client may ask for assistance with either getting in/out of the elevator or using the control buttons. If the client has difficulty with one approach, such as entering forward-facing, he or she may attempt a backward approach.

Changing the Tools to Achieve Independence

Again, the wheelchair may need anti-tip devices, one-arm drive, or adaptations to leg rests. The client who has had a THR may require a reclining wheelchair.

Compensations/Adaptations of Functional Mobility for Clients With Cognitive, Perceptual, or Visual Limitations: Performance Skills/Client Factors

As discussed previously, the AOTA Framework (2014) presents perceptual and cognitive deficits within two sections of the document. The first section addresses basic cognitive skills in the general category of performance skills and the subsections of sensory-perceptual skills and cognitive skills. The Framework (2014) defines these basic cognitive skills as necessary to complete, manage, and modify ADL tasks.

Also as discussed previously, a second section of the AOTA Framework (2014) also addresses cognitive and perceptual deficits. The deficits are discussed under the subsection of client factors called *Body Function Categories.* These body function categories, mental functions, are the affective, perceptual, and additional cognitive skills required to complete ADL tasks.

Specifically, this section will discuss cognitive and perceptual issues as they relate to functional mobility and ADL skills. The format is a brief reader introduction to the topic and examples of compensation/adaptation interventions. Examples of appropriate activities will be listed. For specific definitions, please refer to Chapter 2.

Compensation/Adaptation of Functional Mobility for Cognitive Deficits

See Figure 3-19.

Performance Skills: Cognitive Skills

Table 3-17 briefly presents the subcategories of cognitive skills, as they are typically addressed less formally within most mobility intervention plans.

Client Factors: Body Functions—Global Mental Functions

As stated earlier, global mental functions include consciousness and orientation. Consciousness is further divided to include arousal level and level of consciousness (AOTA, 2014).

Arousal Level

Zoltan (2007) describes arousal level as “alerting,” or a level of alertness that fluctuates (depending upon the state of one’s CNS) and prepares for mobilization to attention.

Occupational therapy intervention at this level is very limited in terms of functional performance. Initially, the client’s level of alertness may be very limited, not allowing for even the simplest of bed mobility training. The therapist may need to see the client for several brief sessions during the day, as able, focusing on sensory stimulation.

Table 3-17

Process Skills and Examples of Compensation/Adaptation Strategies

Process Skill Subcategories (AOTA, 2002a)	Examples of Functional Mobility Compensation/Adaptation Interventions
Energy	
Paces	Provide client with a clock and chart with estimated amount of time required to perform tasks such as transfers, functional ambulation, and transporting objects.
Attends	Refer to Specific Mental Functions category.
Knowledge	
Chooses	Before initiating a transfer, allow client to choose the appropriate assistive device that was used previously.
Uses	Ask client to describe the proper use of the above assistive device.
Handles	After verbally describing the use of the assistive device, ask client to physically demonstrate the use. Monitor for safety.
Heeds	Provide daily checklist to document each time a transfer is completed safely. For example, each time the client reaches back for the chair with both hands.
Inquires	Provide written directions for transfers/functional mobility. Request client to ask one or more questions regarding safety with these tasks.
Temporal Organization	
Initiation	Use external cues such as an audiotape with specific instructions to follow for each step of the transfer. Work with client to develop internal cues to initiate transfers.
Sequencing	Provide client with the written steps for safely completing transfers and functional mobility with/without assistive device, as appropriate.
Organizing Space and Objects	
Searches/ locates	Provide external cuing such as labels or signs to assist with locating assistive device, bathroom, bedroom, etc.
Gathers	Provide checklist of items needed for transporting during functional mobility and transfers by using a walker basket or cart.
Organizes	Ask client to locate items in the environment that may hinder safe functional mobility, such as throw rugs, wet surfaces, or clutter.
Restores	Ask client to verbally instruct caregiver/therapist on how to safely return assistive device and/or transported objects to appropriate places.
Navigates	Teach client techniques for maneuvering in environment and/or around obstacles when using a wheelchair or assistive device.

(continued)

Table 3-17 (continued) **Process Skills and Examples of Compensation/Adaptation Strategies**	
Process Skill Subcategories (AOTA, 2002)	**Examples of Functional Mobility Compensation/Adaptation Interventions**
Adaptation	
Notices/ responds	Grade environmental, nonverbal, or perceptual cues as client notices/does not notice need to maneuver around obstacles.
Accommodates/ adjusts	Problem-solve alternative actions or scenarios with client. For example, client should be able to modify functional mobility skills in order to safely maneuver in many different situations.
Benefits	Assist client/family in problem-solving various functional mobility situations that may occur upon discharge home and plan for adaptations.

Changing the Task to Achieve Independence

The client's level of arousal or ability to participate in the task will dictate the need or readiness to change the method. As stated above, the therapist may need to see the client for several short sessions per day. Depending on the client's response, the physical context may need to be changed. For example, a less distractible environment may allow the client to better attend, or more than likely, a moderate amount of sensory stimulation such as noise/sound may improve the client's level of alertness (e.g., upbeat music).

The client may benefit from simple, very basic, verbal instructions and potentially tactile cuing. Instructions and verbal communication may be upgraded as the client's level of alertness increases.

In order to prepare the client for higher-level skills and encourage sensory stimulation, basic bed mobility tasks may be attempted as the client's level of awareness improves. Refer to the section on bed mobility for more information. Depending on the client's level of alertness and attention span, functional mobility tasks may be graded, starting with simple bed mobility. Tasks such as those that require one- to two-step commands may be attempted such as bridging, rolling, reaching, and sitting upright. The client's level of alertness and attention span will also dictate the client's level of safety awareness and possible insight into his or her abilities.

As levels of alertness increase and the client is able to sit upright in bed, the therapist may begin addressing supine-to-sit transfers to the edge of the bed. While sitting at the edge, if the client's level of alertness allows, simple functional tasks may be attempted such as eating or brushing teeth.

In addition, as levels of alertness and attention improve, the therapist may begin to encourage the client to begin sit-to-stand activities.

Changing the Tools to Achieve Independence

At the most basic levels of bed and functional mobility, it is best to attempt tasks without tools initially. As ability to attend improves, an assistive device may be introduced at the bedside for sit-to-stand activities.

Orientation

Orientation is an individual's awareness of time, person, and/or place. Deficits in orientation may typically present with memory loss and problems with new learning. Because the strategies for improving orientation must be reinforced with all functional mobility skills throughout the day by the entire rehabilitation team and family, the interventions below are presented in general terms. In addition, much of orientation interventions involve visual/verbal cuing and consistency.

Changing the Task to Achieve Independence

While performing bed mobility tasks, the therapist may informally involve orientation training as well. The session may include discussing the client's daily schedule for sitting up, sitting at the edge of the bed, and eventually getting out of bed for functional ambulation. These routines should be discussed and performed daily within the temporal context to encourage consistency and structure as much as possible, particularly as arousal levels improve. The client's physical context should also be well organized and neatly kept.

For example, the therapist may see the client either before or after breakfast, providing verbal orientation to the time of day as related to the functional mobility task. The method may be changed by asking the client basic orientation questions during the task. As another example, the therapist may progress the client to ambulate to the orientation board in order to read the schedule for the day. This should occur throughout the day with the assistance of staff and family.

Changing the Tools to Achieve Independence

As stated previously, basic orientation tools may begin with only a simple calendar or sign of the day and date. The method may be changed by introducing additional orientation boards as level of arousal improves. The boards may incorporate out-of-bed, functional mobility, and therapy schedules/information.

As the client's participation in therapy improves, additional tools may be added to assist with functional mobility such as a walker basket or a cart on wheels.

Client Factors: Body Functions—Specific Mental Functions

Specific mental functions include attention, memory, perception (visuospatial), thought functions (recognition, categorization, generalization), higher-level cognitive functions (judgment, concept formation, time management, problem solving, decision making), and mental functioning (motor planning, specifically dressing apraxia) (AOTA, 2014).

Attention

Attentional deficits may impact the client's ability to learn new functional mobility skills needed as a result of an illness or injury. For example, after sustaining a CVA, a client who needs to use a hemi-walker must have basic attention skills intact in order to be able to learn with higher-level specific mental functions such as memory and problem solving.

Clients who have conditions that affect attention skills must begin functional mobility training with simple tasks, in a short intervention time, which are adapted with progress. It is important for caregivers to speak simply and slowly and allow for processing time (Zoltan, 2007). In addition, distraction should be kept to a minimum although gradually introduced as the client is ready. The physical context should remain the same until the client demonstrates he or she is ready for generalization and/or gradation.

Changing the Task to Achieve Independence

Intervention may begin with bed mobility, progress to sitting at the bedside, and incorporate simple functional skills as attention skills improve. The client may then progress to standing activities and functional ambulation to the bathroom, closet, kitchen, etc. The client may be encouraged to "talk through" each step of the functional mobility activity. For example, the client may plan out the transfer from bed to chair with/without assistance from the therapist before initiating the activity. Before each step of the activity is performed, the client may describe what he or she is going to do and what the safety issues are. The steps and difficulty of the functional mobility activities may be increased as the client is able to attend to task longer.

Changing the Tools to Achieve Independence

With clients being easily distracted, it is important to keep tools at a minimum and simplified. If needed, an assistive mobility device should be introduced first in order to safely initiate functional mobility. Additional tools such as a walker basket or push cart may be added as appropriate and the client's attention improves.

Memory

There are many types of memory and memory deficits; however, this section will focus specifically on intervention strategies related to functional mobility with an adaptive/compensation approach.

Changing the Task to Achieve Independence

Intervention strategies during functional mobility in general may be adapted by providing the client with a functional mobility schedule. Individuals who have limited carry-over should be involved in developing the schedule.

The client may be assessed on a daily basis for carry-over with the steps of functional mobility tasks, getting to and from specific areas, and safety precautions.

Changing the Tools to Achieve Independence

Cuing tools may be used as a strategy to increase memory through the use of signs to locate the bathroom/bedroom, memory notebooks, and labeling of storage areas. An alarm clock may be set to remind the client of his or her out-of-bed, functional ambulation, and therapy schedules. The client may also be encouraged to wear a watch.

The specific mental functions that are addressed less formally and/or less frequently within intervention plans are presented in Table 3-18. Those that require more detail and attention are discussed separately.

Compensation/Adaptation Interventions of Functional Mobility for Perceptual Deficits

As presented in the AOTA Framework document (2014) perception is listed under client factors/specific mental functions; however, particular perceptual topics are not discussed. The topics chosen for discussion below have been determined from the authors' clinical practice as well as current references, which will be presented throughout.

General compensatory/adaptive strategies that apply to clients diagnosed with perceptual deficits center around safety and environmental context. These general strategies include:

- Maximize safety in all situations. Remove unsafe objects as necessary.
- Educate client and all caregivers regarding functional limitations.
- Practice in a variety of physical contexts.

Visual Fixation/Scanning

Visual fixation involves the voluntary ability to sustain gaze while visually attending to a task or an object in the environment. Scanning allows the eye to follow an object without simultaneous head movement. While saccadic eye movement is typically symmetrical (e.g., reading), scanning

Table 3-18

Specific Mental Functions and Examples of Compensation/Adaptation Strategies

Specific Mental Function Subcategories (AOTA, 2002a)	Examples of Compensation/Adaptation Interventions
Thought Functions	
Recognition	During functional mobility session, items needed for bed-to-chair transfer include assistive device, slippers, and bedside chair. Ask client to locate bathroom during functional mobility.
Generalization	Address functional transfers in a variety of possible situations including chairs with/without arms, a couch, low/high surfaces, and a car. Functional mobility may include ambulating on ramps, stairs, grass, and in crowded/cluttered situations.
Higher-Level Cognitive Functions	
Judgment	Teach client to ask for help when unsure of safety. Ask client open-ended questions in order to think out loud before acting.
Concept formation	Keep a daily progress and achievement chart showing amount of assistance needed for transfers and amount of functional mobility achieved. Mark when goals have been achieved.
Time management	Provide out-of-bed and functional mobility daily schedule to encourage increased activity, particularly for discharge environment.
Problem solving	Ask client to assist with modifying environment for increased safety with functional mobility. Set up possible safety issues and ask client to identify them.
Decision-making	Provide client with two or more options for safe and appropriate decision making, before transferring. Allow client to think out loud and verbally state the safe steps of the transfer.

during functional mobility activities, however, involves less predictable patterns that are more complicated (Zoltan, 2007). The client may have difficulty finding his or her way in the environment (topographical orientation), in particular with this deficit, while performing functional mobility tasks.

Changing the Task to Achieve Independence

Provide cuing as needed. Cuing can be verbal or tactile when guiding the client to anchor the initiation of scanning (from left to right) and when controlling the speed of his or her scanning.

Scanning and anchoring tasks may be incorporated into bed mobility tasks when asking the client to roll and sit on one side of the bed, reach for the bed rail, and locate the assistive device and/or chair needed for the transfer.

During transfer activities, the client may be encouraged to scan a small area for the bedside chair and locate the arms of the chair for reaching back to sit. During functional ambulation, the client may scan the room for safety issues/obstacles, find the bathroom door, toilet/shower, and then head back to the bed or chair.

Table 3-19 Body Scheme Disorders and Examples of Compensation/Adaptation Strategies	
Body Scheme Disorders	**Examples of Compensation/Adaptation Interventions: Task and/or Tools Changed**
Somatognosia	During functional mobility activities, use verbal cues to increase awareness of body parts. For example, ask client to pick up the part of the body that holds onto the hemi-walker.
Unilateral body neglect	Educate client on self-monitoring. For example, before standing, client should check to make sure both feet are in place on the floor and hands are pushing off to stand. A daily checklist may be used.
Right-left discrimination	Adapt instructions during functional ambulation training by using left/right directionality at request of client.

Changing the Tools to Achieve Independence

Brightly colored stickers may be placed to the left of doorways in order for the client to anchor upon it and scan to the right without bumping into the side of the door when walking through. The same system may be used for the shower and toilet areas.

Visual Inattention/Neglect

Visual inattention/neglect is most concerning with functional mobility tasks because the client may be at a high risk for bumping into walls or furniture, falling, and/or injury. For those clients who are unable to become aware of the inattention, the therapist will need to modify and simplify the physical context as much as possible.

Changing the Task to Achieve Independence

During all functional mobility activities, encourage the client to increase visual attention by using his or her head and eyes to locate the bed rail, transfer surfaces, doorways, and assistive device. If needed, encourage the client to turn his or her body, as well. Use tactile and/or verbal cuing to encourage awareness of affected side. For example, as the client is walking through a doorway, touch the client's affected UE while verbally cuing to attend to that side and prevent bumping into the doorway. If the client is unable to become aware of inattention, modify and simplify the physical context as much as possible. Gradually grade the tasks as appropriate (e.g., begin by providing all objects/items within the client's intact visual field and grade).

Changing the Tools to Achieve Independence

Encourage the client to wear a watch on the extremity of the affected side as a reminder to attend to that side and prevent bumping into doorways or walls. Attempt to use a mirror during sit-to-stand transfer activities to increase awareness of the affected side.

Body Scheme

Because there are multiple forms of body scheme disorders, and each one cannot be reviewed individually. For this reason, Table 3-19 identifies the most common forms of body scheme disorders as well as examples of compensatory/adaptive interventions for these.

Table 3-20

Visual Discrimination and Examples of Compensation/Adaptation Strategies

Visual Discrimination Disorder	Examples of Compensation/Adaptation Interventions: Task and/or Tools Changed
Depth perception	Adapt the environment by placing neon-colored tape at the edge of stairs and doorknobs.
Figure ground perception	Adapt functional mobility environment to increase cognitive awareness by carefully organizing items in a non-cluttered area. Adapt wheelchair brakes with neon stickers (Zoltan, 2007).
Spatial relations	Store assistive device and other needed items in a consistent manner.
Topographical orientation	Adapt functional mobility environment through the use of easy to read signs, pictures, and familiar landmarks.

Visual Discrimination

Visual discrimination involves the ability to distinguish between various objects or forms in relation to the environment (Zoltan, 2007). Because there are multiple forms of visual discrimination disorders, each one cannot be reviewed individually. For this reason, Table 3-20 identifies the most common forms of visual discrimination disorders as well as examples of compensatory/adaptive interventions for these.

Motor Planning

Motor planning issues may occur in relation to functional mobility with or without the use of assistive devices (tools). The client may have difficulty recognizing that assistive devices are used for functional mobility, even after instruction. In general, clients may also have difficulty negotiating each step involved with functional mobility. In addition, the client with motor planning deficits may present with difficulty following verbal directions when ambulating, which appears to be related to topographical orientation.

Changing the Task to Achieve Independence

- General interventions with all types of functional mobility: The therapist should attempt transfers in several ways. First, the client should be given simple verbal directions with minimal steps involved. If verbal cues are not successful, then tactile cuing may be attempted. The methods may be graded by increasing/decreasing the amount of cuing and steps of the directions involved.

  For deficits that resemble topographical disorientation, the environment may be adapted by simplifying cues for motor planning. For example, simple written cues posted for the client directing him or her toward the bathroom, stairs, chair, etc., may be provided. When supervised, the client may be given simple verbal commands or tactile cues in order to better negotiate the environment.

- Example with transfers from bed to chair with walker: The simplest method with apraxia may be a verbal command that briefly tells the client, "Please go to the chair." A more difficult two-step command may be to say, "Please get out of bed and sit in the chair." Because of physical limitations, the client may not be able to complete the task without the involvement of new learning. For example, if the client has a flaccid LE and UE on the right side, the command of "please go to the chair" will involve much more than it used to. Of course, the client will now need to learn how to negotiate right-sided flaccidity. The next method may be to attempt tactile cuing and physical assistance from the therapist, which is graded based on capabilities (refer to information on transfers in this chapter).
- Example with ambulation to the bathroom with walker: The simplest method may be, again, to ask the client to walk to the bathroom. The therapist would place the walker in front of the client and wait to see if the client will be able to use it appropriately (see below). If the client does not initiate proper use of the walker, the therapist may attempt very simple verbal or tactile commands, as well as demonstration.

Changing the Tools to Achieve Independence

- General interventions for all types of functional mobility: Typically, the use of assistive devices may further confuse a client with apraxia, particularly if ideational apraxia is evident, which affects the ability to use tools. Usually, in terms of functional mobility, clients cannot safely perform tasks without the assistance of a walker, hemi-walker, cane, etc. This poses a significant challenge for the client who requires additional assistance secondary to balance and/or physical limitations, for example. Often, if two individuals are available, the client may do well with handheld assist. This offers the client tactile cuing as well as the guidance and support that may be needed with apraxia, as well as physical challenges.

Compensation/Adaptation Interventions of Functional Mobility for Vision

General Functional Mobility Strategies

- Maximize safety in all situations.
- Educate client and all caregivers regarding functional limitations.
- Practice strategies and adaptations in many possible environments and situations.
- Decrease clutter in environment.
- Use automatic, motion-controlled lighting.
- Control the amount of natural light in environment, as able, in order to decrease glare.
- Provide cuing, as needed.
- Use contrast whenever possible, for example:
  - Use markers on stairs.
  - Place neon-colored stickers on handrail, water knobs (hot, in particular), light switches, and door handles.
  - Use colored toilet seat for contrast.
- Organize belongings in a systematic, predictable routine in order to locate them easily on a daily basis. For example, store bathroom items at a level within safe reach.

- Install carpeting in bathroom to prevent slippage and use bath mat.
- Install grab bars in tub/shower.

Low Vision

When addressing low vision (visual acuity) with a compensation/adaptive approach, the focus is primarily on changing the task within the clients' environment or physical contexts. Again, safety is the priority when considering the client's needs. The occupational therapist may need to refer to a low-vision specialist in order to more specifically train the client on community functional mobility skills.

Changing the Task to Achieve Independence

Maximize contrast as able, as demonstrated in the examples that follow.

- Functional mobility example: When ambulating in the bathroom and bedroom, encourage the client to use a systematic approach when moving in the environment. For example, the client should follow contrast on walls and flooring to maneuver in the environment in the same manner on each attempt.
- Transfer example: When transferring, use a systematic routine for organizing the environment and all transfer surfaces before moving.

Changing the Tools to Achieve Independence

- Adapting walker: Place bright yellow tennis balls or large neon stickers on the bottom of the walker legs in order for the client to easily identify where the walker ends and the floor begins.
- Adapting wheelchair controls: Paint wheelchair brakes and wheels with neon colors.
- Adapting doorknobs: Place neon-colored felt around doorknobs or stickers in the middle of the doorknob.

Visual Field Deficits

Visual fields are the areas of vision that are seen without movement of the eyes or head. Deficits may present on one side of the visual field in one or both eyes (Jacobs & Simon, 2015). Functional mobility is especially challenging for these clients, and all training must consider client safety.

Changing the Task to Achieve Independence

- Functional mobility example: Provide client and caregivers with strategies for cuing the client into affected visual fields in order to prevent bumping into walls, furniture, or doors. Provide supervision during functional mobility whenever safety is not ensured.
- Transferring example: Teach client strategies for locating the transferring surface(s) safely (e.g., remembering to reach back with both hands when sitting).

Changing the Tools to Achieve Independence

During functional mobility, provide all required tools/items with client's intact visual field as in the following examples.

- Transferring example: For a client with a left-field cut, transfer to the right side whenever possible.
- Functional mobility example: For a client with a left-field cut, when turning around during ambulation, encourage the client to turn to the right side.

- Wheelchair mobility: For a client with a left-field cut, encourage the client to stay on the right side of the hallway.

Maintenance for Functional Mobility

Positioning

Proper positioning is a continuous process that is necessary for the skin and joint integrity of all clients, as well as comfort. In addition, good positioning is vital for safe eating/feeding, most functional activities, eye contact, and effective communication. Although positioning is, of course, used with clients who are receiving rehabilitative occupational therapy services, it has been organized under maintenance as it often must or should be implemented long-term.

When considering positioning techniques and use of positioning tools (e.g., pillows, towel rolls, and bolsters), the individual needs of each client must be evaluated. Special attention must be given to clients with decreased/loss of sensation, paralysis, impaired skin integrity, poor nutrition, impaired circulation, and risk of contractures. For example, the therapist must observe areas were bony prominences may be experiencing pressure, causing redness, skin breakdown, eventual ischemia, and necrosis. Protective positioning restraints such as wrist straps should be used only on a short-term basis because their use may cause skin breakdown as well (Fairchild, 2013).

In general, positioning techniques should begin proximally because these techniques may influence the distal musculature (Schell, Gillen, & Scaffa, 2014). For example, tone may be decreased in the distal extremity after positioning the UE properly. Caution should be taken when considering the placement of a pillow under the knee because the position may cause an eventual flexion contracture or deep vein thrombosis (Schell et al., 2014).

Positioning schedules typically require the client's position to be changed approximately every 2 hours in order to prevent skin breakdown. Positions that provide weight-bearing into the involved extremity may assist with normalizing tone and enhance sensory awareness.

Purpose of Proper Positioning

According to Fairchild, the following are specific purposes of proper positioning:

- Prevent contractures and soft tissue injury
- Provide comfort
- Support and stabilize the client
- Allow for efficient function of organ systems
- Provide relief of prolonged pressure through position changes (2013)

In addition, proper positioning allows for greater client interaction with the environment and greater participation in functional activities. Once a decubiti is formed, the client is often restricted in activity, which further emphasizes the importance of proper positioning, either in bed or in a chair. The typical bony prominences that are at risk for pressure ulcers are listed in Table 3-21. When positioning clients, certain precautions should be followed. According to Fairchild (2013), these include the following:

- Observe the skin color.
- Protect the bony prominences listed in Table 3-21.
- Avoid excessive pressure to soft tissue and circulatory or neurological areas.
- Be aware of the special needs of clients with decreased mental status, decreased level of alertness, the frail elderly, individuals with paralysis, individuals with impaired circulation, and individuals with decreased sensation.

Table 3-21

Bony Prominences

Supine	Side-Lying	Sitting
Occipital tuberosity	Lateral ear	Ischial tuberosity
Spine of the scapula	Lateral ribs	Scapular/vertebral prominences
Inferior angle of the scapula	Lateral acromion process	Medial epicondyle of humerus
Spinous processes of vertebrae	Lateral head of humerus	
Posterior iliac crest	Medial/lateral epicondyle of humerus	
Sacrum	Greater trochanter of femur	
Medial epicondyle of humerus	Medial/lateral condyle of femur	
Posterior calcaneus	Malleolus	
Greater trochanter and head of fibula		

Adapted from Pierson, F. M. (1999). *Principles and techniques of patient care* (2nd ed.). Philadelphia, PA: W.B. Saunders.

Table 3-22

Positioning Lying on the Involved Side

The Involved Side	The Uninvolved Side
• Scapular protraction • Shoulder flexion to 90 degrees • Hip flexion • Shoulder external rotation • Full elbow extension • Neutral hip • Slight knee flexion	• Upper extremity positioned alongside the trunk and hip • Knee flexion • The hip and knee are supported with a pilw between them and the involved LE • An additional pillow is placed along the client's back in order to maintain the position

Adapted from Crepeau, E. B., Cohn, E. S., & Schell, B. A. B. (2003). *Willard and Spackman's occupational therapy for physical dysfunction* (10th ed.). Philadelphia, PA: Lippincott Williams & Wilkins.

Positioning in Bed

The typical bed positions include side-lying on the involved side, side-lying on the uninvolved side, and lying supine.

Ideal positioning for the client lying on the involved side is described in Table 3-22 and is depicted in Figure 3-32. These are general guidelines and may need to be adapted for particular clients.

Ideal positioning for the client lying on the uninvolved side is toward prone and is described in Table 3-23 and depicted in Figure 3-33. These are general guidelines and may need to be adapted for particular clients.

Ideal positioning for the client in supine position is described below and depicted in Figure 3-34. These are general guidelines and may need to be adapted to particular clients.

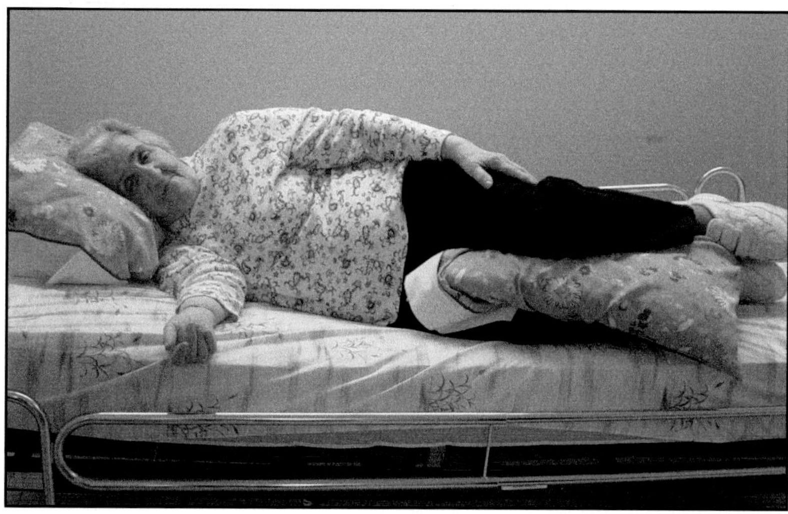

Figure 3-32. Client lying on the involved side.

Table 3-23
Positioning Lying on the Uninvolved Side

Involved Side	Uninvolved Side
• Entire UE supported on a pillow • Scapular protraction • Shoulder flexion to 90 degrees • Elbow flexion up to 90 degrees • Full wrist and finger extension • The hip and knee flexed to 45 degrees • LE supported on a pillow	• UE positioned under a pillow supporting involved UE • LE in slight hip/knee flexion

Adapted from Crepeau, E. B., Cohn, E. S., & Schell, B. A. B. (2003). *Willard and Spackman's occupational therapy for physical dysfunction* (10th ed.). Philadelphia, PA: Lippincott Williams & Wilkins.

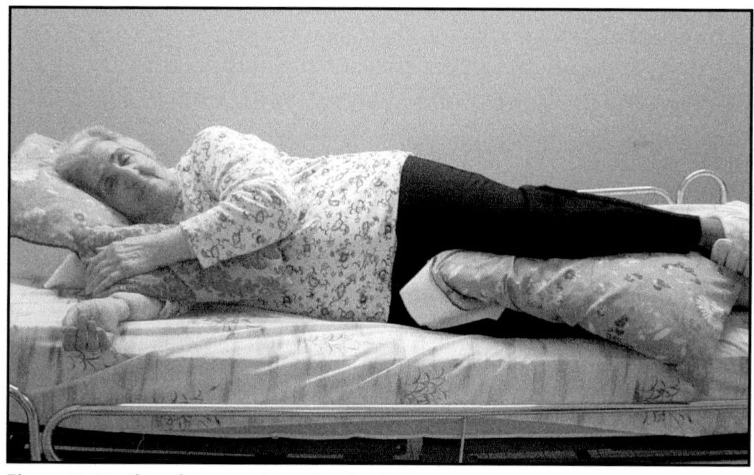

Figure 3-33. Client lying on the uninvolved side.

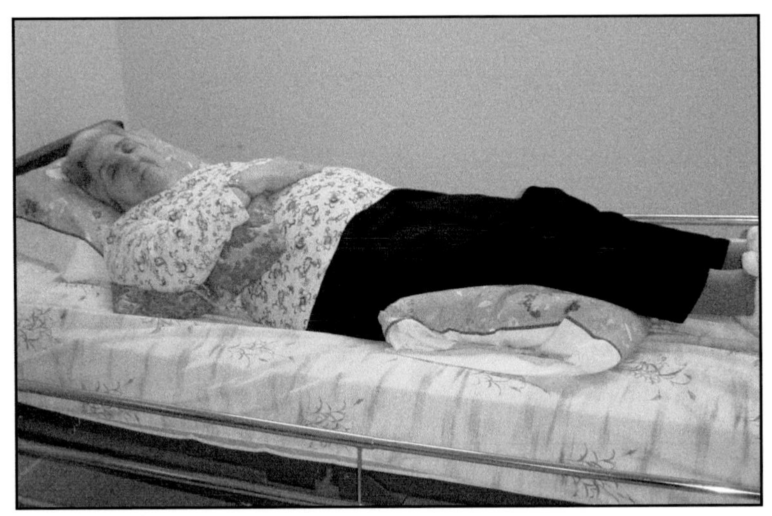

Figure 3-34. Client lying in supine position.

- A pillow positioned under client's involved scapula and hip
- Involved scapula and hip in slight protraction
- Involved shoulder in slight abduction and external rotation
- Involved elbow flexed, wrist and fingers in extension
- Involved hip and knee slightly flexed and positioned in midline

Sitting

Goal setting considerations for sitting should involve the client's medical/physiological status, function and lifestyle, and ultimate goals. Medical considerations include potential for developing contractures, organ function, soft-tissue integrity, and pain/discomfort levels. Functional considerations include the client's tolerance for activity, level of independence, motor control, and communication abilities. Personal and lifestyle considerations may include community involvement and mobility, client roles, environmental issues, and mobility in the home.

Considerations with sitting include promoting trunk stability in an upright midline position while allowing for mobility of the extremities and interaction with the environment. Further considerations include the type of chair chosen. The amount of support given by the chair includes the type of seating surface. For example, special seat cushions are available to prevent skin breakdown for clients with long-term needs. Firm cushions are typically used for prevention of internal hip rotation while in the chair, assisting with trunk stability and support by properly positioning the back and UEs and providing support for sitting balance. Lumbar supports promote anterior pelvic tilt when needed. Proper positioning of the LE includes the hips, knees, and ankles in 90 degrees of flexion when sitting.

Foot stools, adjustable leg rests, wedge cushions, lap boards, adjustable armrests, and straps may be used to enhance symmetrical and supported sitting positions.

Positioning for the Client With a Neurological Injury/Illness

Proper positioning of the client should begin immediately, with all team members and caregivers educated and involved with this process. For example, a client with hemiplegia who initially presents with flaccidity of the involved extremities should be positioned preventing an eventual flexor synergy of hip, which includes external rotation, abduction, and knee flexion. Proper positioning is typically in the opposite pattern of the synergy, although each client must be considered individually. Therefore, positioning a client with a flexor synergy includes knee extension and lateral support of the LE with a pillow or rolled blanket to prevent hip abduction and external rotation.

Extensor synergy occurs when the later stages of hemiplegia cause spasticity of the extensor muscles, which are stronger than the flexors in the affected extremity (Radomski & Latham, 2014). The extensor synergy includes extension and adduction at the hip, knee extension, and ankle plantar flexion. Recommended bed positioning for a client with extensor synergy includes lying supine with slight hip and knee flexion, which may be maintained with a towel roll or small pillow under the knee. In order to prevent adduction and internal rotation, a pillow or rolled blanket may be used to provide medial support between the LEs. While in the supine position, ankle plantar flexion must be prevented through the use of multi-podus boots. Further ankle plantar flexion may be prevented by not allowing tight-fitted sheets/blankets to pull the feet into this position. The affected UE should be positioned to prevent shoulder subluxation, soft-tissue contractures, decreased ROM, and spasticity/flexor synergy resulting in general decreased function. The following positions should be avoided: prolonged shoulder adduction and internal rotation; elbow flexion; supination or pronation; wrist, finger, or thumb flexion; and finger/thumb adduction. Therefore, proper positioning of the affected extremity includes shoulder abduction, external rotation, elbow extension, neutral forearm rotation, slight wrist extension, thumb abduction and extension, finger extension, and slight abduction, all in varying amounts (Fairchild, 2013).

Changing the Tools to Achieve Independence

Positioning may be provided with a pillow, small bolster, rolled towel/blanket, lap tray, or arm trough. The unaffected UE may also assist with positioning, particularly with maintaining the affected extremity in midline.

Caution should also be used with static positioning for long periods of time. Proper positioning and position changes should be alternated with regular ROM and self-ROM exercises (refer to Chapter 2).

Positioning for the Client With a Total Hip Replacement

Precautions With Total Hip Replacement

Position the client in slight hip abduction from midline and neutral rotation. Hip adduction should not be beyond the midline of the body (e.g., do not cross legs). ADL activities with this motion may include crossing legs to don socks and shoes. The listing below describes proper positioning/precautions for clients with THR (Fairchild, 2013).

1. The affected hip should not be extended beyond neutral.
2. While in side-lying, the affected hip should maintain abduction and neutral rotation. The client should be positioned with the affected LE on top of the nonaffected extremity with pillows or a bolster supporting and maintaining the position.
3. Anterior or anterior-lateral approaches must not externally rotate the hip.
4. Posterior or posterior-lateral approaches must not internally rotate the hip.
5. Activities that involve rotation or twisting of the trunk with the LEs fixed must be avoided because these motions involve hip rotation (e.g., standing from the toilet and rotating the trunk around to one side in order to flush).

6. Do not flex the affected hip beyond 90 degrees with a posterior or posterior-lateral approach (e.g., when sitting on the toilet, a raised toilet seat is necessary to avoid 90 degrees of hip flexion).

Additional Precautions With Positioning and Functional Mobility for Total Hip Replacement

- Lying: The client should primarily lie supine while sleeping or resting with a pillow positioned between both UEs, above the knees, to prevent hip adduction. If the client needs to position in side-lying, a pillow should also be placed between the LEs, above the knees.
- Transfers: Scoot to the edge of the bed or chair before standing. Position the affected LE in front of the other when standing from bed or chair. Avoid low surfaces.
- Sitting: Chairs should be higher than knee height and have a firm sitting surface, a straight back, and armrests. Avoid soft chairs, rocking chairs, sofas, and stools. Reclining wheelchairs will accommodate hip precautions by adjusting the backrest.
- Ambulation: Wear well-fitting, supportive, nonskid shoes. Avoid uneven surfaces as able. Follow weight-bearing status. Avoid pivoting on the affected LE. Take small steps when turning.
- Toileting: Use a raised toilet seat or seat above knee height. Avoid twisting for personal hygiene.
- Bathing: Avoid bending or reaching for items, tub controls, etc. Avoid bending or squatting to bathe the LE. Use a long-handled sponge and reacher instead.
- Dressing: Avoid bending over, raising LEs, or crossing legs. Remain seated when donning clothes over feet. Use long-handled devices such as a reacher, dressing stick, and long-handled shoe horn. Use slip-ons or shoes that close with hook-and-loop fasteners or elastic shoelaces.
- Car transfers: Avoid entering the car while standing on a curb or step. Avoid cars with deep or low seats. Use a pillow to raise seat heights.

Issues With Positioning Clients With Rheumatoid Arthritis

Because rheumatoid arthritis is a systemic disease that involves the musculoskeletal system—specifically the joints—prolonged immobilization or positioning should be avoided in order to prevent contractures. Gentle active and passive ROM of involved and uninvolved joints should be performed, as tolerated, on a regular basis. When rheumatoid arthritis is in an exacerbated stage of acute inflammation, extra caution should be taken. Refer to Tables 3-13 through 3-15 for general positioning techniques (Fairchild, 2013).

Issues With Positioning Clients With Burns

Positioning issues with burns include healing of skin, scar tissue development, contractures, and pain. Prolonged immobilization or positioning of affected joints should be avoided, particularly in the "position of comfort." Examples of the position of comfort are prolonged flexion or adduction positions involving the least amount of stress on the burn site or graft. Splinting is the primary positioning technique for burned extremities. Refer to Tables 3-13 through 3-15 for general positioning techniques (Fairchild, 2013).

Issues With Positioning Clients With Amputations

For clients with an above-the-knee amputation, the following positions should be limited or avoided due to risk of contracture of the hip flexor musculature: prolonged hip flexion, elevation of residual limb on a pillow while supine, and sitting limited to 30 minutes at a time. Hip abduction of the residual limb should be avoided to prevent contracture of these muscles. The client should position the pelvis level in order to maintain trunk alignment while supine. This position will also help to prevent back pain and postural issues. When standing, the client should position the residual limb in extension. Occasional prone-lying is recommended to encourage hip and residual limb extension.

Clients with a below-the-knee amputation should avoid the following positions in order to avoid the risk of contractures: prolonged hip and knee flexion and elevation of the residual limb on a pillow while the client is supine. When the residual limb is elevated, the knee should be positioned in extension. The client should not sit longer than 30 minutes at a time in order to decrease the risk of hip flexor and knee contractures. Whenever the client is supine, sitting, or standing, the knee should be positioned in extension. Again, prone-lying is recommended to encourage extension of the residual limb (Fairchild, 2013).

The risk of contracture of the residual limb musculature will limit the client's ability to be fit with and use a prosthetic device; therefore, proper positioning is essential. Refer to Tables 3-13 through 3-15 for general positioning techniques.

Activities of Daily Living: Eating/Dysphagia

Introduction

Before reading this section, it is important to note that the information provided in this text regarding eating/dysphagia is considered entry-level. According to AOTA (2014a), advanced skills are necessary for the occupational therapist to use various assessment or intervention tools safely, such as videofluoroscopic swallowing studies, videoendoscopy, fiberoptic endoscopic assessments, ultrasound, electromyography, and biofeedback. In addition, certain conditions typically require advanced skills, such as for clients with tracheotomies and laryngectomies. The advanced skill levels, which will not be addressed in this text, should build upon the entry-level skills as presented in depth throughout this section. For more information and training regarding advanced skills in eating/dysphagia interventions, refer to the resources provided in Appendix A.

Definitions

AOTA (2014, p. 632) defines swallowing/eating as "keeping and manipulating food/fluid in the mouth and swallowing it." Thus, eating is the ADL skill that is evaluated by the occupational therapist. The deficit that is addressed as a result of difficulty with eating isdysphagia. Dysphagia includes all the stages of swallowing, which will be discussed in depth below. Feeding (as discussed earlier in this chapter) is a distinctly different ADL skill and is defined by AOTA (2014, p. S19) as "bringing food from the plate or cup to the mouth." The difference is that dysphagia intervention addresses oral-motor deficits, whereas feeding intervention addresses the actual skill of feeding oneself. It is common, however, to find deficits in both eating and feeding (AOTA, 2014).

Role of the Occupational Therapist and Occupational Therapy Assistant

Because eating is a basic human need, it is a primary focus of evaluation and intervention of ADLs. According to AOTA, "Both occupational therapist and occupational therapy assistants provide essential services in the comprehensive management of feeding, eating, and swallowing problems" (2014a, pg. 273). Academic institutions provide the basic, entry-level knowledge of eating and feeding issues. The entry-level practitioner may then choose to progress his or her skills to an advanced level while working under the supervision of a therapist experienced in dysphagia.

The role of the occupational therapist is as a dysphagia clinician: performing screenings, assessments, consulting, recommending, reporting, and carrying out the intervention program (AOTA, 2014a). The occupational therapy assistant, under the supervision of the occupational therapist, may contribute to and implement the intervention plan (AOTA, 2014a). For specific details of entry-level and advanced-level knowledge and skills for eating and feeding, refer "Specialized knowledge and skills in eating and feeding for occupational therapy practice" in AOTA (2014a).

Typical Diagnoses Seen With Dysphagia

- Cerebral vascular accidents
- Brain injuries
- Alzheimer's disease
- Huntington's disease
- Brain tumors
- Parkinson's disease
- Multiple sclerosis
- Myasthenia gravis
- Amyotrophic lateral sclerosis
- Developmental disorders
- Guillain-Barré syndrome
- Spinal cord injury
- Pneumonia
- HIV/AIDS
- Facial nerve paralysis
- Head, neck, and oral cancers, as well as the side effects of chemotherapy and/or radiation therapy
- Laryngectomy
- Respiratory issues
- Burns
- Chronic obstructive pulmonary disease
- Nasogastric tubes
- Tracheostomy

- Prolonged mechanical ventilation
- Psychiatric disorders (AOTA, 2010)

Signs and Symptoms of Dysphagia

- Labored breathing/rales
- A wet, "gurgly" voice
- Aspiration
- Pocketing of food
- Coughing while eating/drinking
- Nasal regurgitation
- Rejection of food
- Sensory issues with food
- Open mouth posture
- Drooling
- Increased eating time (chewing and/or swallowing)
- Poor laryngeal elevation
- Poor tongue movement
- Complaints of food stuck in throat
- Painful swallow (Logemann, 1998)

Dysphagia Team

The management of clients with dysphagia is often handled by a multidisciplinary team. Each member of the dysphagia team offers a specific expertise, whether it be in an acute/subacute care, skilled nursing, or home care environment. In addition to the occupational therapist, team members include the following:

- Speech-language pathologist: occupational therapists and speech-language pathologists often work together providing dysphagia evaluation and interventions. In addition, the speech-language pathologist will offer interventions for voice, communication, and cognitive deficits, as appropriate.
- Dietitian: The dietitian's responsibilities include making sure the nutritional and fluid needs of the clients are met. The dietician also creates dysphagia diet levels.
- Physician: The physician determines the diagnosis and writes the referrals for dysphagia evaluations and interventions, specialty referrals, and medications.
- Radiologist: The radiologist conducts and analyzes assessments, which may include video-fluoroscopy and ultrasound.
- Nurse: In addition to providing daily mealtime care for the client, the nurse observes for signs/symptoms of dysphagia and reports information about the client's status to the team.
- Respiratory therapist: The respiratory therapist monitors the client's respiratory status in order to assure that the client's airway and breathing are optimal for eating. This may include clients who are ventilator-dependent or those with tracheotomies.

- Others: Practitioners of other disciplines who may consult with the dysphagia team include physical therapists, pharmacists, dentists, social workers, pulmonologists, and gerontologists.

Phases of the Swallowing Process and Related Deficits

The phases of the swallowing process are the pre-oral phase, oral preparatory phase, oral phase, pharyngeal phase, and esophageal phase. Dysphagia may occur in one or more phases of the swallowing process. The first three phases are assessed through a dysphagia evaluation, while the pharyngeal and esophageal phases are assessed via a modified barium swallow (Avery-Smith, 2003). A basic description of each phase and skills required are as follows:

- Pre-oral phase: The phase of eating when food/fluid is brought to the mouth. This process includes the skills of feeding as well as preparing for the next phases of the swallow (Logemann, 1998).
- Oral preparatory phase: The phase of eating when food is manipulated by the lips, cheeks, tongue, and jaw into a bolus that prepares the food for a safe swallow. Motor as well as sensory (taste, primarily) skills are required at this phase (Logemann, 1998).
- Oral phase: The phase of eating in which the bolus is propelled to the base of the tongue in order to swallow. Skills required include sensation, motor planning, sufficient tongue tone, movement, and coordination. The normal timing of this phase is between 1.0 to 1.5 seconds, after which the phase is considered to have a delay (Logemann, 1998).
- Pharyngeal phase: The phase of eating whereby the swallow is further triggered and initiated. Skills required include proper tongue base movement, closure of the soft palate, bilateral pharyngeal strength, sufficient laryngeal elevation, and sufficient airway closure during the swallow to prevent aspiration. This phase should last less than 1 second (Logemann, 1998).
- Esophageal phase: The phase of eating when the bolus moves from the esophagus into the stomach (Logemann, 1998). Skills required include sufficient esophageal function and motility.

Remediation of Eating/Dysphagia

While the majority of this text discusses adaptation/compensation, remediation will be discussed in this section of eating/dysphagia because both approaches are closely tied to this skill.

Avery-Smith (AOTA, 2010) categorizes remedial eating techniques as indirect interventions related to client factors that may not involve actual eating. These interventions are focused on facilitating and improving the swallow and include range of motion, strength, hypersensitivity, hyposensitivity, and changes in tone, reflexes, and the swallow. Other practitioners have separated interventions into two categories. The first is direct intervention, such as swallowing methods and stimulation of structures. The second is indirect, such as thicker liquids or diet changes (Gupta & Banerjee, 2014).

Decreased Range of Motion

Exercises include passive, active-assisted, active ROM, and self-ROM of the tongue, lips, and cheek. Typically passive ROM may be performed with gloved fingers or the back of a spoon. In addition, laryngeal elevation may be completed by facilitating the Adam's apple into an upward/downward movement. Self-ROM may be performed as a passive or active-assisted form of exercise, as above. Active ROM may be performed in conjunction with passive ROM (as voluntary motion improves) or in isolation. Oral-motor ROM exercises include the following (AOTA, 2010):

- Lip pursing
- Smiling (lip retraction)
- Tongue protrusion/retraction
- Tongue lateralization
- Jaw lateralization

Decreased Oral-Motor Strength

Oral-motor strengthening exercises may be an added intervention as active ROM increases. Decreased oral-motor strength involves resistance applied with fingers or a tongue depressor to the movements as listed in ROM. In addition, lip, cheek, breath, and oral strength may be increased through sucking and blowing exercises using items such as the following (AOTA, 2010):

- Sucking on a straw
- Holding a tongue depressor between the lips
- Popsicles
- Lollipops
- Chewing gum

  Strengthening of pharyngeal and laryngeal movements may also include exercises that facilitate tongue retraction, such as yawning and gargling. In addition, asking the client to raise his or her voice when talking or throat clearing on a regular basis may also increase pharyngeal and laryngeal strength. Note: Contraindications for oral-motor strengthening/resistance may include conditions such as amyotrophic lateral sclerosis and myasthenia gravis because further weakness may be promoted. In addition, it is important to use care with the above tools to prevent aspiration (AOTA, 2010; Avery-Smith, 2003).

- Hypersensitivity: The primary remedial intervention technique for facial and oral hypersensitivity is graded desensitization. Each client will be sensitive to his or her own individual textures, although typically firm textures are most tolerable. Therefore, desensitization techniques should begin with firm textures to the least sensitive areas of the face and/or mouth. Firm textures may include metal utensils, a tongue depressor, or a laryngeal mirror. Grading desensitization to lighter textures will include items such as a gloved finger, toothbrush, disposable oral swabs, and plastic utensils (AOTA, 2010).
- Hyposensitivity: Sensory re-education and sensory stimulation programs are the primary remedial intervention techniques for hyposensitivity. Sensory re-education involves the use of familiar oral-motor objects such as utensils, a toothbrush, and hot/cold items that the client attempts to identify. Examples of sensory stimulation items include the use of a small vibrator, electric toothbrush, popsicles, or ice chips.
- Low tone: Increased tone may be facilitated using techniques such as a small vibrator, electric toothbrush, or a chilled laryngeal mirror applied to the cheeks, lip, and/or oral cavity. Quick stretching may also be used as a facilitation technique.
- High tone: The first remedial attempt at decreasing oral-motor tone should be proper positioning (refer to section on positioning). New techniques and materials should be gradually introduced in order to prevent anxiety, which may further increase tone. In addition, slow passive stretching of the head, neck, and oral-motor area typically decreases tone.

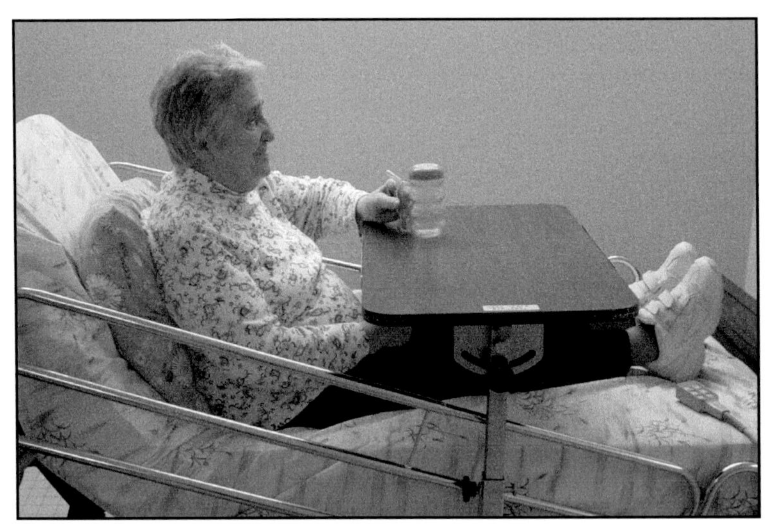

Figure 3-35. Example of proper upright posture at bed level for eating.

- Abnormal reflexes: Once again, proper upright positioning should be the first remedial intervention performed to decrease abnormal reflexes. Items or strategies that promote these reflexes should be avoided. For example, to prevent tonic bite, a metal utensil should not touch the client's teeth (AOTA, 2010; Avery-Smith, 2003).
- Decreased initiation of the swallow: A remedial technique intended to stimulate the swallow is performed with a chilled laryngeal mirror. The faucial pillars are stimulated by the mirror and then the client is asked to dry swallow, and when ready, attempt a specific texture of food or liquid (AOTA, 2010; Avery-Smith, 2003).

Compensation/Adaptation of Eating Deficits/Dysphagia for Clients with Physical Limitations: Performance Skills/Client Factors

Avery-Smith (AOTA, 2010) categorizes the specific process of eating food as direct intervention for dysphagia. Therefore, the actual functional skills involved with eating/dysphagia will be addressed in this compensation/adaptation section. Motor skill deficits and body function limitations may cause choking, malnutrition, dehydration, and eventual aspiration. Prior to addressing dysphagia deficits, the occupational therapist should evaluate the client's ability to sit upright in order to increase safety during eating. See Figure 3-35 for an example of proper upright positioning while eating at bed level. Physical deficits, however, are not the only consideration with dysphagia.

Eating, as a basic human need and satisfaction involves performance patterns such as habits and routines. For example, we often set our clocks by when the next meal will be. The cultural context of eating is also an important consideration when working with clients who have eating dysfunction or dysphagia. For example, many cultures have family gatherings at the Sunday afternoon meal. A client diagnosed with dysphagia who is recommended to be NPO (nothing by mouth) and given a nasogastric or gastric tube can no longer normally engage in these lifelong performance patterns.

In terms of activity demands, eating involves many social experiences. Most of our social activities involve eating, which may cause a client who is NPO to be isolated and embarrassed in these situations. Therefore, while the occupational therapist is facilitating safe and effective

Table 3-24 Diet Levels	
NPO: Nothing by mouth	Secondary to high aspiration risk and/or significant safety issues with eating, it is recommended that the client have an "alternative method of nutrition."
Level 1 Diet: Pureed Diet	The consistency of this diet is similar to pudding, requiring little to no chewing and easy to swallow. Other examples include: mashed potatoes, cottage cheese, nectars, thick milkshakes, sherbet, yogurt, and custard (Dorner, 2002; Jackson Siegelbaum Gastroenterology, 2002).
Level 2 Diet: Mechanical Soft Diet	The consistency of this diet is ground, moist, and semisolid. Dry foods such as crackers and bread are avoided. Appropriate foods should form into a cohesive bolus. Other examples include: ground meats, potatoes, cooked vegetables, canned fruit, scrambled eggs, ripe bananas, and cooked cereals (Dorner, 2002; Jackson Siegelbaum Gastroenterology, 2002).
Level 3 Diet: Advanced Diet	The consistency of this diet is considered soft-solid requiring increased ability to chew. Food is chopped into bite-sized servings. Avoid foods that are dry, sticky, or crunchy. Examples of included foods are chopped meats, potatoes, canned fruit, and cooked vegetables. Soft breads may be allowed (Dorner, 2002; Jackson Siegelbaum Gastroenterology, 2002).
Level 4: Regular Diet	All consistencies allowed.

compensation/adaptations for the physical aspects of dysphagia, he or she should also consider the social, emotional, and cultural impacts of this condition.

Compensation/Adaptation Interventions of Eating Deficits/Dysphagia for Range of Motion, Strength, and Coordination Deficits

ROM, strength, and coordination limitations will impact the client's ability to eat safely without aspiration. Typically, a client with dysphagia will be on an adapted diet, depending on the motor skill or body function limitations. The dysphagia evaluation and modified barium swallow/videoflouroscopy, as appropriate, will help the occupational therapist when recommending a safe diet level for the client.

Diet Levels

The National Dysphagia Diet Task Force (McCullough, Pelletier, & Steel, 2003) has developed national standards for food and fluid consistencies for dysphagia intervention. The four food consistency levels are described in Table 3-24, and fluid consistencies are described in Table 3-25. There are a number of foods that Groher (1997) states are best to avoid when working with clients who are experiencing dysphagia. These are the following:

- Mashed potatoes
- Crackers
- Onions
- Carbonated beverages

Table 3-25 Diet Consistencies for Fluids	
Thick liquids (spoon-thick liquids)	Liquids are thickened to a puree or pudding consistency.* Refer to pureed diet level for examples (Jackson Siegelbaum Gastroenterology, 2002; Dorner, 2002).
Honey consistency liquids	Liquids are thickened to a honey consistency.* (Jackson Siegelbaum Gastroenterology, 2002; Dorner, 2002).
Nectar consistency liquids (medium consistency)	Liquids are thickened to a nectar consistency.* Examples of this consistency are eggnog, nectars, tomato juice, and milk shakes. (Jackson Siegelbaum Gastroenterology, 2002; Dorner, 2002).
Thin liquids	Typical consistency of liquids with no modifications required.

*Commercial thickening agents include Thick n Easy (American International Products, Inc) and Thick-it (Milani Foods, Inc).

- Plums
- Prunes
- Any sticky boluses
- Any boluses that fall apart easily
- Dry boluses
- Mucus producers

With most dysphagia conditions, it is advised to crush medications if possible in applesauce, jelly, custard, or gelatin.

The following section lists ROM, strengthening, and coordination adaptations/compensations for clients with dysphagia.

Changing the Task to Achieve Independence

- Attempt modified swallowing techniques to prevent aspiration, such as chin tuck, head rotation, double swallows, supraglottic swallow (the client holds his or her breath while swallowing and coughs before letting out the breath), and super-supraglottic swallow (the client holds his or her breath, bears down hard, swallows, and coughs after swallowing). Contraindications to the latter two techniques are cardiac or high blood pressure conditions (AOTA, 2010; Logemann, 1998).
- Ask the client to rotate the head and neck toward the affected side when swallowing in order to close off the weak side of the pharynx. This technique allows the unaffected side to propel the bolus and prevents pooling or aspiration (AOTA 2010).
- Ask the client to tuck his or her chin to the chest while swallowing in order to decrease the risk of aspiration with a weak swallow (AOTA, 2010; Logemann, 1998).
- Ask the client to perform "effortful" swallows or swallow hard in order to decrease the risk of accumulating oral residue (AOTA, 2010).
- The Mendelsohn maneuver involves asking the client to hold the tongue into the hard palate while attempting to maintain elevation of the larynx during the swallow (AOTA, 2010; Logemann, 1998).

- Clients with unilateral pharynx weakness may attempt eating in side-lying on the non-affected side if the above techniques fail, as appropriate (AOTA, 2010).
- If a facial droop is present, ask the client to hold the affected side of the lips closed during the oral and swallowing stages to decrease risk of food loss (AOTA, 2010; Logemann, 1998).
- Ask the client to concentrate chewing on the affected side (AOTA, 2010).
- If pocketing of food is a problem, ask the client to sweep his or her cheek(s) with the tongue and/or massage the outside of the cheek in order to move food to the midline of the tongue. The therapist can also rub the outside of the cheek(s) in order to facilitate the clearance of food from the inside (AOTA, 2010).
- Pocketing of food may be prevented by alternating bites of solids with sips of liquid.
- Ask the client to clear the throat and reswallow if voice quality is wet or coughing occurs after drinking/eating.
- For clients who have difficulty with oral clearance, place the bolus at the middle of the tongue and provide tactile cues to the cheek and jaw in order to facilitate tongue movement and initiation of the swallow (AOTA, 2010).
- Present the utensil below the level of the bottom lip in order to prevent hyperextension of the neck, if needed (AOTA, 2010).
- Attempt a swallow, clear throat, and reswallow (double swallow technique) to clear food/liquids.
- Teach clients who have tongue thrust to position food on the posterior aspect of the tongue. Also, backward tilt of the head may help to prevent food from leaving the mouth.
- Sit upright for 30 minutes after meals.

Changing the Tools to Achieve Independence

- Introduce boluses with various characteristics to stimulate the swallow during meals (temperature, size, texture, and taste/flavor) (AOTA, 2010).
- Thicken liquids, as needed, to increase control during the swallow.
- Avoid sticky boluses (AOTA, 2010).
- As above, adapt the diet level per client needs.
- As above, adapt the placement of the utensils to the mouth, as needed.
- Alternate solids/liquids with ice-slush in order to stimulate the swallow (AOTA, 2010).

Compensation/Adaptation Interventions of Eating Deficits/Dysphagia for Sensation Changes and Pain

Clients presenting with decreased sensation in the oral or facial areas must be educated regarding the limitations and safety issues involved (as able) in order to compensate. Examples of potential injuries include biting and hot foods. Adaptations during mealtime may be provided for the client who is unable to comprehend the safety issues involved (AOTA, 2010; Groher, 1997).

Changing the Task to Achieve Independence

- Food should initially be placed in the areas of the mouth with the most intact sensation (AOTA, 2010; Groher, 1997).
- Verbal cues should be given to clear areas where food may tend to pocket.

Changing the Tools to Achieve Independence

- Alternate solids/liquids with ice-slush in order to increase sensation when eating and stimulate the swallow (AOTA, 2010).
- Offer boluses with a variety of sizes, textures, tastes/flavors, smells, and temperatures (AOTA, 2010).
- Offer diet levels that are easy to manage for the client who is experiencing pain, as appropriate.
- A laryngeal mirror may be used to check for pocketing of food (Groher, 1997).
- Clients with hypersensitivity may present with facial grimacing or refusals in reaction to an aversive food/texture.

For clients who are in any type of oral or facial pain, eating may be a negative and very exhausting experience. Groher (1997) recommends the consideration of requesting pain medication or topical antibiotics before or during mealtime. This approach may be contraindicated if oral sensation is further affected, decreasing the ability to safely swallow.

Changing the Task to Achieve Independence

- Create an environment of relaxation and a pleasurable experience at mealtime (e.g., provide relaxing music, decreased noise, and comfort) (AOTA, 2010).
- Clients may tolerate a desensitization program better if they control the situation, such as feeding themselves various textures (Groher, 1997).

Changing the Tools to Achieve Independence

- Provide graded textures of food, utensils, and plates/cups. Typically, desensitization begins with firm touch, such as eating with utensils. Softer objects or textures are introduced last (AOTA, 2010).

Compensation/Adaptation Interventions of Eating Deficits/Dysphagia for Endurance/Energy Deficits

Fatigue or decreased endurance, particularly in clients who have been on prolonged bed rest or recently weaned from a ventilator, will most likely result in weakened oral-motor function. These clients, who typically have a very weak cough as well, are at significant risk of aspiration pneumonia. A weak, ineffective cough will not provide clearance of any aspirated food/liquid, allowing entrance into the airway. By observing the client in order to determine the times of day or conditions that cause decreased endurance, compensations may be implemented, as appropriate (Logemann, 1998).

Changing the Task to Achieve Independence

- Allow the client extended time to complete each meal.
- Adapt mealtime with pacing techniques such as rest periods in between courses or mouthfuls and/or alternating solids/liquids.
- Begin eating with test trays of various textures/liquid consistencies. Progress to small snacks. Then, offer more frequent, smaller meals during the day.
- Provide positioning techniques that increase postural support for better endurance (Logemann, 1998).

Changing the Tools to Achieve Independence

- Adapt diet levels by offering softer foods that take less time and energy to chew.
- Provide a smaller bolus (AOTA, 2010).

Compensations/Adaptations of Eating Deficits/Dysphagia for Performance Skills/Client Factors

See Figure 3-18.

Compensation/Adaptation of Eating Deficits/Dysphagia for Cognitive Deficits

In general, when providing dysphagia intervention for a client who also presents with cognitive deficits, safety and decreasing risk of aspiration is of utmost concern. Examples of conditions that may present with concurrent cognitive deficits include dementia and traumatic or acquired brain injury. Clients who are deemed severely impaired or unsafe to take nutrients by mouth (PO) may be recommended to have an alternative method of nutrition. The medical team would then consider the recommendations, collaborate with the family, and decide on the best nutritional approach for the client, such as a nasogastric tube. This consideration has many medical, cultural, and ethical issues that must not be taken lightly and always at the discretion of the family.

As will be discussed below, cognitive deficits related to dysphagia begin with the basic ability to sustain arousal and attention to task. If these cannot be maintained long enough for safe oral intake, alternative means must be recommended. As higher-level cognitive deficits present, clients may require supervision for safe eating with issues related to impulsivity, pacing, and handling of food, as examples. General intervention techniques may include cuing, hand-over-hand techniques, and visual reminders.

Table 3-26 briefly presents performance skills because they are typically addressed less formally within most dysphagia intervention plans. Only the subcategories that apply to eating deficits/dysphagia have been included in this table.

Client Factors: Body Functions—Global Mental Functions

Global mental functions include consciousness and orientation. As stated earlier, a level of arousal or consciousness must be sufficient to allow for safe eating. Orientation is important when recognizing the time of day, as related to mealtimes. Also with eating, a consistent environment with routines should help to improve orientation, particularly in regard to mealtimes.

Consciousness and Arousal

Changing the Task to Achieve Independence

- Provide small, pureed snacks during heightened level of arousal times.
- Position client as upright as possible. Provide visual and verbal stimulation, such as natural lighting and verbal interactions.

Changing the Tools to Achieve Independence

- During safe levels of arousal, provide client with cold boluses.

Table 3-26
Process Skills and Examples of Compensation/Adaptation Strategies

Process Skill Subcategories (AOTA, 2002a)	Eating Deficit/Dysphagia Compensation/Adaptation Interventions
Energy	
Paces	Introduce one food item at a time. Provide frequent small meals during the day and/or snacks.
Attends	Refer to Specific Mental Functions category
Knowledge	
Chooses	At the beginning of the meal, allow client to choose what he or she would like to eat or drink first, and so on.
Uses	Ask client to describe the proper use of the above assistive devices for safe eating.
Handles	Ask client to demonstrate safe and effective means of eating finger foods as well as handling of utensils. Monitor for safety.
Heeds	Provide daily checklist to document each time aspiration compensations are followed. For example, each time the client double swallows after drinking thickened liquids.
Inquires	Provide written directions for following aspiration precautions. Request client to ask one or more questions regarding safety with these tasks.
Temporal Organization	
Initiation	Use external cues such as an audiotape with specific instructions to follow for each step of the transfer. Work with client to develop internal cues to initiate transfers.
Sequencing	Provide client with the written steps to be followed during mealtime to prevent aspiration and promote safe eating.
Organizing Space and Objects	
Searches/locates	Provide external cuing such as labels, signs, or color-coding of assistive devices in order to locate items before/during meals.
Gathers	Provide checklist of items needed during mealtime, such as thickener for liquids and adapted cup or straw.
Organizes	Ask client to locate items at mealtime that may hinder safety, such as food items that are contraindicated (e.g., unthickened liquids or crackers).
Adaptation	
Notice/responds	Provide cuing or environmental adaptations if observed that client does not notice safety issues at mealtime.
Accommodates/adjusts	Problem-solve alternative compensations during mealtime if chosen interventions do not succeed, such as with swallowing techniques.
Benefits	Assist client/family in problem-solving various mealtime situations that may occur upon discharge home and plan for adaptations.

ORIENTATION

Changing the Task to Achieve Independence

- During mealtimes, review with the client the types of food being served as they relate to the time of day.

Changing the Tools to Achieve Independence

- Provide client with a daily mealtime schedule.
- Provide client with a daily menu from which appropriate foods may be chosen.

Client Factors: Body Functions—Specific Mental Functions

Specific mental functions include attention, memory, perception, thought functions, higher-level cognitive functions, and mental functioning (motor planning) (AOTA, 2014).

ATTENTION

Changing the Task to Achieve Independence

- For the client with attention deficits, massage cheeks to prevent pocketing. Attempt to feed client when he or she is hungry in order to maintain attention. Present one food item at a time with the most nutritious foods first. Assist client as attention decreases during the meal (AOTA, 2010).

Changing the Tools to Achieve Independence

- For the client with attention deficits, provide flavorful foods that the client prefers. Cold foods may sustain attention.

MEMORY

Changing the Task to Achieve Independence

- During mealtimes, ask the client to recall dysphagia techniques taught previously.
- Ask the client to recall what was eaten at the previous meal and use this as a means to improve orientation, as needed.

Changing the Tools to Achieve Independence

- Provide a daily planner for client to record menu, as above.
- Provide visual cues of dysphagia techniques, such as "swallow twice" after each mouthful.
- Provide supervision and verbal cues of dysphagia techniques during meals.
- The specific mental functions that are addressed less formally and/or less frequently within intervention plans are presented in Table 3-27.

In addition, safety issues include those listed in the following section.

Changing the Task to Achieve Independence

- In the case of impulsivity issues, decreased safety, or judgment, provide the client with assistance, supervision, and cuing as needed during meals in order to prevent putting too much food in the mouth, controlling the bolus, and swallowing with each bite.

Table 3-27

Specific Mental Functions and Examples of Compensation/Adaptation Strategies

Specific Mental Function Subcategories (AOTA, 2002a)	Compensation/Adaptation Interventions
Thought Functions	
Recognition	During mealtime, ask client to locate items such as Thick-it, straws, and utensils.
Categorization	If client is alternating liquids and solids for ease of clearance, ask client to categorize which items are liquids and which are solids.
Generalization	When intervention is begun with only small snacks, for example, the compensations used should be generalized to all eventual mealtimes.
Higher-Level Cognitive Functions	
Judgment	Teach client to ask for help when unsure of safety. For example, if client is thickening own liquids, he or she should check with the therapist initially as to whether the consistency is correct. Ask client open-ended questions in order to think out loud before acting.
Concept formation	Keep a daily progress and achievement chart showing amount of assistance needed for correct dysphagia techniques followed. Mark when goals have been achieved.
Time management	Educate client, before discharge, on allowing enough time for meals, particularly if client fatigues easily or eats too quickly.
Problem solving	Set up possible safety issues and ask client to identify them, such as nonoptimal positioning for eating or unthickened liquids.
Decision making	Provide client with two or more options for safe and appropriate decision making before eating. Allow client to think out loud, stating the compensations required for safe and effective swallowing, for example.

- Provide hand-over-hand guidance for the client who may eat too quickly or demonstrate impulsivity. The client may need to be fed if he or she eats too quickly and is at high risk for choking/aspiration.

Changing the Tools to Achieve Independence

- For the client who may eat too fast or demonstrate impulsivity, if a straw is used for liquids, pinch it in order to decrease the amount of fluid with each mouthful.

Compensation/Adaptation Interventions of Eating Deficits/Dysphagia for Perceptual Deficits

See Figure 3-20.

Table 3-28 Body Scheme Disorders and Examples of Compensation/Adaptation Strategies	
Body Scheme Disorder	**Compensation/Adaptation Interventions: Task and/or Tools Changed**
Somatognosia	During mealtime, use verbal cues to increase awareness of body parts with a functional approach. For example, ask client to point to the part of the body that chews food.
Unilateral body neglect	Adapt mealtime by using reminders to chew on the affected side of the body.
Right-left discrimination	During dysphagia intervention, use right-left terminology frequently.

Visual Fixation/Scanning

Changing the Task to Achieve Independence

- Place instructions for dysphagia on a bulletin board (e.g., in the client's room). Ask the client to scan the room in order to find instructions by anchoring to a certain spot on the wall to begin.

Changing the Tools to Achieve Independence

- Provide instructions on neon-colored paper, as above.

Visual Inattention/Neglect

Changing the Task to Achieve Independence

- Place reminders of dysphagia techniques or exercises within the client's visual field.

Changing the Tools to Achieve Independence

- Provide above reminders on colorful paper.

Body Scheme Disorders

Because there are multiple forms of body scheme disorders, each one cannot be reviewed individually. For this reason, Table 3-28 identifies the most common forms of body scheme disorders as well as examples of compensatory/adaptive interventions for these.

Motor Planning

Many individuals with dysphagia present with oral and limb apraxias. These clients with motor planning deficits are typically not able to perform verbal requests upon command, such as "please swallow your food" or "bring the cup to your lips." In general, the intervention plan should provide the client with a natural setting with food as the focus (Groher, 1997).

Changing the Task to Achieve Independence

- The therapist should demonstrate the desired movements. Verbal cues may also be used if proven effective (Groher, 1997).
- Tactile cuing or hand-over-hand guiding should be attempted to initiate eating and then decreased as the client follows through.

Changing the Tools to Achieve Independence

- Initially, the client with apraxia may not be able to use previously familiar tools, such as utensils. Therefore, finger foods may be attempted.

Compensation/Adaptation Interventions of Eating Deficits/Dysphagia for Visual Deficits

See Figure 3-21.

Low Vision

Changing the Task to Achieve Independence

- Most of the examples for low vision and eating/dysphagia are similar to feeding, such as using brightly colored setups for meals and setting up in a predictable manner.
- The therapist may use verbal and tactile cues.

Changing the Tools to Achieve Independence

An audiotape may be used to review dysphagia techniques and instructions specific to the client.

Visual Field

Changing the Task to Achieve Independence

- Teach the client compensation techniques for locating needed objects and instructions.

Changing the Tools to Achieve Independence

- Place instructions for dysphagia techniques and items needed within the client's visual field.

Maintenance Programs

Early in the dysphagia intervention process, it is important to consider whether or not the client will need a maintenance program. Clients who have long-term or chronic conditions such as dementia or cognitive disorders may need this type of program. Maintenance interventions typically involve compensation approaches such as swallowing techniques, positioning, and/or diet changes for chronic or long-term conditions (Logemann, 1998).

Re-evaluation of dysphagia should occur at least every 6 months to a year. For clients with progressively declining conditions, re-evaluation and/or follow-up may be required sooner (Logemann, 1998). In addition to evaluation/re-evaluation, the role of the occupational therapist in maintenance programs is to provide recommendations and caregiver teaching.

Activities of Daily Living: Sexual Activity

Sexual activity is an ADL that is often over looked by occupational therapists. Cheng and Udry (2002) found that fewer women with disabilities were educated regarding sexual activity than women without disabilities. Other research has also concluded that sexual education is too limited among those with disabilities (Travers, Tincani, Whitby, & Bouton, 2014). This lack of education can be due to erroneous assumptions on the part of the therapists, as well as society as a whole. Clients with disabilities are not encouraged to engage in sexual activity by fearful parents and caregivers, as well as others who believe these individuals are not interested (Glass & Soni, 1999). This is true particularly for women with disabilities. As Harilyn Rousso, Director of the New York Networking Project for Disabled Women and Girls, writes,

> So much of the traditional view of female sexuality is based on physical appearance, on meeting Madison Avenue standards of beauty and physical perfection. While disabled women are by no means unattractive, they often differ from these norms. In contrast, male sexuality, which is based less on physical appearance, includes other components, such as income level, status, and type of work; a disability in a man is thus less likely to detract from his sex appeal. (1986, p. 4)

As for the elderly population, there is a societal myth that these individuals no longer participate in sexual activity. The increase in HIV/AIDs in the elderly population is evidence that these assumptions are incorrect (CDC, 2013; Henderson et al., 2004). This is particularly true in elderly populations with physical limitations. One study surveyed clients after stroke and found, "Many stroke survivors experience sexual dysfunction and indicate a desire for additional information and counseling from health care providers" (Stein, Hillinger, Clancy, & Bishop, 2013).

Another reason this topic is not addressed could be the apprehensions of individual therapists. Many therapists are not comfortable with the topic of sexual activity with clients because they are not comfortable with this topic in general. Occupational therapy education regarding sexual activity may be limited (Friedman, 1997), and perceptions regarding the role of occupational therapy remain varied even today (McGrath & Lynch, 2014). In addition, many of today's elderly are not comfortable with the topic of sexuality; therefore, therapists may be even more concerned about broaching this subject. As stereotypes of the elderly are changing, more elderly may ask questions of therapists, and the therapists need to be prepared to respond to these questions. In addition, there are many young adults and middle-aged adults who require the services of occupational therapists, including education regarding sexual activity.

According to the AOTA Framework document, sexual activity is defined as "engagement in activities which result in sexual satisfaction" (2014, p. 19). It is important to note that this definition is not limited to sexual intercourse. Many clients will find sexual satisfaction from activities other than intercourse. The *Gale Encyclopedia of Nursing and Allied Health* defines sexuality to include "body image, self image, gender identities, beliefs, and feelings about sex, capacities for love and friendship, and social behavior as well as overt physical expression of love or sexual desire. A person's sexuality is influenced by ethical, spiritual, cultural and moral concerns" (Gourley, 2013, p. 3004). Because sexual activity includes a variety of issues, education regarding sexual activity is multidimensional. Physical issues related to a disability, psychosocial issues related to social participation, and issues of abuse must all be addressed.

This chapter will address the physical issues related to sexual activity, while Chapter 8 will address the social participation. In addition, some literature has suggested the greatest barrier to sexual activity is self-esteem and self-efficacy, not physical barriers. This should be considered when addressing sexual activity, particularly with young adults (Wiegerink, Stam, Ketelaar, Cohen-Kettenis, & Roebroeck, 2012).

Unlike other ADLs, sexual activity is not an occupation that can be practiced in the clinic. Because intervention is based on education and success of the intervention is very subjective, based on each client, this chapter will focus on compensation/adaptation rather than remediation.

Compensation/Adaptation of Sexual Activity Deficits for Clients With Physical Limitations: Performance Skills/Client Factors: Range of Motion, Strength, Coordination, Sensation/Pain, and Endurance/Energy

Sexual activity can be negatively impacted by motor skill deficits and body function limitations. Limitations in motor functions may create clumsy or uncomfortable situations that clients choose to avoid by avoiding sexual activity as a whole. Body function changes following an injury or illness can result in a decreased desire for sexual activity. Korpelainen, Nieminen, and Myllyla found that "stroke caused a marked decrease in libido among both the patients and their spouses . . ." (1999, p. 716). This may be a result of the illness itself or a result of secondary factors such as decreased body image or impaired sensation. In addition, fear of poor sexual function may limit libido. While this may be true, other authors have studied the importance of proper education to identify and address these issues in order to allow for the occupation of sex (Rosenbaum, Vadas, & Kalichman, 2014).

Performance patterns, context and environment, and activity demands need to be addressed as well. Performance patterns play a very large role in an individual client's sexual activity. As stated in Chapter 1, performance patterns include the client's habits, routines, rituals, and roles (AOTAa, 2014). Client habits and routines can range from an individual who rarely experiences sexual activity to a client who routinely experiences sexual activity. According to the AOTA Framework document, roles "are sets of behaviors expected by society, shaped by culture, and may be further conceptualized and defined by the client" (2014, p. S27). As stated earlier, the socially agreed upon standards and the acceptable code of norms may be based on stereotypes, not the actual code of a particular client. It is important for the occupational therapists to determine the habits, routines, and roles of each client. When examining roles, the role of parent should not be overlooked. Studies have been completed on a number of diagnoses to determine the impact the disability has on sexuality. All of these conclude that the disability has a negative impact, and concerns regarding fertility are an issue among men and women (McAlonan, 1996; Oksel & Gunduzoglu, 2014; Pebdani, Johnson, & Amtmann, 2014; Qaderi & Khoei, 2014).

The areas of context and environment that may impact sexual activity are the client's cultural, spiritual, and social relationships. Culture and spirituality have a long tradition of having an impact on sexual activity. Certain cultures have different expectations of women's and men's sexual interests. Some cultures do not allow sexuality to be discussed as openly as others. For example, according to the Muslim Women's League, an American Muslim organization, sexual education is acceptable (http://www.mwlusa.org/topics/sexuality/sexuality_pos.html). While spirituality does not include religion alone, many religious beliefs will also impact sexual activity. For example, Roman Catholicism holds that sexual activity has a purpose of procreation over recreation. Clients who are widowed may feel guilty about sexual activity outside of a marriage relationship, even if beyond the age of procreation.

Social relationships can be strained because of injury or illness. Concerns over sexuality may put a further strain on these relationships. As stated above, fertility is a large concern for individuals after an injury or long-term diagnosis. Questions of fertility, as well as raising children, need to be addressed with clients so they are well informed of the possibilities. If an adult has to move back in with parents following an injury or illness, this can further limit the individual's social

Table 3-29

PLISSIT Model and Training

PLISSIT	Definitions (Adapted From Wallace, 2004	Training (Adapted From Friedman, 1997)
P	Permission from the client to discuss sexual activity	Therapists are generally sufficiently trained to offer an opportunity for discussion regarding sexual activity
LI	Limited information provided to the client	Adaptations/compensations listed below will provide this information
SS	Specific suggestions provided regarding sexual activity	Some advanced training may be required, depending on the specificity
IT	Intensive therapy regarding issues of sexuality	Not generally provided by OTs unless advanced training has been completed

and sexual activities due to family dynamics. All of these contextual factors offer opportunities for the occupational therapist to open a dialogue with the client and assess the individual's needs.

Activity demands include social demands, required actions, and required body functions and structures. The required actions and required body functions and structures will be discussed. The social demands, as stated earlier, may be unrealistic for individuals with disabilities and for the elderly. Poverty, substance abuse, race, sex, and educational levels can impact expectations. While expectations are important to know, it is more important to assess the particular roles to which an individual client wishes to return.

In general, occupational therapists will be providing information and education to clients who have experienced a physical injury or illness. Some clients who have experienced cognitive or perceptual limitations will also require education. One tool that has been used by occupational therapists and other health care practitioners to organize sexual activity education is PLISSIT. This tool was created in the 1970s, but the validity or reliability of this tool has not been established (Wallace, 2004). Despite this, it is a valuable guide to the level of specificity offered by an occupational therapist. Table 3-29 describes the PLISSIT model and the training required for occupational therapy within this model.

Compensation/Adaptation Interventions of Sexual Activity Deficits for Range of Motion, Strength, and Coordination Deficits

ROM, strength, and coordination limitations will impact positioning during sexual activity. Clients may have difficulty with sexual positions that were preferred in the past. Occupational therapists can discuss positioning without becoming sexually explicit. Examples of this include the following:

- Instruct clients with hemiparesis to adjust positions to find the most comfortable (SRCBulington.net, 2014). For example:
    1. Lie on the affected side, thus allowing the unaffected side to be free for physical contact or additional support.
    2. Discuss positions of comfort with partners in order to avoid being uncomfortable. Request the partner to take a more active role, allowing the client to assume a position that requires less movement.

- Wedges or pillows may be required to support a particular position. General principles can be explained to the client, or if appropriate, specific positions can be reviewed with the client.

Compensation/Adaptation Interventions of Sexual Activity Deficits for Sensation Changes and Pain

As stated earlier, sensory changes can result in a decrease in sensation (hyposensitivity), such as after a CVA, or in increased sensation (hypersensitivity) and pain. For clients with decreased sensation, communication with the partner is vital. The partner can be asked by the client to caress the areas of intact sensation more often, allowing for greater pleasure for the client. If sensation is lacking to the point that pressure areas are a concern, such as after a spinal cord injury, the client should be educated to avoid prolonged positioning and to check the sitting/lying location for objects that can cause pressure or cuts prior to initiating any sexual activity (Friedman, 1997; SRCBurlington.net, 2014).

Decreased sensation can also result in bowel and bladder issues, which can embarrass clients during sexual activity. Clients who are not continent should be instructed to void prior to any sexual activity in order to avoid such situations. These clients should communicate the possibility of incontinence with their partner and be prepared with supplies for clean-up if such an incident occurs (Friedman, 1997; SRCBurlington.net, 2014).

For clients experiencing hypersensitivity or pain, the education is centered on limiting pain so the clients can enjoy the sexual activity. If the pain is positional, such as back pain, clients can communicate with their partner regarding positions of comfort. These positions may be different than what couples are used to, such as sitting rather than lying down; therefore, communication is vital. If the pain is due to contact, such as a burn or amputation of a limb, the client again needs to communicate with the partner regarding what contact causes this pain and how to avoid it.

Pain management techniques can also be incorporated. Massage or meditation prior to sexual activity can reduce pain due to stress or muscle tightness. Sexual activity can be planned when pain medication is most effective (Friedman, 1997). While this limits spontaneity, it will be beneficial for overall enjoyment if pain is absent during sexual activity (Friedman, 1997).

Compensation/Adaptation Interventions of Sexual Activity Deficits for Endurance/Energy Deficits

Decreased endurance can be a result of prolonged hospitalization or lack of activity as well as a particular illness. The elderly are particularly vulnerable to rapid declines in endurance with inactivity and are more likely to experience the most common forms of illness that result in decreased endurance: cardiovascular diseases.

For clients with cardiovascular disease, concerns regarding sexual activity are frequent. According to the American Heart Association (2014) Scientific Statement on Sexual Activity and Cardiovascular Disease (CVD), "Sexual activity is an important component of patient and partner quality of life, and it is reasonable for most patients with CVD to engage in sexual activity." While it is important for clients to discuss concerns with a physician, the occupational therapist can also offer suggestions. Most of these suggestions are general energy conservation principles, such as the following:

- Avoid stressful or rushed environments.
- Avoid sexual activity directly after meals or other physical activity.
- Be aware that fatigue may occur, and that this is normal.
- Seek counseling if issues continue.

For clients with other diagnoses resulting in decreased endurance, such as pulmonary diseases or progressive neurological diseases, these same principles will apply.

Compensation/Adaptation Interventions of Sexual Activity Deficits for Cognitive, Perceptual, or Visual Deficits

While there are some clients who will experience difficulty with sexual activity due to visual loss, this is rare and will not be discussed here. Individuals who experience perceptual deficits may have motor planning difficulties, body scheme disorders, inattention, or certain agnosias that can but do not necessarily have to impact sexual activity. Intervention for these individuals would occur related to the specific deficit if the impact was of concern for the client; however, these deficits are often overcome by clients without intervention.

The appropriateness of education regarding sexual activity for clients with cognitive deficits depends largely on the severity of the deficits. If a client is unable to determine for him- or herself whether a situation is voluntary or not, education regarding avoidance or reporting of abuse may be more appropriate. Rates of sexual abuse have been inconsistent; however, it is widely agreed that those with cognitive disabilities are at a greater risk than other individuals (theARC.org, 2014). For clients with long-standing cognitive deficits, such as adults with developmental disabilities, education may be appropriate, and this is addressed in Chapter 8. Clients with new cognitive disabilities, such as a client with a head injury, will need to be assessed individually to ascertain whether education is appropriate. Education should not be avoided simply because a deficit exists or caregivers do not think it appropriate, but rather based on the safety and competence of each client.

Maintenance of Sexual Activity

Once the client has attained all information requested, these skills will become maintenance because they will remain beyond the time when intervention is being completed with the client. As this is a personal matter, it will be the choice of the client as to whether he or she utilizes the techniques provided or chooses to abstain from sexual activity once education has been completed.

Case 1: Josephine

Josephine is a 75-year-old woman who fell in the garage after tripping over her grandson's skateboard. She sustained a left hip fracture, was admitted to the hospital, and had surgery for a cemented bipolar hip arthroplasty. She was discharged to a short-term rehabilitation facility 5 days after surgery in hopes to finally be discharged home.

Josephine lives in a mother-in-law apartment in her daughter and son-in-law's home. The apartment is above the garage and has 13 steps to enter. Once inside the apartment, there are no architectural barriers except a traditional shower with glass doors. She also has a galley kitchen.

Josephine has a medical history of insulin-dependent diabetes mellitus, osteoarthritis, appendicitis, and a hysterectomy 26 years ago. Prior to this fall, she was independent with all ADLs and IADLs. She did not use any assistive devices and drove short distances. Josephine attends the local senior center where she is active with bingo, line dancing, and water aerobics.

Josephine's goals are to "walk again and go to the senior center." Current status is as follows: (R dominant).

UE ROM	WNL-BUE
UE Strength	BUE grossly 4+/5 to 5/5
Cognition	Occasionally forgetful as to the date, needs cuing for hand placement, hip precautions, and to use assistive device

V/P WNLs
FM Skills WFL-occasional difficulty secondary to arthritis
Functional Mobility and Transfers
Supine-to-sit with cuing and min (a), PWB, sit-to-stand with cuing and mod(a), Ambulates to w/c using RW and CTG
ADL (I) UE bathe/dress; requires adaptive equip for LE ADLs secondary to hip precautions and mod (a) with cuing
Pain 4/5 at rest, 7/10 with mobility

Case 2: Bill

Bill is 44-year-old man who sustained a CVA 1 week ago. He has an unremarkable medical history. He lives in a two-story home with his wife and teenage daughter. As a result of the CVA, he will take a medical leave from his job as an accountant. Although Bill's job requires long hours, he is a devoted husband and father who makes breakfast for the family each morning. His wife works part time as a social worker. Prior to his CVA, Bill enjoyed socializing with his wife and lifelong friends, bowling, and attending his daughter's soccer games.

After initial symptoms of left side numbness and weakness in his left LE, left UE, and left side of face, Bill's wife rushed him to the local ER. While in the ER, the symptoms progressed to full flaccidity in his left UE, difficulty swallowing, and blurred vision. After the ER, he was admitted to the medical ICU for 2 days, then transferred to a neuro step-down unit. His medical team is now evaluating Bill for the intensive rehabilitation unit within the hospital.

Bill's goals are to return to work, cook breakfast, and attend his daughter's soccer games upon discharge.

Current status is as follows: (R dominant)

UE ROM Right: AROM-WNL
Left: PROM WNL, no active motion of LUE noted
UE Strength Right: 5/5 grossly throughout Left-flaccid
Endurance c/o fatigue after 20 minute eval
Sensation
Proprioception RUE-WNL LUE-Impaired
Hot Cold RUE-WNL LUE-WNL
Localization RUE-WNL LUE-Impaired/L side of face, also
FM skills RUE-WNL LUE-Absent secondary to flaccidity
Visual/perceptual Only complains of blurred vision
Cognitive A&O X 3
Tends to have difficulty sequencing simple ADL tasks
Oral-motor Choking with thin liquids, left side of mouth droops
ADL Assist for meal setup, cutting food, and eating sandwiches
Safety: impulsive. Tries to get out of bed on own and out of w/c
Speech clear
Mod (a) with grooming; Max
(a) toileting; Mod (a) bathing
Transfers/functional mobility
Mod (a) supine-to-sit and sit- to-stand; Max (a) stand-pivot with walker.
Mod (a) to maintain sitting balance @ EOB

Affect	Flat, sad, difficult to motivate
Other issues	Moderate subluxation, Left shoulder
Pain	7/10 when shoulder is positioned or moved

Summary Questions

1. Pick one ADL compensation/adaptation method and describe how it is related to one model/theory of occupational therapy.
2. Compare and contrast the remediation and compensation/adaptation approaches to ADL. Give specific examples.
3. Discuss safety issues as related to vision, perception, and cognition in ADLs.
4. Describe one general maintenance strategy in ADLs in relation to dressing techniques.

References

American Occupational Therapy Association. (2010). *Dysphagia care and related feeding concerns for adults self-paced clinical course*, (2nd ed.). Bethesda, MD: AOTA.

American Occupational Therapy Association. (2014). Occupational therapy practice framework: Domain and process (3rd ed.). *American Journal of Occupational Therapy, 68*(Suppl. 1), S1-S48.

American Occupational Therapy Association. (2014a). *The reference manual of the official documents of the American occupational therapy association* (19th ed.). Bethesda, MD: AOTA Press.

American Occupational Therapy Association. (2002b). Roles and responsibilities of the occupational therapist and occupational therapy assistant during the delivery of occupational therapy services. *Occupational Therapy Practice, 7*(15), 9-10.

American Occupational Therapy Association. (2013). Cognition, Cognitive Rehabilitation, and Occupational Performance. *American Journal of Occupational Therapy, 67*(Suppl.), S9-S31.

Arnadottir, G. (1990). *The brain and behavior: Assessing critical dysfunction through activities of daily living (ADL).* St. Louis, MO: Mosby.

Avery-Smith, W. (Ed.) (2003). *Dysphagia care for adults: A self-paced clinical course from AOTA.* Bethesda, MD: AOTA.

Avery-Smith, W. (1998). An occupational therapist-coordinated dysphagia program. *Occupational Therapy Practice, 3*(11), 20-23.

Bowen, A., Hazelton, C. Pollock, A., & Lincoln, N. (2013). Cognitive rehabilitation for spatial neglect following stroke. *The Cochrane Database of Systematic Reviews, 7,* Art. No. CD003586, 1-111.

CDC. (2013). HIV among older Americans. *Centers for Disease Control and Prevention website.* http://www.cdc.gov/hiv/risk/age/olderamericans/index.html. Accessed July 14, 2014.

Cheng, M. M., & Udry, J. R. (2002). Sexual behaviors of physically disabled adolescents in the United States. *Journal of Adolescent Health, 31*(1), 48-48.

Cohen, J. R. (2001). Living with low vision. *Inside M.S., 19*(1), 46-54.

Cole, M. B. (2012). *Group dynamics in occupational therapy* (4th ed.). Thorofare, NJ: SLACK Incorporated.

Dodge, H. H., Kadowski, T., Hayakawa, T., & Yamakawa, M. (2005). Cognitive impairment as a strong predictor of incident disability in specific ADL-IADL tasks among community-dwelling elders: The Azuchi study. *The Gerontologist, 45*(2), 222-231.

Dorner, B. (2002). Promoting an easier swallow. Focus on caregiving. *Provider, 28*(9), 69-70, 73-4.

Fairchild, S. L (2013). *Pierson and Fairchilds principles and techniques of patient care* (5th ed.). St, Louis, MO: Saunders Elsevier.

Fasoli, S. E., Trombly, C. A., Tickle-Degnen, L., & Verfaellie, M. H. (2002). Context and goal-directed movement: the effect of material-based occupation. *Occupational Therapy Journal of Research, 22*(3), 119-128.

Fisher, A. G. (2001). Assessment of motor and process skills (4th ed). Retrieved June 12, 2005, from www.ampsintl.com.

Fisher, A. G. (2002, January). A model for planning and implementing top-down, client-centered, and occupation-based occupational therapy interventions. Short course presented at University of New Hampshire conference.

Friedman, J. D. (1997). Sexual expression: The forgotten component of ADL. *Occupational Therapy Practice, January,* 20-25.

Gibson, J. W., & Schkade, J. K. (1997). Occupational adaptation intervention with patients with cerebrovascular accident: a clinical study. *American Journal of Occupational Therapy, 51*(7), 523-529.

Giles, G. M., Toglia, J., Wolf, T., Radomski, M. V., Champagne, T., Corcoran, M. A., . . . Obermeyer, I. (2013). Cognition, cognitive rehabilitation and occupational performance. *American Journal of Occupational Therapy 67*(6), S9-S31.

Gillen, G. (2011). *Stroke rehabilitation: A function-based approach* (3rd ed.). St. Louis, MO: Elsevier/Mosby.

Glass, C., & Soni, B. (1999). ABC of sexual health sexual problems of disabled patients. *British Medical Journal, 318,* 518-521.

Gourley, M. M. (2002) Sexuality and disability. In K. Krapp (Ed.), *Gale encyclopedia of nursing and allied health* (Vol. 4, p. 2203-2206). Farmington Hills, MI: Thomson Gale Group.

Groher, M. E. (Ed.) (1997). *Dysphagia: Diagnosis and management* (3rd ed.). Boston, MA: Butterworth-Heinemann.

Gupta, H., Banerjee, A. (2014). Recovery of dysphagia in lateral medullary stroke. *Stroke Case Reports in Neurological Medicine 14,* Art. No 40487, 1-4. http://dx.doi.org/10.1155/2014/40487/

Handybar (1999). Avenue Innovations, Inc. http://handybar-shop.com/About-us

Henderson, S. J., Bernstein, L. B., St. George, D. M., Doyle, J. P., Paranjape, A. S., & Corbie-Smith, G. (2004). Older women and HIV: how much do they know and where are they getting their information? *Journal of the American Geriatric Society, 52,* 1549-1553.

Jackson Siegelbaum Gastroenterology. (2002). Dysphagia diet: 5 levels difficulty in swallowing diet. Retrieved on March 20, 2005, from http://www.gicare.com/pated/edtgs07.htm.

Jacobs, K., & Simon, L. (2015). *Quick reference dictionary for occupational therapy* (6th ed.). Thorofare, NJ: SLACK Incorporated.

Kerkhoff, G., & Schenk, T. (2012). Rehabilitation of neglect: An update. *Neuropsychologia, 50*(6), 1072-1079.

Korpelainen, J. T., Nieminen, P., & Myllyla, V. V. (1999). Sexual functioning among stroke patients and their spouses. *Stroke, 30,* 715-719.

Law, M., Baptiste, S., Carswell, A., McColl, M. A., Polatajko, H., & Pollock, N. (1998). *The Canadian occupational performance measure* (3rd ed.). Ottawa, Ontario: Canadian Occupational Therapy Association.

Levine, G. N., Steinke, E. E., Bakaeen, G. G., Bozkurt, B., Cheitlin, M. D., Conti, J. B., . . . Stewart, W. J. (2012). Sexual activity and cardiovascular disease: A scientific statement from the American Heart Association. Circulation retrieved November 7, 2014, from http://circ.ahajournals.org/content/early/2012/01/19/CIR .0b013e3182447787.citation

Liepelt-Scarfone, I., Berger, F. M., Prakash, D., Csoti, I., Graber, S., Maetzler, W., & Berg, D. (2013). Clinical characteristics with an impact on ADL functions of PD patients with cognitive impairments indicative of dementia. *PLoS One, 8*(12), e82902.

Lin, K. (1996). Right-hemispheric activation approaches to neglect rehabilitation post-stroke. *American Journal of Occupational Therapy, 50*(7), 504-515.

Logemann, J. A. (1998). *Evaluation and treatment of swallowing disorders* (2nd ed.). Austin, TX: PRO-ED.

McAlonan, S. (1996). Improving sexual rehabilitation services: The patient's perspective. *American Journal of Occupational Therapy, 50*(10), 826-834.

McCullough, G., Pelletier, C., & Steele, C. (2003). National dysphagia diet: What to swallow? *ASHA Leader, 27,* 16.

McGrath, M., & Lynch, E. (2014) Occupational therapists' perspectives on addressing sexual concerns of older adults in the context of rehabilitation. *Disability and Rehabilitation, 36*(8), 651-657.

Muslim Women's League. (nd). An Islamic Perspective on Sexuality. Retrieved on May 10, 2005, from www.mwlusa.org/publications/positionpapers/sexuality.html

Nagel, M. J., & Rice, M. S. (2001). Cross transfer effects in the upper extremity during an occupationally embedded exercise. *American Journal of Occupational Therapy, 55,* 531-537.

Nelson, D. L., Konosky, K., Fleharty K., Webb, R., Newer, K., & Hazboun, V. P. (1996). The effects of an occupationally embedded exercise on bilateral assisted supination in persons with hemiplegia. *American Journal of Occupational Therapy, 50*, 639-646.

Nosek, M. A., & Howland, C. A. (1998). Abuse and women with disabilities. Retrieved May 31, 2005, from http://www.vaw.umn.edu.

Oksel, E., & Gunduzoglu, N. C. (2014) Investigation of life experiences of women with scleroderma. *Sexuality and Disability, 32*, 15-21.

Omar, M. T. A., Hegazy, F. A., & Mikashi, S. P. (2012) Influences of purposeful activity versus rote exercise on improving pain and hand function in pediatric burn. *Burns, 38*, 261-262.

O'Sullivan, N. (1995). *Dysphagia care: Team approach with acute and long-term care clients* (2nd ed.). Los Angeles, CA: Cottage Square.

Pebdani, R., Johnson, K., & Amtmann, D. (2014) Personal experiences of pregnancy and infertility in individuals with spinal cord injury. *Sexuality and Disability, 32*, 65-74.

Pendleton, H. M., & Schultz-Krohn, W. (Eds.). (2013). *Pedretti's occupational therapy practice skills for physical dysfunction* (7th ed), St. Louis, MO: Elsevier.

Qaderi, K., & Khoei, E. M. (2014). Sexual problems and quality of life in women with multiple sclerosis. *Sexuality and Disability, 32*, 35-43.

Radomski, M. V., & Trombly Latham, C. A. (Eds.). (2014). *Occupational therapy for physical dysfunction* (7th ed.). Philadelphia, PA: Lippincott Williams & Wilkins.

Rogers, J. C., & Holm, M. B. (1994). Performance Assessment of Self-Care Skills (PASS – Home). Version 3.1. Tham, K., Ginsburg, E., Fisher A. G., & Tegner R. (2001). Awareness of disabilities in clients with unilateral neglect. *American Journal of Occupational Therapy, 55*(1), 46-54.

Rosenbaum, T., Vadas, D., & Kalichman, L. (2014) Sexual function in post-stroke patients: Considerations for rehabilitation. *The Journal of Sexual Medicine, (11)*1, 15-21.

Sakakibara, M. M., Miller, W. C., Souza, M., Nikolova, V., & Best, K. (2013) Wheelchair skills training to improve confidence with using a manual wheelchair among older adults. *Physical Medicine and Rehabilitation, 94*(6), 1031-1037.

Schell, B. A., Gillen, G., & Scaffa, M. E. (2014). *Willard and Spackman's occupational therapy* (12th ed.). Philadelphia, PA: Lippincott Williams & Wilkins.

Stein, J., Hillinger, M., Clancy, C., & Bishop, L. (2013). Sexuality after stroke: Patient counseling preferences. *Disability and Rehabilitation, 35* (21), 1842-1847.

TBI help.org (nd). Achieving sexual intimacy after a stroke. Retrieved March 1, 2005 from www.tbihelp.org/sexual_intimacy_after_.htm.

TheARC.org People with Intellectual Disabilities & Sexual Violence. Retrieved October 21, 2015, from http://www.thearc.org/document.doc?id=3657.

Travers, J., Tincani, M. Whitby, P. S., & Boutot, E. A. (2014). Alignment of sexuality education with self determination for people with significant disabilities: A review of research and future directions. *Education and Training in autism and Developmental Disabilities, 49*(2), 232-247.

Uniform Data System for Medical Rehabilitation. (1996). Functional Independence Measure. Amherst, NY, retrieved from www.udsmr.org on June 12, 2005.

Wallace, M. (2004). Sexuality. *MedSurg Nursing, 13*(2), 122.

Wiegerink, D., Stam, H., Ketelaar, M., Cohen-Kettenis, P., & Roebroeck, J. (2012) Personal and environmental factors contributing to participation in romantic relationships and sexual activity of young adults with cerebral palsy. *Disability & Rehabilitation, 34*(17), 1481-1487

Zoltan, B. (2007). Vision, perception, and cognition: A manual for the evaluation and treatment of the adult with acquired brain injury (4th ed.). Thorofare, NJ: SLACK Incorporated.

4

Instrumental Activities of Daily Living

Tracy Van Oss, DHSc, MPH, OTR/L, FAOTA

Chapter Objectives

By the end of this chapter, the student will be able to do the following:

- Define instrumental activities of daily living (IADL) as they pertain to the Occupational Therapy Practice Framework.
- Describe specific models/frames of reference as related to IADLs.
- Comprehend safety issues as related to IADLs.
- Delineate between the roles of the occupational therapist and the occupational therapy assistant as they pertain to the occupation of IADLs.
- Comprehend and identify related social participation as related to decreased independence in IADLs.
- Describe the impact of contextual and environmental factors upon IADLs.
- Identify appropriate IADL intervention strategies based on various performance skills and client factors.
- Identify general IADL remediation strategies.
- Identify specific IADL compensation/adaptation strategies.
- Identify IADL compensation/adaptation intervention strategies related to vision, perception, and cognition.
- Identify general IADL maintenance strategies.

Introduction

According to the Framework, IADLs are defined as, "activities that are oriented toward interacting with the environment and that are often complex (American Occupational Therapy Association [AOTA], 2014). IADL are generally optional in nature, that is, may be delegated to another" (adapted from Rogers & Holm, 1994, pp. 181-202). In general, included in IADLs are the following areas of occupation: home establishment and management, meal preparation, shopping,

Meriano C, Latella D.
Occupational Therapy Interventions: Function and Occupations, Second Edition (pp 249-296).

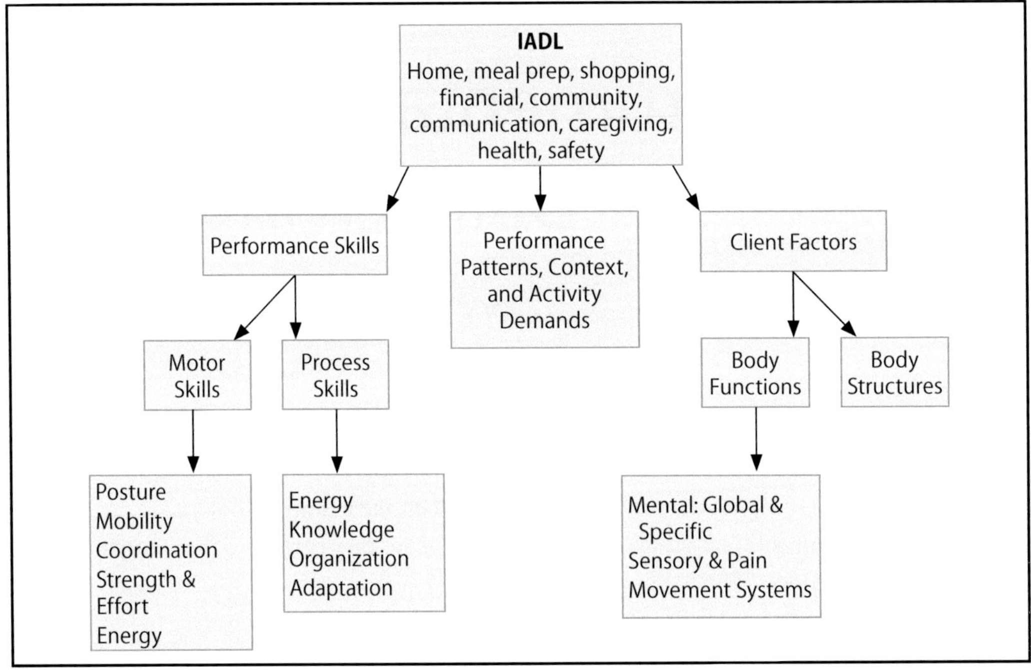

Figure 4-1. Components of IADLs. (Adapted from American Occupational Therapy Association. (2014). Occupational therapy practice framework: Domain and process (3rd ed.). *American Journal of Occupational Therapy, 68*(Suppl. 1), S1-S48.)

financial management, community mobility, communication device use, care of others (including selecting and supervising caregivers), care of pets, child rearing, health management and maintenance, and safety procedures and emergency responses (AOTA, 2014). Intervention in these areas of occupation will be discussed in greater detail throughout this chapter, with the primary focus being on remediation, compensation/adaptation, and maintenance interventions. Frames of reference, safety concerns, implications for the social participation impact on IADLs, context and environment, performance patterns, activity demands, and the role of the occupational therapist assistant will be addressed (Figure 4-1).

Throughout this chapter, the reader will be introduced to the management of clients with neurological, orthopedic, and cognitive/perceptual deficits to facilitate independence with IADLs in the above-mentioned areas of occupation.

The role of the occupational therapist is to facilitate functional independence in all daily activities and participation in life roles to the greatest level of skill. The goal of this chapter is to introduce ways to assist the client in fulfilling both of these goals. As the client is going through the process of remediation of motor skills, process skills, and/or communication/interaction skills, the occupational therapist may offer recommendations for compensation or adaptation to increase the client's independence and safety. At the time that the client becomes capable of participating in IADLs, the occupational therapist must determine whether continuing with the remediation process is appropriate. If so, the client may continue to practice normal movement patterns until mastery is achieved. If not, the therapist will begin instructing the client in compensation and adaptation strategies. For example, if the client is determined to return home alone, he or she will need to become independent with IADLs. If remediation of all skills has not yet been achieved, the client will need to implement compensation/adaptation techniques to facilitate this goal during the ongoing remediation process. If the client was to follow compensatory or adaptive methods from the onset of intervention, the occupational therapist will educate him or her in the most effective strategies to return to independent living. In addition, the goal of this chapter is to educate the occupational therapist in various means of facilitation of a client's functional independence and return to his or her life role.

The AOTA Framework document (2014) has defined various areas of IADLs. These definitions will be the basis for most of this chapter, with additions or clarifications added throughout. The definitions are as listed below.

- Home establishment and maintenance is defined as: "Obtaining and maintaining personal and household possessions and environment (e.g., home, yard, garden, appliances, vehicles), including maintaining and repairing personal possessions (clothing and household items) and knowing how to seek help and whom to contact." Meal preparation and cleanup refers to "planning, preparing, serving well-balanced, nutritional meals, and cleaning up food and utensils after meals" (AOTA, 2014, p. S19).

  Specific tasks within this definition are not listed; however, the most common tasks have been chosen for review in this chapter. These tasks are laundry, light cleaning, outdoor home maintenance, shopping, preparing a meal, setting a table, and washing/drying dishes and putting them away.
- Financial management is defined as "using fiscal resources, including alternate methods of financial transaction and planning and using finances with long-term and short-term goals" (2014, p. S19). In this section, financial management will include check writing, payment by cash, and the use of credit cards.
- Driving and community mobility is defined as, "Planning and moving around in the community and using public or private transportation, such as driving, or accessing buses, taxi cabs, or other public transportation systems" (AOTA, 2014, p. S19). This section will focus on driving and public transportation.
- Communication management is defined as "sending, receiving, and interpreting information using a variety of systems and equipment including writing tools, telephones, keyboards audiovisual recorders, computers or tablets, communication boards, call lights, emergency systems, Braille writers, telecommunication devices for the deaf people, augmentative communication systems and personal digital assistants" (AOTA, 2014, p. S19). This section will focus on everyday use of communication devices, devices or systems for emergency alerting, and adapted devices for the visually impaired.
- Care of pets is defined as "arranging, supervising, or providing care for pets and service animals" (AOTA, 2014, p. S19). This category of IADLs addresses the care of others, including family members and pets.
- Health management and maintenance is defined as "developing, managing, and maintaining routines for health and wellness promotion, such as physical fitness, nutrition, decreasing health risk behaviors, and medication routines" (AOTA, 2014, p. S19).

Table 4-1 reviews the different aspects of each IADL category.

Frame of Reference

Chapter 1 reviewed several frames of reference and models for occupational therapy. As stated in that chapter, occupational therapy has a humanistic philosophy as well as models that are client-centered and systems-based. While a therapist's choice for a frame of reference depends on the setting of intervention, the therapist's preferences, and the needs of the individual client, for purposes

Table 4-1

Components of IADLs

Home establishment and maintenance, meal preparation and clean-up, shopping	• Laundry • Light cleaning • Outdoor home maintenance • Shopping • Preparing a meal • Setting a table • Washing/drying dishes and putting them away
Financial management	• Check writing • Payment by cash • Use of credit cards
Community mobility	• Driving • Use of public transportation or community service transit systems • Mobilizing to bus stops
Communication device use	• Common communication devices (i.e., telephone, computer, pager systems) • Devices or systems for emergency alerting • Adaptive devices for those with visual impairment
Care of others	• Spouse • Children • Parents • Other family members • Friends
Care of pets	• Feeding • Exercise • Health maintenance
Health management and maintenance	• Exercise and fitness • Nutrition • Hygiene • Medication management and compliance

of retraining clients in IADLs in this chapter, the Model of Human Occupation (MOHO) will be discussed. The occupational therapist will be assessing the client's level of volition, habituation, and performance. An occupational profile will be completed and the occupational therapist along with the client will determine the client's goals. Client-centered interventions will be established and executed with the occupational therapy practitioner to achieve the client's optimal ability with IADLs.

In addition to these, therapists using the top-down approach (as discussed in Chapters 1 and 2), may also use frames of reference based on the client's specific situation. For a client who is aging, a developmental frame of reference such as Jung's spiritual stages, Erickson's psychosocial stages, or Levinson's life transitions may be utilized (Cole, 1998).

For a client who has experienced a traumatic brain injury or a cerebral vascular accident (CVA) with behavior changes apparent, a behaviorist theory such as behavior modification may be employed. Behavior modification is based on environmental reinforcers in order to shape behavior (Cole, 1998). This same client may have cognitive deficits and require a cognitive frame of reference such as Toglia and Abreu's cognitive rehabilitation frame of reference. Originally based on learning theory, and now updated by Toglia to include metacognition (insight into own capabilities), this frame of reference emphasizes retraining cognition through hierarchical intervention and brain plasticity (Cole 1998).

Because behavior modification is based on environmental feedback, better carry-over should be demonstrated again with the use of functional activities rather than rote exercise. This is also true of cognitive rehabilitation. According to Cole, "Cognitive strategies are always taught in the context of an activity" (1998, p. 149).

Safety During Instrumental Activities of Daily Living Intervention

According to the Framework, safety procedures and emergency responses include "knowing and performing preventive procedures to maintain a safe environment as well as recognizing sudden, unexpected hazardous situations and initiating emergency action to reduce the threat to health and safety" (AOTA, 2014, p. S20).

The management of clients' performance demands focuses on safety with all aspects of IADLs. Many clients experience age-related physical and sensory changes that may be enhanced by an acute neurological, orthopedic, or cognitive/perceptual event. These acute events may precipitate client factor changes that may affect performance habits and/or performance skills. Driving, using public transportation, and managing medications for self or others are among examples of IADLs that need to be closely monitored with clients, and caregivers must be educated in all safety concerns. Occupational therapists must recognize implications for safety with respect to ADLs prior to facilitating a safe performance with IADLs. Safety concerns will be addressed throughout this chapter with respect to specific areas of IADL intervention.

Implications for Social Participation Impact on Instrumental Activities of Daily Living

Social participation implications are important to consider with each client intervention. The occupational therapist must be sensitive to the mood and affect of the client and assess his or her level of motivation to increase function. A client who was functioning independently at home but now requires supervision to shower and dress may experience feelings of loss of dignity and self-worth. A client who is now unable to drive because of visual changes may experience feelings of sadness and confinement. An individual previously living alone may now need someone to stay with him or her all day or intermittently throughout the day. Changes in performance patterns can result, as the client may need to wait for assistance with self-care, whereas these tasks would have been completed at his or her own convenience prior to the onset of this illness. Home modifications may be required, along with the need to perform everyday occupations within a different context, in order to maintain safety. For example, a client may need to remain on one level of his or her home versus utilizing the upstairs and downstairs as in the past. Changes in a personal natural environment may require time for adjustment as well as psychosocial interventions. Emotions such as sadness, depression, and despondence may be considered normal at first, but if they are prolonged and are interfering with motivation toward independence, psychological intervention may be considered. The occupational therapist must be sensitive to these feelings to the same degree as being aware of the client's physical changes.

The impact of limited performance of a client may also affect family and other interpersonal relationships. The occupational therapist must be sensitive to the dynamics involved as well as offer support and guidance to the family or caregivers. This will facilitate ease and safety in the transition of the client to home in a dignified manner. At times, social work intervention may be indicated, recognized, and initiated even prior to the patient's discharge.

Context and Environment

Context and environment "refers to a variety of interrelated conditions within and surrounding the client that influence performance. Context include cultural, physical, social, personal, temporal, and virtual. The term environment refers to the external physical and social environments that surround the client and in which the client's daily life occupations occur" (AOTA, 2014, p. S28).

Upon initial evaluation, occupational therapists determine the role that context and environment play in occupational performance. For example, culture may play an important role in occupational performance. Some clients may be more receptive to the assistance of others for daily tasks and, therefore, may not be receptive to learning new techniques to advance their independence with IADLs. On the other hand, some clients may refuse the assistance of others or will not allow others in their home to provide them with care. These clients will require rehabilitation to facilitate the return to home in a safe manner.

The physical environment has a direct impact on a client's functional abilities, safety, and productivity (Van Oss, Rivers, Heighton, Macri, & Reid, 2012). Home modifications can improve occupational performance for personal of all ages. Occupational therapy practitioners are trained to perform assessments of human performance while performing functional tasks along with safety within the environment. Particularly with the IADL of cooking, intervention should be provided regarding safety in the kitchen environment, and adaptations should be made as necessary to ensure optimal performance and productivity. Recommendations for adaptations to enhance accessibility of the home can be provided by occupational therapy practitioners. If this is not possible, some success has been seen implementing the virtual context with the use of apps such as Second Life (Linden Lab). For more information on physical context adaptations, see Chapter 3. Table 4-2 lists the areas of context and their impact on IADLs.

Performance Skills

According to the AOTA Framework, performance skills are defined as "observable elements of action that have an implicit functional purpose" (2014, p. S25). Performance skills include motor skills, process skills, and social interactions skills. Table 4-3 lists the performance skill areas and their impact on IADLs.

An acute onset of deficits in the performance skills of motor, process, and social interaction skills will greatly influence functional levels and impact client safety. Clients manifesting deficits in any area of motor performance may be at risk for safety issues unless these areas are remediated or the client demonstrates use of compensation/adaptation strategies to increase independence and

Table 4-2

Contexts and Impact on Instrumental Activities of Daily Living

Contexts (AOTA, 2002)	Impact of Contexts on IADLs and Intervention
Cultural	• Family teaching may be indicated. • Adaptive equipment/durable medical equipment may not be accepted. • ADL/IADLs may be limited to certain times of the day.
Physical	• Home environments may need modifications (i.e., ramps, durable medical equipment, living areas on first floor). • Limitations in mobility in familiar and unfamiliar environments.
Social	• Fear of participating in former social events. • Communication deficits limiting interaction. • Mobility deficits limiting social contexts.
Personal	• Impaired self-image. • Impaired confidence. • Possible limitations with privacy.
Spiritual	• Inability to participate in spiritual services. • Possible loss of faith.
Temporal	• Modifications in daily routine times. • Increased time to complete tasks.
Virtual	• Inability to access the Internet can limit online shopping or communication capabilities.

maintain safety. For example, the client who is able to ambulate safely with a rolling walker but is unable to maintain balance with kitchen tasks that require carrying objects or reaching in low cabinets for items needed may perform these tasks more safely at wheelchair level. A client who may be faced with a kitchen fire and is unable to process the methods of maintaining safety in an efficient and timely manner will not be able to live independently again. A client who comprehends the danger but is unable to communicate via telephone or call out the need for help may benefit from assistive devices for communication to assure safety. The occupational therapist will assess the client's level of safety based on these performance skills and their effect on function for the individual client.

Performance Patterns

The Framework defines performance patterns as "the habits, routines, roles and rituals used in the process of engaging in occupation activities" (AOTA, 2014, p. S27). Table 4-4 lists performance patterns and their impact on IADLs. Habits and routines play a strong role in daily function. An interruption in physical, sensory, or cognitive/perceptual skills may elicit a change in habit or routine to which it may be difficult for the client to adapt. Occupational therapists must remain sensitive to clients' former performance patterns and assist with facilitation and acceptance of new patterns to enhance function. For example, a client who generally awakens and walks outside for the morning paper independently and without an assistive device may need to wait for the assistance

Table 4-3

Performance Patterns and Impact on Instrumental Activities of Daily Living

Category	AOTA Definition (2002, p. 621)	Impact on Instrumental Activities of Daily Living
Motor Skills • Posture • Mobility • Coordination • Strength and effort • Energy	Skills in moving and interacting with task, objects, and environment (Fisher, personal communication, July 9, 2001).	• Poor posture secondary to pain or prolonged use of an assistive device will limit endurance. • Use of walker, cane or crutches may limit ability to carry items. • Impaired fine motor coordination may limit safety with cooking tasks. • Impaired gross motor coordination may limit safety with community mobility. • Increased effort with performance due to muscle weakness may limit muscle energy and endurance for completion of tasks.
Process Skills • Energy • Knowledge • Temporal organization • Organizing space and objects • Adaptation	Skills . . . used in managing and modifying actions en route to the completion of daily life tasks (Fisher & Kielhofner, 1995, p. 120).	• Sustained effort with the motor components of IADL tasks will require pacing and may limit energy available for higher-level problem-solving skills and attention to task. • Impairments may be noted in choosing appropriate tasks, selecting appropriate tools, use of tools, or inability to ask for assistance. • Limitations may be evident in the client's ability to initiate, sequence, continue, and end an IADL task for success. • The client must be able to obtain needed items for a task and organize the environment for task performance as well as return objects to their designated space upon completion. • IADL tasks may often require modifications and adjustments for safe and effective completion.
Communication/ Interaction Skills • Physicality • Information exchange • Relations	Refer to conveying intentions and needs and coordinating social behavior to act together with people (Forsyth & Kielhofner, 1999; Forsyth, Salamy, Simon, & Kielhofner, 1997; Kielhofner, 2002).	• Limitations in range of motion (ROM) and strength may affect ability to communicate verbally or with gesture in the community. • The client may have difficulty requesting information by phone for financial matters. • Social interaction with family or friends may be limited.

Table 4-4

Domain of Occupational Therapy

Category	AOTA Definition (2002, p. 623)	Impact on Instrumental Activities of Daily Living
Habits • Useful habits • Impoverished habits • Dominating habits	Automatic behavior that is integrated into more complex patterns that enable people to function on a day-to-day basis' (Neistadt & Crepeau, 1998, p. 869). Habits can either support or interfere with performance in areas of occupation.	• Selecting and placing clothing out for the next day when needing to be out early. • Forgetting to close kitchen cabinets and drawers. • Smoking.
Routines	Occupations with established sequences (Christiansen & Baum, 1997, p. 6).	Establishing a daily medication schedule.
Roles	A set of behaviors that have some socially agreed upon function and for which there is an accepted code of norms (Christiansen & Baum, 1997, p. 603).	Preparing the evening meal, role of caregiver.

of a caregiver and may need to use a cane or walker for the task. It is often difficult for a client who has been accustomed to certain habits and routines to be receptive to an alternative lifestyle. Further discussion of the role of performance patterns in various areas of occupation will follow.

Activity and Occupational Demands

Activity demands refers to "the components of activities and occupations that occupational therapy practitioners consider during the clinical reasoning process. Depending upon the context and needs of the client, these demands can be deemed barriers to or supports for participation" (AOTA, 2014, p. S32).

The activity demands of IADLs may require more effort and energy than they did previously. Often clients with an acute onset of neurological, orthopedic, and cognitive/perceptual impairments express feelings of fatigue and may be generally deconditioned secondary to prolonged inactivity. Activity and occupational demands include relevance to the client, objects used, space and social demands, sequencing and timing, and required actions, body functions, and structures.

Continuous education in principles of energy conservation and work simplification may assist the client in participating in additional occupations more effectively (White, 2013). An introduction to adaptive equipment and durable medical equipment (DME) would also be indicated at this time. This area will also be addressed in greater detail throughout this section. Table 4-5 summarizes how activity demands can impact IADLs.

Table 4-5

Activity Demands and Impact on Impact on Instrumental Activities of Daily Living

Space demands	Home modifications may be indicated to accommodate assistive devices for gait.
Social demands	Clients may need to entertain within their own home if accessibility to other environments is limited or if community mobility is an issue.
Sequencing and timing	Both skills are needed for clients to be able to prepare a meal in an efficient manner.
Required actions	The client must have the ability to complete all of the required actions necessary for driving to maintain safety.
Required body functions	A client may not participate in outdoor home maintenance activities if he or she demonstrates impaired balance on uneven surfaces.
Required body structures	A client with a nonfunctional UE will be unable to complete tasks requiring bilateral integration such as grasping and holding a laundry basket.

Client Factors

According to the Framework, "Client factors include (1) values, beliefs, and spirituality; (2) body functions; and (3) body structures that reside within the client and may affect performance areas of occupation" (AOTA, 2014, p. S22).

Any change a client may experience within his or her body may influence overall performance. Strength, mobility, ROM, muscle tone, and endurance should be assessed in relation to performance in occupation-based activities. Intervention in the form of remediation or compensation/adaptation will need to occur for the client to achieve independence in IADL. For more information on remediation of these skills, see Chapter 2.

Role of the Occupational Therapy Assistant

The role of the occupational therapy assistant is to facilitate intervention in all aspects of IADL (AOTA, 2013). The occupational therapy assistant, under the supervision of an occupational therapist, may implement an intervention plan utilizing remediation or compensation/adaptation techniques to facilitate independence in home management, financial management, community skills, communication devices, and care of others. For example, in an inpatient rehabilitation setting, the occupational therapy assistant may teach compensation/adaptation techniques to a client with a new CVA to facilitate independence with meal preparation. The occupational therapy assistant may introduce adaptive devices such as a one-handed cutting board, a rocker knife, and/or a walker basket and educate the patient in hemi-techniques. For the client who has undergone a total hip replacement, the occupational therapy assistant may make recommendations for environmental changes within the home. These changes may include rearranging the refrigerator or cabinets to place the client's most frequently used items at waist level or above in order for the client to maintain total hip precautions. An adaptive device such as a reacher may be introduced to assist with certain tasks.

Prior to the intervention of IADL, it is understood that the occupational therapist has evaluated performance skills, performance patterns, and context. As a result of this assessment and interview with the client and/or the client's family, a method of intervention will be selected. A thorough understanding of the client's previous role within the family, the amount of support and assistance available, and quality of socialization outside of the home is important. This will assist the occupational therapist in determining intervention methods. The occupational therapy assistant will discuss with the occupational therapist the findings of the evaluation and interview process in order to recommend intervention. Hence, the occupational therapy assistant will have a thorough understanding of the client's goals and the recommended method of intervention. The occupational therapy assistant may collaborate with the occupational therapist with respect to the client's progress, and together the two will determine new goals when indicated. The occupational therapist will assist the client with recommendations for discharge planning in the inpatient setting and determine the safest plan and the services the client will require upon discharge to home. The occupational therapy assistant possesses the skills to observe the day-to-day progress that a client is making. In the event that the client has demonstrated a change in status, or if the client's set goals seem to be too high or too low, the occupational therapy assistant will need to bring this matter to the attention of the occupational therapist for review.

Evaluation of Instrumental Activities of Daily Living

While the focus of this text is intervention, evaluations will be discussed briefly because they are an important component of the intervention plan. The first step of any evaluation is the completion of an interview or an occupational profile with the client. This allows the therapist to gather information regarding the client's motivating factors, goals, discharge needs, etc. One tool that can quickly and easily be administered to assist in this process is the Canadian Occupational Performance Measure (COPM). This tool is a client-centered, outcome-oriented occupation-based assessment. This tool allows the client to identify areas of occupation in which he or she would like to improve (Law et al., 1998). Using a functional approach, the therapist would then begin to evaluate specific IADLs that the client desires to work on and that are required for discharge planning. While there are many evaluations available, a few examples of formal evaluations include the Performance Assessment of Self-Care Skills (PASS), the Kohlman Evaluation of Living Skills (KELS), the Arnadottir OT-ADL Neurobehavioral Assessment (A-ONE), and the Independent Living Scales (ILS). The PASS and A-ONE were discussed thoroughly in Chapter 3. The KELS, developed by Kohlman and Thomson, is an interview- and activity-based evaluation. The evaluation includes five subsections with money management, transportation, and telephone use relating to IADLs (Thomson, 1992). This tool requires no training, and the evaluation kit is inexpensive. The ILS is a reliable and valid observation-based rating assessment of IADLs. The ILS includes five subsections: memory/orientation, managing money, managing home and transportation, health and safety, and social adjustment. It takes about 45 minutes to administer and can assist in determining appropriate supervision and placement for those with cognitive function limitations (Loeb, 1996).

The Rabideau Kitchen Evaluation can be used to assess a client during a kitchen task (Neistadt, 1992). Of the two types of environmental assessments, the person-environment fit is client-centered while the environmental assessment is more of an audit of the environment. Person fit assessments allow the occupational therapist to view the person, the environment, and the task to create individualized recommendations to improve safety, function, and livability. Refer to Appendix B for additional evaluation tools.

Intervention of Instrumental Activities of Daily Living

Remediation of Impact on Instrumental Activities of Daily Living

In general, remediation of acute impairments involves relearning basic performance skills. Normal movement patterns are necessary for developing independence in all areas of IADL. For example, if a client who is right-hand dominant has experienced a left CVA with resulting right hemiparesis, he or she may be unable to use the right upper extremity (UE) functionally, as in writing a check. By utilizing the remediation approach, the client may develop functional range of motion (ROM), strength, and coordination of the right UE to be able to complete a check-writing task. The client learns to use the affected UE for functional tasks versus learning compensation or adaptation techniques for use of the unaffected UE such as paying by cash or credit card. For more information regarding these foundational skills to IADLs, see Chapter 2.

By the time the client is advanced enough to participate in IADLs, utilizing the remediation approach will have involved practicing each task until mastery has been or is nearly achieved. For example, if the client wishes to manage his or her own checkbook, he or she will have had to practice writing skills to be able to legibly write a check. Basic mathematical skills will also need to be mastered if there is impairment in this area in order to manage money independently.

In conclusion, the remediation approach for clients who are ready to participate in IADLs involves practicing each task until mastery is achieved. The occupational therapist must give careful consideration to the client's allotted rehabilitation benefits as well as the client's disposition plan when working with the client and the rehabilitation team to determine whether or not the remediation approach is the best course for each individual client. The following factors should be considered:

1. The client's overall readiness to learn
2. The client's functional goals
3. The client's prognosis and estimated rate and level of recovery
4. The estimated length of occupational therapy intervention prior to discharge
5. The amount of assistance the client will have upon discharge

With careful consideration of these factors, the client and the rehabilitation team will determine the most appropriate approach for intervention. The selected approach may need to be reconsidered for efficacy if the client is not progressing as efficiently as expected or if recovery has been expedited. It may also be necessary to combine both approaches in order for the client to be discharged to home. Compensation/adaptation techniques may be utilized as the client continues with remediation of deficits. This will allow independence and safety with IADL while continuing to regain function.

Compensation/Adaptation of Impact on Instrumental Activities of Daily Living Deficits for Clients With Physical Limitations: Performance Skills/Client Factors

Limitations a client experiences secondary to impairments in ROM, strength, coordination, sensation, pain, or endurance can greatly affect the client's ability to participate in IADL tasks in a safe and independent manner (Figure 4-2). These clients will have begun occupational therapy intervention once their physicians deemed them medically stable. Therefore, they may have

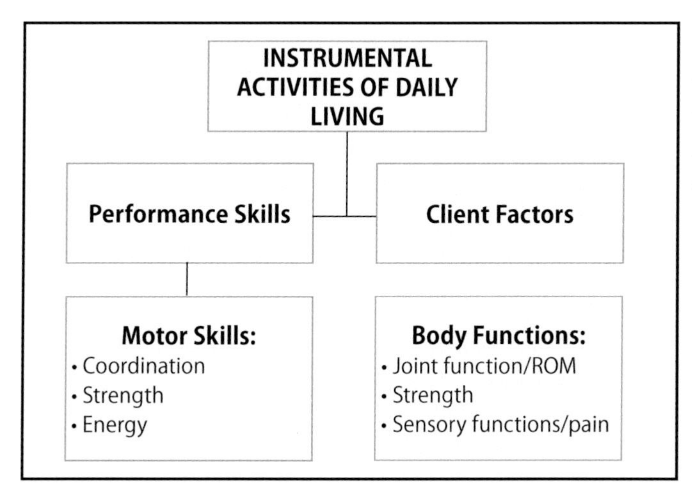

Figure 4-2. Components of performance skills/client factors related to IADLs. (Adapted from American Occupational Therapy Association. (2014). Occupational therapy practice framework: Domain and process (3rd ed.). *American Journal of Occupational Therapy, 68*(Suppl. 1), S1-S48.)

recognized some of the limitations that they will encounter upon discharge to their home early after the onset of their illness.

Physical limitations will dictate the type of task chosen, the manner in which the client performs the task, the assistive devices he or she will need to use to facilitate independence, the level of activity tolerance, and the outcome. The client who is to participate in IADL tasks will need to have achieved a safe functional status through remediation of performance skills, or the client will need to have mastered adequate adaptation/compensation skills to facilitate the same. Whatever the approach, the client and his or her support system, along with the rehabilitation team, will need to determine what goals are feasible for this client.

Compensation/Adaptation Interventions of Impact on Instrumental Activities of Daily Living for Clients With Decreased Performance Skills/Client Factors: ROM, Strength, and Coordination Deficits

Home Management (Home Establishment, Meal Preparation, and Cleanup)

Laundry

Participating in the home management task of doing laundry involves collecting soiled clothing, carrying the load to the washer, separating clothing items, loading the washing machine, adding soap and bleach as indicated, and starting the cycle (Figure 4-3). It then involves removing clothing from the washer and placing it in the dryer, or hanging clothing on a clothes rack or clothesline. Once clothing is dry, the client will fold each piece and place it in a closet or drawer. For some clients, laundry management was a daily chore and for others a chore completed less frequently. Upon initial discharge to home, the client, along with his or her family and/or caregivers, will need to determine the amount of energy the client can allow for this task and still participate in other IADL tasks. It may be determined that the client should complete only one aspect of laundry management initially and gradually work up to full management. Or it may be within the client's tolerance to complete all aspects of this task. Another consideration is the location of the washer and dryer and whether stairs are a factor. For the client with a neurological impairment, navigating stairs may be contraindicated upon initial discharge to home, and therefore completing

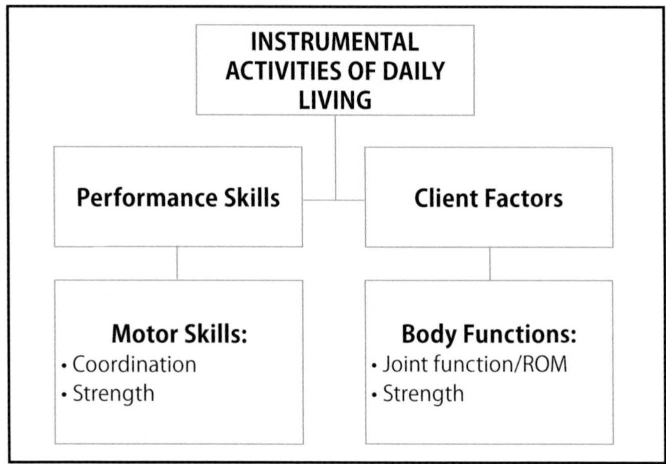

Figure 4-3. Relationship of ROM, strength, and coordination to IADLs. (Adapted from American Occupational Therapy Association. (2002). *Occupational therapy practice framework: Domain and process*. Bethesda, MD: AOTA.)

the full task of laundry management may not be feasible. However, any aspect of the task such as collecting soiled clothing or folding clean laundry may be completed.

Changing the Task to Achieve Independence

Clients with UE physical impairments may experience many performance skill deficits. Some important points discussed are safety, participation level, accessibility, and compensation/adaptation for balance and carrying items. Education in safety is of significant importance, and evaluation of a client's safety should be ongoing. The occupational therapist may need to perform home safety evaluations to assess the environment and make recommendations for modifications. In order to participate in laundry management, the washer and dryer should be easily accessible to the client, especially with the use of an assistive device for gait. Laundry detergent and other laundry needs should be within reach. If hemiparesis is present, the client may need to use one-handed techniques to load the machines and to pour the detergent. Smaller, lighter detergent containers may be indicated for use. The receptacle for soiled clothing may need to be placed near the washer so the client will not need to carry the clothing. If that is not possible, a large duffle bag may be used so that the client can pull it along instead of carrying the clothing.

Placing newly washed laundry in the dryer should be less of a challenge to the client unless balance is an issue. If so, the client may need to remove clothing from the washer and place it on top of the dryer and sit to load clothes into the machine. Once the clothes are dry, the client will need to bring them to a table or other flat surface and fold them via a one-handed technique. The client should then carry small bundles of clothing to the dressers and closets and put them away. If the client is unsteady with gait, the client may need to use a cart to complete this task in a safe and efficient manner. In extreme cases, a wheelchair may be required to maintain safety.

Clients with lower extremity (LE) or trunk limitations will experience different limitations. After joint replacement or back surgery, the client will have limited ROM and also may have to adhere to certain precautions. For example, the client who has undergone back surgery will be limited in bending as well as twisting at the waist. These clients will need to stand for this activity. When sitting, the client may bend forward too far to retrieve the clothing from its place of holding or to load the dryer. For purposes of maintaining precautions and balance, laundry baskets and all other working items should be placed on higher surfaces and not on the floor. Once the task is complete, the client will need to place his or her clothing in a drawer that is higher so as not to bend too far forward at the waist.

Changing the Tools to Achieve Independence

As previously noted, the client may use a duffle bag to carry laundry instead of a laundry basket, which may require the use of both hands, or the client may then pull the duffle bag with one hand. If the client is using a walker, a lighter laundry bag may be attached to the front of the device and the client may need to make more trips to the laundry area. Also, smaller containers of laundry detergent may be indicated as noted above so that it will be easier for the client to grasp and pour with one hand. The use of detergent pods is also an option.

For clients with limited ability to bend, a reacher may be required to assist with placing clothing in the dryer or removing the dry clothing. In addition, for the client with limited weight-bearing status, using a walker or crutches may limit his or her ability to carry clothing to and from the working area. A pushcart may be required so that the client can push the clothes rather than carry them.

Light Cleaning

Light cleaning involves dusting, mopping floors, and organizing the home. Participating in the task of dusting involves bending and reaching to achieve thoroughness, grasping and lifting objects, and manipulation of dust cloths for the task. Mopping floors requires the ability to move furniture to reach all surfaces and to manipulate all required tools for the task. Organizing the home involves sorting important items and placing them in their designated space and eliminating those items that are no longer wanted.

Changing the Task to Achieve Independence

For the client with physical deficits, one-handed techniques once again may be utilized to complete the home management tasks discussed earlier. Utilization of energy conservation techniques may be necessary, as it will take the client a much longer time to complete these tasks. With dusting, the client will move more slowly from one area to the next, particularly if using an assistive device for gait. Removing items with one hand and then dusting and replacing items will take longer, especially if the client must use his or her nondominant hand. The client may be limited to dusting surfaces at waist level or slightly higher or lower if balance is an issue.

Mopping floors is a more challenging task for the client who manifests limited use of one UE and/or a deficit in balance. Light mops that may be pushed with one hand would be an appropriate choice. The client would benefit from mopping a small area at a time, moving slowly to change position.

Organizing the home is a general part of home management. Every client has a comfort level in terms of how his or her home looks. The client with a physical deficit will have to consider all aspects of his or her ability when determining the best way to organize the home. Modifications may be required in order to ensure safety. Regularly used kitchen items, for example, may need to be placed at more safe levels of reach. Items that are normally placed in cabinets or closets may need to be on countertops or on wall racks to assist the client with easier accessibility. Throw rugs may need to be removed, and pet care items will also need to be placed carefully to assure client safety. The client may need assistance at first to reorganize the home, and subsequent organization should be easier. Of consideration to the client will be the level of ability to carry objects from one place to another, as well as maintaining use of the recommended ambulatory device while maintaining balance. It would be beneficial to clients if other members of the household organize their personal items and also maintain general organization to assist the client. If the client lives alone, it should be easier to maintain the home in the way the client desires.

For the postsurgical client who is limited in weight-bearing status on one LE, it may be best to delegate some of the tasks that involve challenging balance to a caregiver. Simple tasks may be accomplished if they do not jeopardize the client's safety. The client may require assistance to set up these tasks and sit while doing so. Once the client is as able to weight-bear as tolerated, he or she may be ready to attempt more involved tasks. The client must also maintain any movement precautions as indicated for total hip replacements, such as avoiding bending beyond 90 degrees either in sitting or in standing, or those precautions for clients who have had back surgery, such as avoiding forward bending or twisting at the waist. Therefore, performing certain tasks at wheelchair level may be contraindicated if they will involve bending forward or twisting at the waist.

Changing the Tools to Achieve Independence

Walker baskets may be indicated to assist with transport of items. A pushcart on wheels may also be an efficient method of transport. The client will need to make good use of adaptive equipment such as a reacher to retrieve items from high or low levels or cleaning tools with extended parts. Depending on the level of deficits and the availability, the client may utilize a wheelchair for these tasks or use outside services to assist with cleaning and organizing the home.

Outdoor Home Maintenance

This activity includes management of lawn, garden, landscaping, and patio. Outdoor home maintenance may be considered one of the more advanced IADLs. Clients may view these tasks as work or leisure. Home therapy intervention by both physical and occupational therapists may be indicated in order to assure that clients maintain safety with each task. Clients must also be realistic in their expectations because these tasks may require a higher-level of endurance and balance.

Changing the Task to Achieve Independence

Clients with limited physical skills may demonstrate impaired balance with gait on uneven surfaces such as grass or sand. It would be beneficial to the client to first practice ambulation on these surfaces and obtain a good level of balance prior to attempting any outdoor home maintenance tasks. Once ambulation is safe, the client may begin the challenge of maintaining the outside of his or her home. The client should be encouraged to choose tasks that are simple at first, yet provide enough of a challenge to feel a sense of accomplishment. Simple weeding tasks may be a good choice, because the client should be able to utilize one-handed techniques to complete this activity, if required. Watering the garden, flowers, or the lawn may also be an appropriate challenge for the client.

Another consideration is the physical space in which the client expects to work. A smaller working area would be indicated initially as the client begins to challenge him or herself with more advanced IADLs.

Lastly, outdoor home maintenance may be a difficult task for clients who are recovering from orthopedic surgery, especially if they maintain a limited weight-bearing status on the affected UE or LE. Of concern also would be limitations in forward bending of the trunk if seated, which would be the position of choice if a client were unable to bear full weight on one LE. Clients who are recovering from total hip replacement surgery or back surgery will be limited in their ability to bend at the waist, which would make gardening from a seated position contraindicated. While the client recovering from orthopedic surgery would need to wait until his or her restrictions are lifted before tackling many of the activities necessary to manage the outdoors, some tasks can be raised to higher surfaces to allow gardening. One example of this would be flowers or vegetables planted in pots on tables or in raised platforms.

Changing the Tools to Achieve Independence

The client may wish to participate in lawn care. Using a riding mower may be the easiest and most energy-efficient method for the client. Assessment of the client's motor skills must first be obtained to assure that the client will have good control of the mower. The client must also be able to step on and off the machine safely. If a riding mower is not available, the client may benefit from pushing a lawn mower if he or she has enough UE strength and enough endurance to tolerate all aspects of the activity. Of consideration would be the client's ability to start the mower with one hand as indicated. If the client does not possess the strength to do so, he or she may require assistance or select a mower with an electric starter.

If the client has the motor skills sufficient to operate a power mower safely, he or she may consider a leaf blower as well to assist with management of leaves and a snow blower to assist with snow removal.

Other tools may include a rolling garden chair with armrests to sit and complete planting or weeding, power equipment versus manual devices to compensate for deficits in motor skills, and garden tools with wider handles for easier grip. Work belts may be considered to carry necessary gardening supplies.

Shopping

The Framework defines shopping as "preparing shopping lists (grocery and other), selecting and purchasing items, selecting method of payment, and completing money transactions" (AOTA, 2014, p. S20). This includes the ability to organize and write or dictate a shopping list and the ability to mobilize in the community safely (discussed later in this chapter). Prior to visiting the store, the client must also determine the method to be used for payment and bring the appropriate money or credit/debit cards to be used. Upon arrival to the store, the client needs to determine what he or she needs to buy, select the necessary items from the shelves, place these items in a basket/cart, and pay for them in an appropriate manner. The client must keep in mind how much he or she is able to buy and carry. This is dependent on the type of transportation being used to bring the client home and the limitations of the client's deficit. After shopping is completed, the client must bring the purchased items into the home and put them away.

Changing the Task to Achieve Independence

A client with physical impairment may demonstrate impaired motor skills. If the client's dominate UE is affected and handwriting is impaired, the client may need to find an alternative method of recording a shopping list. The client can change the task by using the nondominant hand to write the shopping list, investigate technology alternatives for shopping, or participate in home shopping and delivery services. Shopping may be easier for some clients, because most clients find that pushing the shopping cart helps with balance in the store. Endurance will still be an issue for consideration, and this will be addressed later in this section. Clients with LE impairment may have difficulty navigating the store. Also, the use of crutches may limit their ability to push a cart.

Also of consideration may be the limited use of one UE. The client will have to reach for items with the unaffected UE. This may put the client at the risk of unsteadiness and possibly losing balance if he or she has no means of support. It may then be most beneficial for this client to have a companion when shopping. While not ideal, some clients may participate in a Meals on Wheels program to eliminate the need for extensive shopping.

Changing the Tools to Achieve Independence

If using the affected dominant UE, writing devices such as special grips for pens/pencils or other adaptive devices may assist. Figures 4-4 and 4-5 depict examples of adaptive writing devices. If using the unaffected nondominant UE, stabilization of the paper will be a factor to consider. Clipboards may be of assistance or the paper may be taped to the table. Whenever possible, the client using the unaffected UE should be encouraged to use the affected side for stabilization.

Should the activity of writing be deemed not feasible for the client at this time, use of a voice recorder or voice recorder application may be indicated. The client may also be encouraged to

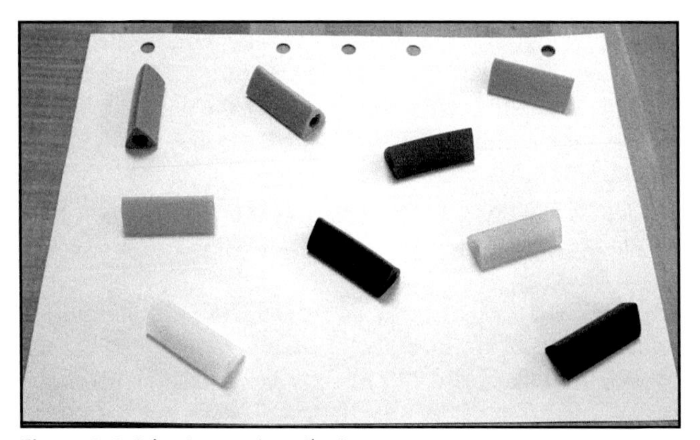

Figure 4-4. Adaptive pen/pencil grips.

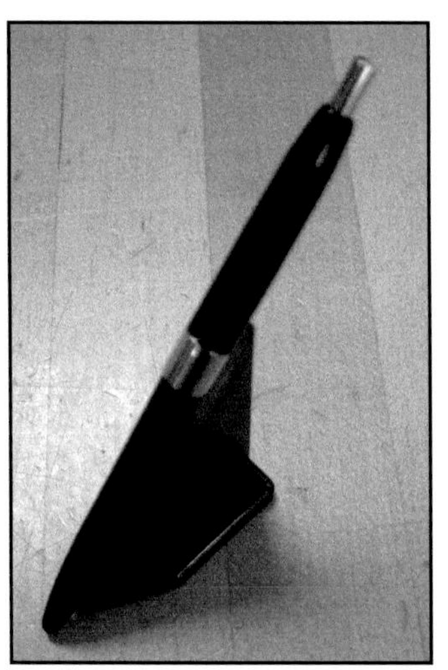

Figure 4-5. Adaptive writing device.

use a computer if he or she is able to manipulate the keys and the mouse with one hand without experiencing frustration. If the client manifests a sufficient gross grasp, he or she may use a stylus to tap the computer keys for writing.

Those clients using a walker and who are not fully weight-bearing on the affected LE will not be able to use the grocery cart to assist with gait. Any of these clients may benefit from an electric riding device or the assistance from friends or family for shopping.

For clients with limited ability to reach items on shelves, a reacher may be utilized. Clients must be informed that items can fall from the reacher and cause injury to them, therefore the reacher should be used for lighter items. If there is a need to retrieve or carry heavier items, this client will need assistance from another individual. Often, grocery store clerks are willing to assist with such tasks, particularly in the smaller neighborhood stores. These clerks may also be available to bring the groceries to the car and load them as well.

Preparing a Meal

Preparation of a meal may have been an important occupation for the client before the onset of an injury or illness. Therefore, it may be very important for this client to be able to return to a level of function that will allow him or her to perform this task safely and as independently as possible once again. According to the AOTA Framework, meal preparation and cleanup includes "planning, preparing, serving well-balanced nutritional meals and cleaning up food and utensils after meals" (2014, p. S20). Setting the table may be included as well.

For preparation of a meal, the client must plan the meal menu, retrieve all ingredients, have the ability to measure them correctly, and follow directions for assembly of the selected recipe. The client will then assemble the ingredients and prepare the dish for cooking or baking. The client must then cook or bake the selected items and set the oven or stove correctly.

Changing the Task to Achieve Independence

The client with physical limitations may have limited use of one UE and/or may need a walker, cane, or crutches to navigate around the kitchen. One-handed techniques may be implemented to assist this client with meal preparation. The client who uses a cane may have the use of one UE to assist with this task but may require increased time and effort to transport items one by one. Kitchen modifications may be indicated so that the client may be able to reach any items needed

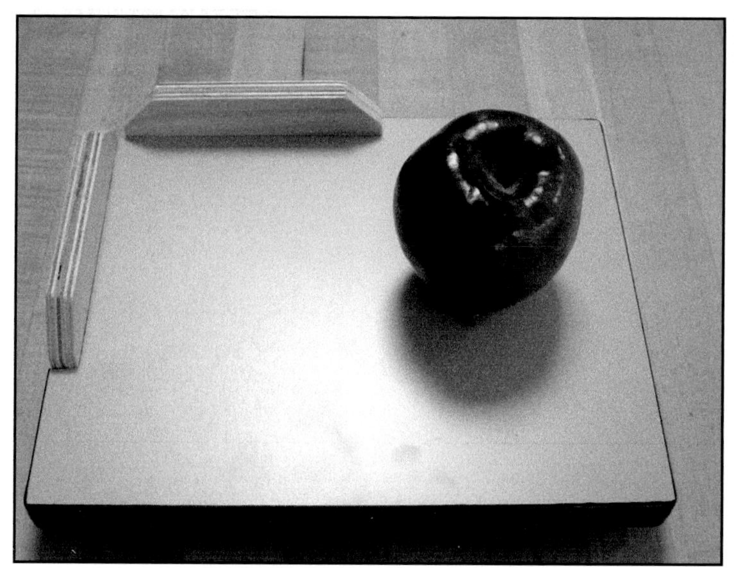

Figure 4-6. Adaptive cutting board.

for meal preparation safely and without loss of balance. For example, frequently used cooking or baking pans normally placed in low cabinets should be placed in cabinets or on countertops at waist level or slightly higher. Refrigerated items should be placed on easily accessible shelves and toward the front. This type of organization is also recommended for the client who is limited in LE or trunk movement.

The client with impaired balance may choose to sit for most of the task of meal preparation. If ambulating and carrying items puts the client at risk for falling, the client may seek help from family. If assistance is not available, the client may choose to use a rolling cart to transport items if doing so is deemed safe by the therapist. Some clients will also choose to move an item along the countertop, walk a few steps, move the item further, etc., until the client and the item have reached the point on the counter where the item is needed.

Changing the Tools to Achieve Independence

The use of adaptive devices will be of great assistance to the client with limited UE use. The use of a walker basket or walker tray, for example, may assist the client with transporting objects from one surface to another. Rocker knives, one-handed cutting boards, and Dycem may also be devices of choice. Figure 4-6 depicts an adaptive cutting board. The occupational therapist working with the client in a rehabilitation setting or in the home must educate the client in the use of these items to facilitate independence with meal preparation. The client with limited UE use will need assistance with placing and removing pans from the oven and the stove. Lighter-weight pots and pans can increase independence, or the client will need to use the microwave or utilize stovetop cooking. If family is available to assist, the client may also ask for assistance with this task in order to maintain safety.

Although not ideal, if meal preparation is not safe, the client may utilize the services offered from others to prepare meals that the client will only need to reheat. Programs that provide hot meals delivered to the home may also be an option for the client to consider in order to eliminate the preparation of one hot meal for the day. Frozen dinners or prepackaged foods may also be used. However, attention must be paid to nutritional content.

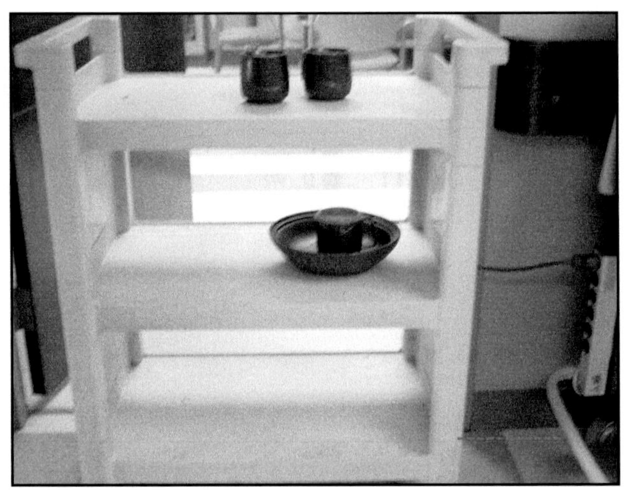

Figure 4-7. Cart utilized for transporting items in the kitchen.

Setting the Table

This task includes retrieving dishes and silverware from cabinets, carrying them to the table, and walking around the table to place the dinnerware at each setting. Napkins, condiments, and drinks must also be retrieved and placed on the table. In addition, the food must be served at the table.

Changing the Task to Achieve Independence

Participating in the task of setting the table is similar to the task of transporting items for meal preparation as outlined above. The client using a cane may be able to carry light items in one hand to the table if he or she demonstrates good balance and good strength of the affected UE since the client will be holding the cane with the unaffected side. This client may have to make several trips to complete the task and avoid lifting heavy objects with just one hand. Once all the necessary items are carried to the table, the client will then need to ambulate around the table and set a place for each family member. The client may complete the task using a wheelchair, if necessary, or may sit to set the table if the table is small enough for the client to reach each setting area from one seat.

Changing the Tools to Achieve Independence

A walker basket, tray, or pushcart may be used to transport some of the table settings (Figure 4-7). Lighter settings may be used, such as paper or plastic plates and cups, to increase ease and safety during transportation of the tableware.

Wash/Dry Dishes and Put Dishes Away

The last task within meal preparation is cleaning and putting away the dishes. This task includes bringing all dishes, pans, and silverware that need to be cleaned to the sink, filling the washbasin, and then adding soap. The client must then wash and rinse all dishes, dry them and put them in their appropriate place. For those clients who use a dishwasher, they will load the dishes and silverware, add soap, and then set and start the device. When dry, the client will remove all items and place them in their appropriate place.

Changing the Task to Achieve Independence

Washing and drying dishes can be completed while standing or sitting. The client may require assistance to carry the items to be washed to the sink. If the client has limited or no functional use of one UE, he or she will have to attempt one-handed techniques for this task. Heavier pans or dishes may have to be left for someone else to wash and dry. If the client is able to use the affected UE, caution must be taken and the stronger arm should bear most of the work. Sensation should be assessed and if there is impairment, the client should be aware to test the water for dish washing with the unaffected hand prior to using the affected side.

In order to manage drying the dishes utilizing a one-handed technique, the client may place a towel on the countertop and place the dish on the towel. With that towel or another, the client can wipe the dishes with one hand.

If the client has a dishwasher in the home, it may be easier to complete this task. The client will need to have good balance to load and unload the machine, especially if working toward the affected side. It may be safer for the client to stand with the machine to his or her unaffected side and load from that position instead of turning toward the affected side to load the dishwasher. If possible, the client can use the affected UE to stabilize him or herself on the countertop while completing the task. To place the dishwasher soap in the machine, the client may use the same positioning technique, stabilizing with the unaffected UE. Use of a raised dishwasher or adjustable-height counters or sink may be beneficial to clients seeking alternative modifications.

To unload the dishwasher or to put hand-dried dishes away, the client should also work with the dishes to his or her unaffected side. The client may stack the dishes first on a counter near where they are to be placed or place each piece in the drawer or cabinet as it is removed from the dishwasher. The client using a walker will place dishes on the countertop and move them along to the cabinet, taking a few steps with the walker after placing the dishes. The client using a cane may use the same technique or may carry the dishes to their destination. As discussed previously, heavy pots, pans, or dishes will have to remain on the countertop until the client has assistance to put them away.

It may be difficult for this client to put dishes away from wheelchair level. If cabinets are high, the client will need to stand to put items away if he or she is able. If not, the client will need to find a new location within reach for these items or wait for assistance.

The clients who must adhere to total hip replacement or spinal surgery precautions may not be able to complete the task of loading and unloading the dishwasher from a standing position because they may need to bend beyond 90 degrees at the hip to complete the task. Attempting this task from a seated position would also be contraindicated, as it would mean bending past 90 degrees. If this client has no assistance, he or she may need to resort to hand-washing and drying of dishes.

The task of putting dishes away may be accomplished if the client can complete the task and maintain the appropriate weight-bearing status/precautions. However, the client will only be able to place dishes in upper cabinets, as he or she will not be able to bend to place any items in the lower cabinets if maintenance of total hip replacement or spinal surgery precautions is required.

Changing the Tools to Achieve Independence

If the client prefers to eliminate this task, paper dishes and plastic silverware may be used. A walker basket, tray, or pushcart may also be utilized for transporting silverware or lighter dinnerware to and from the sink or dishwasher.

Financial Management

Finances are a very important aspect of IADL for all, but especially for those who have been hospitalized and have gone through rehabilitation and for those with chronic illnesses. The cost incurred may be more than the client can put forth if he or she is not covered by insurance. Yet, even if a client is fortunate enough to have appropriate insurance coverage, other expenses may be accrued in an effort to help the client to live safely in his or her own home. A client may require ongoing caregiving to assist with ADLs or IADLs or consider use of personal funds for home modifications or additional DME.

Another consideration would be if the client was the main financial provider for the family or for him or herself. If so, the client may now need assistance with financial planning and budgeting, especially if the client is unable to return to work or to the job he or she left. However, in addition to needing assistance for the long scope of care, the client will need financial assistance for normal day-to-day financial tasks such as paying for groceries and paying monthly bills.

Changing the Task to Achieve Independence

If a client has experienced an injury or illness that has resulted in motor deficits limiting use of the dominant UE, this will make the task of writing difficult. This could impact check writing or any financial matter requiring the client to sign his or her name. The client will need to continue to practice writing skills with the nondominant hand until the highest level of mastery is achieved.

The tasks of managing money and counting bills or change may also be difficult. The client may need to organize his or her bills in a wallet from largest to smallest or fold bills separately within the wallet to make them thicker to grasp from the wallet. In general, most clients can use the unaffected extremity to compensate with little difficulty.

Changing the Tools to Achieve Independence

If the client demonstrates some aspect of strength and coordination of the dominant UE, he or she may be able to relearn writing skills with the dominant hand and use of adaptive devices. Examples of these devices include built-up grips, a weighted pen to stabilize handwriting if tremulous, a weighted holder to slip onto pens for stabilization, or a gliding device that supports a pen or pencil to assist with limited strength or control of the arm. When writing, the client may need to position objects for use on his or her lap or on a tray versus using a table to maintain recommended positioning of the UE or for comfort.

If adaptive devices are not appropriate, the use of cash or debit/credit cards may be more manageable for the client. The client may also benefit from computerized bill paying, which is available through most banks.

For money management, a separate change purse may be utilized so that the client does not have to dig into a purse or pants pockets to locate change.

Community Mobility

Loss of independence in the area of community mobility for the client with a neurological deficit, the client who has experienced orthopedic surgery, or the client with cognitive/perceptual deficits can be debilitating. Limitations in this area may mean a regression from socialization for a client. It may also mean difficulty keeping doctor's appointments, therapy appointments, and other important meetings. A client who is accustomed to going out daily or being free to move about in the community on an as-needed basis may feel restricted with new limitations in this area. For example, in the past, if the client ran out of milk at home, he or she may have easily driven to the store to purchase it. Clients may now have to wait for a family member, caregiver, or friend to take them to the store or to bring the milk to the house. The occupational therapist needs to address the level of importance mobilizing in the community has with each client and determine the best approach toward this goal if it is significant to the individual. The therapist can discuss with clients transportation alternatives, networks of community resources, development of walking programs, or training in the use of public transportation (AOTA, 2012). More information regarding functional mobility intervention can be found in Chapter 3.

The client must determine if he or she wishes to return to driving again, and the therapist must determine if the client is safe enough and manifests the appropriate performance skills to carry out this task. For example, residual deficits in ROM, sensation, vision, endurance, hearing, and higher-level cognitive processing must be evaluated before the client can be referred for a driving examination. If the client manifests the appropriate motor and sensory skills but demonstrates impaired safety and judgment, the therapist should redirect the client's goals and avoid referring the client for a driving examination.

For the client who appears to be ready to begin driving soon after discharge, the therapist should make use of the clinical setting to begin retraining the client in preparation for driving once again. There are some rehabilitation facilities that have an area designated for driving simulation. Often, there is a model car that the client may use to practice the motor components of driving such as placing and turning the key, shifting, steering, and transferring his or her foot from the gas pedal to the brake. It should be noted that driver retraining is not considered an entry-level skill for occupational therapists, and continued education is required prior to initiating this with clients. See Appendix A for further information regarding training.

If driving is unrealistic, the occupational therapist and other members of the rehabilitation team need to address other options with the client and offer suggestions and recommendations for alternative methods of transportation. The client may be fearful at first to use public transportation because the concept may be new to him or her. The elderly client may be concerned about being out alone or may have a fear of selecting the wrong transit system and becoming lost. They may have difficulty with transit fees. Also of concern to any client is the ability to mobilize independently on and off the transit vehicle in a safe manner or walking safely to a bus stop. Weather conditions may also limit the client's ability to use public transportation. The occupational therapist can work with a social worker to determine what means of transportation are available to the client. Some communities offer transportation to and from the home for a minimal fee. If clients are fortunate enough to have family or friends to assist them, they may be sacrificing independence; however, the use of public transportation will be minimal.

Functional mobility within the community must also be addressed with all clients whether they return to driving or decide to utilize an alternative means of transportation. The client must be able to step in and out of a car safely and be able to climb the stairs of a bus or other vehicle independently. Clients recovering from some neurological or orthopedic injuries will need to be transported with their assistive device for gait such as a walker, cane, or wheelchair. If the client has limited or no functional use of one UE, he or she may not be able to use transportation that requires walking up steps secondary to the inability to then carry the walking device and hold on to a rail at the same time.

Changing the Task to Achieve Independence

While clients with a variety of diagnoses will experience difficulty with community mobility, the client with a neurological deficit is the client who needs special consideration for return to driving. After a full interview, assessment, and intervention of the client, the occupational therapist will determine whether the client demonstrates the ability to return to driving in a safe and appropriate manner. As previously discussed, the client will be referred for a driving examination if he or she demonstrates appropriate functional performance in all areas needed to perform the task. If the client does not manifest those performance skills necessary to drive safely, the occupational therapist will work with the client to determine the most effective means of transportation to replace driving. The client who is recovering from orthopedic surgery of the UE or LE may experience the same difficulties with public transportation as the client with a neurological insult. This client, however, should be able to return to driving if he or she wishes, with the consent of the doctor, once sufficiently healed. A driving test would not be indicated.

Changing the Tools to Achieve Independence

The client may rely on family, friends, public transportation, or taxicabs for rides as well as for trips to a shopping center. It is best if the client can select a method of transportation with which he or she can be picked up and dropped off directly at home until achieving more independence with ambulation in the community. Many communities offer low-cost transportation for the elderly as well. The client should use the device that he or she is most safe with for ambulation within the community, even if it is different from the device he or she uses within the home. The client may choose electric riding devices for tasks.

For those clients who are able to return to driving, a certified driving rehabilitation specialist (CRDS) can assist to determine if any adaptive tools are required for driving. Some examples of these are adapted turn signals, foot pedals, or additional mirrors to view surrounding traffic.

Communication Devices

Communication is an extremely important aspect of living. All clients, in order to live at home, will need to be able to communicate their needs and wishes as well as respond appropriately in an emergency situation. For those clients who have experienced impairment in motor, sensory, or cognitive skills, effective communication may be limited without the assistance of an adapted device. The occupational therapist needs to confer with the speech and language pathologist to assess the effectiveness of the client's communication skills prior to making recommendations for discharge.

Changing the Task to Achieve Independence

For the client who has experienced a neurological deficit, communication skills may be strongly impaired. The client may be aphasic or dysarthric, making comprehension of the client's speech difficult. It may also be difficult for the client to express his or her needs. The client may manifest impaired motor skills that will limit efficiency. Any of the above may limit the client's ability to live at home independently or remain at home alone for any period of time.

For the client with aphasia, assessment must be made as to whether the client can perform a task, although he or she may not be able to verbalize the steps of a task. For example, if a client is aphasic and is unable to state the emergency phone number 911, yet when given a telephone the client is able to dial the number appropriately and efficiently, the client may be deemed cognitively capable of recognizing the need for help. If, however, the client's aphasia limits the ability to express him or herself once the call is made, the client may be unsafe. If the client's aphasia is manifested in an inability to dial the phone appropriately, this client may also be deemed unsafe to be alone. The client with dysarthria must be encouraged to speak slowly and clearly when communicating.

A client must be deemed capable of recognizing emergency situations prior to being discharged to home, particularly if 24-hour supervision is not available.

In summary, clients with aphasia and clients manifesting cognitive deficits need to be evaluated carefully in order for an appropriate discharge plan to be made. Clients who manifest with aphasia and cognitive impairment may be most unsafe to be alone.

Changing the Tools to Achieve Independence

Impaired communication may be addressed through the use of portable phones that the clients may have with them at all times. In-home intercoms or pager systems may also be used. If dexterity is impaired, use of one-touch dialing may be beneficial through the use of the unaffected UE if necessary. The client may also use a modified technique for computer use such as one-handed typing or use of a stylus in the affected hand for tapping the computer keys. Communication boards may also be effective in assisting the client with communication of his or her needs. The client may also benefit from an emergency call system in which the touch of one button will alert personnel that he or she is in need of help. There are a variety of apps to facilitate communication if the client is trained to use this technology.

Care of Others and Care of Pets

At times, the client who presents to the rehabilitation team to recover from a neurological insult or from orthopedic surgery has been the sole caregiver of a spouse or a part-time caregiver for grandchildren. It may be necessary to observe this client and recognize any feelings of depression and/or loss of self-worth secondary to limitations in assuming previous roles after rehabilitation. If the client admits to experiencing these feelings, a psychological or psychiatric consultation may be indicated. The social worker assigned to the client must be available to assist the family with arrangements and to provide support to the client as he or she returns home to a new role. AOTA has created a caregiver toolkit to assist family members with a new and often unexpected role. Rehabilitation team members (e.g., nurses, physical therapists, occupational therapists, speech and language pathologists, care managers, and social workers) must educate the client's family prior to discharge as to what they can expect of the client when he or she goes home. If the client was the sole caregiver for a spouse prior to the onset of an injury or illness and this role is no longer safe or appropriate, plans should begin immediately for changes in the client's role upon discharge.

In addition, Baun and McCabe (2003) discuss the impact of a client leaving a pet behind upon admittance to long-term care. The client must relinquish the role of caring for his or her pet, as well as the companionship and unconditional love. As a result, the caregiver must now assume the responsibility of pet care, if able. In turn, the authors also discuss the benefits of the companion animal for the caregiver and the role the pet now takes in terms of comforting the caregiver.

Changing the Task to Achieve Independence

Caring for others in the home may be as simple as supervising medication or as taxing as washing and dressing a spouse. The client and his or her family must discuss what expectations are realistic for the client upon returning home. Recommendations for intervention for the client with neurological deficits or for the client who has undergone orthopedic surgery should reflect the safest environment for all. Clients who have undergone surgical procedures will typically have lifting restrictions, and clients with neurological diagnoses may have residual weakness that will limit their lifting abilities. A client with either neurological or orthopedic deficits may present with balance impairments that may require the use of a device and therefore may restrict the client's ability to care for another.

Child rearing of a younger child may be a particularly difficult task. Family and friends may need to be involved to assist the client and his or her family. Day care centers and after-school programs may be considered to free the clients of some daily activities and supervision to allow them to focus on their own rehabilitation needs. Often, an older child may be interested in being involved in the rehabilitation process and in some of the household management tasks. This will allow the child to feel that he or she is contributing to his or her parent's rehabilitation as well as assist with fulfilling some of the needs of the family.

The client and his or her family must be educated in the importance of the client maintaining his or her own safety and health upon discharge. Often, the client's rehabilitation continues at home. Home physical and occupational therapists should evaluate the client's caregiver role if applicable and determine whether the client and family member are safe. It may be unsafe to discharge a client to home knowing that he or she will be caring for a spouse or other family member in addition to him or herself. At this time, the client and his or her family may choose to acquire additional assistance for a family member in need.

The client who is to return home as caregiver for a pet will need to be evaluated for safety as well. Those clients that have limited balance and are using a device to assist with gait will have to be especially careful of pets crossing their paths and also of any pet toys that may be left on the floor or carpet. The client that is used to bending forward to pick up a pet will have to maintain adherence to any weight-bearing or bending limitations. Placing food or water for the pet may be difficult for clients with an orthopedic diagnosis if they are unable to fully weight-bear on one LE or, as in the case of clients who have had a total hip replacement or spinal surgery, if they are not able to bend to the floor. A client who manifests balance deficits may choose to sit to place food and water on the floor or may choose to place the food on a raised surface. Cats generally will not have difficulty on a raised surface, but this may be problematic for dogs.

Upon the client's arrival home, pets may need to be reintroduced when the client is sitting or lying down and not in a position to be pushed over by an excited pet. Often the client's return home to his or her pet can be very therapeutic and enhance the healing process.

Changing the Tools to Achieve Independence

Pet bowls that are in a raised stand may be useful for clients who are unable to bend to the floor. A reacher may also be used to pick up or put down the bowl. Automatic feeders that need to be filled once per week and automatic litter box cleaners are a possibility to assist clients with limited mobility, strength, and endurance. Pet food may need to be purchased more frequently, in smaller bags, or it may be delivered via online or catalog shopping.

Health Management and Maintenance

This aspect of IADL is of critical importance to the client, and successful management will mean a greater chance for the client to maintain good health and quality of life. Upon initial discharge to home, the client may experience mixed emotions. He or she may be overwhelmed with transitioning from a more secure environment back to home and independent living. Routines must be established early on to assist the client with organization and planning.

The client must first understand the significance of medication compliance and of maintaining appropriate and recommended exercise programs as well as good nutrition and adequate hygiene. Home health care professionals will be available if assistance is needed in generalizing new learning from a rehabilitation setting to the home.

Changing the Task to Achieve Independence

With respect to physical fitness, the clients with neurological or orthopedic impairments will need guidance with developing an individualized exercise program that will promote strength, endurance, and overall good health. The clients should be encouraged to execute the home exercise program that was recommended by the rehabilitation team on a regular basis. Upon discharge from home care services, community exercise programs are also available for continuation of exercise. The client should get approval from the physician before beginning any community exercise program.

Good nutrition is also significant to the healing process. Education should be provided to the client as to what foods are important to consume to reduce any health risks, as well as what foods should be avoided because they are significant contributors to certain health problems. Clients who had been smoking prior to hospitalization should be encouraged to break this habit. We cannot expect all clients to recognize or admit the hazards that accompany smoking, but it is the health care provider's responsibility to provide education to the client concerning these risks.

Clients should also be sure to maintain good hygiene both inside and outside of the home. Improper hygiene is a known cause of spreading infections and of facilitating poor health (Saffari et al., 2013).

Medication management and compliance is an important factor in a client's health and well-being. The client must understand the names and significance of all medications. It is also

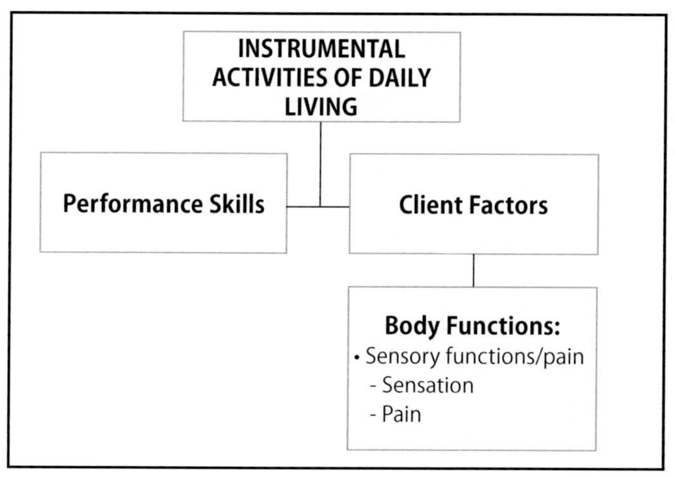

Figure 4-8. Relationship of sensation/pain to IADLs. (Adapted from American Occupational Therapy Association. (2014). Occupational therapy practice framework: Domain and process (3rd ed.). *American Journal of Occupational Therapy, 68*(Suppl. 1), S1-S48.)

important for clients to establish routines to promote medication adherence. This may include specific timing, locations, equipment used, memory aids, and assistance as needed to adhere to medication regimes (Sanders & Van Oss, 2012). Several studies have indicated that clients who begin self-medication prior to discharge from a facility have increased adherence. These clients do not necessarily have increased knowledge; therefore, it is vital that the client understands and is physically/cognitively able to call his or her physician with any questions as well as to reorder prescriptions when needed (Kelly, 1994; Pereles et al., 1996; Webb, Addison, Holman, Saklaki, & Wagner, 1990). In addition, collaboration with other rehabilitation team members regarding medications can improve adherence (Touchard & Berthelot, 1999).

Changing the Tools to Achieve Independence

A client may benefit from using a reacher to retrieve medications that are out of reach. Also to be considered are weekly and monthly medication organizers. The client with a neurological impairment limiting the functional use of one UE may need to have medications placed in uncovered containers or non-childproof containers to allow the client independence in retrieving medication. The client with an orthopedic deficit may need to have medications placed within safe reach. A daily nutrition guide will also be helpful to assist the client in making the most effective food choices.

Sensation Changes and Pain

Impairment in sensation may place a client at risk for injury when taking part in IADL tasks (Figure 4-8). Clients with impaired sensation must have intact cognition in order to be left unsupervised and be educated in the importance of thinking tasks through and concentrating on their performance with each activity. They must also visually focus on the task and guard the affected UE to avoid danger.

The IADL task of meal preparation needs careful attention, particularly when the client is using the stove or microwave and sharp utensils. Tasks involving use of electricity or power equipment also present a concern for the client with impaired sensation. Safety also becomes an issue if the client's impaired sensation affects his or her ability to carry objects such as dinnerware or laundry. The client must also be careful when using cleaning supplies that may include materials that are toxic to the skin.

Generally speaking, the client with either hyposensitivity or hypersensitivity of the UE must be extremely careful with tasks that place him or her at risk of injury. It is wise to use the unaffected

Table 4-6

Summary of Instrumental Activities of Daily Living and Compensation/Adaptations for Sensory Deficits

IADL Task	Compensatory/Adaptive Strategies for Sensation and Pain
Laundry	Use both hands to load/unload washer and dryer.
Light cleaning	Use a dust mitt instead of a cloth that may be frequently dropped.
Outdoor maintenance	Avoid use of sharp objects.
Shopping	Use both hands and/or vision to guide lifting and carrying grocery items.
Meal preparation	Wear an oven mitt to avoid a burn.
Table setting	Visually attend when reaching into drawers for sharp utensils and when carrying and placing them.
Dishes	Check water temperature with the intact hand to avoid a burn.
Financial management	If using a pen or pencil, place a hook-and-loop strip or other textured piece over grip area to enhance the sensation of grasp.
Community mobility	Visually attend to the environment to avoid bumping into objects.
Communication devices	Use the intact hand to control the device, especially in an emergency.
Care of others/pets	Avoid feeding pets by hand to avoid bites. Avoid grooming pet (use a groomer).
Health management	Keep pill bottles opened slightly and use the intact hand to grasp pills. Use wrist weights for UE exercise to avoid losing hold of hand weights.

UE whenever possible to safely complete a task. The client must also be careful when mobilizing in the home or in the community and use visual sense to avoid bumping into objects that may inflict any injury or pain. Table 4-6 summarizes the above IADL tasks as well as the compensatory/adaptive strategies.

Endurance/Energy

As discussed previously with ADLs, a lack of endurance will impact all areas of occupation (Figure 4-9). The inability to sustain activity for a period of time can impact even sedentary IADLs, such as balancing a checkbook. Principles of energy conservation and work simplification are provided to the clients in the form of education and practice in order to increase functional skills without excessive fatigue. These principles include the following:

- Organize work space.
- Organize the task to be completed.
- Select the most appropriate and effective time of day for each task.
- Limit activities to short periods of time on a daily basis.
- Work in areas that are waist level or slightly higher.
- Sit for completion of tasks when possible.

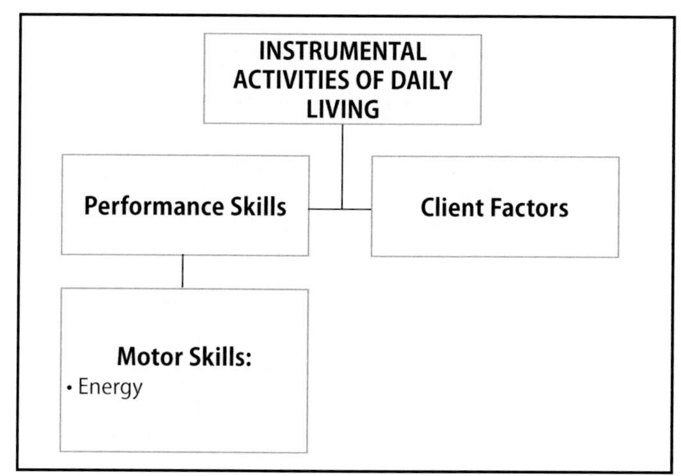

Figure 4-9. Relationship of energy/endurance to IADLs. (Adapted from American Occupational Therapy Association. (2014). Occupational therapy practice framework: Domain and process (3rd ed.). *American Journal of Occupational Therapy, 68*(Suppl. 1), S1-S48.)

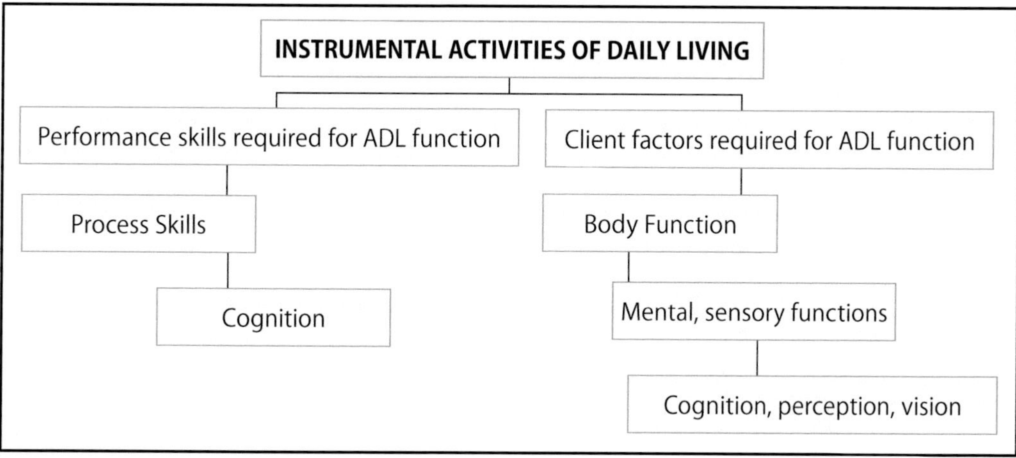

Figure 4-10. Components of performance skills/client factors related to IADLs. (Adapted from American Occupational Therapy Association. (2014). Occupational therapy practice framework: Domain and process (3rd ed.). *American Journal of Occupational Therapy, 68*(Suppl. 1), S1-S48.)

- Use adaptive equipment and DME when indicated.
- Select leisure activities that require less energy to complete.
- Make use of wheelchairs or driving shopping carts for community mobility and shopping tasks, or select stores that are smaller and more easily accessible.
- Use power equipment or tools when indicated.

The clients who incorporate these principles will often find they are more efficient and productive in all everyday tasks. They may have more time and more energy for leisure activities and social events.

Performance Skills/Client Factors

This section will focus on the impact of cognitive, perceptual, and visual deficits upon IADL performance (Figure 4-10). As stated in the ADL chapter, many conditions may lead to these deficits, primarily those of a neurological origin.

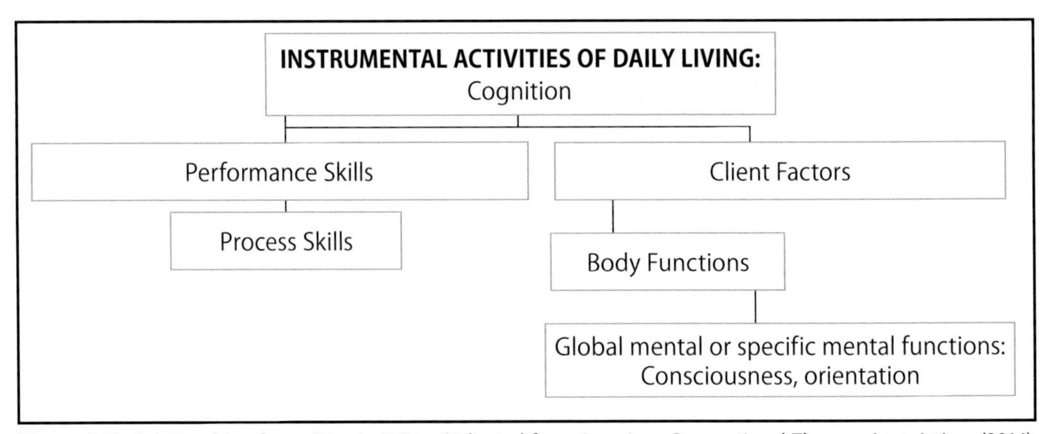

Figure 4-11. Relationship of cognition to IADLs. (Adapted from American Occupational Therapy Association. (2014). Occupational therapy practice framework: Domain and process (3rd ed.). *American Journal of Occupational Therapy, 68*(Suppl. 1), S1-S48.)

The use of cuing, as described in Chapter 1, will also be addressed throughout this chapter in terms of its use for remediation as well as compensation/adaptation. Again, the chapter is organized so that the lowest, foundational skill levels will build upon higher-level skills.

The Framework (AOTA, 2014) presents perceptual and cognitive deficits within two sections of the document. The first section addresses basic cognitive skills in the general category of performance skills. The Framework defines these basic cognitive skills as necessary to complete, manage, and modify ADL tasks.

A second section of the Framework (2014) also addresses cognitive as well as perceptual deficits. The deficits are discussed under the subsection of client factors, called *Body Function Categories.* These body function categories are the affective, perceptual, and additional cognitive skills required to complete ADL tasks. Body function categories are divided into global mental functions and specific mental functions (2014).

- Global mental functions: These include consciousness functions (arousal level and level of consciousness), and orientation.
- Specific mental functions: Attention, memory, perception (visuospatial), thought functions (recognition, categorization, and generalization), higher-level cognitive functions (judgment, concept formation, time management, problem solving, and decision making), and mental functioning (motor planning).

This section will also give examples of compensation/adaptation interventions for each topic. Examples of appropriate activities will be listed. Some IADL examples will not be listed because these tasks may be inappropriate or not possible for a client with these deficits.

A client who has experienced a neurological insult may present with deficits in the areas of cognition, perception and vision, which may limit the client's safety and ability to participate in IADL tasks. Verbal, visual, sensory, and tactile cues may be needed in order for the client to function safely in his or her own home as well as in the community. The occupational therapist must determine the most effective method(s) to increase functional IADL performance. Education must then be provided to the client and his or her family or caregivers.

Cognitive Deficits

See Figure 4-11.

Process Skills

Table 4-7 briefly presents the subcategories of process skills because they are typically addressed in a less formal manner within most IADL intervention plans. Only the subcategories that apply to IADL have been included in this table.

Client Factors: Body Functions, Global Mental Functions

As stated earlier, global mental functions include consciousness and orientation. A client who is to participate in IADLs will need adequate global mental functions in order to complete these higher-level tasks safely and effectively. The client must choose times that he or she is most awake and alert and tasks that are goal-oriented and appropriate for his or her level of motor function. He or she must be sufficiently oriented to the specifics of the task, the demands involved, and the potential outcomes.

Client Factors: Body Functions, Specific Mental Functions

Specific mental functions includes attention, memory, perception (visuospatial), thought functions (recognition, categorization, and generalization), higher-level cognitive functions (judgment, concept formation, time management, problem solving, and decision making), and mental functioning (motor planning, specifically dressing apraxia) (AOTA, 2014).

Attention

Decreased attention skills will affect the client's ability to learn and focus on IADL skills. Attention is a building block for higher-level specific mental functions such as memory and problem solving, and therefore must be addressed first (Zoltan, 2007).

Changing the Task to Achieve Independence

- Light cleaning example: A time schedule may be developed for each task to be completed, with start time and approximate time of completion.
- Outdoor maintenance example: Choose activities that are goal-oriented to the patient to increase attention, rather than tasks that just need to be done.
- Table setting example: Select all items needed before setting the table to deter from distraction and elimination of some items.
- Washing dishes example: Have the client select some favorite music or listen to a favorite television show while completing this task.
- Financial management example: Select time of day when the client is most awake, use good lighting, and have the client sit at a desk or table and maintain good posturing to enhance alertness.

Changing the Tools to Achieve Independence

- Laundry example: If the client does not have a machine that gives an auditory cue when it is done, a timer may be used to signify that the load is done or near completion.
- Shopping example: The client may prepare a list and adhere only to the purchase of those items listed.
- Meal preparation example: Use a timer for cooking and designate specific times for meals to increase attentiveness to task.

Table 4-7 Process Skills and Sample Adaptations/Compensations	
Process Skill Subcategories (AOTA, 2002)	**Examples of IADL Compensation/Adaptation Interventions**
Energy	
Paces	Assist the client in preparing a list of home management activities and develop a daily/weekly schedule for these tasks.
Attends	Refer to Specific Mental Functions category.
Knowledge	
Chooses	Ask the client to choose a dinner recipe for the week.
Uses	Have the client select from the recipe the items he or she needs to purchase at the store.
Handles	Observe the client in preparation of the meal.
Heeds	Create a list of safety measures the client must adhere to when preparing a meal and ask him or her to check off each item as completed.
Inquires	Encourage the client to ask questions regarding preparation of the meal when unsure.
Temporal Organization	
Initiation	Give the client a time frame in which the meal preparation needs to be completed. Use a sounding device to signal time to begin the task.
Sequencing	Ask the client to read the recipe in the sequence that it needs to be completed and number each step.
Organizing Space and Objects	
Searches/locates	Select one cabinet for laundry supplies such as detergent, bleach, fabric softener, and dryer sheets.
Gathers	Have the client use two laundry receptacles that are appropriate for transporting, one for dark clothing and one for whites and gather and sort clothing appropriately.
Organizes	Devise a checklist with the client for all needed steps for laundry management in the recommended order and have him or her check off each step as completed.
Restores	Create a list of steps with the client to complete after the laundry is done in order to restore the machines and working area to the pre-working state (i.e., clean out dryer filter, return laundry receptacles to appropriate place, put away supplies).
Navigates	Educate the client in the safest carrying techniques for all needed supplies to complete the task. *(continued)*

Table 4-7 (continued)

Process Skills and Sample Adaptations/Compensations

Process Skill Subcategories (AOTA, 2002)	Examples of IADL Compensation/Adaptation Interventions
Adaptation	
Notices/responds	Observe the client's performance with managing laundry and gradually substitute visual checklists with verbal cues as needed as the task becomes more automatic to the client.
Accommodates/adjusts	Problem solve with the client how to determine whether a laundry load is small, medium, or large and adjust the amount of detergent, bleach, etc. needed.
Benefits	Discuss with the client the benefits of following the directions for loading the machine and for adding laundry detergent, bleach, and/or fabric softener and ask the client to discuss safety issues that may develop if instructions are not followed.

- Community mobility example: If using the city bus line, a written note of the client's destination can be provided to the bus driver in case the client loses his or her attention while traveling.
- Communication device example: Visual reminders such as flashing lights or auditory cues can remind the client to charge batteries. Daily calendar reminders would be helpful as well.
- Care of others/pets example: The client may benefit from a written schedule, an alarm, or a timer as reminders.
- Health management example: Daily nutrition guides and medication dividers will be helpful.
- Exercise videos/DVDs may also enhance attention.

Memory

Although there are many types of memory and memory deficits, this section will focus specifically on intervention strategies related to ADLs with an adaptive/compensation approach.

Changing the Task to Achieve Independence

Intervention strategies during IADLs, in general, may be adapted by providing the client with a schedule. For individuals who have limited carry-over, involve him or her in developing the schedule. The same strategy may be implemented for creating lists of items needed for cooking, shopping, and cleaning, as well as basic instructions for carrying out IADLs.

- Light cleaning example: For each task, provide a list of instructions on how to complete, materials needed, and designate one day for each task and write on calendar.
- Outdoor home maintenance: Have the client review the instructions for all equipment, state safety precautions, and demonstrate use first.
- Table setting example: Draw a picture of a table setting for the client to follow and list all needed dinnerware.
- Washing dishes example: Provide verbal cues.

- Financial management example: Keep bills in one area, select a day of the month for payment, and write on calendar.
- Community mobility example: Have the client write down his or her destination, the name of the transit system he or she is taking, and the time of arrival and departure.
- Communication devices example: List all instructions for use of devices near the equipment and list all important phone numbers.

Changing the Tools to Achieve Independence

- Laundry example: Provide a checklist with all steps listed, designate 1 or 2 days a week as laundry days, and mark on a calendar.
- Shopping example: Have the client keep an ongoing list of items needed and use the list when at the store.
- Meal preparation example: Use written recipes and timers when cooking or baking and hang a sign over the stove to remind the client to turn it off.
- Care of others/pets example: Prepare a daily schedule of tasks and check off as they are completed.
- Health management example: Utilize daily nutrition guides, medication sorters, and written exercise programs. Write all appointments on calendars.

The specific mental functions, which are addressed less formally and/or less frequently within intervention plans, are presented in Table 4-8.

Perceptual Deficits

See Figure 4-12.

Visual Fixation/Scanning

Clients who present with perceptual deficits involving visual fixation and limited ability to scan the environment will need continued practice and adaptation/compensation strategies in order to complete IADL tasks. The following compensatory/adaptive strategies may be implemented to assist the client. The client must first recognize that a deficit exists and be receptive to new strategies. Continued practice and repetition of purposeful activities should enhance the client's performance.

Changing the Task to Achieve Independence

- Laundry example: Have the client turn his or her head when reaching for and placing clothing. Place items far enough apart to encourage more head movement.
- Light cleaning example: When mopping or sweeping, give the client a point of visual focus to the left and right and tell him or her to stop once he or she has reached each point and move in the other direction.
- Outdoor home maintenance example: If the client is sweeping or raking, instruct him or her to visually attend to the broom or rake and follow the movements with his or her head and eyes; encourage wide and long strokes.
- Shopping example: The client will need to scan for all items he or she wishes to purchase; verbal cuing for a start and end point will be indicated.
- Meal preparation example: Ask the client to state the ingredient needed and ask him or her to locate the area in which it can be found, and then visually attend to that place.

Table 4-8

Specific Mental Functions and Examples of Compensation/Adaptation Strategies

Specific Mental Functions Subcategories (AOTA, 2002)	Examples of Compensation/Adaptation Interventions
Thought Functions	
Recognition	Given all adaptive devices, the client will select those appropriate for each IADL task to be performed. Choice selection can be graded beginning with a choice of two and increasing as appropriate.
Categorization	Given all cleaning supplies, the client will select those items needed for each specific task. Color coding may be useful using tape or marker with a general list (i.e., red for laundry supplies, blue for dishes, etc.).
Generalization	Discuss the principles of self-care that the client has learned and create a list of ways he or she can generalize this new learning to the care of others.
Higher-Level Cognitive Functions	
Judgment	Discuss vignettes that may lead to unsafe conditions and ask the client to identify appropriate methods of handling them. Create a list of people the client may call with specific questions before acting if he or she is unsure of what to do.
Concept formation	Determine goals with respect to IADLs and chart progress weekly. Have the client state what accomplishments he or she has achieved.
Time management	Provide the client with a daily time schedule and ask him or her to plan the day incorporating daily routines as well as tasks or appointments that are specific to that day.
Problem solving	Ask the client to identify problems that he or she has encountered in the past and identify the solution that worked best. Have the client refer to this learning when encountering a new challenge.
Decision making	Have the client discuss the pros and cons of each choice he or she is to make and then select the best choice and determine the reasoning behind this choice for future decision making.

- Table setting example: Instruct the client as to how many places need to be set.
- Washing dishes example: When loading or unloading the dishwasher, remind the client to turn his or her head when reaching and placing dishes.
- Financial management example: When balancing a checkbook, have the figures the client needs to add and subtract placed horizontally rather than vertically to encourage scanning from left to right with verbal cues if needed.
- Community mobility example: The client will need supervision for community mobility, with verbal cuing to turn his or her head in each direction to scan the environment. It would be helpful if the client remains with the most visual and auditory stimulation to his or her impaired side.

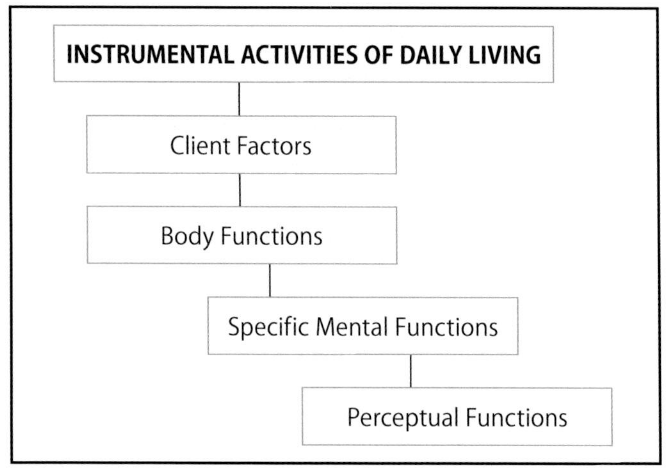

Figure 4-12. Relationship of perception to IADLs. (Adapted from American Occupational Therapy Association. (2014). Occupational therapy practice framework: Domain and process (3rd ed.). *American Journal of Occupational Therapy, 68*(Suppl. 1), S1-S48.)

- Care of others/pets example: Have the client exercise the dog or play catch to trigger visual scanning and release fixation.
- Health management example: Have the client scan the calendar daily for any appointments or important matters for that day.

Changing the Tools to Achieve Independence

- Communication devices example: Raised surfaces for control buttons would be helpful so that the client can use his or her tactile sense while scanning to find the appropriate button.

Visual Inattention and Neglect

For clients who are unaware of inattention deficits, the therapist will need to modify and simplify the physical context of IADLs as much as possible. Gradual grading of activities will also be required. For example, begin by providing all objects/items within the client's intact visual field; incorporate visual scanning through head as well as eye movements during functional activities, etc.

Changing the Task to Achieve Independence

- Laundry example: Have the client with left inattention/neglect stand to the right of the washer and dryer if possible and turn to the left to load the machines.
- Light cleaning example: Cue the client to reach all four corners of the counter or table when cleaning and count as he or she reaches them.
- Outdoor home maintenance example: Place marker points at each side of the garden as points of reference when the client is weeding.
- Shopping example: Identify one item in the aisle that the client needs and ask him or her to look toward the impaired side of vision to locate it.
- Meal preparation example: Place all adaptive cooking devices to the impaired visual side of the client's working area, and place commonly used spices in cabinets to the client's impaired visual side.
- Table setting example: Have the client set the table clockwise or counter-clockwise depending on which visual field is impaired (e.g., clockwise for right inattention/neglect and counter-clockwise for inattention/neglect to the left).

Table 4-9 Body Scheme Disorders and Sample Compensation/Adaptation Strategies	
Body Scheme Disorder	**Compensation/Adaptation Interventions Strategies: Task and/or Tools Changed**
Unilateral body neglect	Use verbal cuing as well as visual demonstration to encourage bilateral integration with meal preparation.
Right-left discrimination	Have the client wear a ring or bracelet on the dominant hand and use this as a point of reference when performing IADL activities.

- Washing dishes example: Stack soiled dishes to impaired side, and have the client stand with the dishwasher on his or her impaired visual side.
- Financial management example: Place a border on each check on the side of the client's visual impairment.
- Community mobility example: The client will need to rely on family or community transportation.
- Care of others/pets example: Have feeding dishes and food placed on the client's impaired visual side.
- Health management example: Place all medications or health supplies in cabinets to the client's impaired visual side.

Changing the Tools to Achieve Independence

- Communication devices example: Raised surfaces to enhance tactile sensation will assist the client in finding control buttons.

Experience of Self and Time/Body Scheme

Body scheme is a foundation skill that uses sensory or internal awareness of the body and the spatial relationship of the body parts to one another (Jacobs & Simon, 2015; Zoltan, 2007). Because there are multiple forms of body scheme disorders, each one cannot be reviewed individually. For this reason, Table 4-9 identifies the most common forms of body scheme disorders as well as examples of IADL compensatory/adaptive interventions for these.

Visual Discrimination

Visual discrimination refers to the ability to detect differences and similarities between objects, thereby determining whether they are alike or different (Okkema, 1993). The client who wishes to return to the tasks of IADLs will need to learn compensation/adaptation strategies in order to participate in an independent and safe manner. Caregivers will need to be educated in the specifics of the client's deficit and how it will relate to the client's ability to function. Education will need to be provided as to what can be expected of the client and what strategies he or she will need to perform in order to complete the tasks. The client will need to possess intact cognitive skills such as deduction and reasoning in order to learn to compensate and adapt to functional activities (Okkema, 1993). Table 4-10 describes sample compensation/adaptation strategies for visual discrimination disorders.

Table 4-10 Visual Discrimination and Sample Compensation/Adaptation Strategies	
Visual Discrimination Disorder	**Compensation/Adaptation Interventions: Task and/or Tools Changed**
Form discrimination	Have client sort laundry by similar items and by color (i.e., white T-shirts, black socks, etc.).
Depth perception	Instruct the client to utilize the sense of touch and feel for surfaces and boundaries when attempting tasks such as pouring liquids or batters or placing items in containers.
Figure ground perception	Adapt containers holding most commonly used spices and other meal preparation items with colors to distinguish them from other items in cabinets.
Spatial relations	Color-code cleaning supplies and cabinets in which they belong and ask client to return all supplies as used.
Topographical orientation	Label cabinets or use picture representations of items to be found inside. Identify place settings by placemats.

Motor Planning

Motor planning involves the individual's ability to organize and perform movements in order to carry out purposeful activity (Jacobs & Simon, 2015). Apraxia is a category of motor planning deficits whereby impairments of purposeful movement or skills do not involve in-coordination, sensory deficits, visual/perceptual issues, language deficits, or cognitive deficits alone (Schell, Gillen, & Scaffa, 2014).

Zoltan (2007) states that a client with apraxia will present with errors in performance skills such as perseveration, inability to perform upon command, and limitations in tool usage. In general, apraxia may be addressed through adapting the environment, limiting tool usage, hand-over-hand activities, chaining, using familiar activities for interventions, presenting activities in small steps, and limiting verbal commands.

Changing the Task to Achieve Independence

- Laundry example: If laundry is a familiar task for the client, begin with backward chaining and offer hand-over-hand assistance versus verbal cuing.
- Shopping example: Reintroduce shopping in a familiar but small store, such as a neighborhood market or drug store. Begin with only a short list of familiar items. Offer hand-over-hand assistance when necessary.
- Washing dishes example: Provide hand-over-hand assistance and backward or forward chaining activity as needed. Eliminate glass items and sharp objects as necessary.

Changing the Tools to Achieve Independence

- Light cleaning example: If this task is familiar to the client, begin with using cleaning supplies that may be familiar to the client, such as a sponge or feather duster. Add more tools as client improves.

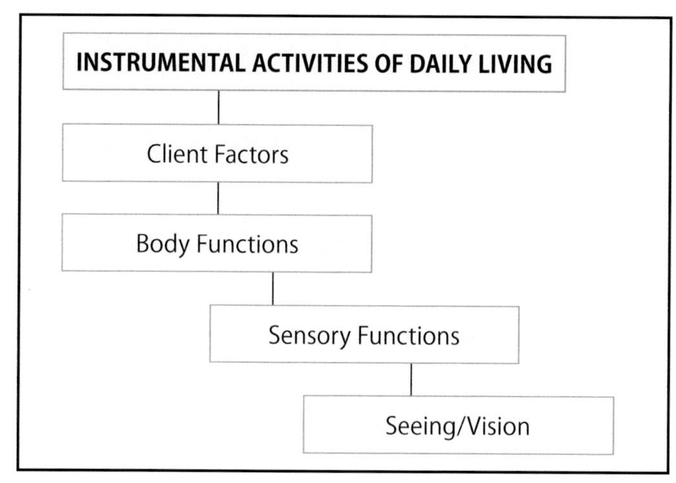

Figure 4-13. Relationship of vision to IADLs. (Adapted from American Occupational Therapy Association. (2014). Occupational therapy practice framework: Domain and process (3rd ed.). *American Journal of Occupational Therapy, 68*(Suppl. 1), S1-S48.)

- Meal preparation example: Begin activity with having the client prepare a simple sandwich or snack that does not require the use of kitchen tools. As the client improves, gradually implement the use of a simple, safe utensil, such as a spoon or butter knife.
- Table setting example: Begin activity by setting the table for one person with only a few items such as a plate and spoon or plastic fork. Add more place settings or utensils as able. Use backward chaining to set the table, as needed (adaptation of task).

Vision

See Figure 4-13.

Low Vision and Visual Field Deficits

Because these deficits tend to have similar issues in relation to IADLs, they are presented below in a general compensation/adaptation approach.

A client who has experienced a neurological deficit may also manifest changes in vision. These changes may include double vision, otherwise known as diplopia, a visual field cut, and/or deficits in depth perception. Any change in vision will impact IADL in some way. The client will need to learn to compensate or adapt to these changes in order to regain functional independence. Recommendation should be made for the client to see an ophthalmologist or an optometrist specializing in neurological deficits, especially if he or she wishes to participate in IADLs. Deficits may be more evident in these activities than were noted in basic ADLs. Upon evaluation, it may be determined that the client may benefit from specially made glasses containing prism to assist with facilitation of normal vision. Visual training may also be indicated. The occupational therapist should instruct the client in visual compensation techniques until the client is able to visualize in a normal manner. These include the following:

- Position materials in the unaffected visual field to assist with reading or identifying objects.
- Use magnifiers or magnifying lamps to enhance reading (Figure 4-14).
- Memorize the phone dial, use one-touch or speed dialing, or purchase a telephone with larger, easier-to-read numbers.
- Utilize audible rather than visual devices such as talking clocks/watches, temperature scales, and calculators (Figure 4-15).
- Use tactile aids that raise surfaces of appliance controls.

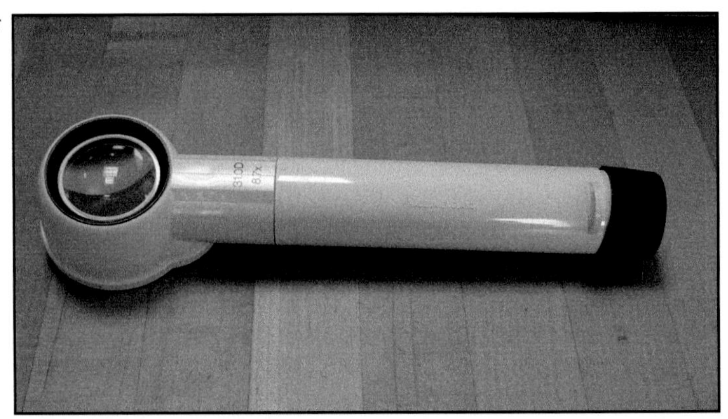

Figure 4-14. Magnification lamp for reading.

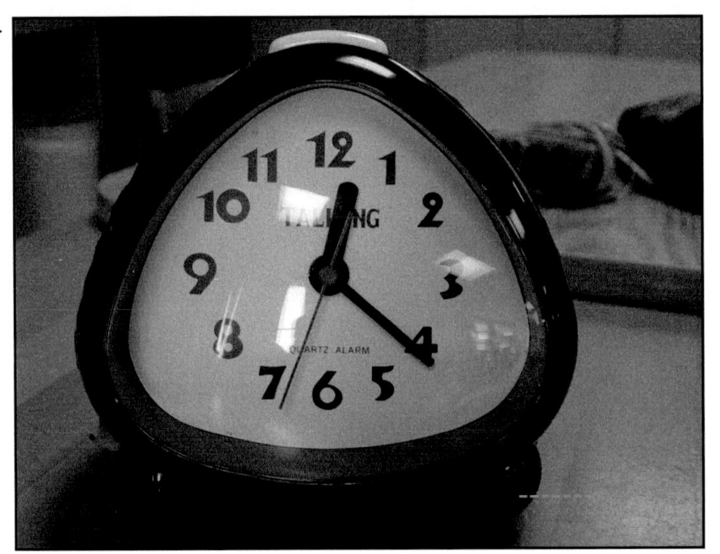

Figure 4-15. Talking clock.

- Maintain proper lighting with all mobility and avoid sun glare by using eye shades and shades or curtains in the home.
- Reposition the head to scan the environment of the affected side.
- Use bright tape to mark each step of a flight of stairs.
- Listen to books on tape or invest in large-print magazines.
- Visit a low-vision store for various cooking and leisure activity items specifically made for clients with low vision.
- Avoid working with hot surfaces, sharp objects, or toxic materials.
- Use tactile sense whenever possible to enhance vision.
- Modify the home to eliminate clutter and try to keep furniture and other items in the same place.

Maintenance of Instrumental Activities of Daily Living

One of the basic precursors for IADL maintenance is a good understanding of all teaching and the necessities of compensation or adaptation techniques to maintain safety along with independence for all areas of IADLs. The client must be educated regularly throughout rehabilitation, both in a facility and subsequently in the home. Generalization of new learning to the home setting may at times be challenging. It is important, therefore, that the client have continued rehabilitation to assure that new techniques are being generalized. Practice is also important in order for new techniques to become automatic to the client. With a good basis for relearning of performance skills, new performance patterns and habits should become inherent in the client's behavior. The client will then have the opportunity to generalize this new behavior to many contexts.

Case Study 1: Jim C., CVA

Jim C. is a 57-year-old single man who lives alone. A very close group of friends noted significant changes in his mental status one day as they were visiting. These friends subsequently reported that Jim was having trouble expressing himself for 2 or 3 days prior to this, although he refused to seek medical evaluation. Emergency medical service was called on this particular day, and Jim was found to have an elevated blood pressure of 240/120 mm Hg. He was brought to the emergency department of the local hospital and was diagnosed by head CT as having a left parietal lobe infarct, with no bleeding. Jim had recently been discharged from the hospital for treatment of bilateral LE cellulites, which was also noted to be present at the time of this admission. He was noted to be aphasic. After evaluation, Jim was admitted to the hospital for treatment of the cellulites and control of his high blood pressure, along with monitoring and intervention of his acute left CVA.

Jim's medical history is significant for hypertension and chronic LE edema and cellulites. He lives alone in a one-level home with one step to enter. He was independent with all ADLs and IADLs prior to admission, including dressing changes of his LEs. He was driving and working part time at a local restaurant. His family was limited to one distant relative who lived out of the area.

Jim was evaluated by physical, occupational, and speech therapy after his admission to the hospital. His overall strength of the UEs and LEs was graded at 4 of 5; however, the question was raised as to whether or not the client was stronger, as he was noted to have difficulty following commands. He demonstrated no deficits with coordination or sensation of the UEs or LEs. He ambulated without a device with contact guard assistance initially. He was alert; however, orientation was difficult to assess as the patient manifested severe receptive and expressive aphasia of the Wernicke type. He was able to follow simple one-step commands intermittently with visual and tactile cues as needed.

The speech therapist's evaluation results found Jim to be severely aphasic. He demonstrated deficits in auditory comprehension, conversational speech, and the ability for new learning. Jim often used sound substitutions in naming objects. For example, he would say "bable" instead of "table." He would often substitute words saying "shoe" for "sock" or "chair" for "table." Often Jim fabricated words in conversation, and he was found to have perseverative speech as well. The occupational therapist's evaluation found Jim to be pleasant and cooperative, requiring maximum verbal, visual, and tactile cuing for testing and subsequently for treatment. He was noted to be at supervision level to shower and dress, with contact guard assistance for functional transfers using grabber assistance when available.

As previously noted, Jim manifested overall functional strength. He demonstrated good balance and physical therapy intervention focused on higher-level balance skills and community mobility. He was able to navigate stairs without difficulty and he required no assistive devices for gait. Physical therapy intervention also focused on management of Jim's LE wounds and subsequent infection.

Interdisciplinary intervention was based on cognitive retraining, auditory comprehension, following commands, identifying objects appropriately, wound care, strengthening, and facilitating independence with BADLs and IADLs in a safe manner. Jim was evaluated shortly after his hospital admission for transfer to the hospital's intensive rehabilitation unit, as he was deemed unsafe to be discharged home alone.

Jim was admitted to the intensive rehabilitation unit 5 days after initial admission. Upon evaluation by physical, occupational, and speech therapy, he demonstrated approximately the same status as was noted upon acute care evaluation. He received daily physical and occupational therapy, and speech therapy was administered approximately three to four times per week. Occupational therapy's main focus in the rehabilitation setting was on safety and cognitive retraining for IADLs because the client was soon independent in BADLs. Physical therapy's focus was on strengthening, gait, and mobility within the hospital community, higher-level balance skills, and wound care for the LE cellulites. Speech therapy focused also on cognitive retraining, but the main focus was the client's aphasia. Simple object identification tasks and following simple one-step commands was the intervention of choice initially.

Although Jim was progressing well with the motor and functional aspects of therapy, safety remained a primary concern. Jim was not functioning in an unsafe manner within the rehabilitation unit; however, the concern was that he would be unsafe if discharged home to an uncontrolled, unsupervised environment. Jim's safety deficits revolved around his aphasia. He was unable to dial 911 correctly on a consistent basis, and even when he did, he was unable to state appropriately his problem or his address. He was independently managing his finances prior to his CVA, yet he was now unable to perform simple money management tasks accurately.

Occupational therapy intervention initially focused on remediation of cognitive skills. It appeared it would be a long process to complete, and in the interim, Jim needed to be able to function at home. Intervention was re-evaluated, and focus was placed on compensation/adaptation techniques. These will be further addressed. Although improvement was seen, it was still evident that Jim was going to require some assistance throughout the day for some IADL tasks.

The occupational therapist focused on the performance areas of safety and financial management during the course of Jim's rehabilitation stay. To assess safety with meal preparation, Jim was given the cooking task of baking corn muffins. He prepared the muffins with supervision and no verbal cuing except to direct him to where the needed items could be found in the occupational therapy kitchen, as this setting provided a new context in which to perform. Although Jim verbalized the instructions incorrectly when reading them from the box, he prepared the mixture with 100% accuracy and no cuing. He safely placed the muffins in the oven, needing assistance only to set the oven timer. When they were ready to come out, he removed the pan safely and remembered to turn the oven off. Jim completed the task of clean-up appropriately, utilizing good safety. Throughout this meal preparation task, Jim executed appropriate performance skills requiring mobility and processing; however, he was noted to have continued impairment in communication/interaction skills. The demands of the activity were appropriate for his level of performance, and all client factors were noted to be within functional limits. The occupational therapist deemed him safe for performance in the kitchen.

Throughout his rehabilitation stay, Jim was independent in making his bed and doing his own laundry. He functioned safely and appropriately, but his aphasia persisted and certain cognitive deficits still needed to be addressed.

Financial management was a greater challenge for Jim. He had difficulty naming coins and identifying their value. The occupational therapist created a guide for Jim, with the individual coins taped to a sheet of paper and their names and money denominations written next to them. Continued drills in naming the money types as well as problem-solving the tasks of making change and giving the correct amount needed for a purchase were performed. Ultimately, Jim improved and was able to provide the correct coin or bill upon request 90% of the time. He was also able to select the appropriate monies needed upon request. For example, if the occupational therapist asked Jim to give her $2.54, Jim was able to do so. When Jim was told that he made a purchase of $8.64 and gave the clerk $10, he was able to make the correct change with minimal cuing 100% of the time. Check writing was not a normal habit for Jim, nor was the use of credit cards. He paid only by cash. Therefore, it was essential that money management intervention focused on cash management skills.

The occupational therapist also worked on creating a grocery shopping list with Jim, to identify items by name and to calculate the cost. He was able to write the list appropriately, copying the names of items from a store flyer. Jim required maximum assistance with the problem-solving aspects of this task. For example, he was asked how much it would cost if he wanted to purchase 2 pounds of bananas at 69 cents per pound. He was unable to add or multiply to obtain the correct answer.

The occupational therapist took Jim to the hospital cafeteria to assess generalization of the newly relearned money management skills. They went at a time when the cafeteria was quiet to minimize the stress of the task. Jim selected an item for purchase, and upon arriving at the cashier he was able to provide the correct amount of money for payment. Both Jim and the occupational therapist were pleased at his ability to perform this task in a new context where activity demands were different and slightly greater for him.

Intervention of home safety and client safety revealed that Jim was unable to state the 911 emergency phone number consistently and upon demand. The occupational therapist provided Jim with a telephone and asked him what he would do in the case of an emergency such as a fire. Jim responded that he would run out of the house, but was unable to state the emergency number consistently. The occupational therapist worked with Jim on dialing the number and he quickly was able to do so; however, difficulty was noted in verbalizing his needs, his name, or his address secondary to his aphasia. The occupational therapist designed a written dialogue for Jim to recite stating that he had aphasia, what his name was, where he lives, and that he needed help. Jim practiced continually with this dialogue, but was still inconsistent with his verbalizations. The occupational therapist challenged Jim with various emergency vignettes and was pleased that Jim was able to at least recognize danger even though his verbal response to it was limited. She felt confident that he would be able to remove himself from any danger if needed, yet she was concerned that he would have difficulty stating his needs if medical attention was indicated. It was recommended that Jim purchase an emergency call system to assure his safety in a time of emergency. He said he would consider it.

Jim's discharge plan was an issue secondary to his limited insurance and subsequent inability to receive home health care or home therapy. He remained on the rehabilitation unit for an extended period of 3 weeks. The care manager/discharge planner in charge of Jim's case was in touch with his distant relative on a regular basis, and he was insistent that Jim would need further rehabilitation until arrangements were made for him to be eligible for home services. Jim was in the process of applying for Medicaid. He was not happy with the recommendation that he could not go home, because he felt that he would be fine. He stated that friends would be there to assist with cooking and transportation as needed. This was confirmed by the occupational therapist and the care manager after discussion with these friends. Jim stated he would not drive. He had concerns about his home because the weather was changing from early to late fall during his admission. He was expecting his last paycheck and wondering if it had come and if so, where it was. His social work representative had been contacted and was in the process of assisting Jim with his financial concerns and his family was notified about his concerns regarding his home.

Despite the above interventions, Jim decided that he was unwilling to transfer to a short-term rehabilitation facility and he signed himself out of the intensive rehabilitation unit one evening against medical advice. Contact was made with Jim the next day to be sure that he would visit his primary physician for continued monitoring of his blood pressure and his chronic cellulites. Subsequent contact with the client found him to be functioning fairly well at home alone, with improvement noted in certain aspects of his speech. The rehabilitation team hoped that Jim followed through with all recommendations and that he was educated sufficiently to maintain his safety at home.

Case Study 2: Annie D., Parkinson's Disease and Fractured Humerus

Annie D. is a 75-year-old married woman with known history of Parkinson's disease. She lives with her husband on the second floor of a three-level home. Annie was independent with all ADLs and most IADLs prior to her recent fall and subsequent fractured rib and fractured left humerus. She ambulated with a straight cane but also owned a walker. Annie and her husband have one married daughter and one granddaughter who live out of state. Annie's daughter and son-in-law come into town often and assist Annie and her husband with grocery shopping and with transportation to appointments because neither Annie nor her husband drive. Annie's husband is not well and requires assistance from a home health aide for ADL, although he participates in cooking tasks with Annie. He has been in and out of the hospital frequently, and on one particular evening he fell at home. Annie rushed from her bed to assist him and consequently fell. Annie had an emergency call system and was able to call for help. She was taken to the hospital where she was diagnosed with a fractured rib and a left humerus fracture.

Annie had been discharged from the hospital a few months earlier after treatment for dehydration and frequent falls. She was admitted for rehabilitation and discharged home at her current level of function. Annie's husband remained at home during Annie's hospital stays with home health aide assistance as well as assistance from his daughter and son-in-law.

Annie's medical history is significant for Parkinson's disease, coronary artery disease, hypertension, coronary stent placement, myocardial infarction, noninsulin dependent diabetes mellitus, osteoarthritis, bilateral LE cellulites, and pneumonia. Outward symptoms of her Parkinson's were noted to be slight hand tremors and gait imbalance.

Annie was admitted to surgery for an open reduction internal fixation of the left humerus. Her postoperative orders indicated that Annie was non-weight-bearing on her left UE. When medically stable, she was evaluated by physical and occupational therapy. Annie was noted to be alert and oriented to self, time, place, and situation and followed all commands appropriately. She was able to make her needs known. She complained of pain in her rib area and in the left UE for which she was receiving medication.

Annie was right-hand dominant. Right UE strength was assessed to be 4- of 5 throughout. Passive ROM and strength of the left UE were unable to be assessed secondary to pain. She was noted to have edema of the left hand and was given a compression glove for edema control. Annie was instructed in the purpose of the glove and she was educated in further edema control techniques including positioning of the left UE in elevation and active fisting exercises. Annie was receptive and compliant with all teaching. Coordination and sensation of the right UE was intact. Left UE coordination was unable to be assessed, and Annie complained of numbness and tingling of the third through fifth digits of the left hand. Functional evaluation involved assessment of Annie's ability to don her hospital booties. She was noted to require maximal assistance for this task.

Physical therapy evaluation noted that Annie's LE strength was assessed at 4 of 5 bilaterally with intact coordination and sensation. Neither the physical therapist nor the occupational therapist was able to assess mobility upon initial evaluation secondary to Annie's complaints of pain. Upon treatment of Annie, it was noted that she required maximal assistance of two for bed mobility and moderate assistance of one for sit-to-stand transfers.

It was determined that Annie would once again need intensive rehabilitation prior to returning home secondary to her impaired motor skills and new and challenging activity demands. Annie needed to relearn independence with ADLs and IADLs with training within the context of the intensive rehabilitation unit and consequent generalization to living in her own home again.

Upon admission to the rehabilitation unit, Annie was re-evaluated by physical and occupational therapy. Her functional status was approximately the same as it was upon initial hospital assessment. Annie was able to tolerate assessment now of her left UE. She was able to complete active shoulder flexion against gravity to approximately 90 degrees and was assessed at 3- of 5 strength. Elbow and forearm strength were unable to be assessed secondary to the fracture. Left wrist flexion/extension and left grip were also assessed at 3- of 5.

Because Annie had received therapy services at the rehabilitation unit in the past, she was familiar with rehabilitation and the benefits of physical and occupational therapy. Initial occupational therapy goals for Annie were the following:

1. Increase Annie's ability to perform bathing and dressing with minimal assistance and adaptive equipment as needed.
2. Complete toilet transfers with minimal assistance and grabber as needed.
3. Increase right UE strength to 4+ to 5 of 5 and left shoulder and wrist strength to 3 of 5.
4. Decrease left hand edema to none.
5. Increase left hand grip to 4 of 5.

Annie's orthopedic physician recommended active ROM activities of the left UE to facilitate increased extension of the elbow. He also recommended passive stretching of the left elbow into extension. Annie did not tolerate the stretching too well because of the pain it elicited, despite receiving pain medication prior to stretching. Therefore, she was encouraged to actively use the left UE for functional tasks. She remained non-weight-bearing on that arm.

Upon first weekly assessment by occupational therapy, Annie had achieved minimal assistance level for grooming and bathing; however, she continued to require maximal assistance for dressing. She had been provided with a reacher but required continued practice. She was not receptive to a sock aid, although she had one at home, because she was unable to manipulate it well enough secondary to the motor limitations of her left arm. Toilet transfers were now with contact guard assistance with right grabber. Right UE strength was increased to 5 of 5 throughout; however, left UE shoulder, wrist, and grip strength remained at 3- of 5. She no longer manifested any edema of the left hand but was encouraged to maintain elevated positioning when sitting or sleeping. Annie was ambulating 75 feet with a straight cane and minimal assistance.

Occupational therapy intervention continued to focus on increasing Annie's independence with bathing, dressing, and grooming, as well as with functional mobility. At week 2, introduction was also made to intervention of simple home management tasks and increasing ROM of the left elbow. Annie was fitted for a progressive extension splint as recommended by her physician. The occupational therapist educated Annie and the nursing staff in donning and doffing techniques and in the method of adjusting the splint. Prior to discharge, Annie's daughter was also instructed verbally in these techniques, and written instructions were provided. Although Annie made good attempts at donning the splint, she was unable to do so. Her husband would be unable to help her upon discharge home. It was then determined that Annie would wear the splint only when her daughter was there, unless the home health aide provided for her upon discharge could be instructed in placing the splint. The tension was preset, with Annie only able to tolerate the lowest level of tension. She and her daughter were instructed to allow the home therapist to adjust the tension and gradually increase it if Annie was able to tolerate more.

By the end of week 2, Annie had shown further progress. She was now able to shower because the staples in her left arm had been removed. She completed a tub transfer with right grabber with contact guard assistance. She showered with minimal assistance for thoroughness secondary to limitations in motor performance of the left arm. Annie was now able to complete upper body dressing with minimal assistance, including both button-down and pullover tops, and completed donning of her underwear and skirt with supervision. She remained dependent for her socks, but was able to don her shoes with hook-and-loop fasteners with supervision. Toilet transfers were now completed independently, and Annie was ambulating 125 feet with the straight cane and supervision. Left shoulder flexion remained at 3- of 5 strength; however, left wrist and grip strength increased to 3 of 5. Left elbow ROM was assessed at -40 degrees extension to 105 degrees of flexion, a minimal change from her original status.

Home management tasks were an excellent choice of intervention for Annie because she enjoyed them and they were part of her habits and routine patterns prior her admission. Also, Annie used her left UE volitionally with light baking tasks, kitchen cleaning and organization, folding her laundry, and also in decorating the rehabilitation unit's Christmas tree. The occupational therapist noted greater use and extension of the left UE with all home management tasks.

Annie was considered to be safe with all aspects of ADL and IADL evaluated within the rehabilitation setting. Of concern was her discharge to home and her role in caring for her husband. These concerns were discussed with her family, who assured the rehabilitation team that Annie would not be responsible for her husband's care, but only for herself.

Annie was discharged to home approximately 3 weeks after admission to the intensive rehabilitation unit. As previously stated, her daughter was invited in for teaching in the use of the extension splint. The care manager/discharge planner in charge of organizing Annie's home services was looking into the possibility of Annie receiving home health aide services in the evening to assist with donning the splint prior to Annie retiring to bed. Annie's daughter was willing to educate the home health aide in donning the splint. If it were not feasible, Annie would resort to wearing the splint only when her daughter was there to help, and she was instructed to inform her orthopedic surgeon of this upon discharge.

Annie was ambulating within her room and to and from the bathroom with the straight cane at an independent level. Toilet transfers, hygiene, and clothing management were all performed independently upon discharge. Tub transfer remained at contact guard assistance, and it was recommended to Annie that she wait for her daughter or the home health aide before showering. Annie verbalized understanding of this recommendation. Bathing abilities were advanced to supervision level, and dressing abilities remained at minimal assistance, except Annie was still dependent for donning her socks. Grooming abilities were assessed at independent level. Annie required assistance with meal preparation with the lifting and transporting of heavier items. She was able to perform cleanup tasks using the right UE for grasping most items and assisting with the left.

Right UE strength remained 5 of 5 throughout. Left UE shoulder and wrist flexion/extension was assessed at 3 of 5, and Annie was now able to complete pronation and supination of the left forearm with 2+ to 3- of 5 strength. Left elbow PROM was assessed at -40 degrees of extension to +95 degrees of flexion, demonstrating slight improvement.

Annie demonstrated good advancement toward her IADL goals of independent living once again. However, she was unable to care for her husband without assistance.

Summary Questions

1. Discuss how contextual factors affect IADLs and give at least two specific examples.
2. Discuss how psychological implications may impact IADL performance.
3. Describe the role of the occupational therapy assistant in IADL intervention.
4. Discuss how three body function categories, if impaired, may affect IADL.

References

American Occupational Therapy Association. (2014). Occupational therapy practice framework: Domain and process (3rd ed.). *American Journal of Occupational Therapy, 68*(Suppl. 1), S1-S48.

American Occupational Therapy Association. (2013). *The reference manual of the official documents of the American Occupational Therapy Association* (18th ed.). Bethesda: MD: AOTA.

American Occupational Therapy Association (2012). The Occupational Therapy Role in Driving and Community Mobility Across the Lifespan. Retrieved from http://www.aota.org/Older-Driver/Professionals/CE/Toolkit/Professional/Brochures-and-Fact-Sheets/41773.aspx

Baun, M., & McCabe, B. (2003). Companion animals and persons with dementia of the Alzheimer's type. *American Behavioral Scientist, 47*(1), 42-51.

Boyt Schell, B. A., Gillen, G., & Scaffa, M. (2014). Glossary. In B. A. Boyt Schell, G. Gillen, & M. Scaffa (Eds.), *Willard and Spackman's occupational therapy* (12th ed.) (pp. 1229-1243). Philadelphia, PA: Lippincott Williams & Wilkins.

Christiansen, C., & Baum, C. (Eds.) (1991). *Occupational therapy: Overcoming human performance deficits.* Thorofare, NJ: SLACK Incorporated.

Cole, M. B., (1998). *Group dynamics in occupational therapy* (2nd ed.). Thorofare, NJ: SLACK Incorporated.

Jacobs, K., & Simon, L. (2015). *Quick reference dictionary for occupational therapy* (6th ed.). Thorofare, NJ: SLACK Incorporated.

Kelly, J. M. (1994). Implementing a patient self-medication program. *Rehabilitation Nursing, 19*(2), 87-90.

Law, M., Baptiste, S., Carswell, A., McColl, M. A., Polatajko, H., & Pollock, N. (1998). *The Canadian Occupational Performance Measure* (3rd ed.). Ottawa, ON: Canadian Occupational Therapy Association.

Loeb, P. A. (1996). *Independent living scales.* San Antonio, TX: Psychological Corp.

Logan, P. A., Gladman, J. R. F., Avery, A., Walker, M. F., Dyas, J., & Groom, L. (1994). Randomised controlled trial of an occupational therapy intervention to increase outdoor mobility after stroke. *British Medical Journal, 329*, 1372-1374.

Okkema, K. (1993). *Cognition and perception in the stroke patient: A guide to functional outcomes in occupational therapy.* Gaithersburg, MD: Aspen.

Pereles, L., Romonko, L., Murzyn, T., Hogan, D., Silvius, J., Stokes, E., Long, S., & Fung, T. (1996). Evaluation of a self-medication program. *Journal of the American Geriatric Society, 44*(2), 161-165.

Saffari, M., Koenig, H. G., Pakpour, A. H., Sanaeinasab, H., Janah, H. R., & Sehlo, M. G. (2013). Personal hygiene among military Personnel: Developing and testing a self-administered scale. *Environmental Health and Preventive Medicine, 19*(2), 135-142.

Sanders, M., & Van Oss, T. (2012). Using daily routines to promote medication adherence in older adults. *American Journal of Occupational Therapy, 67*(1), 91-99.

Schell, B. A. B., Gillen, G., Scaffa, M. E. (2014). *Willard and Spackman's occupational therapy for physical dysfunction* (12th ed.). Philadelphia, PA: Lippincott Williams & Wilkins.

Thomson, L. K. (1992). *The Kohlman evaluation of living skills* (3rd ed.). Bethesda, MD: AOTA.

Touchard, B. M., & Berthelot, K. (1999). Collaborative home practice: nursing and occupational therapy ensure appropriate medication administration. *Home Health Nurse, 17*(1), 45-51.

Van Oss, T., Rivers, M., Heigton, B., Macri, C., & Reid, B. (2012). Bathroom Safety: Environmental modifications to enhance bathing and aging in place in the elderly. *OT Practice, 17*(16), 14-16, 19.
Webb, C., Addison, C., Holman, H., Saklaki, B., & Wagner A. (1990). Self-medication for elderly patients. *Nursing Times, 86*(16), 46-49.
White, K. M. (2013). Occupational therapy interventions for people living with advanced lung cancer. *Lung Cancer Management, 2*(2), 121-124.
Zhang, L., Abreu, B. C., Seale, M. S., Masel, B., Christiansen, C. H., & Ottenbacher, K. J. (2003). A virtual reality environment for evaluation of a daily living skill in brain injury rehabilitation: reliability and validity. *Archives of Physical Medicine and Rehabilitation, 84*(8), 1118-1124.
Zoltan, B. (2007). *Vision, perception, and cognition* (4th ed.). Thorofare, NJ: SLACK Incorporated.

5 Education

Kimberly D. Hartmann, PhD, MHS, OTR/L, FAOTA

Chapter Objectives

By the end of this chapter, the student will be able to do the following:

- Define education according to the Occupational Therapy Practice Framework.
- List the types of postsecondary education options for students with disabilities.
- Describe the educational methods that be allow increased accessibility to education for students with disabilities.
- Describe the impact of Section 504 of the Rehabilitation Act of 1973 and the Americans with Disabilities Act on postsecondary education for students with disabilities.
- Describe the process for verification as an adult student with a disability.
- Differentiate essential functions and reasonable accommodations.
- List four guiding factors in the postsecondary disability services.
- Describe the influence of adult learning theories on services for students with disabilities in postsecondary education.
- Define education as an occupation.
- Describe the skill set of occupational therapy practitioners in postsecondary education.
- List possible roles for occupational therapy in postsecondary education.
- Describe universal design as a concept for accessing education.
- Discuss strategies for environmental modification in postsecondary education settings.
- Define the roles of assistive technology for adult students with disabilities.

Introduction

The early philosopher Aristotle wrote that education was central to a fulfilled person, to human flourishing, and to the actual doing of learning (Barnes, 1982). Education as both a formal and informal process leading to three major categories of learning: theoretical, practical, and technical.

Meriano C, Latella D.
Occupational Therapy Interventions: Function and Occupations, Second Edition (pp 297-324).

These categories remain a foundation for education today. Postsecondary education (PSE), any educational process that occurs after high school, often represents increased opportunities for employment, expanded potential for higher socioeconomic status (Unger, 1994), and improved concepts of both self-advocacy and self-determination (Kertcher, 2014). PSE for adult students with disabilities can expand learning as thinking, practical learning, and technical learning.

These tenets in education support the definitions and categories of education found in the Occupational Therapy Practice Framework: Domain and Process (American Occupational Therapy Association, 2014). Education as an occupation is defined as "activities involved in learning and participating in the educational environment" (AOTA, 2014, p. S42). Education may also be considered a type of intervention practitioners in occupational therapy utilize in all areas of occupation. "Education as an intervention is the use of activities that impact knowledge and information about occupation, health, well-being, and participation, resulting in the acquisition by the client of helpful behaviors, habits, and routines that may or may not require the application at the time of the intervention session" (AOTA, 2014, p. S42).

The purpose of this chapter is to discuss the roles of occupational therapy practitioners in facilitating and supporting adult clients-students as they pursue PSE. The chapter will provide a framework for working as a team member in a variety of PSE environments, evaluating the client's functional needs, selecting appropriate interventions to promote success with educational goals, and to provide resources that may prevent future barriers to successful performance in the PSE environments. For the purposes of this chapter, education as an occupation will be examined for clients or students who are 21 years of age and older. The occupational therapy client will be referred to as either *client* or *student* throughout this chapter.

Defining Postsecondary Education

Postsecondary education has become more critical for all adults and in particular for adults with disabilities. In the late 1950s only about 20% of American workers needed some type of postsecondary education, with a dramatic increase to 56% needing such an education in 2000. The National Center for Special Education Research estimates that a person with a college degree will earn $1 million more over a lifetime than a person with only a high school education (National Center for Special Education Research, 2011). As the need for increased knowledge and skills to compete in the workforce grows, there is an increasing interest in all forms of PSE by adult students with disabilities (Barnard-Brak, Lechtenberger, & Lan, 2010). Learning, however, is not just an economic issue; it is also important for social and cultural growth. Education provides important information about societal norms and helps to expose individuals to information that might not be obtained simply in going about daily life. Some students are able to study abroad or meet students from other countries studying in the United States and further broaden their knowledge base. Some adults will seek educational opportunities for leisure purposes, such as a cooking or art class. Others may seek education, such as attending college, because of the leisure opportunities educational environments can provide such as sports, clubs, and organizations. The significance of adult education or PSE in a client's life, either for the continued pursuit of knowledge or for the leisure opportunities it offers, is important for occupational therapy practitioners to recognize and take into consideration during intervention planning. PSE in any of the extended options available today can be a powerful experience for developing occupational skills in cognition, social participation, leisure, teamwork, work ethic, communication, and problem solving.

Postsecondary education options and opportunities continue to develop and grow. Including the traditional programs in higher education, specialized educational options have developed to meet the needs of identified populations such as adult students with intellectual challenges,

Table 5-1

Postsecondary Education Options for Adults With Disabilities

Options	Goals of the Program
Four-year colleges and universities	Broad undergraduate education and a major Professional, career, or graduate focus Need to meet admissions criteria Need to meet the essential functions or technical standards of specific program or major with or without accommodations May have residential options on campus Need to self-disclose disability to determine reasonable accommodations
Two-year colleges	Focus on technical or vocational careers Will require some general education courses Admissions criteria open Need to meet the essential functions or technical standards of specific program or major with or without accommodations Can earn an associate degree or a certificate Need to self-disclose disability to access reasonable accommodations
Continuing education (CE) programs	Can access classes without admissions criteria Typically ungraded Series of CE may lead to a certificate in a skill area Can focus on leisure, academics, or skill development
Dual enrollment	Part of a transition plan from high school under age 21 Combined high school and college experience

learning disabilities, and mobility issues, and for a variety of supported learning-living communities. Adult students with disabilities have an increased number of PSE options (Table 5-1), allowing for a more accurate match of the adult student with disabilities (ASWD) with the most appropriate PSE for success (Barnard-Brak, Lechtenberger, & Lan, 2010, 2010; Kertcher, 2014). As the types of PSE options have increased, so has the diversity of educational methods (Table 5-2) found in most PSE options today (Bragg & Townsend, 2007). Satellite campuses and the array of times when courses are offered provide more flexibility in terms of location and time. This can allow the ASWD to select an education option based on transportation needs, best time of day for learning, or best location or time of day depending on any personal support needed for success. The plethora of teaching-learning methods supports the ASWD. The student can select a traditional class setting, online teaching, or a blended format in real time or at the student's pace to support the individual learning style or as an accommodation to a specific disability. Multimedia advances, Internet-based video resources, e-text, and built-in assistive technology options allow for improved flexibility in the delivery of content, completion of assignments, support resources, and access to text. All of these options are critical to consider when developing an intervention plan for success in the occupation of education.

Table 5-2

Diverse Methods Education to Meet Needs of Adult Students

Diverse Education Methods	Description
Satellite campuses	Access to public transportation Shorter driving distances In local community for increased support
Time of course offerings	Day, weekend, evening Allow for part-time employment Allow options for support personnel to attend
Teaching methods	Face-to-face in-class experience Online synchronized for real time at a distance Online asynchronized for anytime and extended time access Blended face-to-face and online Multimedia
Assistive technology	Accessibility options are built into websites E-texts allow for modification or converting text to speech Tablet and smartphone apps increase customization
Student support services	Available for extended hours Available in video-based tutorials Student support services, 504 and ADA Counseling Specialized on-site services for veterans, employment support, career services, and study skills

Adapted from Balestreri, 2008; Bragg & Durham, 2012; Bragg & Townsend, 2007; Oertle & Bragg, 2014.

Legal Rights of Adults With Disabilities, Definition and Statistics of Students With Disabilities in Postsecondary Education Environments

Basic Legal Review

Adults with disabilities have certain civil rights that enable them to attend postsecondary institutions. These rights are a result of primarily two acts: Section 504 of the Rehabilitation Act of 1973 (PL 93-112) and the Americans with Disability Act of 1990 (ADA, 1990, PL 101-336). Because of these acts, postsecondary institutions cannot discriminate on the basis of disability and must allow equal access for individuals with disabilities otherwise qualified to attend classes as long as they meet the academic and technical standards for admission and participation (Madaus, 2005). Students accepted into the institution have the right to reasonable accommodations, program accessibility, and auxiliary aids/services (Brinckerhoff, McGuire, & Shaw, 2002). Section 504 of the Rehabilitation Act of 1973, a civil rights legislation, prohibits discrimination on the basis of disability in programs and activities that receive federal financial assistance: "No otherwise qualified person with a disability in the United States . . . shall solely by reason of . . . disability, be excluded from participation in, be denied the benefits of, or be subjected to discrimination under any program or activity receiving federal financial assistance" (http://www2.ed.gov/about/officie/list/ocr/504faq.html, March 2, 2015).

Section 504 applies to all colleges and universities because for the most part they all receive federal funds. At these institutions, individuals with disabilities have the right to access and/or the opportunity to participate in the same programs and activities as other students with the use of supplementary aids and services as needed (www.section508.gov). In Section 504, an individual with a disability is one who meets the following definition:

1. Has a physical or mental impairment that substantially limits one or more major life activities.
2. Has a record of such impairment.
3. Is regarded as having such an impairment.
4. At the postsecondary level, the Office of Civil Rights interprets a qualified student with a disability to be a student with a disability who meets the academic and technical standards for admission or participation in the educational program or learning activity (U.S. Department of Health and Human Services, http://www2.ed.gov/about/officie/list/ocr/504faq.html, March 2, 2015).

The ADA created new and comprehensive civil rights protections for individuals with disabilities. It prohibits discrimination on the basis of disability in private employment (Title I), all state and local government agencies (Title II), and places of public accommodation such as museums, restaurants, and theaters (Title III), and mandates accessibility to communication services for people who are deaf, hard of hearing, or speech-impaired (Title IV) (Americans with Disabilities Act, 1990). While public colleges/universities are covered under Title II, most private colleges/universities have activities for the public and are covered under Title III. In 2010, ADA regulations were revised including its ADA Standards for Accessible Design (http://www.ada.gov/2010ADAstandards_index.htm).

Process for Verifying a Disability for Accommodations

Under Section 504 and the ADA, institutions may require adequate documentation/verification of a disability and the need for accommodations before such accommodations are made.

Before an accommodation will be provided by the academic institution, the following steps must be accomplished:

1. Students must apply to the academic institution (which includes meeting the essential functions if applicable).
2. Students must disclose their disability.
3. Students must provide documentation to verify the disability.

Verification is usually required in the form of a medical or psychological evaluation or statement. However, evaluations from vocational rehabilitation agencies or formal/informal evaluations from the institution's disability support services officer or coordinator may be accepted as verification of a disability (University of Kansas Institute for Adult Studies, 1998, p. 54).

The Association of Higher Education and Disability (2012) suggested that three sources of information be considered to verify a disability: the student's self-report and self-disclosure, observation and interactions, and information from external sources (Figure 5-1). The sources of documentation should lead to the final determination of disability understanding that typically, a disability is a lifelong eligibility factor and thus the recent nature of the document should not be considered as the most critical factor. The documentation should meet three tests for verification including being nonburdensome so as to support student disclosure, being common sense in

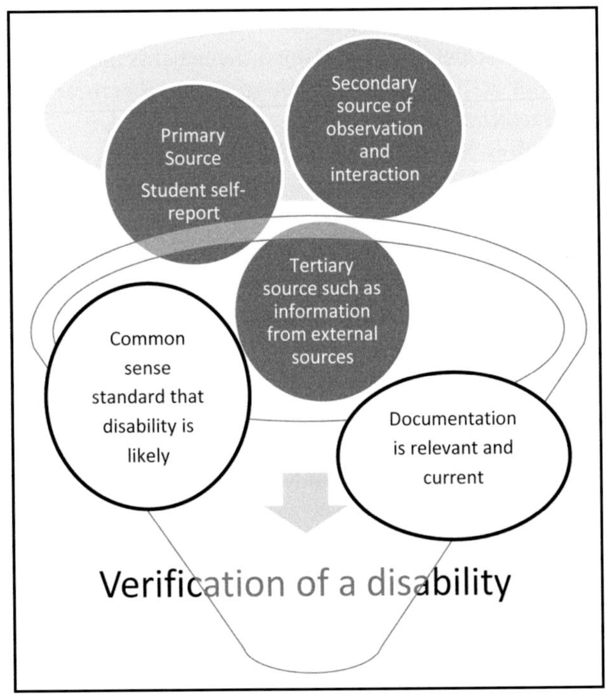

Figure 5-1. Key elements in disability documentation.

nature such that a reasonable person would conclude that a disability exists given the information, and being current and relevant. The definition of current documentation does not have a mandated time period because most disabilities are permanent (AHEAD, 2012; Cory, 2011). If above criteria are met and a student's disability is verified, then the student will be eligible for accommodations and will begin to work with the disabilities coordinator at the academic institution to establish an accommodation plan and to determine whether the accommodations are reasonable for the specific courses or program of study.

Essential Functions and Technical Standards: Accommodations and Auxiliary Supports

Two important concepts associated with the legal rights of an ASWD are essential functions or technical standards and accommodations or auxiliary supports. In addition to meeting entry requirements, adult students with disabilities must meet any essential functions or technical standards associated with their courses, programs of study, or other learning activities within the PSE. Essential functions and technical standards are often used interchangeably and are similar to those designating a specific job performance in the realm of employment. These are different than academic standards (such as grades, quality point average, successful completion of specific program requirements) and may refer to the cognitive, physical, and behavioral abilities that are necessary for satisfactory completion of a course or program curriculum. The essential functions can be completed with or without accommodations or auxiliary supports (Association of the American Medical Colleges, 1993, 29CFR1630.2). Colleges and universities that establish essential functions typically share these on a program website or in an educational catalog or program description. The ASWD may be asked to read and sign a statement that they believe they can meet the essential functions prior to beginning an academic program. This ensures that the student has been duly informed of the program or course requirements. Essential functions are typically associated with academic programs of a professional nature and are rarely a prerequisite for continuing education programs. Essential functions are usually described within several categories including sensory and observational skills, cognitive skills, motor skills, behavioral and social skills, communication skills, and intellectual/conceptual abilities. Occasionally, and depending on the type of educational program, endurance, coordination, and emotional health may also be included.

For adult students with disabilities, auxiliary supports may include assistive technology or other tools that allow the student to circumvent the disability and meet the essential functions of the course or program.

> Accommodation means any change to a classroom environment or task that permits a qualified student with a disability to participate in the classroom process, to perform the essential tasks of the class, or to enjoy benefits and privileges of classroom participation equal to those enjoyed by adult learners without disabilities. (University of Kansas Institute for Adult Studies, 1998, p. 54)

Typically formal program support for the faculty is not considered an accommodation or auxiliary support, and PSE systems do not usually provide personal care attendants or other personnel that may be required in a course or the program (Kallio & Owens, 2012). Some ASWD may not request or require accommodations or auxiliary supports to meet the eligibility for admissions or to meet the essential functions. The student may also independently design an individual strategy or tool that meets their needs. In other situations, an ASWD may request an accommodation, at which time the Office of Students with Disabilities will work with the student and other professionals to determine whether a requested accommodation is reasonable. The final determination of reasonableness for accommodations may be within the purview of the PSE institution. However, there are some benchmarks to use to facilitate the determination as to whether or not an accommodation is reasonable (Higher Education and the ADA, 1997; Jarrow, 2015). It can be clearer to define what may not be considered reasonable, again understanding that each PSE institution may modify their requirements and procedures.

1. An accommodation is not reasonable if it poses a direct threat to the safety or health of people other than the ASWD. The higher education institution bears the responsibility to document the risk of harm to others.
2. An accommodation in not reasonable if it will require a substantial change in a primary element of a course, the program, the curriculum, or learning activity. In some circumstances, the institution may decide that the accommodation is not reasonable if the method in which the course is conducted or services are provided is substantially changed.
3. The final criterion to consider is that an accommodation may not be considered reasonable if it poses an undue financial or administrative burden. Here again the PSE institution needs to provide the proof or documentation of such a burden, and the final check and balance relates to the intent of the laws: to assure that access to opportunities for education is maintained for adult students with disabilities who are otherwise qualified to participate (Higher Education and the ADA, 1997; Jarrow, 2015).

The importance of accommodations and auxiliary aids is supported in the literature (Dowrick, 2005; Gregg, 2011; Holmes & Silvestri, 2012; Mull & Sitlington, 2003). However support personnel are also of critical value (Dowrick, 2005; Oertle & Bragg, 2014). The occupational therapy practitioner should understand that ASWD are underutilizing all accommodations and supports because they are either not seeking out these supports and accommodations or they are seeking the support personnel and accommodations too late in the educational experience (Barnard-Bark, Lechtenberger, & Lan, 2010). This may be due to several factors associated with self-disclosure of a disability, the first step in acquiring supports and accommodations (Corrigan & Matthews, 2003; Petronio, 2002; Smart, 1999; Torkelson, Lynch, & Gussel, 1996). Taking this information into consideration, the occupational therapy practitioner as a member of the ASWD postsecondary educational faculty and program support team should obtain a foundational knowledge of those items of utmost importance to the students themselves regarding accommodations and supports, including the following:

1. Be student-centered. Understand the student's concerns related to self-disclosure and stigma, coordinating student support services, and developing natural supports within the program of study or in social venues (AHEAD, 2012; Dowrick, Anderson, Heyer, & Acosta, 2005). Begin early in the PSE process to plan learning and educational outcomes and review these regularly as part of the advisement or mentoring process (Bragg & Durham, 2012; Huger, 2011).
2. Plan transitions. Transitions occur in postsecondary education from secondary to postsecondary, within elements of the postsecondary learning experience such as from classroom learning to field or experiential learning, and in the transition to employment. Each time there is transition planning and dialogue as to the changes to be expected and the reasonable accommodations, especially those related to assistive technology (Dowrick et al., 2005; Garrison-Wade & Lehman, 2009; Oretle & Bragg, 2014).
3. Consider universal design for learning. The application of these principles develop good teaching-learning methods for all students. This will increase the natural supports in the classroom and possibly decrease the stigma of accommodations (Beck, Diaz del Castillo, Fovet, Mole, & Noga, 2014; Oretle & Bragg, 2014; Quick, Lehmann, & Deniston, 2003).
4. Re-evaluate and reconsider the roles of assistive technology. Assistive technology is increasingly more available, and features of common technology can be modified to allow for easier access by ASWDs. Technology utilization varies in different environments and needs to be re-evaluated for effectiveness and appropriateness on a regular basis (Graham-Smith & Lafayette, 2004; Holmes & Silvestri, 2012; Mull & Sitlington, 2003; Oretle & Bragg, 2014).

These four concepts may in fact be guiding factors for the occupational therapy practitioners in service delivery for adult students with disabilities in postsecondary educational settings.

Statistics on Adult Students With Disabilities in Higher Education and Employment

Statistics on ASWD in PSE are related to the concept of self-disclosure, meaning the statistics are only as accurate as the rate of self-disclosure of a disability. ASWD also enter a variety of PSE environments from different systems, such as from secondary education, as a veteran, or from other systems in which the disability was acquired after high school.

The high school graduation rate for students with disabilities was 62% in the years 2012-2013 (U.S. Department of Education National Center for Education Statistics, 2015). The rate of graduation varies tremendously by state and among African Americans and Hispanics (Diament, 2015). The graduation rate increased 3% over 2 years, increasing students' eligibility to enter PSE institutions.

The U.S. Department of Education, National Center for Education Statistics (2013) reported that 11% of all undergraduate students enrolled in postsecondary institutions reported a disability (the data set was from 2007 to 2008). The average age of ASWD was 27 years, compared to the average age of students not reporting a disability, which was 23.4 years. Veterans constituted a larger percentage of undergraduate students with disabilities than of undergraduates without disabilities (4.6% vs 3.2%). The U.S. Department of Education, National Center for Education Statistics, Postsecondary Education Quick Information System (PEQIS) (2009) reported that the largest percentage of ASWD had learning disabilities (31%), attention deficit disorder (18%), and mental illness or a psychological or psychiatric condition (15%) (U.S. Department of Education, 2011, p. 8).

Postsecondary education is correlated with employment (Barnard-Brak, Lechtenberger, & Lan, 2010; Quick et al., 2003) as well as development in many other life areas including social participation, leisure pursuits, and interpersonal development. The economic connection to PSE continues to be strong as evidenced by the fact that students with disabilities and an earned bachelor's degree have jobs in areas closely related to their degree and have similar full-time starting salaries compared to students without disabilities (National Center for Educational Statistics, 1999, and 2009). However, in 2013 the unemployment rate for people with disabilities was 13.2%, whereas the unemployment rate for people without disabilities was 7.1% (Bureau of Labor Statistics, 2014). In the same report, 34% of workers with a disability were employed part time as compared to 19% of people without disabilities. Thus, the rate of employment of people with disabilities continues to be lower than that for people without disabilities, and possible inclusion of ASWD in one or more of the PSE options may increase their preparation for employment in the future. The statistics for ASWD in PSE and the employment data indicate the importance of using all mechanisms to encourage students with disabilities to select and actively participate in one or more options in PSE. As practitioners, applying the theories of adult education with the power of occupational performance analysis and compensatory strategies will help ensure an equal opportunity for students with disabilities to be successful.

Applying Basic Adult Learning Theory

Occupational therapy practitioners can use the information from Chapter 1 on occupational therapy theories in conjunction with the theoretical knowledge presented in this chapter, as well as their own professional experiences, to form an approach for working with adults wishing to pursue PSE. Theories related to adult learning will be discussed under the following categories: behaviorist, cognitive, humanist, and social learning.

The basic assumptions of the behaviorist theory include the belief that learning is manifested by a change in behavior, and learning is determined by the environment rather than the learner (Merriam & Caffarella, 1991). Early theorists include Watson, Thorndike, Pavlov, Guthrie, and Skinner. In the behaviorist theory, the purpose of education is to promote a desirable behavioral change, the teacher has ultimate authority, and the learner is a passive listener. Incentives, feedback, and emphasis on mastery and competence describe the basic approaches and methods of learning (Cole, 1998; Merriam & Caffarella, 1991). Learning activities may include hints, cues, or consequences that guide students to desired behaviors.

In contrast, the cognitive theory views learning as a process occurring inside the learner in an attempt to make sense of the world and give meaning to experiences. Some of the major theorists include Piaget, Bruner, and Ausubel. Gestalt learning theorists include Wertheimer, Kohler, Koffka, and Lewin. In the cognitive theory, the purpose of adult learning is knowledge acquisition. Instructors create the proper conditions for learning, and the learner is actively involved in the learning process (Cole, 1998; Merriam & Caffarella, 1991). Learning will include challenging learners beyond their current ability but within their potential level of development, thus allowing the material to be internalized.

While the cognitive theories examine the mental processing of information and the behaviorist theories focus on the environment shaping observable behavior, the humanist theories examine the potential for growth as a motivation for learning (Merriam & Caffarella, 1991). Key theorists include Maslow, Rogers, and Knowles. In the humanistic perspective, experience separates adults from youth when learning. The purpose of education is to enhance personal growth, development, and self-actualization. In the humanist perspective, students learn how to learn, and there is a relationship between the facilitator of learning and the learner. Learning activities may include group discussion, self-directed learning, and experiential learning (Cole, 1998; Merriam & Caffarella, 1991).

Finally, the social learning theories suggest that people learn by observing other people. Key theorists include Bandura and Rotter. The purpose of learning in the social theories is to promote desirable changes in knowledge, attitudes, and behavior. The role of the learner is one of an observer, decision maker, and processor of information, while the instructor serves as a model or provider of models as well as a facilitator. Approaches to learning may include demonstration, modeling, apprenticeships and mentoring, tutorials, peer partnerships, and on-the-job training (Merriam & Cafarrella, 1991).

Each of the theory groupings discussed have very different assumptions about the way adults learn. Occupational therapy practitioners should identify the most appropriate theory of learning based on each client and the context of intervention in order to develop strategies that will enhance their client's learning in therapy. Occupational therapy practitioners working with adults in an education setting must be familiar with the key theories of learning for adults. They also must be able to identify the learning styles of their clients to better assist them in attaining their educational goals. Understanding how adult students learn will be important when working with other professionals assisting the client, such as the disabilities services coordinator at the school or university, professors, and any other professional assisting with the client's goal of attending PSE classes. Understanding this information will assist the occupational therapy practitioner in problem solving and offering suggestions to both professionals and the client as it relates to the client's physical disability. Merriam and Caffarella (1991) suggest learning as a process (rather than an end product), focusing on what happens when learning takes place. Lastly, the occupational therapy practitioner should determine the client's primary method of learning. Everyone has a particular style of learning that he or she prefers. This will be especially important for clients whose physical limitations include cognitive impairments. A preferred learning style does not indicate how intelligent a person is but defines how a person's brain works best and most efficiently when attempting to learn new information (Halsne, 2002). Understanding personal learning styles can assist with success during any type of educational activity. Occasionally, depending on the reason a client is being seen in occupational therapy, a preferred learning style may not be possible any longer, and assisting the client with adapting to a new learning style may be necessary. Learning styles have traditionally been classified as auditory, visual, and tactile/kinesthetic (Halsne, 2002). This classification is one of the simplest forms, and it is suggested that those interested in further study on learning styles review the literature for the many theories and classifications that exist.

As the name would suggest, auditory learners prefer learning by hearing such as listening to a live lecture or audiotape. Visual learners, on the other hand, prefer to learn new information by reading or viewing a demonstration. Learners who prefer to manipulate materials when first being introduced to them are often classified as tactile/kinesthetic learners. Tactile/kinesthetic learners prefer to learn by doing, with hands-on practice being the best way for this type of learner to master a concept (Halsne, 2002).

Defining Education as an Occupation

Education, a life activity, is one of the primary occupations identified in the Occupational Therapy Practice Framework (AOTA, 2014). As a category of occupation, education is defined as "activities needed for learning and participating in the educational environment" (AOTA, 2014). Education can be defined as formal, informal personal education or interest exploration, or participation in informal personal education (AOTA, 2014). All of the categories of PSE options as described earlier in this chapter can be included within these subsets as defined in the

Table 5-3

Education as Occupation: Definitions and Examples

*Education Category	*Definition	Examples
*Formal participation	Academics	4-year or 2-year college classes, labs, service learning professional behaviors
	Nonacademics	Dorm life, obtaining meals transportation
	Extracurricular	Clubs, exercise, leisure, sororities/fraternities life, social participation, making choices
	Vocational	Work study, volunteering, teaching assistant, work
*Informal personal or Interests exploration	Identification of topics	Exploration of majors degrees and careers
	Methods for obtaining information	Ways for obtaining knowledge and skills: shadowing, coaching, learning and career support centers, faculty advisor relationships
*Informal personal education participation	Informal classes or programs provide instruction or training	Continuing education short noncredit courses skill training certifications

*Adapted from American Occupational Therapy Association. (2014) *Occupational therapy practice framework: Domain & process* (3rd ed., p. S20). Bethesda, MD: AOTA Press/American Occupational Therapy Association.

Occupational Therapy Practice Framework (Table 5-3). PSE provides rich opportunities for development not only in planned programs of study or major but also in areas of occupation such as social participation, leisure pursuits, and managing activities of daily living in new environments (AOTA, 2013). Thus, occupational therapy practitioners may have a variety of roles in working with ASWD. A unique ability of occupational therapists is that they in fact can actually transition with the ASWD across service delivery systems and institutions. If the student is transitioning from secondary environment, from rehabilitation in the case of a newly acquired disability, or from a veterans medical institution; the occupational therapist is mobile and adaptable and can serve as a case manager, advocate, educator, consultant, or interventionist depending on the ASWD occupational profile, goals, and needs in the education environments.

Occupational Therapy Skill Set and Roles in Postsecondary Education

Although there is minimal discussion in the literature regarding occupational therapy practitioners working to attain adult educational goals, practitioners can use their unique skills in a variety of ways. Occupational therapists working with clients in PSE will likely work with students who have a disability and are transitioning from high school, who have a newly acquired disability and are transitioning from a rehabilitation environment or a veterans medical system, or who are returning to PSE to develop a new or refined skill and knowledge set. Although this text focuses on adults with physical disabilities, the coexistence of disabilities across areas other than physical should not be minimized, and it may be those invisible disabilities that create some of the most significant challenges in PSE (AOTA, 2013; Gutman, 2008). In all of the venues, the occupational therapist would be involved in the evaluation and intervention process as established as best practice (AOTA, 2014). The occupational therapist may always be involved with an ASWD in health

Table 5-4

Skill Set of Occupational Therapy Appropriate to Postsecondary Education

Skills That Cross All Intervention Methods
Therapeutic use of self Consultant
Specific Areas of Intervention
Occupations and activities Preparatory methods in assistive technology Preparatory methods in environmental modification Education and training Advocacy and self-advocacy

care or rehabilitation settings; however, the unique role in the PSE options and environments is the connection between the practice of occupational therapy and the intent and the letter of the laws supporting the ASWD. Therefore, the approaches to intervention may primarily focus on assisting the ASWD to establish, maintain, and modify the skills or abilities in order to be as successful as possible in the PSE institutions (AOTA, 2013, 2014). The focus of occupations and activities for independence in PSE allows for matching of specific tasks in PSE with the needs of the individual student in terms of specific adaptations, accommodations, and auxiliary supports.

The skill set of occupational therapists (Table 5-4) positions them to be leaders in assisting ASWD to adapt in PSE. The skill set of the occupational therapist is broad, with two skills that are useful in the roles of case manager: therapeutic use of self and consultation. The occupational therapist can use communication skills, role-modeling and role-playing, coordination, facilitation of self-determination, and self-advocacy skills and coaching on how to develop productive habits and routines (AOTA, 2013). The occupational therapist is also skilled in applying the principles of universal design and activity analysis of the environmental accessibility and assistive technology, allowing the occupational therapist to assist the ASWD to develop lifelong skills to maximize the opportunities in higher education. As occupational therapists, our roles should focus on assisting students with disabilities to be successful, focusing on factors for success: practicing successful ways of positive self-disclosure, understanding the tasks of the PSE programs and matching those to reasonable accommodations and supports, and minimizing any stigmas or stereotypes about the student's individual disability (Barnard-Bark, Lechtenberger, & Lan, 2010). As outlined earlier in this chapter, the occupational therapist should consider the four guiding factors from the literature when working with a client in PSE environments. These are student centeredness, planning ahead for transitions, applying principles of universal design, and re-reviewing options for assistive technology.

Role of Occupational Therapist as Evaluator

The Occupational Therapy Practice Framework (3rd ed.) clearly articulates the evaluation process in the profession: "The evaluation process is focused on finding out what a client wants and needs to do; determining what a client can do and has done; and identifying supports and barriers" (AOTA, 2014, p. S13).

Table 5-5

Occupational Therapy Profile Questions Adapted for Postsecondary Education

General Guiding Questions
• What are your goals for entering the postsecondary setting, the program, or the course of study? • What supports or accommodations allowed you to be successful in other educational settings? • What are the immediate goals and longer goals for entering this postsecondary setting? • Are you comfortable, ready, and prepared to self-disclose your disability? What might you need to feel prepared to self-disclose? • How would you describe your strongest learning style (e.g., auditory, visual, hands-on)?
Adapted from *Occupational Therapy Practice Framework: Domain and Process* (3rd ed.), 2014, AOTA Press, p. S13.
Questions Related to the Educational Context and Environment
• What are the activities and behavioral standards and expectations of your PSE setting, program, or courses (cultural context)? • Do you have any non–disability-related personal attributes that may need to be considered in the postsecondary environment (personal context)? • How will the timing of your daily activities or routines integrate with the timing of the activities in your new educational setting (temporal context)? • How might the physical environment of the educational setting influence your participation? Are the support service offices, classes, labs, off-campus learning, and social areas accessible? Can you use all of the learning materials in each educational event (physical environment)? • When in this educational setting will you want points of social participation or connection or engagement? What supports may be necessary for these to be meaningful (social context)?
Adapted from Occupational Therapy Practice Framework: Domain and Process (3rd ed.), 2014, AOTA Press, p. S28.

ASWD in PSE environments are focused on discovering what they want in education and need to accomplish to be successful and obtaining appropriate supports or accommodations to meet the educational requirements. Thus, occupational therapy can be an important member of the team is assisting ASWD. The occupational therapy knowledge and skills in interviewing the student in occupation, the contextual variables influencing the occupation, and the activity demands of the occupation will target specific areas for support and possible accommodation. The occupational therapist working in conjunction with the office of students with disabilities or the ADA compliance office may be able to design a more complete plan of the supports that may improve access to educational opportunities.

The occupational profile, the first step in the evaluation process, can be instrumental. The occupational profile focused on education infuses the therapeutic use of self in a student-centered manner to facilitate a discussion of activities in the educational environment that are important, the influence of contextual variables, and what supports may be most appropriate (Table 5-5).

The therapist can engage in data collection from the student using the guiding areas of the occupational profile, questions related to an analysis of the context variables (cultural, personal, temporal, physical, and social contexts), and questions related to the activities involved in the occupation of education. The information gathered will be useful in targeting student outcomes and determining the roles of the occupational therapist in planning transition, case management, education or training in universal design, designing accessibility, and implementing the use of assistive technology.

Roles for the Occupational Therapist in Transition From High School

The transition from high school to PSE is included as part of the Individuals with Disabilities Education Act (IDEA) Amendments of 1997 (P. L. 105-117). As a member of the transition team, the occupational therapist makes recommendations based on the students' needs and abilities, and makes predictions regarding possible areas of challenge in the postsecondary environment. However, once discharged from the school-based services or graduation from high school, the high school student no longer has access to these school-based professionals in a formal manner (Kardos & White, 2005). However, there are multiple roles the occupational therapist can assume prior to the discharge or graduation, especially in a consultant role, educating the high school education team, student, and family in ways to decrease barriers and provide equal opportunity to participate in learning activities. A critical area for education is recognizing differences between secondary and postsecondary education environments, the importance of transition planning, the barriers to student self-disclosure and need for support to development self-advocacy, and the power of a team approach.

Transition from any environment to PSE can be challenging. However, when the transition is from a secondary to a postsecondary environment, the ASWD needs to have some preparation, which can be woven into the occupational therapy interventions. There are several basic reasons why the transition from high school to PSE is challenging: the laws governing rights of ASWD are different than when in high school; the ASWD is in fact an adult and must practice self-advocacy; the institutional responsibilities do not focus on remediation or rehabilitation (which is the norm in secondary education); and the student has a significant level of responsibility (Kallio & Owens, 2012; Oertle & Bragg, 2014). The occupational therapist can work with the high school team to educate the student and family about the key differences between high school and PSE.

1. The high school team works to develop an individualized educational plan. The PSE environment has a disability support office, and the student must self-identify to the office and request accommodations.
2. A high school is responsible for testing a student to identify any disability. The student must provide documentation to verify both eligibility to attend the PSE program and to verify disability.
3. In high school, accommodations, services, supports, and assistive technology are provided to meet the individualized educational plan. In the PSE environment, services and reasonable accommodations may be provided in order to provide equal access to participate in the college programs.
4. High schools are often required to provide personnel to support the student in the high school environment. The PSE setting does not have to provide personal care or paraprofessionals or other support personnel.
5. In the high school environment, the educational team is required to provide educational services that will allow the student to meet the educational goals. In the PSE environment, the student must reach out to the office of disability. Once accommodations are established, the ASWD is responsible for communicating with faculty and meeting the requirements of the educational courses or programs.

The transition from high school, where the laws and services can be classified as entitlements, to those of the PSE environment, or one of eligibility, can be challenging (AHEAD, 2012; Cory, 2011; Kallio & Owens, 2012; Oertle & Bragg, 2014). A role for occupational therapy may be to educate the student with a disability while in the high school environment about the changes and provide opportunities for the student to develop self-advocacy and self-empowerment behaviors to prepare for a successful transition to PSE.

Role of Occupational Therapist as Case Manager

The occupational therapist's role as case manager is debated (Daykin, 2001; Lamb, 2003). Social workers and nurses are most often placed in the role of case manager. Social workers receive training in social policy, community organization, and community resources to help them most effectively provide resources for their clients (Case-Smith, 1991). Nurses too have played an important role in case management, particularly in acute care settings (Lohman, 1999). Occupational therapists, however, also receive education on health care, social, educational, governmental, and community systems as they relate to the practice of occupational therapy (ACOTE, 2015). Despite the community debate, AOTA's Scope of Practice (2004) includes case management as an appropriate occupational therapy intervention.

In some settings, it is a natural extension of the occupational therapy practitioner's roles and responsibilities. For example, early intervention services recognize occupational and physical therapists as potential case managers (Case-Smith, 1991). As students approach graduation, occupational therapy practitioners have participated in the transition-planning phase of high school as discussed earlier. Transition services are included as part of the IDEA Amendments of 1997 (IDEA: Public Law, 105-17). These services are designed to facilitate the move from high school to postsecondary activities, including PSE. The participation of the occupational therapist in transition planning is critical for the success of the student (Asher, 2003; Davidson & Fitzgerald, 2001; O'Reilly, 2000).

Occupational therapy practitioners working with adult clients also serve as case managers. Occupational therapy practitioners in geriatric, outpatient, mental health, and acute care settings all may find themselves taking on the role of case manager (Jacobs, 2002; Lamb, 2003; Lohman, 1999). Mental health centers use occupational therapy practitioners as case managers, either as part of their role as occupational therapist or with the job title of case manager (Jacobs, 2002; Lamb, 2003). In other settings, case management responsibilities may require more specialized training. For example, in an acute care setting, the occupational therapist may have to participate in advanced training classes on medical processes and medical economics in order to effectively perform the duties of a case manager (Lohman, 1999).

The services available to students seeking PSE are both university- and community-based. For a student with a disability, understanding and making sense of these services can be difficult and overwhelming. As case managers, occupational therapists can assist by facilitating connections with these supports and/or coordinating communication between these services. Occupational therapists have specialized training in the grading of activity and occupation and in the use of this strategy to promote independence. A more adaptive or compensatory approach, is one in which the occupational therapist serves as the catalyst for maintaining support access and usage and coordinating the communication between services to assist the client with meeting educational goals. Again, this strategy is one in which occupational therapists receive specialized training. They are able to determine the need for compensation, as opposed to remediation, and are skilled in the therapeutic use of self in practice. These strategies can be used both with adult students with developmental or physical disabilities who have transitioned from high school to PSE and with individuals who have experienced a new diagnosis or impairment and are attempting to return to college or a university.

Role of Occupational Therapy in Education and Training in Principles of Universal Design

Universal design was originally a term related to the design of the physical environment (Universal Design Summit, 2013). The key concepts applied to learning are *universal design for learning* (Rose & Gravel, 2010) and *universal design for instruction*, a proactive approach to teaching that uses inclusive instructional strategies that benefit a broad range of learners, including students with disabilities (Scott, McGuire, & Embry, 2002). A review of all three sets of principles yields an underlying concept: that environments and practices in those environments can empower and enable ASWD or create barriers for ASWD (Swain, French, Barnes, & Thomas, 2004). The direct connections of universal design (UD) to both learning and instruction are not often clear but allow for a framework to increase accessibility for students with disabilities. In addition, UD places a responsibility on disability service providers and other educational professionals to reflect on PSE programs and practices and to design access initially in the development phase of courses and programs and holds that reflective feedback from postsecondary students with and without disabilities can provide higher education providers with a deeper understanding of accessibility for all (Beck et al., 2014; Rose, Meyer, & Hitchcock, 2005).

> The nine Principles of UDI [universal design for instruction] provide a framework for college faculty to use when designing or revising instruction to be responsive to diverse student learners and to minimize the need for 'special' accommodations and retrofitted changes to the learning environment. UDI operates on the premise that the planning and delivery of instruction as well as the evaluation of learning can incorporate inclusive attributes that embrace diversity in learners without compromising academic standards. (Scott, McGuire, & Embry, 2002, p. 1)

The occupational therapist has a working knowledge of universal design principles in environmental design and accessibility. The focus of these nine principles is to improve accessibility of the educational environment to diverse learners, or as in the focus of this text and chapter, ASWD.

The nine principles of universal design for instruction are based on the principles of universal design and effective instruction and were developed as part of a federal grant from the U.S. Department of Education at the University of Connecticut's Center on Postsecondary Education and Disability (Scott, McGuire, & Embry, 2002). They are defined as follows:

1. Equitable use: Instruction is designed to be useful to and accessible by people with diverse abilities. Provide the same means of use for all students—identical whenever possible, equivalent when not.
2. Flexibility in use: Instruction is designed to accommodate a wide range of individual abilities. Provide choice in methods of use.
3. Simple and intuitive: Instruction is designed in a straightforward and predictable manner, regardless of the student's experience, knowledge, language skills, or current concentration level. Eliminate unnecessary complexity.
4. Perceptible information: Instruction is designed so that necessary information is communicated effectively to the student, regardless of ambient conditions or the student's sensory abilities.
5. Tolerance for error: Instruction anticipates variation in individual student learning pace and prerequisite skills.
6. Low physical effort: Instruction is designed to minimize nonessential physical effort in order to allow maximum attention to learning. Note: This principle does not apply when physical effort is integral to essential requirements of a course.

7. Size and space for approach and use: Instruction is designed with consideration for appropriate size and space for approach, reach, manipulations, and use regardless of a student's body size, posture, mobility, and communication needs.
8. A community of learners: The instructional environment promotes interaction and communication among students and between students and faculty.
9. Instructional climate: Instruction is designed to be welcoming and inclusive. High expectations are espoused for all students (Scott, McGuire, & Shaw, 2003).

As technology becomes embedded in higher education pedagogy and teaching-learning methodology, the principles of universal design for instruction will have more options to meet its purpose: increased accessibility for all. The occupational therapist with knowledge and skills in activity demand analysis (AOTA, 2014, p. S13), performance skill analysis (AOTA, 2014, p. S25), and preparatory methods such as environmental design and assistive technology (AOTA, 2014, p. S29) can play a critical role as a team member in disability services for students with disabilities in higher education environments.

Role of Occupational Therapy in Environmental Modification

Accessibility is one of the barriers that students with physical disabilities in particular may face once deciding to enter, return, or continue with PSE or adult education programs. Structural accessibility includes the accessibility of physical facilities including ramps, automatic doors, elevators, accessible restrooms, classrooms, laboratories, libraries, computer centers, and cafeterias. The broad intent is also to consider physical accessibility to any of the learning opportunities associated with the ASWD's course of study or degree program. In some situations that may include access to other structures, for example: a pond for a course on the environment or a kiln for a fine arts class. In addition, the presence of the following will impact many students with disabilities: curb cuts, handicapped parking, and adaptive on-campus transportation or shuttle services in all buildings and on all campuses. Additionally, structural accessibility includes nontraditional methods of accessing campus services such as the various options available through online learning.

One important role that occupational therapists play when working with clients is the role of educator. Educating our clients about acceptable methods of program accessibility in educational institutions is an important foundation to provide. Both Title II of the ADA and Section 504 of the Rehabilitation Act require educational programs that are accessible and usable by individuals with disabilities (Scott, 1994). Structures built after January 26, 1992, must follow the ADA standards for accessible design. These newer buildings, therefore, usually do not pose a problem to individuals with physical disabilities. However, many educational institutions operate in older buildings, which make structural modifications difficult. In these cases, schools can meet accessibility accommodations through nonstructural methods. Although these methods are not considered ideal and must not result in any type of segregation of students with disabilities, they can be effective in providing a student's access. Some examples of remedial and adaptation/compensation accommodations are listed subsequently. In addition, occupational therapists need to consider the possible barriers clients with physical disabilities may face when attending events in specialty classrooms such as labs, theaters, and gymnasiums. Although most of these types of classrooms will be in compliance with the ADA standards for accessible design, there will be cases in which they are not, and the occupational therapy practitioner should problem-solve with the client on the preferred method for accessibility. Academic accessibility, or access to classroom information, also includes the institution's ability to satisfy necessary accommodations, such as extended time for examinations and assignments, note takers, and doing work in a different way or in a different place.

There are also multiple methods of achieving accessibility through nonstructural changes in the environment, such as the following:

- Reassignment of services or classrooms to an accessible location such as the ground floor of a building or relocation to completely different building
- Moving computers in libraries and computer labs to an accessible location
- Providing accessible workstations
- Modifying hardware on doors to allow for access

Role of Occupational Therapy in Assistive Technology

Assistive technology is considered a compensatory approach, allowing technology to circumvent the disability to maximize access to learning opportunities for increased function and maximum independence. While there are many ways to define assistive technology, the definition that has been most widely accepted by professionals is from the Assistive Technology Act of 1998. It states that an assistive technology device is: "Any item, piece of equipment or product system whether acquired commercially off the shelf, modified, or customized which is used to increase or improve functional capabilities of individuals with disabilities." The act further states that assistive technology service means: "Any service which directly assists individuals with a disability in the selection, acquisition, or use of an assistive technology device" (Assistive Technology Act, 105-394, S. 2432, 1998).

This term also includes the following:

- The evaluation of the needs of individuals with a disability
- The purchasing, leasing, or provision of the device
- The selection, designing, fitting, customizing, adapting, applying, maintaining, repairing, or replacing of the device
- Coordinating and using other therapies, interventions, or services such as those associated with education and rehabilitation plans and programs
- Training and technical assistance for the person with a disability, or if appropriate, the family of the person
- Training or technical assistance for professionals, including individuals providing education or rehabilitation service, employers, or other individuals who are substantially involved in the major life functions of individuals with disabilities (Assistive Technology Act, 105-394, S. 2432, 1998)

As described previously, Section 504 is accessed by the student and accommodations are primarily student driven. The role of the occupational therapy practitioner in addressing assistive technology issues in a PSE environment would likely be to provide information on, and access to, the most beneficial assistive technology for the student within the PSE. It is the occupational therapist's role to work in a collaborative model with the student to determine the best fit for assistive technology. It may also be the role of the occupational therapist to work directly in collaboration with the disability services coordinator on site at the educational institution to advocate for the most appropriate device. It is also possible that a school, required only to provide equipment within reasonable accommodation guidelines (according to Section 104.44 part D of The Rehabilitation Act of 1973, Section 504), will provide a more complex and perhaps more appropriate piece of equipment if it is recommended by a qualified professional such as an occupational therapy practitioner. Technology as a tool is part of everyday life, but for a student with a disability it is a tool for liberation: "Technology is a lot like freedom . . . Once it is uncorked, there is no putting it back. Its fruits are there for everyone's enjoyment and benefit. It is often said that assistive technology is liberating [for the individual with a disability] and that is certainly the case. But it is time to be clear that assistive technology is liberating not just for the individual with a disability but indeed for America as a whole" (Williams, 1991).

Assistive technology tools or devices can be categorized from low to high (Cook & Polgar, 2015; Edyburn, 2003; Sweeney, 2007). The categories of technology are associated with the increasing complexity of the tool and complexity of the training process to use the tool and may include the associated cost of the tool. One goal for the occupational therapist is to have as few technology tools as possible for the greatest number of functions as possible. In this manner, the ASWD will have fewer tools to manage and more functional needs met. Additional goals for the practitioner in the matching process of student to technology are noted in the literature, as follows:

1. Focus on the assistive technology to reduce the ASWD reliance on others and thus depend on the assistive technology to circumvent the disability (Day & Edwards, 1996; Margolis & Michaels, 1994).
2. Review the selection of the assistive technology to ensure that the student's needs are met while meeting the demands of the PSE curriculum and requirements (Mull & Sitlington, 2003).
3. When possible, consider technology platforms that are the same as those used by students without disabilities in the same PSE setting in order to provide natural peer support systems.
4. Explore the accessibility features of a computer operating system for adaptations that may assist students with physical, visual, and hearing disabilities.
5. Assistive technology can be expensive, so education of the ASWD as to resources for funding is critical.
6. Prevent technology abandonment by training the ASWD in the use of the tools for the clearly identified purpose and ensure successful utilization through follow-up training reviews (Todis, 1996).

Technology is not to be a stand-alone tool but instead integrated with the ASWD occupational profile, goals in the PSE, the environmental context variables, and universal design for instruction and assistive technology. As each one of these variables change or develop then the assistive technology will require a review and a possible adaptation.

One model that supports integrating these variables is human activity assistive technology (HAAT). This model integrates the attributes of the individual, the activity, and the contexts in order to determine the assistive technology (Cook & Polgar, 2015). The contextual component of this model is broad in order to encompass the inherent aspects of an activity and to include the context variables associated with the occupational therapy (AOTA, 2014) such as the physical environment, temporal, social, cultural, and personal contexts. Thus the contextual aspects of the environment in which the activity occurs is a critical concept to be considered in order to provide appropriate supports to the use of the technology (Figure 5-2).

Because assistive technology in some service systems may include seating systems, powered mobility, adapted driving, and adaptive tools for personal activities of daily living, it is important to focus on the utilization of assistive technology for educating adults in PSE environments. In this specific setting, assistive technology as provided by the institution may be limited to those tools related to reasonable accommodations that provide equal access to educational opportunities. An understanding of assistive technology tools can be achieved by classifying those tools according to the functions they can serve (Table 5-6) for the ASWD (Gregg, 2011; Holmes & Silvestri, 2012) including accessibility to information, producing educational assignments, scheduling and time management, organization and memory, attention and concentration (Cook & Polgar, 2015; Gregg, 2011; Holmes & Silvestri, 2012; Mull & Sitlington, 2003). Accessibility features are built-in

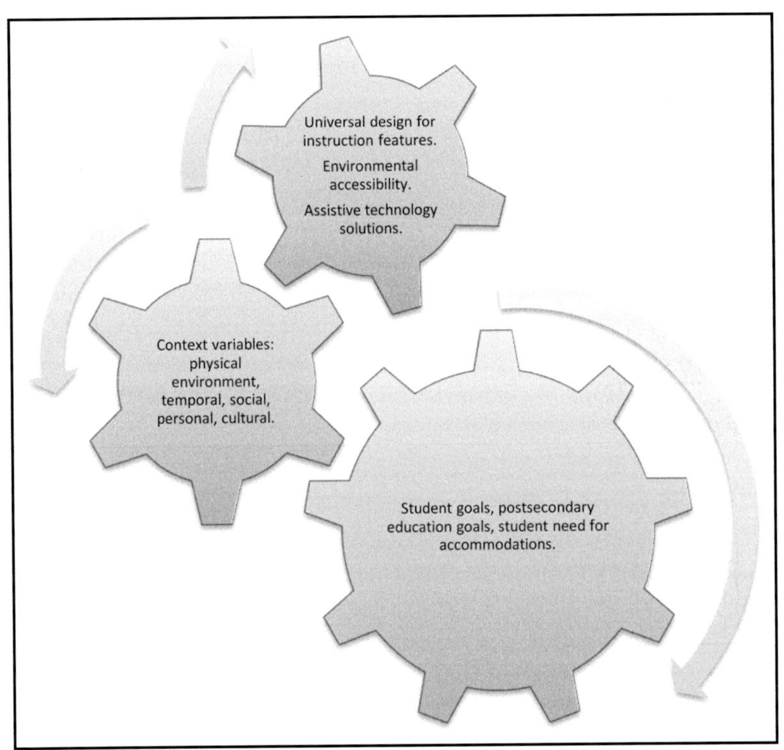

Figure 5-2. Integration of assistive technology: student-environment context-universal design and assistive technology.

components of a computer, tablet, or smartphone operating system. In addition, word processing software programs also have accessibility features built in. The practitioner can learn about accessibility features through the operating system or settings section of the technology or through searching for accessibility features via the help command in a software program. Accessibility features (Table 5-7) allow the student to circumvent physical, sensory, or learning challenges in order to more efficiently use the hardware or software. Access features may also allow the faculty to create more user-friendly documents by adding alternative size and color text or images to represent content, having the text read by the computer (synthetic speech), or having the faculty actually record a voice-over for the text. These access features are used to adapt the text or the screen to implementing universal design for instruction concepts as discussed earlier in this chapter.

Tablet and smartphone technology has accessibility features built in that can be found under the control panel, settings, or general tab. The number of apps available for both tablets and smartphones is growing rapidly and does require careful consideration when being used as an accommodation in PSE. The most common shortfall is the extensive number of apps, leaving the occupational therapist and student to match the app to the specific activity for the educational environment (Batista & Gaglani, 2013; Erickson, 2015; Mosa, Yoo, & Sheets, 2012). Physical access via touch/swipe/pinch as well as the bilateral skill of object stabilization may require tools to hold the tablet or smartphone or use of features such as voice control. Vision may be essential, and the small screen size limits magnification. A consistent benefit of using a tablet or smartphone is portability. Two possible issues are physical access and vision. As with all assistive technology as previously described, the occupational therapist is a vital member of the team to assist the ASWD to match activity demands of the PSE environment, the context variables including the physical

Table 5-6

Sample Assistive Technologies According to Functional Purposes in Postsecondary Education

Functional Activity	Assistive Technology	Web Resources
Access to information	Alternative keyboards	https://www.enablemart.com/computer-accessibility
	Optical character recognition	http://finereader.abbyy.com/about_ocr/whatis_ocr/
	Text to speech	http://www.naturalreaders.com
	Font adjustments: size and color	Use help command on your computer to find built-in features
	Cursor adjustments	Use help command on your computer to find built-in features
	Personal FW system	http://gofrontrow.com
	Closed captioning	http://www.3playmedia.com
	Access features	Search: "access features" in computer operating system
Produce assignments	Keyboarding shortcuts: Abbreviation expansion Word prediction Electronic dictionary Templates	Search: Conduct Internet search by computer brand
	Outlining software	http://lifehacker.com/5419988/five-best-outlining-tools
	Mind mapping software	http://www.digitaltrends.com/computing
	Voice recognition or voice to text	http://www.nuance.com
	Access feature voice to text	Search: "access features" in computer operating system
Organization and memory	Access features	Search: "access features" in computer operating system
	Electronic organizers and calendars	Search: "electronic calendar organizer" on www.amazon.com
	Personal tape recorders	Search: "digital voice recorders" on www.bestbuy.com
Attention and concentration	White noise	Search: "white noise machine" on www.sharperimage.com
	Noise-cancelling headset	http://www.bose.com/

Note: Products and resources listed do not constitute author endorsement. Instead, the resources listed are a place to begin exploring assistive technology. Conducting a general search through your preferred Web browser will uncover a plethora of products.

Table 5-7

Descriptions of Accessibility Features

Accessibility Feature	Description
Auditory Assist	
Sound sentry	Generates a visual display when a sound occurs
Show sounds	Displays captions for speech and sound
Narrator	Reads aloud the text on the screen
Visual Assist	
High contrast	Changes background and font color
Cursor options	Changes the rate of cursor blinking Changes width of cursor
Pointer	Change size, color, and type of pointer Trailing leaves visible path of pointer movement
Tool bar functions	Highlighting tool Font style and size function On-screen scaling Insert pictures, clip art, smart art, hyperlinks
Magnifier	Magnifies entire screen or selected portion
Alternative Keyboard Access	
Filter keys	Slows or eliminates repeat function of a key
On-screen keyboard	Allows for keyboarding by pointing and clicking with a mouse or other cursor control device
Speech recognition	Allows student to talk and the computer will type
Touch screen	Option available when purchasing a monitor or screen
Mouse keys	Use arrow keys instead of a mouse to move the pointer or cursor
Note: Not all of the features listed above are available in all operating systems or software. In addition, others not listed may be available. Check the help command or computer control panel settings for a complete list of available options.	

environment, the performance skills of the ASWD, and the mobile devices such as tablets and smartphones (Erickson, 2015).

Case Examples

Case Example: Leann

Background

Leann is a 19-year-old woman who sustained a traumatic brain injury at the age of 16. She was a passenger in a car that slid on black ice and ran into a ditch. After 3 weeks in a coma, Leann began the long process of rehabilitation. She missed her junior year of high school, though she returned the following year. She was eligible for special education services and completed high school successfully with the support of the education team and the individualized education program.

Following graduation, Leann underwent two surgeries, one to increase her speech volume and one to address a severe contracture in her left elbow. She was referred to outpatient occupational therapy following the surgeries. The occupational therapist evaluated her and determined she has limited functional use of both upper extremities due to bilateral paresis, decreased mobility due to limited ambulation, poor balance, and poor endurance, and almost inaudible speech, even following the surgery. She has intact cognition and perceptual skills, though she reports that sometimes she needs to hear information more than once to "get it all." She uses a power wheelchair independently and can walk for limited distances. She is independent in toileting and feeding light finger foods but requires help lifting a heavy beverage.

Occupational Profile and Performance Related to Postsecondary Education

Upon interview to determine her occupational profile, Leann decided to attend the local community college with a focus on general education in social services. Her dream is to be a social worker working with families. She deeply values many points of engagement with others and indicated that she needs support in advocating for herself as an adult.

An observation of her performance in the high school environment and then at the community college saw her patterns of performance. Leann is easily fatigued, especially when using her arms excessively. She needs assistance with writing, page turning, carrying and manipulating textbooks, opening doors, and drinking beverages. She also will need alternative test-taking methods, and perhaps extra time for assignments. Leann needs extra time to travel between classes, meals, and social events due to wheelchair use.

Occupational Therapy Roles

Educator

The occupational therapist can enlist one member of the team to review the difference in student responsibilities from high school to the postsecondary setting. Using the therapeutic use of self, the occupational therapist can role-model and role-play with Leann about the most appropriate methods to self-disclose her disability status to the office of disability services. Because Leann indicated in her profile that she enjoys people and wants to focus on social work, the occupational therapist may also educate Leann on options for co-curricular activity involvement at the community college.

Case Management Services

The occupational therapist takes a facilitatory role, believing Leann can take over her own case management once she has connected with necessary services. She contacts the disability services office (DSO) and arranges for an intake meeting with Leann and a counselor in that office. The occupational therapist reviews the course list with Leann, and they contact the registrar to determine where the classes are held, the distance between classes, and the amount of time between classes. The occupational therapist may practice navigating the community college environment and develop strategies for inclement weather, parking changes, and changes in course locations. Once the disability office has reviewed Leann's documentation and approved accommodations, the occupational therapist and Leann again can role-play how to discuss those accommodations with faculty and peers.

Accessibility

The occupational therapist and Leann go to the campus together and assess her mobility, including access to buildings, the student center, and bathrooms. They discover the bathroom doors are too heavy for her to open independently and refer this to the DSO, which agrees to have the in-class note taker assist with bathroom access in between classes. All other campus facilities are accessible.

Assistive Technology

The occupational therapist recommends the following:

1. A laptop computer for the in-class note taker to use
2. Software to read text aloud so Leann can listen to lecture notes if she becomes fatigued
3. Voice-activated software for converting speech to text for completing assignments and computer control
4. The occupational therapist may work with Leann's physical therapist and the wheelchair vendor to determine the safest and most reliable method for mounting or securing the laptop to the wheelchair for ease of transport and ease of computer setup.
5. Recommendations for other assistance include extended and alternative test-taking strategies, texts on CD so her computer can read aloud, and student readers if necessary for texts that are not available on CD.

Case Example: Raymond

Background

Raymond is a 21-year-old man who recently completed his junior year at an Ivy League college. Raymond's major is pre-law, and he has been on the dean's list since his freshman year. He is a popular student who has served in various student leadership roles on campus. He was named captain of the football team for his upcoming senior year and has been a star player since high school. Over the summer, he was brought into the emergency room by his football teammates when he could not participate in a practice session due to extreme numbness and tingling in his UEs and double vision. Once a complete battery of tests was completed, Raymond was diagnosed with multiple sclerosis. When a complete history was taken, it was discovered that Raymond had been having symptoms for the past 6 months. He had been ignoring the symptoms, which included frequent numbness and tingling in his extremities as well as fatigue and other visual disturbances, because he believed they were due to his academic lifestyle and the demands football had placed on his body.

Occupational Profile and Performance

Raymond was referred to outpatient occupational therapy. Raymond described his values as being fiercely independent, enjoying apartment living, wanting the freedom to use a car as he wished to visit family and friends. He did not feel comfortable discussing his limitations and often hid his symptoms from family and physicians. He expressed fear of becoming depressed and longing for his previous life roles. Once engaged in conversation about his former roles, he becomes most animated when discussing his academic and athletic accomplishments and appears to have a desire to return to school. His physicians all indicate good potential to return to and be successful in college, and Raymond's parents are supportive of this goal. Raymond is hesitant because he feels his ability to participate in college as he once did is gone and he is embarrassed to be in class and not be able to participate.

His most recent occupational therapy evaluation revealed significant visual deficits, diminished short-term memory, and noticeable spasticity in both arms. He is having difficulty initiating movement and cannot use his hands and fingers in a coordinated manner. These are all impacting his daily life: the low vision is limiting his ability to use a computer and read books, magazines, and newspapers; his short-term memory loss is affecting his ability to remember to take his medication effectively, and his arm weakness and spasticity is limiting his ability to perform self-care tasks (e.g., dressing, bathing, hygiene) and writing and computer-related tasks (e.g., he can no longer write or type effectively due to weak grasp and finger incoordination). During the occupational therapy evaluation, Raymond expressed concern that he is becoming increasingly depressed.

Case Study Questions

- What are the roles of the outpatient occupational therapist as related to Raymond's educational status?
- If Raymond decides he would like to attempt to return to school, what resources would need to be recruited and why?
- What evaluation/assessment procedures would need to be completed if the occupational therapy practitioner wants to assist him in returning to his former educational role?
- What assistive technology would be most appropriate for Raymond and how might the occupational therapy practitioner assist him in attaining it?
- What are the boundaries and limitations of which the occupational therapy practitioner must be aware if Raymond returns to school while still being treated in the outpatient setting?

Chapter Summary Questions

1. What is the definition of education according to the Occupational Therapy Practice Framework?
2. What are three types of PSE options for students with disabilities?
3. What are two current educational methods that will allow increased accessibility to education for students with disabilities?
4. What are the two primary laws that govern and support equal opportunity for education for ASWD?
5. In a role as a transition planner, how will you describe the process for verification as an ASWD to your client?
6. Describe when an accommodation is considered reasonable.
7. List four guiding factors in the postsecondary disability services.
8. What are four possible roles for occupational therapy in PSE?
9. What are five strategies for environmental modification in PSE settings?
10. What types of assistive technology for ASWD will provide alternative access to the computer, increase ease of completing academic assignments, or provide access to educational information for students with disabilities?

REFERENCES

Accreditation Council for Occupational Therapy Education (ACOTE) Standards and Interpretive Guide. (2015).

American Occupational Therapy Association. (2004). Occupational therapy scope of practice. *American Journal of Occupational Therapy, 58.*

American Occupational Therapy Association. (2010). Specialized knowledge and skills in technology and environmental interventions for occupational therapy practice. *American Journal of Occupational Therapy, 64*(6), S44-S56.

American Occupational Therapy Association. (2013). Students with Disabilities in postsecondary education settings: How occupational therapy can help. Fact Sheet. Retrieved from www.aota.org.

American Occupational Therapy Association. (2014). Occupational therapy practice framework: Domain and process (3rd ed.). *The American Journal of Occupational Therapy, 68*(Suppl. 1).

Americans with Disabilities Act. 42 U.S.C. §12101 (1990).

Americans with Disabilities Act. 42 U.S.C. §12111 (1990).

Americans with Disability Act, 34 C.F.R. §104 (1999).

Asher, A. (2003). From student to employee: helping students with disabilities make the transition. *Developmental Disabilities: Special Interest Section Quarterly, 26*(4), 1-4.

Assistive Technology Act. (1998). Public Law, 105-394, S. 2432.

Association on Higher Education and Disability. (2012). Supporting accommodation requests: Guidance on documentation practices. Retrieved from www.ahead.org.

Barnard-Brak, L., Lechtenberger, D., & Lan, W. Y. (2010). Accommodation strategies of college students with disabilities. *The Qualitative Report, 15*(2), 411-429.

Barnes, J. (1982). *A lively and concise introduction to Aristotle's work.* Oxford, United Kingdom:Oxford University Press.

Batista, M. A., & Gaglani, S. M. (2013). The future of smartphones in healthcare. *Virtual Mentor, 15*(11), 947-950.

Baum, C. (Ed.), *Occupational therapy: Enabling function and well-being* (2nd ed.). Thorofare, NJ: SLACK Incorporated.

Beck, T., Diaz del Castillo, P., Fovet, F., Mole, H., & Noga, B. (2014). Applying universal design to disability service provision: Outcome analysis of a universal design (UD) audit. *Journal of Postsecondary Education and Disability, 27*(2), 209-222.

Bragg, D. D., & Durham, B. (2012). Perspectives on access and equality in the era of college completion. *Community College Review, 40*, 106-125.

Bragg, D. D., & Townsend, B. (2007). ASHE reader on community colleges in the 21st century: Introduction. In B. Townsend & D. Bragg (Eds.), *ASHE reader on community colleges* (pp. xix-xxviii). Boston, MA: Pearson.

Bureau of Labor Statistics. (2014). Persons with a disability: Labor Force Characteristics-2013. Retrieved from www.bls.gov/cps.

Case-Smith, J. (1991). Occupational and physical therapists as case managers in early intervention. *Physical and Occupational Therapy in Practice, 11*(1), 53-70.

Cook, A., & Polgar, J. (2015). *Assistive technologies: Principles and practice* (4th ed.). Sacramento, CA: Mosby.

Corrigan, P. W., & Matthews, A. K. (2003). Stigma and disclosure: Implications for coming out of the closet. *Journal of Mental Health, 12*(3), 235-248

Cory, C. R. (2011). Disability services offices fort students with disabilities: A campus Resource. *New Directions for Higher Education, 154*, 27-36.

Davidson, D. A., & Fitzgerald, L. (2001). Transition planning for students. *OT Practice, 6*(17), 17-20.

Day, S. L., & Edwards, B. J. (1996). Assistive technology postsecondary students with learning disabilities. *Journal of Learning Disabilities, 29*, 486-492, 503.

Daykin, W. (2001). Yet another role: the community occupational therapist as care manager. *British Journal of Occupational Therapy, 54*(1), 46.

Diament, M. (2015). Graduation rates inch up for students with disabilities. Disability Scoop. Retrieved from http://www.disabilityscoop.com.

Dowrick, P. W. Anderson, J., Heyer, K., & Acosta, J. (2005). Postsecondary education across the USA: Experiences of adults with disabilities. *Journal of Vocational Rehabilitation, 22*(1), 41-47.

Edyburn, D. L. (2002). Models, theories and frameworks: contributions to understanding special education technology. *Special Education Technology Practice, 4*(2), 16-24.

Erickson, K. (2015). Evidence considerations for mobile devices in the occupational therapy process. *The Open Journal of Occupational Therapy, 3*(2), Article 7.

Friederich, A., Bernd, T., & De Witte, L. (2010). Methods for the selection of assistive technology in neurological rehabilitation practice. *Scandinavian Journal of Occupational Therapy, 17*(4), 308-318.

Garrison-Wade, D. F., & Lehmann, J. P., (2009). A conceptual framework for understanding students' with disabilities transition to community college. *Community College Journal of Research and Practice, 33*, 415-443.

Graham-Smith, S., & Lafayette, S., (2004). Quality disability support for promoting belonging and academic success within the college community. *College Student Journal, 38*, 90-99.

Gregg, N. (2012). Increasing access to learning for the adult basic education learner with learning disabilities: Evidence-based accommodation research. *Journal Learning Disabilities, 45*(1), 47-63.

Gutman, S. A. (2008). Supported education for adults with psychiatric disabilities. *Psychiatric Services, 59*(3), 326-327.

Halsne, A. (2002). Online versus traditionally-delivered instruction: A descriptive study of learner characteristics in a community college setting. (ERIC document Reproduction Services No. ED465534). Retrieved March 30, 2005, from EDRS Online.

Holmes, A., & Silvestri, R. (2012). Assistive technology use by students with LD in postsecondary education: A case of application before investigation? *Canadian Journal of School Psychology*, 1-17.

Huger, M. S. (2011). Fostering a disability-friendly institutional climate. *New Directions for Student Services, 134*, 3-11.

Individuals with Disabilities Education Act Amendments of 1990 (Public Law 101-476). 20 U.S.C., 400 et seq.

Individuals with Disabilities Education Act Amendments of 1997 (Public Law 105-17). 20 U.S.C., 1400 et seq.

Jacobs, K. (2002). Navigating the road ahead. *OT Practice, June*, 24-30.

Jarrow, J. (2000, October). Students with disabilities in higher education: Confirmations and cautions from the Boston University lawsuit. Retrieved April 9, 2005, from http://www.janejarrow.com/tv_station/bu/maintext.html.

Jarrow, J. (2015). What is a reasonable accommodation? Pepperdine Disability Services. Retrieved from http://www.pepperdine.edu/disabilityservices/faculty/articles/whatisreason.htm.

Kallio, A., & Owens, L. (2012). Opening doors to postsecondary education and training. Wisconsin Department of Public Instruction. Retrieved from https://pubsales.dpi.wi.gov/product/opening-doors-to-postsecondary-education.

Kardos, M., & White, B. P. (2005). The role of school-based occupational therapist in secondary education transition planning: A pilot survey study. *The American Journal of Occupational Therapy, 59*(2), 173-180.

Kertcher, E. (2014). Postsecondary education for students with intellectual disabilities: An emerging practice area for occupational therapy practitioners. *OT Practice, 19*(21) CE1-CE8.

Lamb, M. (2003). Case management for a geriatric outreach program in British Columbia. *Occupational Therapy Now, Sept/Oct*, 30.

Lohman, H. (1999). What will it take for more occupational therapists to become case managers? Implications for education, practice, and policy. *American Journal of Occupational Therapy, 53*(1), 111-13.

Madaus, J. W. (2005). Navigating the college transition maze: a guide for students with learning disabilities. *Teaching Exceptional Children, 37*(3), 32-37.

Margolis, V. H., & Michaels, C. A. (1994). Technology: The personal computer as a resource tool. In C. A. Michaels (Ed.), *Transition strategies for persons with learning disabilities* (pp. 239-269). San Diego, CA: Singular.

Merriam, S. B., & Caffarella, R. S. (1991). *Learning in adulthood.* San Francisco, CA: Jossey-Bass.

Michaels, E. (2004). Campus inclusion. *OT Practice*, 10-13.

Mull, C., & Sitlington, P. L. (2003). The role of technology in the transition to postsecondary education of students with learning disabilities. *The Journal of Special Education, 37*(1), 26-32.

Mull, C., Sitlington, P. L., & Alper, S. (2001). Postsecondary education for students with learning disabilities: A synthesis of the literature. *Exceptional Children, 68*(1), 97-118.

National Center for Education Statistics. (1999). Students with disabilities in postsecondary education: A profile of preparation, participation, and outcomes, NCES 1999–187. Washington DC: Office of Educational Research and Improvements.

National Center for Education Statistics. (2011). Students with disabilities at degree-granting postsecondary institutions. US Department of Education. Retrieved from http://nces.ed.gov.

Newman, L., Wagner, M., Knokey, A, M., Marger, C., Nagle, K., Shaver, D., Wei, X. (2011). The post high school outcomes of young adults with disabilities up to 8 years after high school. A report from the National Longitudinal Transition Study-2 (NLTS2) (NCSER 2011-3005). Menlo Park, CA: SRI International.

O'Reilly, A. (2000). Transition services planning and the school-based services. *OT Practice, 5*(20), 16-17.

Oertle, K. M., & Bragg, D. D. (2014). Transitioning students with disabilities: Community college policies and practices. *Journal of Disability Policy Studies, 25*(1), 59-67.

Petronio, S. (2002). Boundaries of privacy: *Dialectics of disclosure*. Albany, NY: State University of New York Press.

Quick, D., Lehman, J., & Deniston, T. (2003). Opening doors for students with disabilities on community college campuses: What have we learned? What do we still need to know? *Community College Journal of Research and Practice, 27*, 815-827.

Rehabilitation Act of 1973. Section 504, 29 U.S.C. §794 (1977). Rehabilitation Act of 1973, Section 504, 28 C.F.R. §35

Rose, D. H., & Gravel, J. W. (2010). Universal design for learning. In E. Baker, P. Peterson, & B. McGaw (Eds.), *International encyclopedia of education* (3rd ed). Oxford, United Kingdom: Elsevier.

Rose, D. H. Meyer, A., & Hitchcock, C. (2005). *The universally designed classroom: Accessible curriculum and digital technologies*. Cambridge, MA: Harvard Education Press.

Scott, S., McGuire, J. M., & Embry, P. (2002). *Universal design for instruction fact sheet*. Storrs, CT: University of Connecticut, Center on Postsecondary Education and Disability.

Scott, S., McGuire, J., & Shaw, S. (2003). Universal Design for Instruction: A new paradigm for teaching adults in postsecondary education. *Remedial and Special Education, 24*(6), 369-379.

Section 504 of the rehabilitation act. (n.d.). Retrieved from www.section508.gov on June 8, 2005.

Swain, J., French, S., Barnes, C., & Thomas, C. (Eds.). (2004). *Disability barriers enabling environments* (2nd ed.). London, United Kingdom: Sage.

Todis, B. (1996). Tools for the task? Perspectives on assistive technology in educational settings. *Journal of Special Education Technology, 12*(2), 49-61.

Torkelson Lynch, R., & Gussel, L. (1996). Disclosure an self-advocacy regarding disability related needs: Strategies to maximize integrations in postsecondary education. *Journal of Counseling & Development, 74*, 352-357.

Unger, K. (1994). Access to educational programs and its effect on employability. *Psychosocial Rehabilitation Journal, 17*(3), 117-126.

Universal Design Summit 5 (2013). Proceedings of the national conference on universal design May 6-8. Retrieved from http://udsummit.net.

University of Kansas Institute for Adult Studies. (1998). *Accommodating adults with disabilities in adult education programs*. Lawrence, KS: University of Kansas for Research on Learning.

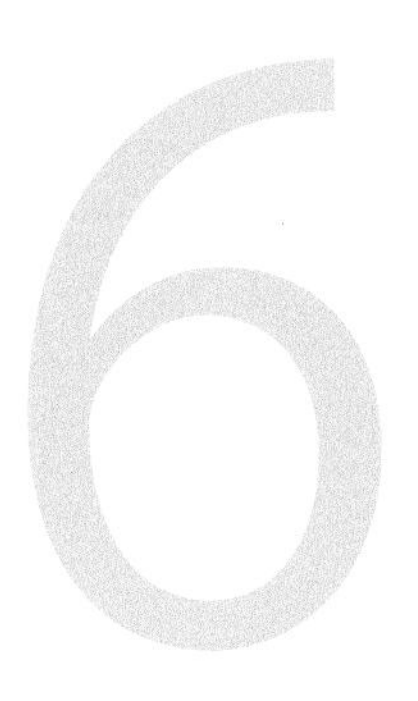

Work

Martha J. Sanders, PhD, MSOSH, OTR/L, CPE
Robert Wright, OTR/L

Chapter Objectives

By the end of this chapter, the student will be able to do the following:

- Define work as it pertains to the Occupational Therapy Practice Framework.
- Describe specific models/frames of reference as related to work.
- Comprehend safety issues as related to work.
- Delineate between the roles of the occupational therapist and the occupational therapy assistant as they pertain to the occupation of work.
- Identify psychological implications as related to decreased independence in work.
- Comprehend issues related to ergonomics, industrial rehabilitation, work hardening, and work conditioning.
- Describe the impact of contextual and environmental factors upon work.
- Identify specific work compensation/adaptation strategies.
- Identify general work remediation strategies.
- Identify work compensation/adaptation intervention strategies related to vision, cognition, and musculoskeletal systems.
- Identify general work maintenance strategies.

Definition of Work

Work is central to human existence as a means of providing sustenance, self-worth, and self-identity (Bing, 1989). Although the meaning attributed to work may vary according to the individual worker, occupational therapy has acknowledged the health-promoting purpose of work since its inception (Harvey-Krefting, 1985). The profession of occupational therapy has been instrumental in using work as an intervention to enable physical and psychiatric rehabilitation as well as an outcome for industrial rehabilitation following work-related injuries (Harvey-Krefting, 1985; Stein & Cutler, 1998). Thus, work is both a means for promoting health and an end for sustaining our

Meriano C, Latella D.
Occupational Therapy Interventions: Function and Occupations, Second Edition (pp 325-361).

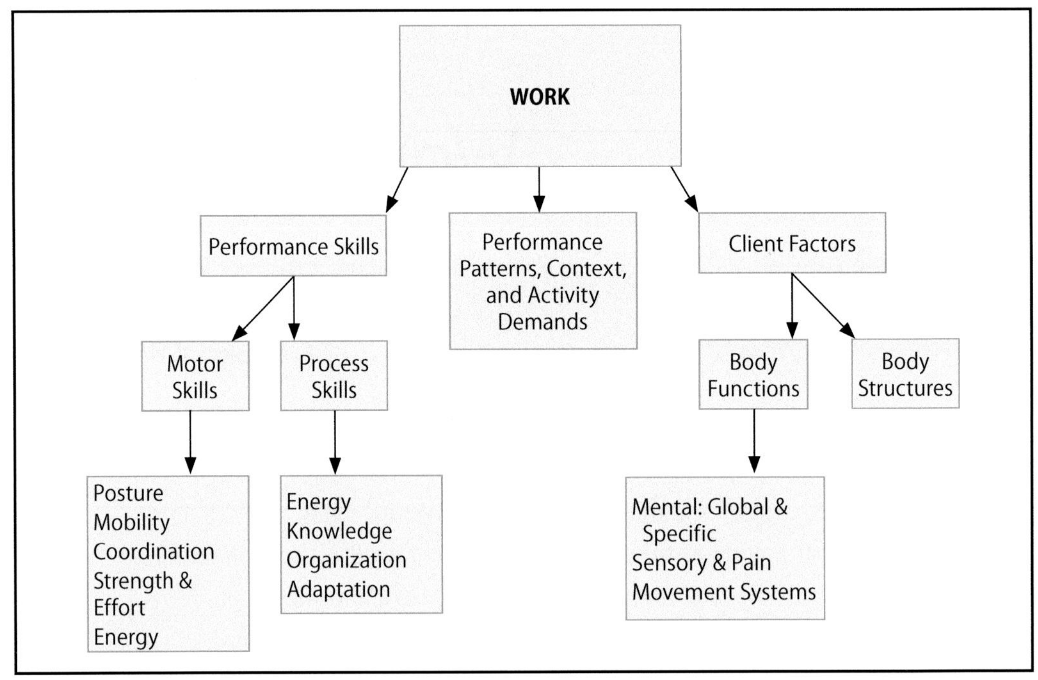

Figure 6-1. Components of work. (American Occupational Therapy Association. [2014]. Occupational therapy practice framework: Domain and process (3rd ed.). *American Journal of Occupational Therapy, 68*(Suppl. 1), S1-S48.)

existence. Work is an important performance area of occupation as identified in the Framework (American Occupational Therapy Association [AOTA], 2014) (Figure 6-1).

According to the Framework (AOTA, 2014), work is "labor or exertion; to make, construct, manufacture, form, fashion, or shape objects; to organize, plan, or evaluate services or processes of living or governing; committed occupations that are performed with or without financial reward" (Christiansen & Townsend, 2010, p. 423). Work therefore includes all activities required to perform the role of a worker or volunteer both inside and outside of the home. The specific content areas included in the work performance domain are employment interests and pursuits, employment seeking and acquisition, job performance, retirement preparation and adjustment, and volunteering, both exploring and participating (AOTA, 2014).

Employment interests and pursuits include identifying work interests based on an individual's skills, abilities, interests, and the opportunities available. The process of identifying employment interests actually begins with the imitative play of young children who simulate the actions of adult role models and heroes. Young children learn about the world of work through school and home responsibilities that provide both internal and external rewards for productivity, goal achievement, and leadership. Career choices become gradually crystallized throughout adolescence and young adulthood as individuals identify their strengths, specific skills, and the job opportunities available to them (Erikson, 1997).

Prevocational planning may utilize standardized and nonstandardized skills assessments, vocational interest tests, and career inventories to promote self-discovery. Vocational interest tests provide potential career options for individuals based on the similarity of their responses to those who have demonstrated success in a particular field (Trombly & Radomski, 2014).

Employment seeking and acquisition refers to the process of identifying employment opportunities, developing a resumé, completing a job application, preparing for the interview, completing the interview, and negotiating terms of employment (AOTA, 2014). This process is undertaken and practiced as adolescents seek various part-time or temporary jobs. These skills become further honed as individuals search for jobs in which their personal subsistence and future career are related to job performance. They may be repeated as older workers enter "bridge employment" or post-career part-time jobs.

Job performance, the focus of this chapter, includes developing work habits, learning and performing job tasks, and continually updating skills, as well as assimilating into the norms or culture of the work setting (AOTA, 2014). Part-time work in adolescence often serves as a means to learn about and establish such fundamental work habits as punctuality, attendance, learning a task, and relating to supervisors and peers (Atwood, 1992). Although adolescents readily become competent at basic job tasks, the interactional aspects of the job, such as coping with angry customers (e.g., in the food service industry) and communicating with supervisors, are not well-developed at this age without specific training (Atwood, 1992). This chapter will focus on work hardening and ergonomic modification, because these areas are typical practice areas for work programming. Retirement and volunteering aspects of work programming will be addressed in Chapter 7.

Components of Work According to the Framework

Effective intervention for work involves a thorough examination of client factors that impact the client's ability to meet the demands of the workplace. Client factors include body functions (such as specific and global mental functions, sensory functions, neuromuscular, muscle movement, and cardiovascular functions) and body structures that support these functions. Clients who have been injured on the job might have limitations in neuromuscular and muscle functions that make some aspect of the job difficult or unsafe to perform. For example, a client with low back pain may be unable to perform a manual material handling job that requires frequent lifting from the floor and decreased trunk motion, due to limited strength, flexibility, and pain. Another client with carpal tunnel syndrome may have difficulty performing fine motor assembly tasks due to a weak pincer grasp, deficits in finger coordination, or sensory discrimination deficits caused by changes in the sensory cortex over a long period of time (Prosser & Conolly, 2003).

Performance skills refer to the functional components of performing the job. Performance skills are composed of motor skills, process skills, and social interaction skills that enable successful job performance. Motor skills include one's posture during work and use of proper body mechanics while performing the task (AOTA, 2014). Motor skills also include the myriad of motions that workers assume while performing job tasks, such as reaching for an object, squatting to change a tire, walking to shelve items, or standing at a cash register. Coordination relates to manipulative activities integral to most assembly, computer, and fine motor tasks. Individuals use muscle power to move objects during the course of work when lifting, pushing, and pulling objects or loads. One's ability to pace oneself at work in order to complete the required amount of work becomes increasingly important with age.

Process skills, based on cognition and executive functions, enable individuals to correctly sequence, organize, prioritize, and modify job tasks for a successful outcome (AOTA, 2014). While such tasks become automatic for highly skilled or experienced workers, those who are returning to work, learning a new job, or learning a new technique may need retraining or practice to resume their previous levels of productivity. For example, a butcher who has returned to work following wrist tendonitis may decide to use an ergonomic knife to improve his or her wrist position while working. However, the individual may need to adapt his or her usual hand position and movement patterns to accommodate the change in handle position. Workers with psychiatric disabilities may also need assistance in organizational aspects of the job (Stein & Cutler, 1998).

Social interaction skills may be well-established in seasoned workers. However, as stated, younger workers (Atwood, 1992), workers with psychiatric disabilities (Stein & Cutler, 1998) and young adults with learning disabilities, attention deficit disorder, or an autism spectrum disorder (Stacey, 2001) may not have developed strong interactional or coping skills in responding to authority figures, taking feedback (particularly criticism), making "small talk," and following the formal and informal rules of the workplace. One aspect of coping with customer service work, emotion regulation, the ability to manage one's emotions in the workplace and perceive others' emotions (Goleman, 1998), is considered to be a key factor in the success of collaborative workplaces and effectively functioning work teams.

The activity demands in the workplace refer to the environmental, physical, and social demands of the workplace that would commonly be included in a job analysis (Ellexson, 2004). Occupational therapists who work with clients returning to a job from an injury or from an illness (e.g., stroke or heart disease) need to understand the job demands in order to develop goals that will enable clients to safely perform their jobs. The activity demands will include the objects or equipment workers use, the environmental conditions (such as the size of the workspace, the illumination levels, noise levels, temperature, and flooring, among others), the required actions, sequence, and productivity demands (AOTA, 2014). A task analysis will provide the required performance skills, body structures, and body functions for the job.

The social demands of a job may refer to the informal (unspoken) means of working together as a team, the type of dress code for "dress-down days," the attitudes toward injured workers on disability, or the informal rules common to a group or culture of workers. The social demands of the workplace are considered to be critical to an individual's success in a particular job (Sanders, 2004; Stein & Cutler, 1998).

Performance patterns refer to the habits, routines, and roles that support one's job (AOTA, 2014). Habits may include organizing oneself for the day by writing a to-do list (or using a related app), keeping folders orderly, or clearing one's desk before leaving for the day. Habits are considered to be integral to time management skills (Stein & Cutler, 1998) and become particularly important in prevocational skills development. Routines are broader sequences that include embedded habits. For example, as a routine for beginning a workday for a manufacturing supervisor may include checking e-mails in the morning while drinking a morning coffee, checking a production log, and donning personal protective equipment before going to the shop floor and making rounds to check on each operation. An end-of-shift procedure for a grocery clerk "cashing out" might include counting money, reconciling a register, and then locking up, or other established sequences performed on a regular basis.

The context refers to the overall conditions related to the job. The physical context, or the environment, refers to the lighting, air quality, noise level, temperature, and overall quality of space in which the worker is employed. The social context refers (broadly) to the level of support among workers and supervisors, role status of particular work positions, and the influence of union membership, among others. The social context may also include any changes to the organization such as downsizing or expanding, which change the overall climate of the workplace. Cultural aspects of the job may include the background of workers or the work group cultures formed by individuals who perform a particular job skill, trade, or occupation. The cultural backgrounds of the workers may impact their means of relating to authority, their educational level, and their career goals. The culture of a work group impacts their definition of quality of work, attitudes toward disability, ways of organizing their day, and the informal "ways of doing things" that are critical to mastery over one's job. The closely related personal context may refer to an individual's training or educational background for the job and age-related changes relative to performing the job.

Frames of Reference

Frames of reference that are commonly applied to work programming are the biomechanical frame of reference, person-environment-occupation-performance (PEOP; Law et al., 1996), and the rehabilitative/acquisitional frame of reference for those returning to work following and injury. The biomechanical frame of reference focuses on maximizing human movement in order to facilitate occupational performance (Green & Roberts, 1999; Trombly & Radomski, 2014). Impairments in body structures due to injury, disease, or pain may cause dysfunction in the movement system. According to the biomechanical frame of reference, human movement is enabled through adaptations or modifications that increase an individual's strength, endurance, and range of motion (ROM) (LeVeau, 1992). The fundamental concepts of kinetics (study of forces) and kinematics (the study of human movement) are applied to workplace interventions to maximize the workers' capacities. For example, work heights may be adjusted to enable proper positioning for lifting or hand use, and workloads may be decreased to minimize the forces necessary to accomplish the job. As discussed in Chapter 2, interventions under the biomechanical frame of reference commonly include exercises or techniques that gradually increase an individuals' strength and ROM such as pulleys, aquatics, use of weights or exercise equipment, or aerobic activities. In work hardening, job simulations are used to increase individuals' endurance or tolerance to job tasks (refer to section on Industrial Rehabilitation).

The biomechanical frame of reference is not a client-centered approach, and therefore needs to be used in conjunction with an approach that integrates individuals' needs and personal goals into the intervention plan. The rehabilitative approach, also called acquisitional, focuses on enabling an individual to function as independently as possible after an injury (Trombly & Radomski, 2014). Within this approach, environmental modifications and adaptive equipment are used to compensate for deficits that limit effective functioning. The rehabilitative approach supports the individual's need to work in order to support him- or herself. Interventions therefore focus on means by which to restore work-related skills and prevent further dysfunction through education, purposeful activity, and active problem solving. Finally PEOP (Law et al., 1996) clearly addresses the relationship and interface between the individual and the environment, which becomes a focus of ergonomics particularly for prevention and for return-to-work modifications needed for the job.

Role of the Occupational Therapy Assistant

The role of the occupational therapy assistant in the performance area of work parallels other intervention areas. Occupational therapy assistants may work alongside the occupational therapy to carry out work-hardening interventions, education, and ergonomic modifications, provided they have demonstrated competency in that skill. Occupational therapy assistants may also contribute to work evaluations by completing standardized aspects of a functional capacity evaluation (FCE) or a job analysis for which they have demonstrated competence. However, the occupational therapy is responsible for interpreting results of the FCE and job analysis and developing a plan with the client to meet his or her vocational goals.

Safety Issues

Worker Safety

Concerns for client safety are paramount in work programming. The Occupational Safety and Health Administration Act (OSHA) of 1970 was promulgated in order to provide a safe workplace for all workers. To that end, employers identify the safety regulations relevant to that work environment and develop safety procedures to which workers are expected to comply.

Safe practices for the workplace begin with using the proper technique to perform one's job. The proper technique refers to using motor and cognitive skills such as choosing the proper tools for the job, sequencing aspects of the job, positioning one's body correctly, using personal protective equipment, such as safety glasses and steel-toed shoes, and implementing the proper work methods. Personal protective equipment refers to garments that act as a barrier to protect the body from potential harm (Kjellen, 2000). The degree to which the environment is well-maintained and free from electrical (cords), mechanical (machines properly guarded or locked), air quality, and chemical hazards, among others, greatly impacts worker safety.

Organizational and individual worker variables also impact workplace safety. Individual behaviors may include worker knowledge, training, level of fatigue, and risk-taking behaviors. Over a period of time, workers may develop "shortcuts," or quicker ways of performing a task that circumvent safety practices and increase the risk of developing further injuries (Kjellen, 2000). Thus, therapists and supervisors need to be constantly vigilant about reinforcing safety rules. Workers must acknowledge the impact of physical or psychological deficits or chronic illness on the ability to safely perform a job. At the worksite, ergonomic modifications or treatment-related interventions such as splints must not interfere with job performance and job safety.

Therapist Safety

Although most therapists focus on the safety of their clients, therapists need to acknowledge their own safety when working at a job site or in the clinic. In the clinic, therapists need to acknowledge electrical safety when working with frying pans filled with water or multiple appliances plugged into one fuse or circuit (Bracciano, 2007). Ground-fault circuit interrupters should always be installed to prevent short-circuiting of faulty equipment.

Thermal electrical equipment may cause burns if precautions are not taken to protect oneself from heat guns, hot packs, or hot water from splinting pans or hydroculators. Similar to industrial workers, therapists should develop safe practices when using potentially hazardous equipment, such as using tongs (not fingers) to remove hot packs, turning off a heat gun when not in use, and positioning oneself correctly when using a razor blade knife (to prevent the knife from injuring the thigh on a follow-through swipe). Proper maintenance of equipment helps to prevent unnecessary mechanical malfunctions.

The importance of therapists using proper body mechanics for assisting clients in using job simulation equipment cannot be underestimated. Darragh, Huddleston, and King (2009) found that a sample of occupational therapists working in physical management were developing injuries while treating clients at a rate of 16.5 per 100 workers for 1 year, a rate as high for workers in heavy manufacturing. Further, therapists tend to underestimate their musculoskeletal risk while working with clients. Thus, the body mechanics principles recommended for clients (maintaining an upright posture, using the body in a symmetrical manner, and keeping the load close to the body) should be rigorously followed by therapists themselves. In particular, when performing therapies from the standing position (such as assisting with job simulation activities) the occupational therapist should avoid a half-leaning posture, with the trunk flexed over the client, as this places significant strain on the low back. In such a case, practitioners should move closer to the client (or object) to prevent awkward forward-bending postures. Therapists will need to learn the proper body mechanics for using a hand truck, assisting a client with transfers, and using tools correctly. Finally, therapists performing on-site ergonomic evaluations are expected to abide by the same personal protective equipment mandates as the workers.

Ergonomic Modifications

Introduction

Ergonomics addresses the interaction between the work and the worker so that jobs can be performed in the safest, most productive, and most comfortable manner possible (Bridger, 2009; Kroemer, 2008). While the broad field of ergonomics includes many specialty areas, such as designing health care equipment, industrial tools, computer systems, and controls and displays (e.g., pilot cockpits and car dashboards), most occupational therapists work in the area of musculoskeletal ergonomics (Jacobs, 2008). This area of ergonomics focuses on the prevention of work-related musculoskeletal disorders (MSDs) in business and industry. More recently, ergonomics has been applied to nonwork activities such as leisure, housework, and across the lifespan caring for children and older adults in various settings (Lueder & Rice, 2008; Sanders, 2004; Sanders & Morse, 2005).

The simplest definition of ergonomics, fitting the work to the worker, implies the client-centered nature of ergonomics and the focus on designing work tasks and equipment to be used without difficulty by the worker or "end user." In a proactive manner, ergonomic design is a health-promoting intervention that improves the efficiency, energy, and ease of use for all workers performing a certain job task (Bridger, 2009; Kroemer, 2008). Tasks that are ergonomically designed attempt to minimize, if not eliminate, hazardous exposures for workers performing that task. More often, however, ergonomic interventions are modifications or adaptations that are applied retroactively to work tasks or work processes that have contributed to a diagnosed MSD in individuals or groups of clients. In this regard, ergonomic interventions focus on modifying the work tasks, the work environments, and the organization of work in order to minimize risks that may contribute to musculoskeletal pain.

In ergonomics, the terms *adaptation* and *modification* are similar and therefore will be addressed together.

This chapter will focus on intervention strategies for the workplace involving ergonomic adaptations (such as the use of specialized ergonomic tools) and ergonomic compensations, referred to as *assists* (such as lifting tables to minimize heavy forces to the low back). Accurate worksite evaluations are necessary to determine the intervention required.

Goals and History

As stated, the goals of ergonomics are to decrease musculoskeletal discomfort and increase work productivity, efficiency, and comfort. Although these goals may seem distinct, in actuality, a worker who is more comfortable is also more productive. Comprehensive ergonomic intervention programs can increase worker productivity while decreasing health care costs, workers' compensation costs, and the risk for developing an MSD (Kroemer, 2008; Oxenburgh, 1997). In fact, the cost-benefit ratios of ergonomics for manufacturing sector companies are reportedly up to 15:1, meaning that for every $1 on ergonomic programming, a company saves $15 in direct savings, with savings sometimes realized within 1 year (also called *return on investment*) (Goggins, Spielholz, & Nothstein, 2008; Tompa, Dolinschi, de Olivera, Amick, & Irvin, 2010). Thus, ergonomic intervention benefits both the employee and the employer.

History of Ergonomics

The science of ergonomics dates back to as early as 1717, when Ramazzini, the father of occupational medicine, speculated on factors within the work environment that contributed to his patients' illnesses. Ramazzini described the "violent and irregular motions," "bent posture," and "tonic strain on the muscles" as factors that contributed to musculoskeletal pain in his patients (in Wright, 1940). In fact, he documented the same fundamental physical and psychological risk factors found to contribute to MSDs today.

As the Industrial Revolution took hold, Frederick Taylor and Frank and Lillian Gilbreth revolutionized the organization of work by applying scientific methods to modern factory management in order to make work more efficient. Taylor broke down entire jobs to a series of repetitive tasks performed by individual workers. While the job tasks became more efficient, workers were repetitively using the same body part to accomplish a task. The tasks became monotonous and distanced workers from the overall goal and feeling of accomplishment of completing the entire product. Not surprisingly, Workers' Compensation Boards were developed in the 1930s to address work-related injuries. Taylor promoted assembly-line pacing, motion and time measurements for each job, and paying workers according to production standards and incentives—typical factory, assembly-line models used today (Sanders & McCormick, 1993).

The era following World War II was a time of considerable growth in ergonomics as technology was applied to military procedures and equipment. An appreciation for the "human element" as the weak link in a mechanical operation was recognized. The Human Factors and Ergonomics Society was formed in 1957 and advanced the science of ergonomics among civilian companies producing pharmaceuticals, automobiles, and consumer products. In the 1980s and 1990s, burgeoning computer use became the focus of many ergonomic studies. However, the disasters at Three Mile Island nuclear plant in Pennsylvania and the Union Carbide pesticide plant in Bhopal, India, underscored the critical importance of human factors in worker safety today (Sanders & McCormick, 1993).

Legislation Affecting Ergonomics

Presently, no federal ergonomic standard exists, although an ergonomic standard has been in the making for over two decades. The recent history of ergonomic regulations began in the early 1980s when OSHA began to issue voluntary guidelines designed to assist industry with controlling the increasing number of MSDs in the workplace. In 1981, the National Institute of Occupational Safety and Health (NIOSH), the agency performing research on occupational safety and health, developed the Work Practices Guide for Manual Lifting, which provided industry with analytical procedures used to determine the amount of weight employees could safety lift in a given situation. In 1991, these lifting calculations were revised and widely distributed for use in industry (NIOSH, 1994a). In 1991, OSHA also introduced the Ergonomics Program Management Guidelines for Meatpacking Plants in response to skyrocketing rates of MSDs (OSHA, 1991). This manual outlined a comprehensive ergonomics program designed to prevent upper extremity (UE) injuries in the meatpacking industry. In 1997, the Elements of Ergonomics Programs was developed and distributed by NIOSH to enable managers to perform ergonomic workplace evaluations and devise ergonomic programming to decrease MSDs in all industries (NIOSH, 1997).

In 2001, a federal ergonomic standard was passed and subsequently rescinded in 2002 with a change of governmental offices. Although the standard survived only a few months, the act sensitized employers to the importance of ergonomic interventions in managing employees' injuries and provided a comprehensive written ergonomics program for industry to emulate. Proactive approaches are now aimed at combining ergonomics programming with workplace health promotion initiatives to promote Total Worker Health, a NIOSH initiative (Punnett, Cherniack, Henning, Morse, & Fagri, 2009).

At present, industries can be cited for obvious and willful ergonomics violations under the "general duty clause" of the OSH Act (5a)(1) of 1970. This clause states that every employer must "furnish to each of its employees employment and a place of employment which is free from recognized hazards which are causing or likely to cause death or serious physical harm." Therefore, companies who repeatedly ignore obvious ergonomic hazards can be cited and fined for not providing a safe workplace for its workers (OSHA, n.d.).

A Model of Ergonomics and the Development of Musculoskeletal Disorders

Although ergonomics has traditionally focused on the physical or biomechanical aspects of performing a job, such as the tools, the postures, and forces, the psychosocial aspects of work play strong roles in the development of MSDs (Warren, 2004). Further, injuries may still occur even when the most well-designed equipment is utilized (Bridger, 2009; Sanders, 2004).

Consider the following scenario:

Joe is a 37-year-old man who works as an instructional technologies programmer at a local college. Joe works 6 to 7 hours per day on the computer and plays video games at lunch. Joe has monthly deadlines necessitating that he work overtime toward the end of the month in order to meet these deadlines. Joe moved into a new work area that was equipped with an ergonomic keyboard, adjustable chair, adjustable keyboard tray, and ergonomic mouse. Joe's workstation was adjusted to his height of 5'6" and to his body dimensions. Joe was given stretches to perform every hour and a free pass to the gym at lunch. However, after 1 month of working in the new workstation, he began to complain of numbness, tingling, and paresthesias in his right hand, and elbow pain in his left arm. An occupational therapist observed him at his workstation and found he had moved his computer to the right corner of the desk (to give him more room), and he was sitting on the edge of his chair with one foot tucked under his body. He had brought his personal laptop computer to work and was working on two computers simultaneously. He therefore spent much of his day twisting his body and keying in a manner that placed pressure on his wrists. Further inquiries about his hobbies revealed that he played the drums 2 nights per week.

This case reveals that the design of the tools and equipment are not the sole components of an ergonomics plan. Joe was given the proper ingredients for an ergonomically correct workstation. However, he was not educated in proper use of the equipment and personalized his workstation in a manner that negated the intent of the original setup of the equipment. Nor did Joe understand the impact of all activities on the development of MSDs, including playing video games on his computer at lunch and playing the drums at home.

The National Research Council (1998), in its extensive review of the scientific research relevant to MSDs, outlined a broad conceptual framework to examine all the factors that contribute to MSDs in the workplace (Figure 6-2). MSD refers to injuries that develop gradually over time due to repeated stressors to a particular part of the body (NIOSH, 1997). MSDs include lateral epicondylitis, deQuervain's disease, rotator cuff tendonitis, and wrist tendonitis. MSDs may also include nerve entrapments such as carpal tunnel syndrome and Guyon's canal syndrome (NIOSH, 1997; Prosser & Conolly, 2003). The model suggests that the primary factors in the initial development of an MSD are physiologic loads that are placed on body tissues throughout the day. Body tissues respond to these loads by gradually strengthening and becoming conditioned, or by fatiguing and becoming injured, depending on the condition of the tissue, extent of the loads, and opportunity for rest. Signs and symptoms of MSDs, such as pain or inflammation, may progress to a disabling condition if intervention is not provided.

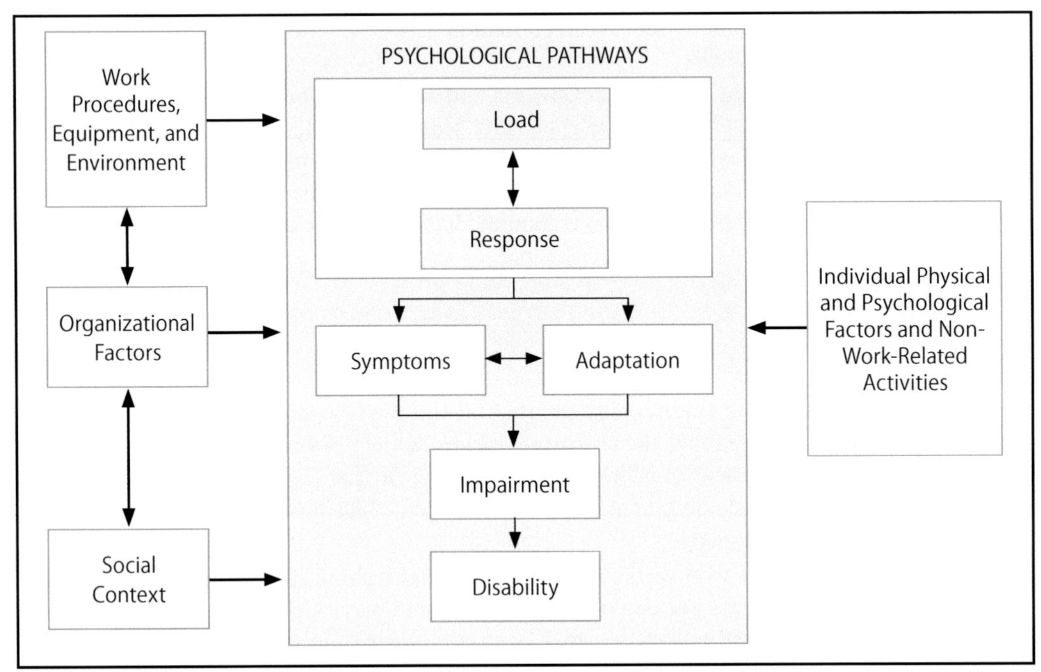

Figure 6-2. Factors that contribute to MSDs in the workplace. (Adapted from National Research Council. [1998]. Work-related musculoskeletal disorders: A review of the evidence. Washington, DC: National Academy Press.)

As the model indicates, factors in the home and work environments contribute to the development of MSDs in varying degrees. In the workplace, the type of tools used, height of the equipment, and forces used on the job all impact tissue loads. Organizational factors such as the pace of the job, the necessity for overtime, and workers' abilities to exert control over their job tasks also influence the development of MSDs. In fact, strong causal relationships exist between the development of cardiovascular disease and high job strains (high job demands with low control over the job) (Karasek & Theorell, 1990; Warren, 2004). Further, psychosocial issues such as the degree of social support, relationships with authority and peers, and organizational culture may influence the development or perception of illness. For example, piece-rate incentives may motivate employees to work faster and longer hours but contribute to overuse of muscle groups.

In the model, the individual worker's physical and psychological factors that influence the development of MSDs refer to client factors such as the worker's health history, level of physical conditioning, stress, attitude, personal work style, and the performance of hobbies or nonwork-related activities. Table 6-1 delineates the areas that are addressed by ergonomics.

In short, ergonomics addresses not only the activity demands of the workplace (work tasks and procedures), but also the psychosocial components of the job including work organization and personal or individual characteristics such as size, work style, home and work stressors, hobbies, and other responsibilities. Individuals have a higher risk for developing an MSD when both biomechanical and psychosocial factors are present in a job or non-work situation (NIOSH, 1997).

Occupational therapists are in a unique position to address all these factors because they are trained to analyze tasks, systems, and individual characteristics as related to overall health. The following section will discuss biomechanical factors, as they tend to be the initial focus of risk factor reduction.

Table 6-1 Areas Addressed by Ergonomics
Work Tasks (Physical)
• Work procedures • Work tasks • Tools • Work environment
Workplace Organization (Psychosocial)
• Job content • Organizational factors • Worker support • Work culture
Worker Contributions (Individual)
• Personal stress level • Homework responsibilities • Personal size • Worker style • Hobbies

Biomechanical Risk Factors

The biomechanical risks inherent in work tasks were the initial focus of research in the industrial arena. The primary biomechanical risk factors are considered to be repetition, force, awkward postures, static postures, contact stresses, and vibration. Modifying factors of cold or hot temperatures, acceleration of forces, and duration of the task interact with the primary risk factors.

- Repetition: Repetition refers to performing the same motions over and over within a given time period. Jobs are typically classified according to the percentage of similar motions performed within a certain cycle time. Jobs are characterized as low repetitive if similar movements are repeated less than 50% of the time. Jobs are considered to be highly repetitive if similar movements are performed more than 50% of the time (Silverstein, Fine, & Armstrong, 1987).
- Force: Force is commonly expressed as the amount of effort required by a worker to overcome external loads by pushing, pulling, grasping, or handling objects. In reality, two types of force exist: external forces are the loads exerted on the body during work-related activities; internal forces are the amount of muscle tension developed to overcome external loads. In industry, external forces are usually the reference point. A high-force job is considered to be one in which workers use more than 10% to 15% of their maximal strength during a job task or a grip force, averaging more than 4 kg on a sustained basis (Kroemer, 2008; Silverstein et al., 1987).
- Awkward postures: Awkward postures are those that deviate from a neutral posture. A neutral posture is one in which muscle forces are approximately balanced throughout the body so the head is upright, shoulders at one's side, elbows flexed to 90 degrees, forearms in mid-position of supination and pronation, back straight, and knees slightly flexed. The ears, neck, shoulders, hips, knees, and ankles should be approximately aligned from a lateral view (Leveau, 1992). Awkward postures are associated with the gradual development of MSDs due to an

imbalance of musculature and cumulative strain. The postures include neck flexion, shoulder protraction, shoulder flexion and abduction greater than 30 degrees, elbow flexion greater than 100 degrees or less than 60, trunk flexion, and wrist flexion, extension, and deviation greater than 30 degrees (NIOSH, 1997). The greater the deviation, the greater the risk to the body. Therapists should understand that muscles and tendons must generate increased internal forces to accomplish a task when working in an awkward position versus when working in a neutral posture (Leveau, 1992).

- Static postures: Static postures are those maintained in the same position for greater than 20 minutes. Static postures stabilize the body proximally, resist the force of gravity, and allow for distal mobility. Static positions create sustained muscle contractions that limit blood flow to contracted muscles. Thus, fatigue rapidly develops in statically contracted muscles even at low workloads (Bridger, 2009). Static postures commonly occur when individuals perform repetitive and tedious work with hands while stabilizing the body proximally, such as in computer work or assembly line and machining operations.
- Contact stresses: Contact stress is pressure placed on the skin and underlying soft-tissue structures. Contact stresses may contribute to tendon, nerve, and other soft-tissue injuries over a period of time. Compression can occur from the edges of desks, work surfaces, tool edges, tool handles, or other workstation components (Kroemer, 2008).
- Vibration: Prolonged exposure to vibration from vibrating hand tools or surfaces may contributes to hand-arm vibration syndrome (HAVS) or vibration white finger (VWF), in an workers who use vibrating tools with high-frequency vibration beyond the recommended time period for the job (NIOSH, 1989).

Ergonomic Evaluations

Ergonomic evaluations identify the risk factors involved in performing the job tasks along with the organizational and individual factors impacting job performance. Ergonomic evaluations should be completed on the individual worker performing the job because each individual performs a job in a slightly different manner. Ideally, the evaluation should prioritize which risks pose the greatest risk to an individual, then interventions should be planned accordingly.

Ergonomic evaluations for work task–related (also called biomechanical) risks may take the form of observations, direct measurement, or standardized tests in addition to self-reported surveys and simple checklists. Surveys and checklists provide a quick means of identifying which jobs may be hazardous and should be analyzed further. Direct observation and measurement can provide more specific information that may be necessary (NIOSH, 1997; Sanders, 2004). OSHA and NIOSH provide multiple resources for public use including ergonomic checklists and the NIOSH lifting equation. The NIOSH lifting equation is widely used in manual material-handling jobs when workers are lifting, handling, and carrying equipment or product on a regular basis (NIOSH, 1994).

A job analysis must be performed prior to analyzing risk factors. A job analysis, similar to an activity analysis, breaks down the job into the specific components. The job analysis identifies the steps to the tasks, the physical and cognitive demands, the posture and motions involved, equipment or product used (size and weight), and durations involved in lifting, carrying, and manipulating objects (for a complete discussion see Ellexson, 2004).

Ergonomic Interventions

Anthropometric Principles

Anthropometrics is the study of human body dimensions, such as height, limb length, foot size, hand size, and even head circumference. Anthropometrics also includes physical capacities such as the ability to lift, carry, and grasp objects (Pheasant, 2001). When designing a workspace for an individual or a group, knowledge of anthropometrics is a starting point for ergonomic interventions. Clients' sizes and typical capacities need to be identified in order to design equipment or tasks that "fit" the worker.

Ideally, each type of equipment would be designed to fit the size of each worker. Realistically, however, managers in industry purchase equipment and plan workstations to accommodate most workers, including the largest man (95th percentile) and the smallest woman (5th percentile) in order to keep costs reasonable. Anthropometric charts provide reference data on the sizes of typical worker populations. However, this information may not capture all sizes of today's increasingly diverse workforce of women, older adults, workers with disabilities, obese workers, and workers from different backgrounds. Thus, therapists must identify specific workforce characteristics and take direct measurements when feasible.

The process of planning a work area for workers (or users) incorporates knowledge of anthropometric data and worker requirements. For example, if a factory decides to buy chairs for all shop workers including lab technicians, assembly persons, and clerical workers, the procurement specialist must identify who will be using the chairs and the distinct needs or criteria for each work group. The lab technicians may need a chair with height adjustment that will accommodate a high lab bench; the assembly workers may need a sit/stand chair to allow alternate positions; and the clerical workers need lumbar and thoracic support for comfort in a seated position all day. All workers' chairs need to accommodate their particular body sizes and functional demands.

The following four main categories of anthropometric criteria are used in designing ergonomic workstations:

- Clearance refers to planning enough space for headroom, legroom, and elbow room.
- Reach refers to locating controls, materials, and equipment within close proximity to a worker.
- Posture refers to organizing the job so that a worker can assume a neutral posture relative to the work surface and controls.
- Strength refers to the muscle strength and grip strength related to lifting or carrying weighted loads.

In order to accommodate the largest range of users, clearances should be designed for the largest user (needing the most space), whereas reaches should be designed for the smallest user (user with the shortest reach) (Pheasant, 2001).

Categories of Interventions

Ergonomic interventions modify, adapt, and in some cases compensate for hazardous job tasks that present excessive physical stresses to the body. Ergonomic interventions, called *controls* by OSHA, are categorized in terms of whether the intervention changes the design of the job (engineering controls), changes the way the job is performed (administrative controls), and/or offers a means to protect a worker while performing the job (work practice controls). Although design changes are considered to be the most effective, recommendations from all categories of interventions are offered in order to thoroughly manage the problem. Each of these will be discussed below.

Engineering Controls

The ideal ergonomic solutions are those that will improve the design of the workstation or job task for all those performing the job. Engineering controls are recommendations for the design of the equipment, workstation layout, work processes, transport of materials, design of the tools, and mechanical assists that will minimize inherent risks in the job. Engineering controls are considered to be the preferred way to solve or mitigate problems (NIOSH, 1997). The OSHA website offers design control recommendations for numerous occupational groups including nurses' aides, electricians, carpenters, and computer workers, among others.

Standing Workstations

The design of both sitting and standing workstations is based on anthropometry and principles of body mechanics during dynamic tasks. Optimal heights of standing workstations depend not only on the height of the individual performing the task but also on the type of work performed. Kroemer (2008) suggests that workers who perform precision work while standing should work at surfaces whose heights are 2 to 4 inches above the elbow, with the elbow flexed to about 90 degrees. This height allows for proximal stability while performing detailed work. For light assembly, workstation surfaces are typically 2 to 4 inches below elbow height; heavy work surfaces are 4 to 5 inches below the elbow to allow for additional force or effort from the shoulders and trunk to assist in the work.

Other intervention considerations for standing workstations are the flooring and prolonged standing position. Workstations should provide supportive or cushioned flooring in order to minimize stress to the low back and prevent leg and foot fatigue. Anti-fatigue mats can cover hard flooring at individual workstations where necessary. Rails or stools elevate one foot, allowing workers to alleviate strain from the lower back. Sit-stand chairs allow workers the option to change postures or lean against the chair while standing (Kroemer, 2008).

When standing stations are used for lifting and packaging, mechanical assists can compensate for a worker's muscle strength and thus minimize worker fatigue and injury. Conveyor systems and carts or containers with wheels can decrease the need for carrying items. Mechanical assists such as pallet jacks, cranes, and other mechanical hoists can lift a product to an optimal position to be handled or bring products to desired destination.

Sitting Workstations

Workers in seated workstations strive for a neutral sitting posture with options for variability and movement. The neck should be upright, shoulders at one's side, hips flexed greater than 90 degrees (90 to 100 degrees), elbows flexed close to 90 degrees, wrists in neutral without deviation, lumbar curve supported, and feet flat on floor (see Figure 6-4).

The comfort of sitting workstations is highly dependent upon the design, fit, and adjustability of a chair. Many variations in chair designs exist; however, all ergonomic chairs should have the following adjustable features:

- Adjustable chair height: Individuals who share workstations will need to adjust their chairs at the start of a shift. Workers may also change chair heights during the day according to the work surface height and task. Generally, the chair height should be adjusted so that the elbows are level with the work surface or slightly higher.
- Seat angle: An individual should be fully seated on the chair with the hips 90 to 100 degrees of hip flexion. This position will minimize pressure on the discs of the spine yet still allow for use of the hands. Individuals should be able to lean back in their chairs periodically to alleviate pressures on the low back.

- Seat pan: The seat pan should be wide enough and deep enough to support the thighs without touching the posterior aspect of the knees. The edges of the seat pan should be rounded with padding to distribute the pressure of the ischial tuberosities.
- Back rest: The backrest should support both the lumbar curve and thoracic region. This support is especially important for office workers who spend the majority of time at their desks.
- Footrests: Feet need to be resting on the floor or on footrests in order to relieve pressure on the thigh and low back. Inexpensive footrests can be purchased or made from wooden platforms.
- Armrests: Armrests may support the arms when they are held in the same position for much of the task. However, armrests may interfere with getting close to the desk and keyboard for office workers. While individual situations dictate, in general office workers tend not to use armrests while keying because this forces the trunk into a forward flexed position. Armrests may be used while talking on the phone or during pause breaks.
- Base: The chair base should have five points or casters for the greatest stability.

Computer Workstations

The criteria for ergonomic computer workstations encompass those discussed for sitting workstations, in addition to further guidelines for interfaces with the keyboard and monitor. The worker should be directly facing the monitor and viewing the screen with a downward gaze of about 15 degrees. The monitor should be positioned about an arm's length away from the worker. Those with bifocals and progressive lenses may find sitting in a more reclined posture (110 degrees of hip flexion) with the monitor tilted slightly backwards will enable them to view the monitor without straining their necks (Hedge, 2004).

Workers should use their wrists in a neutral (straight) position for keying in order to avoid compression to the median nerve. Keyboards are commonly positioned in a "negative tilt" in order to accommodate this position, which means that the keyboard is slightly tilted away from the user. Document holders should be used when inputting data or text from a paper. Use of a document holder minimizes eye and neck movements required to shift between the documents and the computer screen. The document holder should be placed as close to the monitor as comfortably possible. The mouse should be positioned close to the keyboard, within easy reach of the user (for further information on computer workstation ergonomics, refer to Hedge, 2004; Sanders, 2004).

Tool Design

Ergonomic tools must be designed to fit the anatomical structures of the hand while fulfilling the functions of the task. Many traditional tools place pressure on the soft-tissue structures of the hand, which may contribute to injury over a period of time. Traditional pliers, for example, are designed with a short handle that places pressure on the thenar eminence near the thenar branch of the median nerve. Over a period of time, such pressure may injure the median nerve. Many other tools, such as traditional scissors and can openers, place pressure on neurovascular structures lateral to each finger. Tools such as hammers, saws, wrenches, and screwdrivers cause the worker to assume an ulnarly deviated position of the wrist during use. This position places further stresses on the forearm musculature because a worker must generate more force to accomplish the job using this deviated position (Bridger, 2009; Kroemer, 2008)

Ergonomic tools are now being designed to distribute pressure across a larger area of the hand and improve the position of the hand and wrist. Ergonomic pliers, for example, extend the handle through the palm and provide coated rubber padding to the handles. Saws, knives, and other tools are being designed with a "pistol grip," which includes a vertical handle design that places the wrist in neutral relative to the working area of the tool (Figure 6-3). Table 6-2 provides a list of design principles that should be incorporated into ergonomic tools.

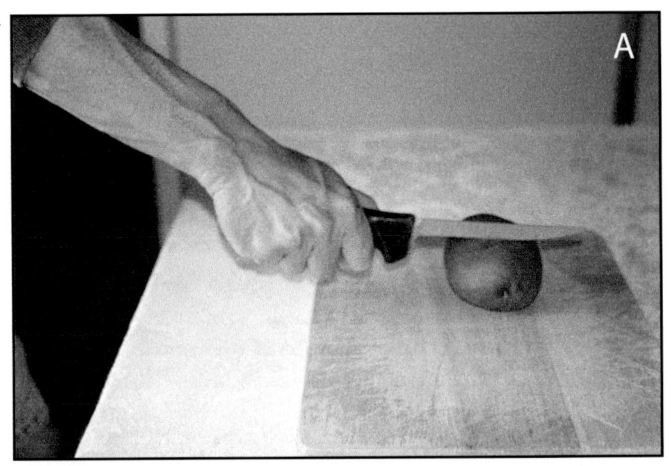

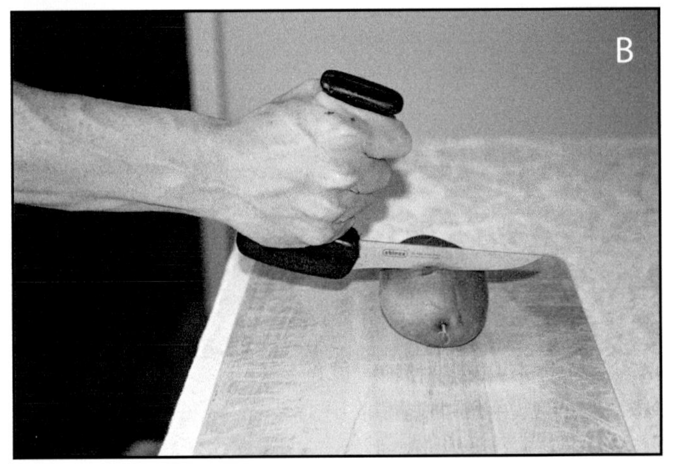

Figure 6-3. (A) Standard knife. (B) Pistol-grip knife.

TABLE 6-2

DESIGN PRINCIPLES THAT SHOULD BE INCORPORATED INTO ERGONOMIC TOOLS

- Handles with round edges and rubber coating
- Tool handles that extend through palm
- Loop handle designs with spring openings
- Pistol grip for vertical surface
- Inline grip for horizontal surface
- Balanced tools to avoid excess torque during use
- A trigger strip rather than a trigger button
- Tools designed for either hand (right or left)

Principles to Reduce Force

The quip "Power with motors rather than muscles" holds true for ergonomic design. Efforts to reduce the force in a task focus on decreasing the resistance a worker must overcome in order to

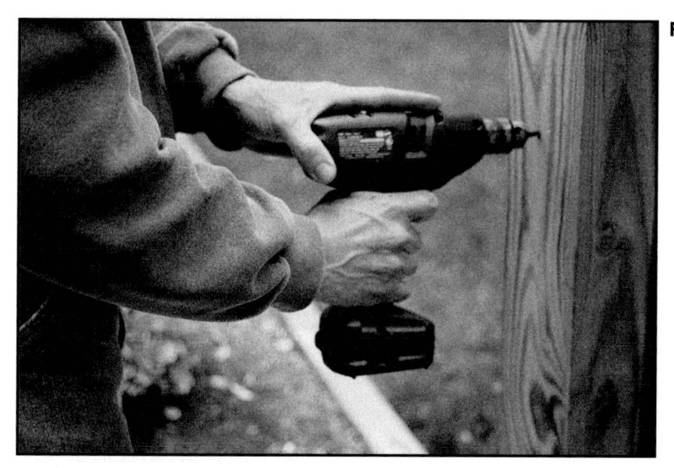

Figure 6-4. Power drill with pistol grip.

TABLE 6-3
COMMON MEANS TO REDUCE FORCE

- Use mechanical assists such as conveyor systems, pallet jacks, and overhead cranes to transport items.
- Use handles or hand slots to improve ability to carry containers or packages.
- Use a counterbalance sling support to hold a tool in place while using the tool.
- Keep the center of gravity of tools closest to worker.
- Break down a heavy load into smaller loads if possible (although this practice may increase the repetitions).
- Reduce handle slipperiness by increasing the coefficient of friction on the handle.
- Clean and maintain controls in order to minimize resistance during operation.

complete a task. This may involve decreasing the weight of loads, decreasing the resistance to operate a machine, or decreasing the weight of a tool during use. While decreasing loads may requires more repetitions (or trips if a large load is broken into smaller loads), this is still preferable to lifting, pushing, or carrying loads larger than one can safely assume. Figure 6-4 shows a power drill with a pistol grip. Table 6-3 identifies common means to reduce force.

Principles to Reduce Repetition

Repetition is difficult to minimize without the use of automation. However, efforts can be made to decrease repetitive exposures to each individual by enlarging the job tasks so an individual is not performing a repetitive cycle or job all day or enlisting another worker to assist. Some examples of means to reduce repetition in a job are provided in Table 6-4.

Principles to Reduce Awkward Postures

Work in awkward positions places excess stress on musculature and may entrap muscles and tendons against bony structures or soft-tissue structures. Awkward postures are most apparent when workers perform tasks requiring forward bending and twisting of the back, using the hands above the shoulders, lifting with a load away from the body, or deviating the wrist while using a tool. The adage "Bend the handle instead of the wrist" implies that good equipment and workstation design can minimize poor body positions (Figure 6-5). Many jobs can be modified so the

TABLE 6-4
COMMON MEANS TO REDUCE REPETITION

- Enlarge job tasks to include more variety of movements and components.
- Mechanize using power tools.
- Automate the job.
- Enlist other workers to assist in the job.

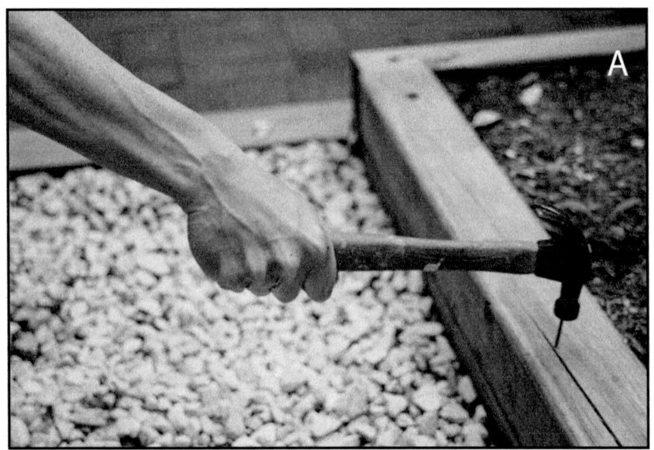

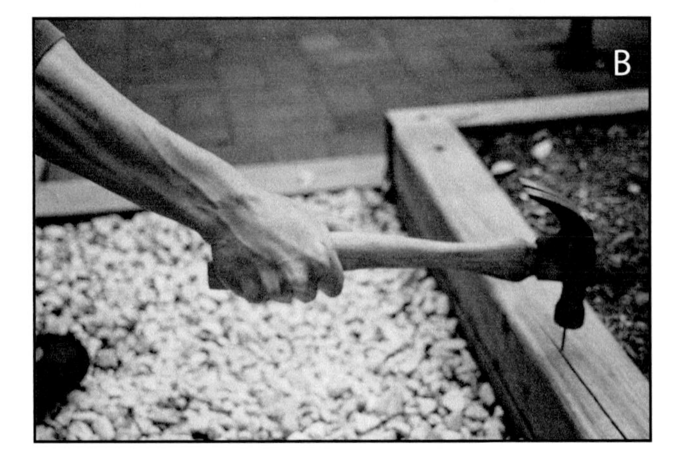

Figure 6-5. (A) Poor and (B) good hammer design.

product or process is positioned at elbow or waist height. Typical recommendations are provided in Table 6-5.

ADMINISTRATIVE CONTROLS

Situations exist in which the work equipment or work environment cannot be changed, although hazards (or risks) still exist. In such cases, administrative controls may become the primary source of interventions. Administrative controls are management approaches to organizing the job so that worker risks are reduced. These controls may include providing proper training for the workers (in safe procedures), making sure the equipment and work area is maintained properly

Table 6-5 Typical Workplace Recommendations
• Use fixtures to tilt parts such as vice grips. • Adjust the work height to avoid forward bending at the waist. • Use turntables to hold the work. • Rotate the part so that the wrist is straight. • Position work close to elbow height.

(such as knives sharpened), or rotating workers among tasks to minimize exposure to one particularly difficult job (NIOSH, 1997).

Administrative controls should be used in conjunction with engineering and work practice controls in order to effectively manage a safe work environment. While administrative controls address how the job is organized and workers trained, the overall culture of the workplace also impacts the degree to which supervisors, managers, and workers will support safety and ergonomic interventions. A culture of workplace safety will prioritize safe worker practices over extremely high work productivity standards, recognizing that healthy workers are key to a viable business (Melnik, 2004). Further, jobs that are designed to use a variety of skills, provide new learning, and offer the worker control over the job are considered to be healthier and equated with fewer chronic conditions (Karasek & Theorell, 1990). The following recommendations help to minimize hazardous workplace exposures and situations for individual workers.

- Train workers properly for the job.
- Allow the worker to control the pace of the job.
- Enlarge the job to include a variety of workers' skills.
- Rotate workers through hazardous jobs if workers' skills are comparable.
- Maintain the equipment regularly.
- Schedule breaks to allow for rest and recovery.
- Provide a new employee conditioning period.
- Educate workers on risk factors and symptoms of overuse.
- Monitor workers' symptoms regularly.
- Offer modified duty programs for injured workers.

Work Practice Controls

Work practice controls are those measures a worker can take to protect him- or herself on the job. Such controls include not only using personal protective equipment, but also utilizing the correct body mechanics, sitting posture, and proper technique that was provided through training, and stretching regularly. Work practice controls are important in industries that have fewer options for changing the task design.

Work practice controls focus on means by which individual workers can take responsibility for protecting themselves. Whereas a company can provide optimum equipment and tools, breaks, and job variety, the individual worker must be committed to using and adjusting the equipment properly and following body mechanics programs. Most workers have good intentions of working injury-free and following company guidelines when first beginning a job. However, over time, some workers tend to take shortcuts or rearrange a workstation in order to hasten job completion.

These changes often increase the risk of injury. Workers benefit from ongoing reminders, training sessions, or "tool-box talks" to emphasize the importance of adherence to safe practices (Melnik, 2004).

Principles to Reduce Static Postures: Stretching

As mentioned, static postures can contribute to muscle fatigue and musculoskeletal pain over a period of time. Stretching exercises have been found to decrease back and neck musculoskeletal pain in computer workers when performed regularly throughout the day, using either software reminders or hard-copy programs (Kietrysa, Galperb, & Vernoc, 2007; Marangoni, 2010). Recommendations for stretching frequency vary; however, a general goal is to move every 20 minutes (change body positions) and stretch every hour for at least 2 to 3 minutes.

The following work practice controls are important for workers to follow:

- Use personal protective equipment: gloves, safety glasses, helmets, knee pads.
- Follow correct body mechanics.
- Stretch throughout the day.
- Use proper work technique.
- Adjust workstations as needed.

Other Interventions

Occupational therapists are well aware of individual worker differences that can impact a job. For example, those who work with greater speed and intensity at work tend to be at higher risk for MSDs (Feurerstein,1996). Since MSDs result from the accumulation of strains throughout the day and over time, a worker's hobbies, home responsibilities, and level of stress may contribute to the development of MSDs (Sanders, 2004). Thus, occupational therapy practitioners should examine the impact of all activities in a typical day on a person's health relative to the workplace.

The occupational therapist's understanding of a worker's injury and lifestyle can also contribute greatly to success in return-to-work programs (please see the next section). Occupational therapists may educate and train workers in using the least amount of force to accomplish a job (such as computing for video display terminal workers, scaling for dental hygienists, or over-tightening screws for electricians). Occupational therapists can help workers identify sources of stress and offer stress reduction programs to enhance work and home coping. Finally, occupational therapists can also encourage a healthy lifestyle including good physical and mental health in an overall workplace wellness approach.

A Comprehensive Ergonomics Program

The overturned ergonomics standard provided recommendations about comprehensive management of MSDs through ergonomic intervention. An ergonomics program should include identification of worker hazards or risk factors, means to control the risks, and training on proper work procedures, use of body mechanics, and safety precautions. Additionally, early reporting of MSD symptoms, medical intervention, and a return-to-work program are effective means of limiting the severity of injury and keeping the worker engaged in the worker role even during rehabilitation. These program components are presented in Figure 6-6 surrounding an ergonomics committee consisting of management and hourly personnel that provides input to all facets of the program.

Melnik (2004) provides strategies for keeping an ongoing ergonomics program viable, active, and visible to all employees. Such strategies include management commitment and employee involvement in program planning and execution. Occupational therapists need to understand the

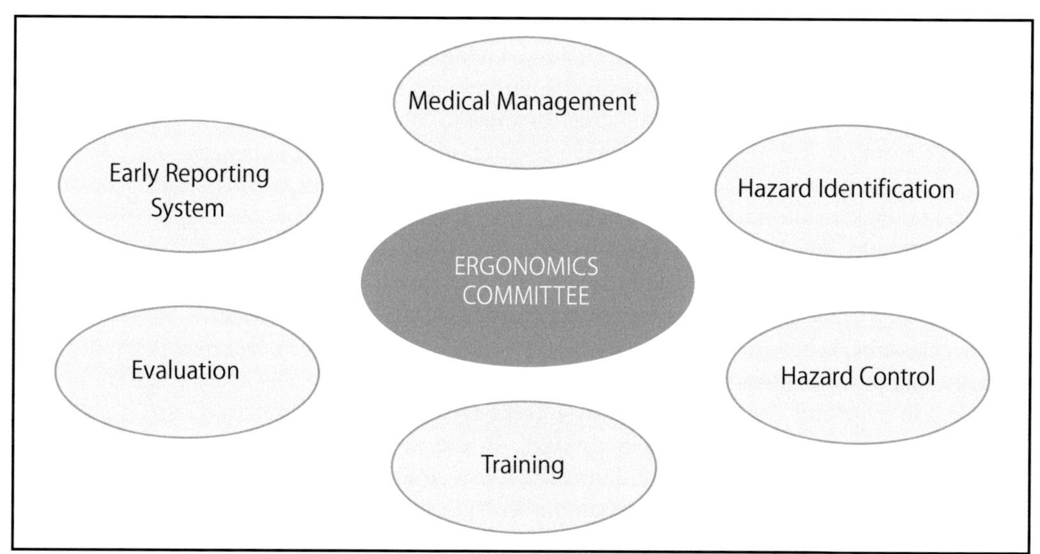

Figure 6-6. Ergonomics committee. (Adapted from Warren, N. [2004]. The expanded definition of ergonomics. In M. Sanders (Ed.), *Ergonomics and the management of musculoskeletal disorders*. St. Louis: Butterworth-Heinemann.)

culture of the company and develop ergonomic programs that are flexible and creative in order to maintain ongoing support of its employees.

Ergonomic Trends for Special Populations

Older Workers

The participation of older adults in the workforce (aged 55 and older) has steadily increased from 55% in 1982 to almost 65% by 2012, so that almost 25% of the workforce will be older workers. The labor force participation rate of older adults is expected to continue its steady pace until at least 2018, with women and workers over aged 75 showing the greatest increases (Toossi, 2013). While the rates of labor participation are increasing, many employers have not recognized the physical or social needs of older workers, their unique motives for working, and the experience that they can offer to a younger workforce. In fact, a study of over 2,000 retirees conducted by the American Association of Retired Persons (AARP) (2003) found that the major reasons retirees work or seek employment are to remain productive (73%), stay mentally (68%) and physically (61%) active, earn money (51%), do something enjoyable (49%), be around people (47%), help people (44%), and learn new things (20%). Additionally, at least 70% of the retirees seek a work environment where they can engage in new work experiences and interact with other people. Hence, older adults are motivated to work by social and health reasons rather than income alone.

This section will outline some changes associated with aging that may impact the workplace. It will offer interventions that can modify and compensate for physical losses associated with aging.

Impact of Aging on Work Capacities

Age-related losses in physical and functional capacities vary greatly among older adults. The extent to which changes in capacities affect work performance depends to a great extent on the work being performed. In general, older adults meet job demands despite age-related changes in sensory, cognitive, and neuromuscular status. Challenges may further exist when chronic conditions are superimposed on age-related changes.

Visual changes may include decreased near vision, difficulty focusing, blurred vision, problems with color discrimination, difficulty recognizing moving objects, and difficulty seeing at low levels of illumination. These changes impact work environments that have glare due to direct lighting or shiny surfaces, low levels of illumination, or work tasks that require careful scanning, precision, discriminating features of a task or even reading work schematics or instructions. Most older adults will need glasses or visual correction for near vision. Visual impairments such as cataracts and macular degeneration make such changes more pronounced.

Hearing ability may become diminished for higher frequencies and for speech recognition. In work situations with high background noise and high demands for rapid communication, deficits in hearing may be more pronounced and impact work performance (Wegman & McGee, 2004).

Musculoskeletal changes occur in muscle and tendon tensile strength, ligament flexibility, joint mobility, and posture. Muscle strength in older adults noticeably declines around age 60 due to a decreased number and size of skeletal muscle fibers. However, older adults who remain physically active show only moderate declines in strength. In the workplace, changes in muscle strength impact the amount of loads that should be safely lifted for older workers, since older workers will be using a higher percentage of their maximum strength to lift loads. They will require more time to recover from lifting and may walk at a slower speed and have decreased endurance for large-muscle, aerobic tasks (Wegman & McGee, 2004).

Although past research has documented the gradual decline of cognitive abilities with increasing age, current research is finding that cognition for older adults is not a single construct that maintains or declines as a whole. Research studies suggest that older adults are able to solve simple everyday problems and arithmetic problems with the same accuracy as younger adults. However, they tend to be slower at solving more complex tasks than younger adults. Older adults seem to have difficulty holding many items in working memory and retaining knowledge of word processing commands. They benefit from being challenged in a cognitive task and improve performance over time in order to match job demands. Most researchers suggest, however, that these deficits seem to be at the high range of intellectual capabilities and may not impact everyday work-related tasks (Chueng & Strough, 2004; Schooler, Mulatu, & Oates, 1999).

Ergonomic Interventions for Older Workers

With these physical changes in mind, the following interventions focus on specific adaptations for older adults, acknowledging that these design changes universally increase the ease of work performance for all workers.

Engineering Controls

Older workers should make use of mechanical assists to assist with lifting and seek to minimize lifting manual loads when possible. Work environments should be well-lit, following the higher illumination ranges suggested for older workers in various tasks (approximately 25% to 30% higher than for younger workers) (Kroemer, 2008). Ergonomic tools should be considered in order to reduce the hand forces needed and promote an improved hand position. Other ergonomic aids such as ergonomic box cutters, glare filters, and an ergonomic mouse should be individually adapted to the worker.

Workers with visual changes should have many low-vision aids available that are relevant to the workplace including magnification, clocks, watches, measuring devices, task lighting, signage, and large-font numbers or typeface. Employers should design offices with appropriate contrast in colors, hand-rail support, and nonslip flooring to enhance the safety and work performance of workers and minimize the chances of falling (Sanders et al., 2014; Wegman & McGee, 2004).

Because most older workers will be using the computer for some aspect of work, software design should be older-worker–friendly in order to minimize eye fatigue and improve the speed and retention of computer skills. Fisk, Rogers, Charness, Czaja, and Sharit (2009) recommend a software screen setup that enlarges critical information and minimizes distractions. Software should place minimal demands on working memory by keeping directions simple and visually available, providing drop-down menus, minimizing switching from one screen to another, and limiting visual searches.

Administrative Controls

The AARP (2003) specifically addressed the preferred work environment for an older worker. An elder-friendly work culture is one in which the experiences and opinions of older adult workers are respected and valued. Such workplaces should provide flexible or part-time scheduling so older adults can take off time to care for relatives as needed or go to doctors' appointments.

Fisk et al. (2009) suggest that training for older adults should be thorough yet self-paced, with ample time to learn and practice tasks prior to performing them on the job. Training programs should build on previous experiences of older workers to enable them to make cognitive associations for new job tasks. Cuing, ongoing visual instructions, and developing new work habits may assist in compensating for any cognitive deficits in speed or working memory. The process of progressing an older worker from simple to complex tasks in a training program may facilitate the older worker's adaptation to new work environments. Periodic updating, retraining, and learning new skills will benefit both the older worker and the company.

The job should be designed so that older workers work alongside other colleagues in teams to experience social support. Jobs should be designed so that older workers use a variety of skills and update skills in order to challenge themselves and feel personal control over the job. Ideally, older workers can mentor younger workers to pass along job-specific knowledge and enjoy the opportunity for intergenerational contact (Sanders & McCready, 2010). As for any worker, the job should allow for creativity and personal growth.

In order to minimize fatigue, companies should allow workers to pace job tasks throughout the day, alternate sitting and standing, and take pause breaks to conserve energy (Leighten et al., 2013; Ng & Law, 2014; Sanders & McCready, 2009). Lifting policies for older workers may include lift teams or decreasing the maximum loads lifted by 20% for the older worker (Haight & Belwal, 2006).

Work Practice Controls

Older adult workers need to take the same precautions as younger workers to protect themselves, being especially vigilant in executing proper body mechanics and pacing themselves throughout the day to maximize their endurance. They may consider joint protection techniques for the body and hands or purchasing prescription eye safety wear. Since older workers have a higher risk of developing a chronic disease than younger workers, older workers need to consider the impact of medications on their workday performance and gradual return to work following an illness.

Ergonomics can improve the experience of older workers so work is a productive and self-fulfilling experience that goes beyond implications for material income. Occupational therapists can promote respect for the unique individual qualities that each older worker brings to the workplace.

Obese Workers

A further demographic trend impacting work performance is the increasing rate of obesity in the adult population. In the United States, 35.7% of the adult population aged 20 years and older is either overweight or obese (CDC, 2010). Obesity is associated with increased health care costs due to greater risk for diabetes, heart disease, stroke, and certain types of cancer. Further, obese workers who are injured are less likely to return to work after 3 months than nonobese counterparts due to illness-related work disability (Lilley, Davie, Ameratunga, & Derret, 2012).

Workplaces must ensure that work equipment and vehicles are the correct fit for the worker who is obese, as for any worker. For example, a standard work chair is typically rated for a load of 280 lbs; a ladder is typically rated to accommodate persons up to 350 lbs; a truck bench or back hoe seat is only rated for a load of 350 lbs. Workplaces need to ensure that equipment is safe for all members of the workforce. Additionally, some jobs have constraints of size relative to the space in which they work such as the width of a trench, the circumference of a manhole, the width of a bus or plane aisle, etc. Such workplace demands may impact employment options. In health care environments, individuals caring for clients who are obese need to use lifting equipment and seek assistance for any moving or transfers of clients. Importantly, occupational therapy practitioners need to remind employers of needs associated with rescue responses for all workers such as hoists, stretchers, or safety lines.

Industrial Rehabilitation

History of Industrial Rehabilitation and Occupational Therapy

Dr. Leonard Matheson is considered to be one of the founding fathers of industrial rehabilitation. Dr. Matheson renewed our interest in work interventions during the 1970s by incorporating clinical expertise related to specific diagnoses with task analysis and work environments (www.ot.wustl.edu). He transformed the clinic into a shop or factory, allowing for more effective reproduction of critical job duties and therapeutic intervention to facilitate recovery of lost work skills, abilities, and tolerances. Injured workers would present themselves daily for up to 12 weeks and engage in functional work tasks designed and graded to advance the ability and tolerance of the given injured worker. In time, this gave way to many forms of industrial rehabilitation that have grown and changed to meet the needs of today's injured worker (www.ot.wustl.edu).

Components of an Industrial Rehabilitation Program

Industrial rehabilitation refers to work programs whose goals are to remediate a client's injury in order to return to the workforce. Industrial rehabilitation may be appropriate for workers who have psychiatric and/or physical disabilities. Although the focus of this chapter is physical disabilities, psychosocial issues are recognized as critical and thus addressed. Individuals with psychiatric issues may benefit from retraining relative to the time structuring and interactional aspects of the job. Rehabilitation may include means to increase clients' overall strength, endurance, and job-specific skills as well as prevocational skills such as punctuality and following directions. Programs may include compensation for deficits in skills such as teaching clients to use lifting aids to compensate for limited strength.

Safety Restrictions and Concerns

Prior to engaging a worker in the work-hardening process, the worker should be cleared medically. Concerns that should be considered are tachycardia, resting heart rate above 110 BPM, blood pressure significantly above 140 systolic and 90 diastolic mm Hg, and other unstable medical conditions, such as recent development of kidney stones (Demers, 1992).

Implications for the Americans with Disabilities Act

The worker's ability to meet the critical job demands determines the individual's ability to return to performing the job. The Americans with Disabilities Act (ADA) suggests that a worker protected under the ADA can perform the essential job functions (29 C.F.R. § 1630.2[m]), or those functions that cannot be completed by another employee, with reasonable accommodation. According to the ADA, reasonable accommodations may include environmental modifications, job modifications, or the use of specific equipment that will allow the employee to perform the essential job functions (ADA, 1990, 42 U.S.C. § 12111[9]). These accommodations must be requested by the employee and must not cause undue hardship for the employer (42 U.S.C. § 12111[10]). The determination of undue hardship is relative, based on the size of a given company. Reasonable accommodation to a small company could mean provision of a small inexpensive cart that could be pushed so loads did not need to be carried. Reasonable accommodations for a larger company could mean installing a hoist and crane system to automatically transport an object so the product is not manually handled. The occupational therapist serves as an expert at assisting employers in adapting actual vocational demands and means of accommodation.

The ADA was amended in 2008, with the amendments going into effect in January 2009. The focus of the amended ADA was ensuring that employers provide adequate modifications for people with disabilities instead of the unintended focus since 1990 on "proving" or "disproving" that individuals had a covered disability. The amendments have been put in place to assure that employers have fulfilled their obligations under the ADA. Additionally, it assures that an "interactive process" has been offered to protected individuals with a logical exploration of reasonable accommodations (Lindeman, 2009).

This process is a ready-made entry point for occupational therapists as their training and skill sets are ideal for identifying challenge, barrier, and adaptive means to remedy the situation. An example of such a process would be a limitation of floor-level lifting for worker who lacked necessary knee range of motion to provide material handling efforts at floor level. The identified problem can be reasonably solved by stacking and securing three pallets together for a lifting platform or by building a lightweight 18" high pallet so that a given load is now 18" off of the floor at a height where the worker is able to negotiate the given load effectively. The implications of the amendments are being seen as legal cases play out with the amendments being integral relative to workers' compensation matters.

Acute Rehabilitation

Therapy delivered by occupational therapists at the acute stage of industrial rehabilitation focuses on the recovery of body structures such as soft-tissue injuries, joint trauma, ligamentous sprains, and muscle strains. Injuries are typically treated the day of injury or as soon as medically appropriate. The acute phase of care can last up to 3 months; such interventions typically occur in an outpatient clinic setting. Early but appropriately controlled movement allows for effective control of symptoms and avoidance of chronic conditions (Prosser & Conolly, 2003).

As explained in Chapter 2, various modalities including ice, heat, iontophoresis, and electrical stimulation are utilized by the therapist to control inflammation, pain, and swelling. Manual therapies, muscle energy, and myofascial and craniosacral therapy may also be used to address painful symptoms (Bracciano, 2007). It should be noted that some interventions stated above require continuing education beyond entry-level skills. Special care should be taken to assure that the normal joint and tissue integrity above and below the site of treatment is maintained. Functional activity is graded to offer enough stress to facilitate proper healing, not exacerbate the injury. The focus of intervention is expedited care to allow the worker to resume performance skills and normal work routines.

Therapists should make an effort to understand the worker's personal belief mechanisms about injury and recovery and educate him or her as to the most effective process for recovery. Addressing the emotional content of the injury is equally as important as treating the worker's actual physical complaints. The worker may have competing advice from medical, legal, and work arenas, all of which impact recovery. Concerns outside of the worker's actual injury may include pressure from decreased financial resources as well as chronic pain. New roles (homemaker or child care provider) may become a barrier to returning to work or exploring alternate means of employment.

Often, the worker cannot readily resume full duty upon returning to work and may need a modified duty job for a short time. Occupational therapists assist physicians in determining the extent of limitations. Simple functional evaluations or more formal functional capacity evaluations (see next section) provide objective data for this process (Isernhagen, 1995). It is crucial that the therapist encourage the worker to take responsibility for his or her own well-being. Health club membership or other effective means of fitness training, weight loss, tobacco cessation, and ergonomic equipment should all be encouraged as a normal part of healthy living.

On-Site Programs

The birth of on-site programs was stimulated from the need to offer more effective means of intervention to larger corporations. The concept is to offer effective intervention with the least amount of lost time (Key, 1995; Yassi, 2005). Depending on the company size and injury, on-site care can range from the provision of an occupational health nurse and therapist onsite for 3 days per week to larger offerings including X-ray equipment and daily rehabilitation. The on-site facility offers the injured worker immediate care, follow-up intervention, and rehabilitation without having to visit an off-site clinic during work hours (Isernhagen, 1995). The continuity of care from clinic to worksite can hasten both return to work for clients and resumption of the worker role.

A benefit of on-site therapy is that the therapist is able to directly assess the worker's ability to engage in given work tasks, understand the factors that contribute to injury, and effectively plan intervention toward returning to previous work capacity. All care providers at on-site facilities are keenly aware of the work environment and work nature. This is especially important when decisions are being made about work readiness, modified duty, and ergonomic modifications. On-site programs typically offer more direct communication between medical provider, employer, therapist, and worker. The venue creates more effective understanding and limits information delay.

Subacute Rehabilitation

Subacute intervention begins typically after resolution and healing of an injury, somewhere between 3 and 6 months after injury. The injury itself is stable, although it may have become a persistent or chronic condition. At this stage, the elapsed time since injury may present with ramifications that are as significant as the original injury. For example, workers may have become deconditioned and may present with guarding of the involved extremity due to prolonged painful conditions.

Occupational therapy intervention scenarios focus on addressing long-term complaints, specific work activities that may exacerbate the condition, and new manifestations that are born from long-standing conditions. Therapists may continue to utilize preparatory modalities appropriate for subacute conditions (e.g., continuous ultrasound, moist heat, and transcutaneous electrical stimulation) to ready clients for functional use. Updated home exercise programs also facilitate recovery. More likely, the therapist will need to focus on regaining time-limited ROM, joint excursion quality, and pain management (Isernhagen, 1995).

Return-to-Work Fitness

Following subacute therapy, a worker may need to be placed in a brief program intended to build tolerance, stamina, and strength. A return-to-work fitness program offers the worker a supervised fitness program that targets specific needs and weaknesses in order to transition back to work. Partial engagement of actual duties in the form of modified duty may be beneficial and be included in the work fitness program. The program prescribes fitness activities graded to the worker's level of physical capacity and offers recommendations for a program that can be followed independently at a local fitness facility, community center, home gym, or home exercise program. The worker should understand the balance between sustaining adequate fitness to insure tolerance to work and overtraining, which further stresses musculature.

Work Hardening and Work Conditioning

Work Hardening

Work hardening incorporates work fitness but focuses further on improving the functional limitations that have developed from a given injury. Work hardening typically consists of injury intervention, specific fitness training, specific work act simulation, conditioning, body mechanics training, and safe work practice training. The objective is to reestablish a sense of normal work momentum by fabricating an environment that simulates the eventual full work demands that will be expected of the worker. Workers simulate tasks to build up a tolerance to the stresses associated with work performance. With time, the worker can readily tolerate the stresses without setback or exacerbation of injury (Demers, 1992; Goss, Christopher, Faulk, & Moore, 2009).

The client in a work-hardening program is expected to resume normal activities of daily living and prework rituals prior to participation in the program. Specifically, the worker is expected to rise, shower, dress, and eat breakfast as would be expected prior to going to work. The worker is then expected to arrive to work hardening on time and ready to invest in the program. A typical work-hardening program can be 5 days a week and 8 hours long but may vary according to the clinic and insurance.

Work hardening is generally provided in a group setting by a multidisciplinary team of providers. The team typically consists of occupational therapists, physical therapists, medical providers, rehabilitation nurses, case managers, and may also include psychology and sociology professionals. The team works collaboratively to provide consistent intervention in all facets of the program (Demers, 1992). Work hardening is designed to return an injured worker to the most optimal level of functional ability where employment opportunity readily exists. Outcome studies on the return-to-work status of clients in work-hardening programs suggest 50% to 88% of all workers return to work and remain at work at least 6 months after discharge from a program and show significant pre-post test functional gains (Goss et al., 2009; Scully-Palmer, 2000).

Work-hardening equipment typically incorporates actual work samples from industry as well as equipment that simulate job motions. Work samples may include actual kegs of beer, saws, hammers, plumbing, or electrical tools that allow workers to practice their trade in a clinical environment. Job simulation equipment simulates specific tasks using computerized equipment that provides numerous attachments and adjustments to enable practice in similar positions and resistance levels as the actual job. Low-tech work samples, ramps, lift boxes, work frames, and assembly kits are also seen across the country. Figure 6-7 identifies a client simulating a plumbing task that resembles the motions and equipment that he would need to perform on the job. Figures 6-8 through 6-10 provide additional examples and descriptions.

The work-hardening program assesses the worker's injury and current functional status using a baseline evaluation called a functional capacity evaluation (FCE). The goal of the FCE is to identify the functional attributes of an injured worker, compare these skills with the known job demands, and determine whether the worker can perform the essential job functions fully, with restrictions, or not at all. Essential functions, as stated earlier, are those tasks that must be completed in order for the worker to be wholly competent in terms of performing his or her job. Essential functions are composed of critical demands that constitute the physical nature and quantities of work associated

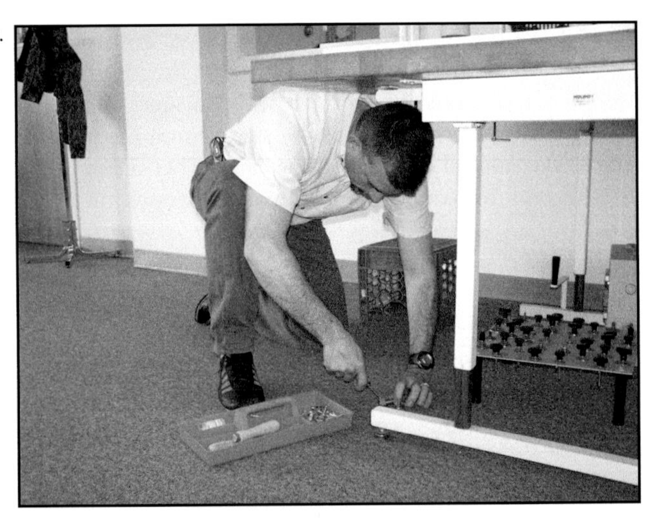

Figure 6-7. Client simulating plumbing task.

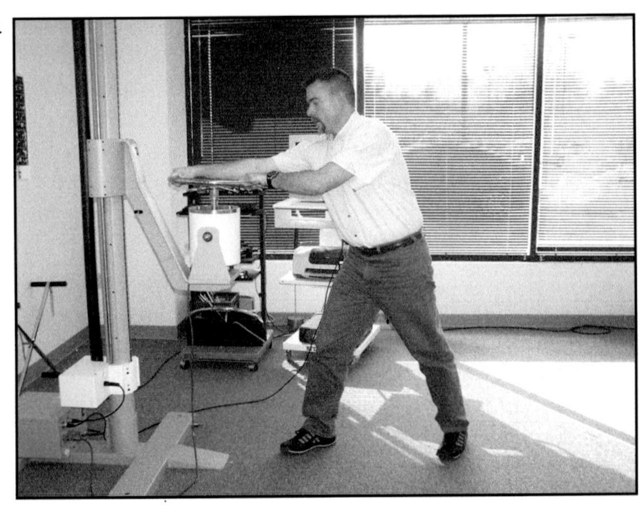

Figure 6-8. Client simulating plumbing task.

with the essential functions. Work is also often composed of nonessential functions and demands that are typically associated with a given duty but are not criteria for competence.

The results of the FCE are compared to the demands of the job in order to develop an intervention plan that will increase the client's functional status to the level necessary to resume normal work participation. The FCE specifically defines an individual's ability to perform work-related performance skills and performance patterns (Isernhagan, 1995). Various FCEs evaluate cognition, vision, and mentality; however, most FCEs directly relate to the workers' compensation focus on a worker's physical ability. For example, a carpenter who recently underwent a rotator cuff repair would need to strengthen his shoulder in order to hammer overhead, ascend a ladder, and operate a circular reciprocating saw. The carpenter, given the time away from work, would likely also need to recover his overall aerobic capacity and general work tolerance. The occupational therapist would offer the carpenter functional and exercise-based activities to address these issues so that the worker could resume his past job. Table 6-6 identifies the basic components of a FCE. The most simplistic subtests of an FCE are typically universal, but variations in procedure, methodology, and test components exist. The FCE components will be specific to evaluator philosophy,

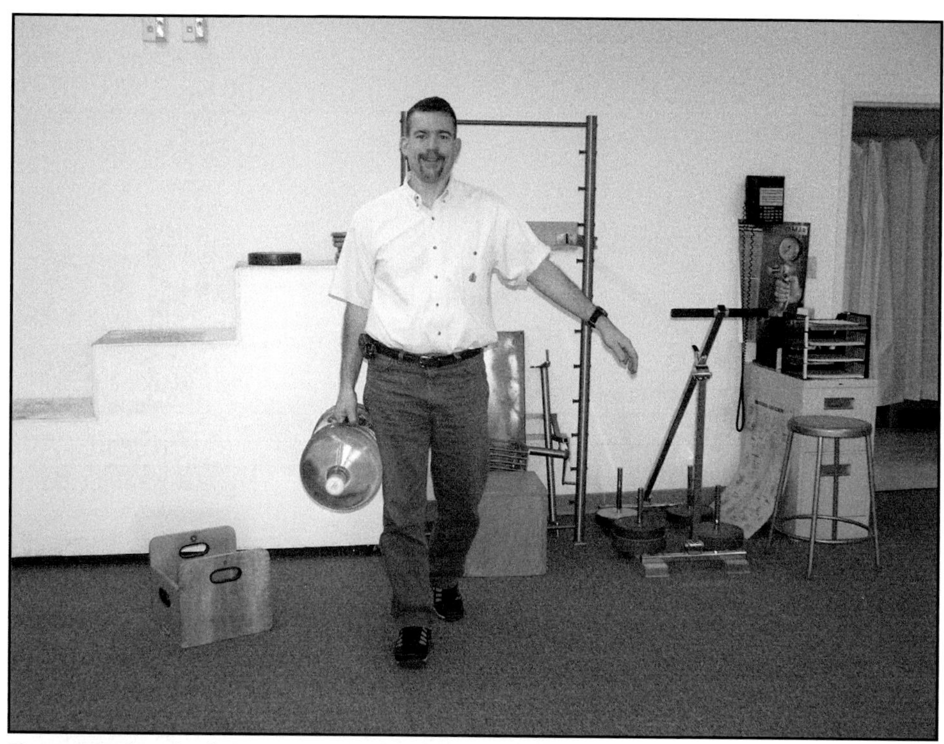

Figure 6-9. Client simulating common work task.

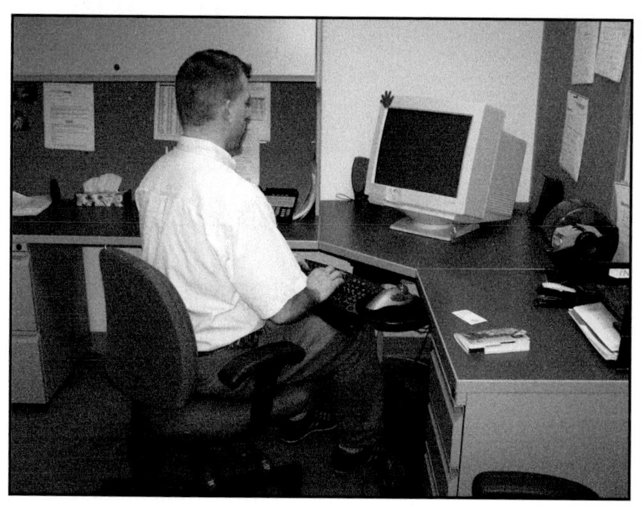

Figure 6-10. Client simulating computer-based task. Note neutral posture in sitting.

job demands, and intervention approach. Figure 6-11 shows a client performing a weighted lifting component from the floor to mid-thigh height.

Aspects of the FCE can also be used as part of normal occupational therapy evaluation and intervention, especially in the industrial rehabilitation arena, where a progressive understanding of the worker's functional abilities is needed to know how to adjust, update, or advance therapy. Specific FCE subtests (bending, squatting, reaching, lifting, etc.) can be used to provide meaningful information to medical providers relative to establishing "recuperative posts" or "temporary alternate work" opportunities.

Table 6-6 Basic Components of a Functional Capacity Evaluation
• Health interview and physical exam • Grip/pinch/dexterity tests • Posture and activity tests • Manual material handling/weighted negotiation (lifting) • Job simulation • Cardiovascular tests were relevant • Behavior profile • Reliability of effort determination

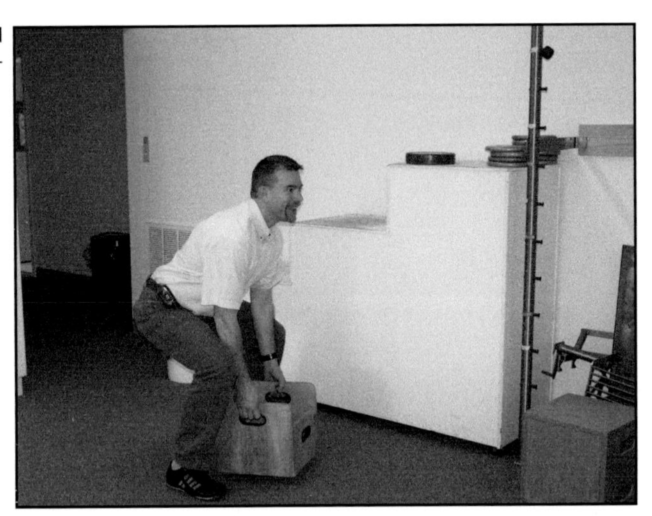

Figure 6-11. Client performing a weighted lifting component from the floor to mid-thigh height.

Overall, the work-hardening program should instill a sense of growing independence so that the occupational therapist offers more encouragement than direction by the end of the program. The worker is ready and able to return to the rigors of employment with the needed fitness, conditioning, and mindset to address the dynamics of full-time work participation and the physical dynamics of the actual work itself.

Work Conditioning

Work conditioning differs from work hardening in that typically no team is present to collaboratively treat the worker. According to Jacobs and Simon, work conditioning is defined as "an intensive work-related, goal-oriented conditioning program designed specifically to restore systemic neuromuscular functions (e.g., strength endurance, movement, flexibility, motor control) and cardiopulmonary functions. The objective of a work conditioning program is to restore physical capacity and function to enable the patient/client to return to work" (2015, p. 318). Workers engaged in work conditioning generally engage in a combination of physical exercise, stretching, fitness, aerobic conditioning, body mechanics training, and some limited involvement in work-related functional tasks. Work conditioning can occur either as an individual program or in a group setting with several workers completing the program together. The workers may not share similar work demands but are encouraged to offer each other positive reinforcement and an effective level of competition or peer pressure. Work conditioning often lasts 2 to 4 hours per day and may occur several days per week.

Work conditioning does not require an extensive clinical environment in terms of exercise equipment to be successful: a treadmill, some weights, BTE (Intertek Testing Services), and a floor mat are typical of many programs. Similar to work hardening, the work conditioning program instills within the worker the importance of continuing the daily fitness and exercise routines that have been established. However, less work simulation is performed prior to returning to the job.

The provision of work hardening and work conditioning services present both challenges and growth opportunities depending on the economy and the local job environment. This finding is due to the effect of reimbursement dollars for service benefit. When jobs are plentiful, there is a clear path taking an injured worker from workplace injury to return to a specific job, with work hardening as the intervention. In such cases, reimbursement for work conditioning and work hardening programs are available and supportive. However, when workers are without specific employment opportunities, there is less support to fund a program, especially when specific work demands are not clear and when employment is not guaranteed. The occupational therapist should understand the community economy and reimbursement trends (Peskin, 2012).

Body Mechanics Training

Both work hardening and conditioning share as part of their intervention strategies health promotion activities such as education and training specific to body mechanics and safe work practice. Body mechanics focuses on teaching workers to use their bodies effectively and safely. Training focuses on teaching workers how heavy loads affect their bodies, possible consequences of cumulative stress, and anatomy and kinesiology of the back and shoulders (Melnik, 2004).

Many approaches to body mechanics exist. Common lifting techniques for lifting objects from the ground include semi-squatting and stooping (Melnik, 2004; Straker, 2003). Although positions vary, most approaches maintain that lumbar lordosis, or "locking in the spine," is the safest position for the back. Principles include keeping the load close to the body, keeping the back straight, and avoiding twisting the back. Because twisting places significant torque on the back, workers are trained to move with the load taking small steps, pivoting their feet, or stance shifting instead of fixing their feet and twisting from their low back. Workers must anticipate the weight of the load and expect load shifting for unsecured objects (Greene & Roberts, 2002). Workers in health care such as certified nursing assistants must learn how to apply lifting principles to transferring clients in health care facilities. However, use of lifting assists (such as Hoyer lifts or stand-tilt stations) are strongly encouraged to prevent health care worker injury.

Although most body mechanics programs focus on proper use of the low back, shoulders also present with lifting concerns. Overuse of the shoulder may cause tendonitis, which may lead eventually to a rotator cuff tear. In order to prevent this sequela, workers are trained to keep loads close to the body and avoid reaching with loads. Positions that place excessive torque on the shoulders are lifting above chest level or greater than 90 degrees of shoulder flexion/abduction. The worker's hand coupling (relationship of hand to object to be lifted/moved) may be modified to identify the most effective means to handle loads in a given lift.

Safe Work Practice

Safe work practice advances body mechanics training to the entire behaviors associated with meaningful work. The worker is taught to consider every aspect of the given job in terms of physical stress and the opportunity to physically respond to the stress by ideal work practice and/or adaptation of the demand. Advanced problem solving is encouraged to allow a level of preparedness for the possible outcomes of a given demand. Workers are trained to remain in full attention to their physical acts. Therapy can set the stage for safe work practice by providing dynamic activity that does not follow a routine or level of repeatability. A simple training tool is having the worker respond to weighted medicine balls that are caught in various scenarios off rebounding equipment. Workers must anticipate the trajectory and decelerate the ball, all the while maintaining proper spinal and shoulder posture. Safe work practice inherently includes body mechanics training but goes further to instill a sense of general safety for all vocational participation within the workplace context.

Pain Management

Another extension of work hardening and work conditioning is the arena of pain management. This intervention is focused on workers whose pain issues supersede the actual functional implications of their given injury or injuries. Two intervention approaches exist to address this issue: behavioral and functional.

Behavioral Intervention

Behavioral intervention is typically a team-oriented intervention composed of the same professionals as a formal work hardening program. Intervention consists of work hardening and work conditioning, except the worker's identified pain behaviors are literally "disacknowledged" by the team. The worker with pain is rewarded only for functional gains and assertive dialogue about any symptoms. According to this approach, the worker is weaned off of all pain medications, as it has been determined the worker's pain is present despite pain medication and the medication is no longer therapeutic. Additionally, intervention extends beyond the worker to the worker's family or support network, such that family and significant others are trained to not enable the worker's current pain paradigm. This program is demanding and can be stressful to both the worker and the therapist. The worker elects to adopt wellness behaviors or fails the program by not adopting healthful beliefs. The therapist needs to fully understand the end goal in order to encourage functional and therapeutic activity despite the worker's pain (Guzman et al., 2001).

Functional Restoration

The goal of functional restoration is to offer a safe environment for the worker to resume normal movement, activity, and vocational/avocational involvement. Strategies are provided to offer effective pain management such as ice, pacing, and conditioning. The worker's medical provider may offer strategic medications to maximize the worker's tolerance and pain modulation to facilitate success in the program. Ideally, the worker will graduate from the program with a renewed sense of self and ability. Pain modulation should be a personal concern and no longer a public one, with effective pain therapy being made available to the worker.

As in work conditioning, functional restoration focuses on maximizing physical ability through exercise, aerobics, weighted activity, and activities that promote normal movement patterns. The worker's pain issues are not denied but rather intellectualized so that workers can understand how to use their bodies despite the pain. Permission is given to work through pain or to accept pain. Many of these workers are overtly fearful that their pain somehow represents some level of fragility or structural instability within their bodies. This creates a tendency to minimize activity in order to avoid pain. This strategy may be effective during the acute phase of injury but remains counterproductive in the chronic phase because the decreased movement and activity results in range limitations that continue a cycle of pain (Schonstein, Kenny, Keating, & Koes, 2003).

As with all forms of intervention, it is paramount that the occupational therapist be able to instill a sense of importance in the worker about maintenance of skills and ongoing fitness and health. Many clinics offer some form of "after care" where the worker can return informally and use the clinic as a health club and check in with the care team. This service offers a good bridge upon completion of a formal program but should be time limited so that workers ultimately take full responsibility for themselves.

Implications for Psychosocial Issues

As stated, the majority of clients are referred to industrial rehabilitation with a physical injury resulting in pain, functional deficits, and inability to work. However, social and psychological issues may disrupt the family and impact quality of life for many workers undergoing a work-related injury (Kirsh & McKee, 2003). In some situations, the multiple perspectives of stakeholders create a tone of frustration among the health care providers, work supervisors, human resource personnel, compensation systems, and workers. Each player has a different perspective when interacting with the injured worker. For example, supervisors may want a quick return to work to maintain productivity, human resource personnel may be concerned with insurance costs, health care providers want to avoid re-injury and promote functional return, while workers need a full paycheck and a sense of self-worth. Because chronic pain is not a visible injury, workers feel they must legitimize the pain. Research studies report that injured workers feel misunderstood and not respected by employers, society, their community, and coworkers (Kirsh & McKee, 2003). Occupational therapy practitioners can minimize some issues by keeping open communication with stakeholders and focusing on preparing a client physically and psychologically to return to work.

Outcomes of Work Hardening Programs

Work hardening programs strive to prepare a worker to return to the job. However, if the worker does not achieve the physical capacities necessary for the workplace, the employer may further use discharge assessments or FCEs to understand how to modify the relevant work area or job process in order to allow the worker to be competent. The worker may also be referred to vocational retraining, which attempts to retrain the worker for potential vocations at the physical demand levels identified by the completed FCE. A final scenario is that the worker may never return to employment and use the FCE to gauge a financial award to the worker to compensate him or her for any suffered injury or condition.

Occupational Therapist's Expanded Role in Work as Consultant and Expert Witness

Occupational therapists have served as consultants and experts in many capacities. In ergonomics, a consultation model is common in that occupational therapy practitioners provide ergonomic evaluations and recommendation, case-based interventions, and educational services (such a prevention programs) to companies on a short-term basis with periodic follow-up (Sanders, 2004). In industrial rehabilitation, services follow a more traditional intervention model, with individuals attending work hardening and work conditioning programs until goals are achieved or insurance limits reached. Now, however, opportunities for consultation in the industrial work arena have expanded. Traditional industrial consultation service included reviewing fellow occupational therapy care provisions, documentation, and demonstration of expertise. Now, expert venues are associated with expertise in the ADA, functional status, behavior, work site accommodation, adaptive provisions, etc., as our occupational arena entails. Opportunity to provide this expertise ranges from simple chart and care reviews and consulting demands to informal and formal legal proceedings (Allen, Ainsworth, & Long, 2010).

In summary, ergonomics can improve the experience of workers so work is a productive and self-fulfilling experience that goes beyond implications for material income. The overall goal is that the worker experiences a satisfying job or career that promotes personal satisfaction and competency in a healthful work environment. Ergonomic and industrial rehabilitation services can offer prevention, modification, and remediation services to promote worker health. Dr. Matheson eloquently captures this sentiment when he says, "After you save a person's life, the only thing that is more profound is to re-establish competency at work" (personal communication, 2005).

Summary Questions

1. Define ergonomics and its relation to occupation.
2. Discuss the difference between work hardening and work conditioning.
3. Discuss compensation/adaptation strategies for older workers.
4. How might a visual or perceptual deficit impact the safety of a worker? Discussion a specific example of a profession in the discussion.

References

Allen, S., Ownsworth, T., Carlson, G., & Strong, S. (2010). Occupational therapists as expert witnesses on work capacity. *Australian Occupational Therapy Journal, 57*(2), 88-94.

American Association of Retired Persons. (2003). Staying ahead of the curve: The AARP working in retirement study. AARP Knowledge Management: Washington, DC.

American Occupational Therapy Association. (2014). Occupational therapy practice: Domain and process (3rd ed.). *American Journal of Occupational Therapy, 68*(Suppl. 1), S1-S48.

Americans with Disabilities Act, 34 C.F.R. §1630 (1999). Americans with Disabilities Act. 42 U.S.C. §12111 (1990).

Atwood, M. J. (1992). Adolescent learning in two environments. *Work, 2*(2), 61-81.

Bing, R. K. (1989). Work is a four-letter word! A historical perspective. In S. Hertfelder, & C. Gwin (Eds.), *Work in progress: Occupational therapy in work programs*. Rockville, MD: AOTA.

Bracciano, A. G. (2007). *Physical agent modalities* (2nd ed.). Thoroughfare, NJ: SLACK Incorporated.

Brady, S., Mayer, T. G., & Gatchel, R. J. (1994). Physical progress and residual impairment quantification after functional restoration, Part II: Isokinetic trunk strength. *Spine, 19*, 395-400.

Bridger, R. S. (2009). *Introduction to ergonomics* (3rd ed.) New York, NY: CRC Press.

Centers for Disease Control (2010). Adult Obesity facts. Retrieved at: http://www.cdc.gov/obesity/data/adult.html.

Chueng, S., & Strough, J. (2004). A comparison of collaborative and individual everyday problem-solving in younger and older adults. *International Journal of Aging and Human Development, 58*(3), 167-195.

Christiansen, C., & Townsend, E. (2010). *Introduction to occupation: The art of science and living* (2nd ed.). Thorofare, NJ: Prentice Hall.

Darragh, A. R., Huddleston, W., & King, P. (2009). Work-related musculoskeletal injuries and disorders among occupational and physical therapists. *American Journal of Occupational Therapy, 63*, 351-362

Demers, L. (1992). Work hardening: A practical guide. Boston: Andover Medical Publishers.

Ellexson, M. (2004). Job analysis and worksite assessment. In M. Sanders (Ed.), *Ergonomics and the management of musculoskeletal disorders* (pp. 283-298). St. Louis, MO: Butterworth-Heinemann.

Erikson, E. (1997). *The life cycle completed: Extended version*. New York, NY: W. W. Norton & Co.

Feuerstein, M. (1996). Workstyle: Definition, empirical support, and implications for prevention, evaluation, and rehabilitation of occupational upper-extremity disorders. In S. D. Moon, & S. L. Sauter (Eds.), *Beyond biomechanics: Psychosocial aspects of musculoskeletal disorders in office work*. Bristol, PA: Taylor and Francis.

Fisk, A. D., Rogers, W. A., Charness, N., Czaja, S. J., & Sharit, J. (2009). *Designing for older adults* (2nd ed.). New York, NY: CRC Press.

Goggins, R., Spielholz, P., & Nothstein, G. L. (2008). Estimating the effectiveness of ergonomics interventions through case studies: Implications for predictive cost-benefit analysis. *Journal of Safety Research, 39*, 339-344.

Goleman, D. (1998). Working with emotional intelligence. New York: Bantam Books.

Goss, D. L., Christopher, G. E., Faulk, R. T., Moore, J. (2009). Functional training program bridges rehabilitation and return to duty. *Journal of Special Operations Medicine, 9*(2), 29-35.

Green, D. P., & Roberts, S. L. (1999). *Kinesiology: Movement in the context of activity.* St. Louis, MO: Mosby.

Guzman, J., Esmail, R., Karjalainen, K., Malmivaara, A., Irvin, E., & Bombardier, C. (2001). Multidisciplinary rehabilitation for chronic low back pain: systematic review. *BMJ, 322*, 1511-1516.

Haight, J. M., & Belwal, U. (2006). Designing for an aging workforce. *Professional Safety, 30*, 20-33.

Harvey-Krefting, L. (1985). The concept of work in occupational therapy: A historical review. *American Journal of Occupational Therapy, 39*, 301-307.

Hedge, A. (2004). Ergonomic guidelines for arranging a computer workstation: 10 steps for users. Retrieved at http://ergo.human.cornell.edu/ergoguide.html on Nov. 1, 2004.

Isernhagen, S. J. (1995). *Work injury management.* Gaithersburg, MD: Aspen Publishers.

Jacobs, K., (Ed.) (2008). *Ergonomics for therapists* (3rd ed.). St. Louis, MO: Mosby Elsevier.

Jacobs, K., & Simon, L. (2015). *Quick reference dictionary for occupational therapy* (6th ed.). Thorofare, NJ: SLACK Incorporated.

Karasek, R., & Theorell, T. (1990). *Healthy work: Stress, productivity and the reconstruction of working life.* New York, NY: Basic Books.

Key, G. L. (Ed.). (1995). Industrial therapy. Philadelphia: Elsevier/Mosby.

Kietrysa, D., Galperb, J. S., & Vernoc, V.(2007). Effects of at-work exercises on computer Operators. *Work, 28*, 67–75,

Kirsh, B., & McKee, P. (2003). The needs an experiences of injured workers: A participatory research study. *Work, 21*, 221-231.

Kjellen, U. (2000). *Prevention of accidents through experience feedback.* New York, NY: Taylor & Francis.

Kroemer, K. H. E. (2008). *Fitting the human: Introduction to ergonomics* (6th ed.). Boca Raton, FL: CRC Press.

Law, M., Cooper, B. A., Strong, S., Stewart, S., Rigby, P., & Letts, L. (1996). The person-environment-occupation model: A transactive approach to occupational performance. *Canadian Journal of Occupational Therapy, 63*, 9-23.

Leijten, F., Heuvel, S., Geuskens, G., Ybema, J., Wind, A., Burdorf, A., & Robroek, S. (2013). How do older employees with health problems remain productive at work?: A qualitative study. *Journal of Occupational Rehabilitation, 23*(1), 115-124.

Leveau, B. F. (1992). *Williams's and Lissner's biomechanics of human motion* (3rd ed.). Philadelphia, PA: WB Saunders.

Lilley, R., Davie, G., Ameratunga, S., & Derret, S. (2012). Factors predicting work status 3 months after injury: Results from the prospective outcomes of injury study. *British Medical Journal Open Access, 2.*

Lindeman, D. L. (2009). What the new ADA Amendments Have to Do with You: A Brief Guide for HR Managers. Retrieved at http://greenwaldllp.com/files%5C20090916185129_The-New-ADA-Amendments.pdf.

Lueder, R., & Rick, V. B. (2008). *Ergonomics for children.* London, United Kingdom: Taylor & Francis.

Marangoni, A. (2010). Effects of intermittent stretching exercises at work on musculoskeletal pain associated with the use of a personal computer and the influence of media on outcomes. *Work, 36*, (27) 27–37.

Matheson, L. (1988). How do you know that he tried his best? The reliability crisis in Industrial Rehabilitation. *Industrial Rehabilitation Quarterly, Spring.*

Marras, W. (2012). The complex spine: The multidimensional systems of causal pathways for low-back disorders. *Human Factors, 54*(6), 881-889.

Matheson, L., Dodson, M., & Wolf, T. (2011, March). Executive dysfunction and work: Tying it all together. *Work & Industry Special Interest Section Quarterly, 25*(1), 1–4.

Mayer, T., Taber, J., Bovasso, E., & Gatchel, R. J. (1994). Physical progress and residual impairment quantification after functional restoration, Part I: Lumbar mobility. *Spine, 19*, 389-394.

Melnik, M. (2004). Implementing an effective injury prevention process. In M. Sanders (Ed.), *Ergonomics and the management of musculoskeletal disorders* (pp. 242-360). St. Louis, MO: Butterworth Heinemann.

Moon, S. D., & Sauter, S. L. (Eds.). (1996). *Beyond biomechanics: Psychosocial aspects of musculoskeletal disorders in office work* (pp. 23-42). Bristol, PA: Taylor and Francis.

National Institute of Occupational Safety and Health. (1994). Applications manual for the revised NIOSH lifting equation, DHHS (NIOSH) Publication No. 94-110. Cincinnati, OH: NIOSH Publications Dissemination.

National Institute of Occupational Safety and Health. (1994). Elements of Ergonomic programs: A primer based on workplace evaluations of musculoskeletal disorders. DHHS(NIOSH) Publication No. 97-117. Cincinnati, OH: NIOSH Publications Dissemination.

National Institute of Occupational Safety and Health. (1997). Musculoskeletal disorders and workplace factors: A critical review of epidemiologic evidence for work-related musculoskeletal disorders of the neck, upper extremity and low back. US Department of Health and Human Services DHHS (NIOSH) Publication No. 97-141.

National Institute of Occupational Safety and Health. (1989). Occupational exposure to hand-arm vibration [DHHS pub no. 89-106]. Cincinnati: US Department of Health and Human Services.

National Research Council. (1998). *Work-related musculoskeletal disorders: A review of the evidence.* Washington, DC: National Academy Press.

Ng, E. S., & Law, A. (2014). Keeping Up! Older Workers' Adaptation in the Workplace after Age 55. *Canadian Journal on Aging, 33*(1), 1-14.

Occupational Safety and Health Administration. (1991). Ergonomics program management guidelines for meatpacking plants. Retrieved at http://www.ergoweb.com/resources/reference/guidelines/meatpacking.cfm on Feb. 16, 2005.

Occupational Safety and Health Administration. (n.d.). Home page. Retrieved at http://www.osha.gov/SLTC/etools/computerworkstations/positions.html.

Oxenburgh, M. (1997). Cost-benefit analysis of ergonomics programs. *American Industrial Hygiene Association Journal, 58*,150-156.

Peskin, S. (2012). Managed care reimbursement: Hardened hearts. Retrieved at http://www.managedcaremag.com/category/topics/reimbursement.

Pheasant, S. (2001). *Bodyspace.* London, United Kingdom: Taylor-Francis.

Prosser, R., & Conolly, W. B. (2003). *Rehabilitation of the hand and upper extremity.* St. Louis, MO: Butterworth-Heinmann.

Punnett, L., Cherniack, M., Henning, R., Morse, T., & Faghri, P. D. (2009). CPH-NEW Research Team. A conceptual framework for integrating workplace health promotion and occupational ergonomics programs. *Public Health Rep., Jul-Aug*;124 Suppl 1:16-25.

Ramazzini, B. (1717). De morbis artificum diatriba. In W. Wright (Trans, 1940), *The diseases of workers.* Chicago: University of Chicago Press.

Sanders, M. (Ed.). (2004). *Ergonomics and the management of musculoskeletal disorders.* St. Louis, MO: Butterworth-Heinemann.

Sanders, M., & Morse, T. F. (2005). Ergonomics of caring for children: An exploratory study. *American Journal of Occupational Therapy, 59*(3), 285-295.

Sanders, M., & McCready, J. W. (2010). Does work contribute to successful aging in older workers? *The International Journal of Aging and Human Development, 71*(3), 209-229.

Sanders, M., & McCready, J. (2009). A qualitative study of two older workers' adaptation to physically demanding jobs. *Work, 32*(2), 111-122.

Sanders, M. S., & McCormick, E. J. (1993). *Human factors in engineering and design.* New York, NY: McGraw-Hill, Inc.

Schonstein, E., Kenny, D. T., Keating, J., & Koes, B. W. (2003). Work conditioning, work hardening and functional restoration for workers with back and neck pain. Cochrane Database Syst Rev., 1, CD001822.

Schooler, C., Mulatu, M. S., & Oates, G. (1999). The continuing effects of substantively complex work on the intellectual functioning of older workers. *Psychology and Aging, 4*(3), 483-506.

Scully-Palmer, C. (2000). Outcome study: An industrial rehabilitation program. *Work, 15*, 21-23.

Silverstein, B. A., Fine, L. J., & Armstrong, T. J. (1987). Occupational factors and carpal tunnel syndrome. *American Journal of Industrial Medicine, 11*, 343-358.

Stacey, W. (2001). The stress of progression from school to work for adolescents with disabilities . . . What about life progress? *Work, 17*(3), 175-182.

Stein, F., & Cutler, S. K. (1998). *Psychosocial occupational therapy.* San Diego: Singular Publishing.

Straker, L. M. (2003). A review of research on techniques for lifting low-lying objects: 2. Evidence for a correct technique. *Work, 20*, 83-96.

Tompa, E., Dolinschi, R., de Olivera, C., Amick, B. C., & Irvin, E. (2010). A systematic review of workplace ergonomic interventions with economic analyses. *Journal of Occupational Rehabilitation, 20*, 220-234.

Toossi, M. (2013). Employment outlook: 2008-18. Labor force projections to 2018: Older workers staying more active. *Monthly Labor Review*, November, 132, 30—51.

Trombly, C., & Radomski M. (Ed.). (2014). *Occupational therapy for physical dysfunction* (7th ed.). Philadelphia, PA: Lippincott Williams & Wilkins.

Warren, N. (2004). The expanded definition of ergonomics. In M. Sanders (Ed.), *Ergonomics and the management of musculoskeletal disorders*. St. Louis, MO: Butterworth-Heinemann.

Washington University in St. Louis. (2005). Meet the faculty. Retrieved at www.ot.wustl.edu on June 12, 2005.

Wegman, D. H., & McGee, J . P. (2004). *Health and safety needs of older workers*. Washington, DC: The National Academies Press.

Yassi, A. (2005). Health promotion in the workplace—The merging of the paradigms. *Methods of Information in Medicine, 44*(2), 278-84.

7

Retirement, Volunteering, and End-of-Life Issues

Marilyn B. Cole, MS, OTR/L, FAOTA

Chapter Objectives

By the end of this chapter, the student will be able to:

- Define retirement and volunteerism as they pertain to the Occupational Therapy Practice Framework.
- Describe specific models/frames of reference as related to retirement and volunteerism.
- Comprehend common problems noted in the retirement process.
- Delineate between the roles of the occupational therapist and the occupational therapy assistant (OTA) as they pertain to the occupations of retirement and volunteerism.
- Comprehend and identify related physical and psychological implications as related to decreased independence in retirement and volunteerism.
- Describe the impact of contextual factors upon retirement and volunteerism.
- Identify appropriate retirement and volunteerism intervention strategies based on various performance skills and client factors.
- Identify general retirement and volunteerism remediation strategies.
- Identify compensation/adaptation intervention strategies related to retirement planning.
- Identify specific volunteerism compensation/adaptation strategies.
- Identify general retirement and volunteerism maintenance strategies.

Retirement Defined

Retirement Definitions

Retirement may be defined as the cessation of paid work (Warner, Hayward, & Hardy, 2010). Although usually associated with older adulthood (ages 60 to 65 years), retirement may occur at

Meriano C, Latella D.
Occupational Therapy Interventions: Function and Occupations, Second Edition (pp 363–401).

any age and for a variety of reasons. A retirement age of 65 was first proclaimed by Chancellor Bismarck of Germany in 1889. He chose this age by adding 20 years to the average life expectancy for his day, which was 45. In 1935, the U.S. government adopted age 65 as the age at which older adults became eligible for retirement pensions (Social Security). Individuals in 1900 spent 3% of their lives in retirement, as compared to 25% to 35% or 20 to 35 years today (Chop, 1999; Warner, Hayward, & Hardy, 2010). Part of the reason for this change is a longer life expectancy, currently 83 years for men and 85 for women (Precis, 2012).

Attempts to define the "typical" retirement life course in America have found current retirement patterns more diverse than in previous years. Using the National Institute on Aging Health and Retirement Study (2008), a large longitudinal study based in the U.S., Warner et al. (2010) found that men aged 50 years can expect to spend half their remaining lives (16 years) working for pay; for women aged 50 years, can expect to spend one third of their remaining lives working for pay, or approximately 12 years. These researchers identified seven retirement-related transitions between employment, retirement, work disability, (including possible multiple re-entries into the labor force), and mortality. Some general patterns include the following:

- A significant spike in numbers of those retiring at age 62, the earliest eligible age for Social Security benefits, although many "retirement events" occur before that age.
- 50% of all men in the study have retired by age 63.
- 16% of men will die while still employed.
- 29% of men who retire will re-enter the work force at least once.
- 35% of women who retire will re-enter the work force at least once.
- For women at age 60, 53% are still working, 8% work disabled, and 33% have retired.
- Significantly fewer women die while employed (7%), and few become work disabled (8%).
- Women's retirement patterns are highly variable and do not coincide with Social Security eligibility.

Another way of viewing the evidence from the Health and Retirement Study (2008) is that permanent retirement is currently the exception rather than the rule (Cahill, Glamdrea & Quinn, 2012). These researchers defined *retirement* as exiting from full-time career employment (10+ years with same job). They found that most retirement is more gradual, often includes "bridge" jobs (60%) or part-time employment and may involve multiple re-entries and exits. This large scale study confirms that today's retirement patterns are many and varied, and that retirement from a career job is not a one-time event but a process that takes place over time for the majority of older Americans. A significant trend among baby boomers recently dubbed the *aging boom* (Azer, 2008) is the emergence of "encore careers" combining purpose, passion, and a paycheck (MetLife Foundation, 2005). This surge of retirement-eligible elders reports that they (1) want to do work that helps others, now and in retirement; (2) need continued income in retirement; (3) want greater flexibility in retirement jobs; and (4) advocate for changes in public policy to remove obstacles for community-oriented second (encore) careers.

These changing patterns have major implications for occupational therapists seeking to design appropriate interventions for retirement transitions. The roles defined by the American Occupational Therapy Association's (AOTA) Occupational Therapy Practice Framework (2014) may need to be altered to include other options in the retirement transition, such as adapting employment and guiding retirees in selecting bridge jobs or seeking other employment alternatives to supplement inadequate income. For baby boomers, encore careers are paid or unpaid positions with social impact (Mercer, 2011) They can represent anything from starting a business, working part time in public service, or returning to school for training in an entirely different career (Cahill et al., 2012).

Retirement preparation and adjustment currently appears under the work area of occupation in the AOTA Framework III (2014). The role of occupational therapy in this area includes "determining aptitudes, developing interests and skills, and selecting appropriate avocational pursuits" (AOTA, 2014, p. S20). This implies the need to replace the worker role by restructuring one's time (temporal organization) and establishing new performance patterns, routines, and roles. Logical outcomes of this process might be linked with occupational therapy's role in the areas of leisure and volunteerism, as well as exploring the possibility of returning to paid work (see Chapter 6 for interventions with older workers).

Retirement and Health

A well-planned retirement for persons in relatively good health usually results in an improvement in mental health and well-being (Mandal & Roe, 2008). However, many people today retire in less than ideal circumstances. Research correlates retirement with increased risk for a broad range of health conditions, including increased stress (Lo & Brown, 1999; Perreira & Sloan, 2001; Sharpley, 1997), depressive symptoms (Szinovacz & Davey, 2004), alcohol consumption (Lin, Guerrieri, & Moore, 2011; Perreira & Sloan, 2001), declines in both physical and mental conditions (Gallo, Bradley, Siegel, & Kasl, 2000), suicide (Di Mauro, Leotta, Giuffrida, Distefano, & Grasso, 2003), and a significantly increased risk of mortality (Morris, Cook, & Shaper, 1994). Variables affecting health in retirement identified by researchers include marital status (Szinovacz & Davey, 2004), socioeconomic status (Wilson, 2001), health insurance (Baker, Sudano, Albert, Borawski, & Dor, 2002), social security retirement incentives (Gruber & Wise, 1999), mental attitude (Fletcher & Hansson, 1991; Mayring, 2000; Reitzes & Mutran, 2004), gender (Geerts, Ponjaert-Kristoffersen, Verbandt & Verte, 1999; Hanson & Wapner, 1994; Quick & Moen, 1998), and life narratives and coping style (Jonsson, 2011; Jonsson, Josephsson, & Kielhofner, 2001).

Health studies at the national level have focused on the factors that interfere with ability to work for those older than 50 years (NIA, 2010). A report entitled "Growing Older in America" summarizes the health findings as follows:

- The top five chronic health conditions for those 55 years and older are (1) arthritis, (2) hypertension, (3) psychiatric/emotional, (4) heart diseases, and (5) diabetes.
- Lifestyle factors significantly increased health risks, including smoking, heavy drinking, obesity, and lack of physical exercise.
- Cognitive health declines with age (10% of those older than 70 years have moderate to severe cognitive impairments), and this places substantial burden on family caregiving.
- Health varies by socioeconomic status and ethnicity. Higher educational level translates to better health, while African American and Hispanics report poorer health than whites (NIA, 2010).

Much medically oriented research has demonstrated the continued competence of older adults, as well as both their inclination and suitability for continued employment or other productive occupations. The Well Elderly study, a well-known randomized controlled trial, and its subsequent replications (Clark et al., 1997, 2011; Jackson et al., 1998; Mountain & Craig, 2011) supports occupational therapy interventions that help community-living older adults to stay active and involved. A recent systematic review of occupational engagement and health outcomes further confirms that a wide variety of occupations and activities can facilitate continued health and well-being for community-dwelling older adults (Stav, Hallenen, Lane, & Arbesman, 2012). These authors suggest increased roles for occupational therapy practitioners in wellness and prevention for this population.

Retirement and Productive Aging

The concept of productive aging, brought into mainstream gerontology in 1982 by Pulitzer Prize winner Richard Butler, challenges the significance of retirement alone as a way to understand the changes in occupational engagement in older adulthood. *Productivity* refers to occupations, both paid and unpaid, that contribute to the "maintenance or advancement of society as well as to the individual's own survival or development" (Creek, 1997, p. 34). This term opens the door for occupational science to define the productive occupations of older adulthood. Knight et al. (2007) identified the five most commonly held productivity roles for older adults. They are home manager, caregiver, volunteer, paid worker, and lifelong learner. An additional role of self-manager, which includes autonomy, self-care, and self-advocacy, is considered productive because it prevents elders from becoming dependent and a "premature social burden" (Donati, Moorfoot, & Deans, 2004). These roles have also been supported by multiple qualitative research studies over the last decade (Carr & Manning, 2010).

Theories of Retirement and Older Adulthood

Most theories addressing the retirement transition are derived from the developmental theories of older adulthood. Historically, Jung and Erikson first proposed that development continues throughout life, and contemporary theories support this notion. Theories of evolution and continuity have replaced ages and stages, and clearly there is little correlation in older adulthood between chronological and developmental ages. Older theories are summarized in Table 7-1.

Continuity Theory

Atchley (1989) suggests that as adults age, they make adaptive choices that tend to preserve existing internal and external structures and strive to maintain their self-identity and existing perceptions of self and the world. Some aspects of Atchley's theory have been validated in more recent studies (Atchley & Baruch, 2004; Reitzes & Mutran, 2004).

Theories of social support and identity have also confirmed that continuing one's social connections and self-categorization as members of specific social groups contributes to older adults' maintaining health and well-being and increased ability to cope with changes later in life (Jetten, Haslam, & Haslam, 2012). This theory supports occupational therapy's use of group interventions with this population, and promotes the importance of occupational therapy interventions that enable older clients to continue their participation with social groups of their own choosing.

The Third Age and Other Contemporary Theories

Peter Laslett's (1989, 1997) idea of separating young retirees from the older ones has growing credibility in light of recent research. Laslett divided life into the following four stages:

- 1: Childhood and preparation for work
- 2: Employment and raising one's family
- 3: Third age beginning with retirement and ending with the onset of disability
- 4: Begins when elder becomes dependent in at least one activity of daily living

The term *third age* represents a change in the culture of aging based on the reality of an extended life expectancy and a delayed onset of age-related functional decline (Carr, 2009; Weiss & Bass, 2002). The third age concept has spawned a worldwide plan of action on aging: to provide for continued growth and education for successful aging to the "young old" and to better prepare them for the "fourth age" of dependency and physical decline (Baltes & Smith, 2001). To accomplish this, thousands of Universities of the Third Age (U3As) have opened across the globe, beginning with the

Table 7-1

Older Developmental Theories of Aging

Theory, Authors, References	Main Concepts
Carl Jung, 1933	Afternoon of Life
Eric Erikson, 1963, 1997	Generativity vs. Stagnation Integrity vs. Despair Transcendence
Activity Theory of Aging, Havighurst, 1961	Keeping busy after retirement preserves health and well being for older adults
Disengagement Theory, Cumming & Henry, 1961	Retirees gradually withdraw from social and work obligations, and narrow social contacts as they age
Atchley's Stages of Retirement, 1975, 1976	1. Honeymoon phase—new retirees actively pursue projects previously precluded by employment, such as traveling or remodeling their homes 2. Disenchantment phase—realization that retirement hasn't worked out as they had hoped, requiring retirees to cope with the negative realities of retirement such as loss of income 3. Re-orientation phase—re-evaluation of life leads to restructuring of one's lifestyle, including a search for meaningful occupations and establishing a new daily routine 4. Termination—advanced aging and the onset of disability necessitate dependence on others

University of Toulouse in 1973, the two major archetypes being French and British U3A models (Formosa, 1996). Most offer educational programs based on the preference of members, including instruction in crochet, dressmaking, bridge, and wine appreciation as well as the study of a broad range of age-related topics dubbed *educational gerontology* (Withnall, 2002). Participants (students) tend to fall within the 60- to 70-year age cohort (Formosa, University of Malta, retrieved April 22, 2005).

For the past two decades, the field of gerontology has embraced the "era of the third age" as the "new paradigm for qualitative research in the United States" (Carr & Manning, 2010, p. 16). This extensive review of productive aging studies leaves little doubt that the emergence of the third age has completely changed the landscape of older adulthood, focusing on late-life productivity, self-development, meaningful engagement in activities, and other positive aspects of aging.

Baltes' Selection, Optimization, and Compensation Theory

Baltes' theory of selection, optimization, and compensation applies both biological and psychosocial theories of aging across the lifespan (Baltes, 1997). Its holistic nature makes this theory especially compatible with occupational therapy.

- *Selection* refers to both biological and cultural factors. Biological selection focuses on maximizing sexual maturation in youth and shifts to the functions of cell repair and maintenance in later life. Cultural influences may promote engagement in specific occupations, such as education, sports, and vocational training during adolescence, which shifts to other occupations at each subsequent life stage. In advanced aging, prioritizing occupational goals becomes more significant as energy resources decrease.

- *Optimization* is the goal-directed allocation of resources; it shifts over the lifespan as one's priorities change. For example, the occupations involved with building a career require the middle adult's full attention and energy, while retirement focuses on finding meaning and self-fulfillment in other productive occupations.
- *Compensation* is the use of environmental factors to support the functions for which people choose not to expend energy and takes place throughout life. For example, older adults may focus on volunteer and leisure occupations and use the assistance of others to compensate for their lack of time spent in home maintenance.

Common Problems in Retirement

The literature on retirement discusses a broad range of positive and negative consequences. Many older adults view retirement as a long-awaited liberation from responsibility, an increase in leisure time, and an opportunity to pursue more creative endeavors (Cohen, 1999). This may indeed be true when retirement is voluntary, accompanied by adequate financial and social pre-planning, and the retiree remains healthy and energetic. However, even the most healthy and well-prepared retirees seem destined to struggle with the transition to retirement. As Clark et al. (1997) predicted, the process requires an active involvement in the redesign of one's lifestyle. The following is a summary of some of the predictable problems with adjusting to retirement:

- Loss of the worker role
- Lack of time structure
- Changes in social interactions and relationships
- Loss of purpose or daily meaning
- Financial factors, loss of income
- Increased stress
- Decline in social status

Loss of the Worker Role

Working involves more than bringing home a paycheck. For many, working becomes very much a part of one's identity. In leaving work after many years of employment, the new retiree may also be leaving behind a vast social network that provided a major source of social and emotional support. People in Western cultures incorporate a strong work ethic that sustains them through educational programs, vocational training, and their income-earning years. However, this same ethic provides little incentive for learning to relax and enjoy life, causing most to arrive at retirement largely unprepared.

Lack of Time Structure

This may be the biggest challenge of all. Work provides a daily structure for most of one's life, through a more or less routine activity (performance) pattern. The Framework defines performance patterns (habits) as "automatic behavior that is integrated into more complex patterns that enable people to function on a day-to-day basis" (AOTA, 2014, p. 27). Younger adults who manage their time effectively often spend 75% to 90% of their day in routines (Cole, 1998). In effect, the loss of these well-learned routines necessitates a large investment of energy in restructuring one's time in ways that are satisfying and meaningful. Assisting retirees in redesigning their lifestyle is an important role for occupational therapists working with this age group.

Changes in Social Interactions and Relationships

After many years of interaction with colleagues and coworkers, retirees often find themselves suddenly disconnected from important social networks. When family relationships and friendships outside of work have not been nurtured along the way, retirement often involves the need to rebuild one's social circles. People who attempt to continue connections with former coworkers often find these relationships unfulfilling. Retirees may need the assistance of occupational therapists in finding new occupations within which to build shared experiences with others.

Loss of Purpose or Daily Meaning

Retirees whose identity is highly invested in their worker role are more likely to experience feelings of depression after leaving work. The loss of pleasure in daily activities can lead to a loss of self-worth accompanied by feelings of helplessness and hopelessness. Part of retirement planning needs to address the exploration of leisure interests and potential volunteer roles that the client finds engaging and meaningful. The types of occupations retired individuals find meaningful vary widely. According to Warr, Butcher, and Robertson (2004), occupations in the "family and social" and "church and charity" domains most highly correlate with affective well-being and life satisfaction. The Jonsson, Josephsson, and Kielhofner (2001) study confirms the importance of "engaging occupations" in the achievement of life satisfaction in retirement. An engaging occupation is one infused with meaning, enjoyment, challenge, intensity, and a commitment or connection with others (the community) (Jonsson, 2011). This finding gives positive guidance for occupational therapy interventions with those anticipating or transitioning into retirement.

Financial Factors and Loss of Income

Statistics tell us that many baby boomers reaching retirement age in the next 3 to 10 years will not be financially prepared (Hershey & Mowen, 2000). For others, retirement will be accompanied by pensions or lump-sum retirement plan payouts that will need careful management in order to provide sufficient monthly income to sustain retirees for another 20 to 25 years. Major marketing efforts in the U.S. focus on this trend, offering investments, financial advisement, long-term care insurance, and retirement community housing options in many appealing locations. Still, a large percentage of retirees will need assistance with adjusting their lifestyle to a lower or fixed income. The AOTA Framework (2014) defines financial management as "using fiscal resources, including alternate methods of financial transaction and planning and using finances with long-term and short-term goals" (p. S19). Finances have a profound effect on one's lifestyle. Occupational therapists may need to assist retirees in restructuring their living arrangements, daily habits, and activity patterns to accommodate changes in economic resources.

Increased Stress

On Holmes' (1978) social readjustment rating scale, retirement ranks number 10 out of 43 stressful life events, yielding a stress score of 43 out of 100. Sharpley (1997) used a self-perceived stress in retirement scale to study the effects of stress on retirees from 6 months to 5 years after retirement. Three factors were found to produce stress: (1) missing work, (2) personal health, and (3) relationship issues. Parsons (2003) looked at the effects of stress on overall lifespan. He noted that the longevity of "well nourished humans of the modern era" cannot be entirely explained by the propensity for stress resistance, and that evolutionary theories of aging need to be considered. Krause (1986) found that older women living alone are more vulnerable to the effects of chronic life strain and stressful life events. McAndrew (2002) notes that many stressful life events can coincide with retirement, having a cumulative effect on the older adult. For example, retirement (stress score 45), may be accompanied by a personal injury or illness (53), a change in financial status (38), a change in the number of marital arguments (35), a change in living conditions (25), and revision of personal habits (24), yielding an overwhelming level of stress for the retiree. Occupational therapists may be called upon the assist clients in identifying stressors, developing or supporting coping mechanisms, and establishing new routines to reduce or manage stress.

Decline in Social Status

Work often provides a basis for social status, not only because of the income generated, but also because of one's position within the work organization. Persons having a powerful position within a corporation or professional organization enjoy a feeling of control over others and their own working conditions and environment. This feeling of control may be difficult to duplicate in avocational pursuits after retirement. Because of the strong work ethic of Western cultures, gainful employment in any capacity implies a higher level of social status than that of unemployment. After retirement, it is inevitable that some older adults will be viewed differently by others in their social circles and communities. The third age movement has done much to counteract the negative stigma of retirement. Ageism in society still creates barriers for older adults seeking continued career growth or experiences in lifelong learning. Occupational therapists can evaluate social contexts in the immediate, community, and institutional environments and assist clients with overcoming these barriers to continued participation through engagement in meaningful occupations with others.

Retirement Interventions

While much has been written about occupational therapist's role with the elderly, little attention has been given to retirement specifically. This section will review individual and group approaches to the various aspects of retirement.

Early Retirement

The incidence of early retirement in the U.S. has declined in recent years, partly due to an increasing scarcity of younger workers. Of those who retire early, approximately 30% do so because of ill health. For these individuals, a decrease in financial wealth due to loss of income has a statistical relationship with a worsening of disability and an increased need for health services (Disney, Grundy, & Johnson, 1994).

Prevention

There is evidence that interventions that promote worker adaptation and employer accommodation following the onset of a health impairment may enable workers to keep their jobs or continue to be gainfully employed (Daly & Bound, 1996). Recent studies show that presenteeism, or working while sick, can affect a worker's productivity even more than its opposite, absenteeism (Precis, 2012). In a review of the effectiveness of workplace health promotion programs, researchers found little consistency in results, suggesting that more care be taken to adjust the programs to workers actual fitness and health needs (Cancelliere et al., 2012). One 6-month occupational health intervention program for workers (aged 50+ years) at risk for early retirement demonstrated a 50% reduction in early retirement (de Boer, van Beck, Durinek, Verback, & van Dijk, 2004). Clients whose illness or injury has caused a leave of absence from their current jobs with the expectation of returning to work may be good candidates for such prevention programs.

Client use of strategies such as incorporating relaxation or exercise into work routines or changing the movements used to accomplish work tasks are examples of worker adaptations. Using adaptive equipment such as sound-enhanced telephones or adapted computer keyboards may be initiated by either client or employer. Examples of accommodations made by the employer might be flexible working hours to accommodate rest or exercise breaks, physical changes in positioning such as ergonomic office chairs, or changes in task demand such as conference calls replacing on-site meetings. Occupational therapists may play a consulting or advisory role with clients and their employers to make mutually beneficial adjustments to the work situation in order to prevent the necessity of early retirement.

Self-assessed poor health has been found to be a strong predictor of early retirement due to mental disorders, musculoskeletal disorders, and cardiovascular diseases (Karpansalo, Manninen, Kauhanen, Lakka, & Salonen, 2004). Workers with chronic low back pain, anxiety, and the perception of control by others contributed significantly to the incidence of early retirement (Harkapaa, 1992). In another study, a positive link was found between cigarette smoking and early retirement due to permanent disability (Rothenbacher et al., 1998). These findings provide evidence of the need for group preventive programs in the workplace.

Establishing, Remediating, and Maintaining Work Functions

When illness or injury causes temporary inability to work, the occupational therapist's role in rehabilitation may focus on work readiness. Specific interventions may be designed to build skills related to an identified work role, as well as building range of motion, strength, and endurance while performing simulated work tasks. See Chapter 6 for specific strategies for work adaptations.

Compensation (Modifying/Adapting)

When health conditions prevent a return to former employment, the occupational therapist's role is somewhat similar to working with an older retiree. Persons facing early retirement need help in making the transition to a new life structure. An assessment of skills and aptitudes may lead to recommendations for volunteer work, alternative part-time work, and/or participation in community organizations. However, there are some essential differences occupational therapists must consider when working with early retirees.

A younger retiree may wish to continue family or social roles that are different from those of an older adult. New areas of socialization with peers of a similar age group may be needed. When working with a younger retiree, special attention should be given to the client's life stage and the occupations that can facilitate continued growth and development. For example, a single or divorced young adult for whom dancing and bicycling are no longer physically possible could participate in discussion groups or organizational fundraising with others in his or her age group. Persons with a specific health condition, such as being a cancer survivor, might find it meaningful to volunteer to help others with a similar condition.

Middle-aged retirees might find meaningfulness in volunteer caregiving roles or roles that utilize their special skills and talents in more creative ways. For example, Debi worked as a nursing supervisor in a busy surgical unit prior to her stroke at age 47. Afterwards, she discovered that she had a latex allergy, one that was exacerbated by the routine use of latex gloves and other equipment during medical procedures. In the year of rehabilitation following her stroke, Debi used her computer to establish an online information center for others with a latex allergy, a role that allowed her to use her medical background to help others by managing the website from the comfort of her home.

Retirement Planning in Older Adulthood

Many older adults do not plan ahead for the time when they will be dependent on others for their care, probably for the same reasons that they do not plan for retirement, being unable or unwilling to visualize their future. With baby boomers reaching retirement age soon, many marketing efforts focus on planning for long-term care, but these efforts focus mostly on investment in retirement communities and purchasing long-term care insurance.

Most sources agree that pre-planning has a positive effect on smoothing the transition into retirement (Nuttman-Shwartz, 2004) as well as life satisfaction afterwards (Reitzes & Mutran, 2004). Some of the factors associated with a successful retirement include a feeling of well-being, relatively good health, continued social interactions, and an optimistic outlook (Mayring, 2000).

Prevention

Hershey and Mowen (2000) examined financial pre-planning skills through the use of hypothetical retirement scenarios requiring the participant to apply problem-solving and decision-making strategies. They concluded that both financial knowledge and personality constructors predicted the extent of pre-retirement planning. One of the most significant findings of this study for occupational therapists is the need for future orientation and an ability to visualize the future. Thus, in addition the need for education and training with regard to financial planning, occupational therapy prevention groups can be designed to focus on the ability to visualize personal future scenarios, to predict the consequences of alternative modes of behavior, and to make conscious choices regarding steps required to achieve one's goals. Furthermore, these researchers suggest that different pre-planning strategies may be required for different personality types. Occupational therapists are well-prepared to develop group activities utilizing different learning styles to promote these essential skills for adequate retirement planning.

Transitions at Retirement: Establishing, Restoring, or Maintaining (Remediating) the Occupational Areas, Skills, and Patterns for Health and Well-Being

Considering recent theoretical developments and research with regard to retirement, clients in the third age must be treated differently from those of the 80+ age group. The preponderance of evidence points toward a continuation of active involvement in occupations and interactions with others as the key to successful retirement for the 60 to 80 age group (Rowe & Kahn, 1998). Occupational therapists need to recognize that the transition to retirement is a process, one that many retirees handle poorly without professional help. Several adult developmental theories can guide occupational therapy interventions for this age group. Some of the tasks are reappraising the past, re-examining one's values and goals, evaluating and nurturing selected social connections, recognizing age- and health-related adaptations, rebalancing one's time, and redesigning one's lifestyle.

Reappraising the Past

In individual work, the occupational therapist may facilitate this process by asking thoughtful questions or through evaluation activities. One useful tool in looking back over one's life is to create a timeline (Figure 7-1). The client identifies significant life events along a continuum from birth to the present. Extending the timeline 10 years into the future will give the occupational therapist an indication of the client's future time perspective.

In one case example, several major changes cluster around specific years creating a pattern of crisis and recovery, with work being the main means of coping. As this individual approaches retirement, pacing the changes and establishing alternate coping strategies is critical.

Reminiscence is another way occupational therapists may facilitate life reappraisal (Parker, 1995). The occupational therapy perspective in planning reminiscence groups (unlike recreational groups) should focus specifically on the client's perceptions of life's accomplishments and

The following is a time line beginning the year you were born and continuing to 10 years from today. Please place an X along this line to record each major event of your life, including year.

- Birth
- Graduations
- Marriage
- Moving to new location
- Birth of children
- Employment changes
- Retirement
- Personal injury or illness
- Specific leisure pursuits begun
- Important volunteer positions initiated or ended
- Any other important life events

X____X _______________X
Birth Now Death

Figure 7-1. Timeline evaluation at retirement with future perspectives (Created by Marli Cole-Shiraldi).

disappointments and on identifying client coping strategies that have failed or succeeded in the past. This group activity may assist clients in identifying the unmet goals and meaningful occupations that will be continued into retirement.

Re-Examining One's Priorities

A natural outgrowth of the reevaluation process may be to affirm or change one's life goals. The value of building wealth leads young adults to spend most of their time and energy advancing their career. In retirement, clients will need to redirect their energy toward other meaningful pursuits, such as deepening their relationships with others or contributing to their communities. Identifying enduring values builds a foundation for setting occupational priorities after retirement, such as joining community organizations (socialization), volunteering for social causes (altruism), engaging in health-promoting or creative activities (physical and mental health), or becoming more active grandparents (meaningful family relationships). Raising awareness of one's values and beliefs increases the likelihood that clients will set occupational priorities that are meaningful and satisfying in their retirement years. Occupational therapists may examine values as a part of the evaluation process or create individual or group interventions that focus on awareness of one's values.

Social Networks: The Importance of Staying Connected

Continued social participation is critical to maintaining older adults' mental and physical well-being and successful aging (Rowe & Kahn, 1998). In a landmark national study funded by the National Institutes of Health, researchers identified some of the patterns of socialization for older adults, finding differing social connections at different ages and specific transitions, such as retirement (Cornwell, Laumann, & Schumm, 2008). To summarize, they found that (1) younger retirees had larger social networks, with less closeness and more non-family members; (2) older retirees' networks were smaller but closer, and involved more frequent socialization with neighbors, religious participation, and volunteering; and (3) some life transitions, such as retirement and bereavement, actually increased social connectedness. In a critically appraised review of occupation- and activity-based interventions, occupational therapy researchers found "strong evidence

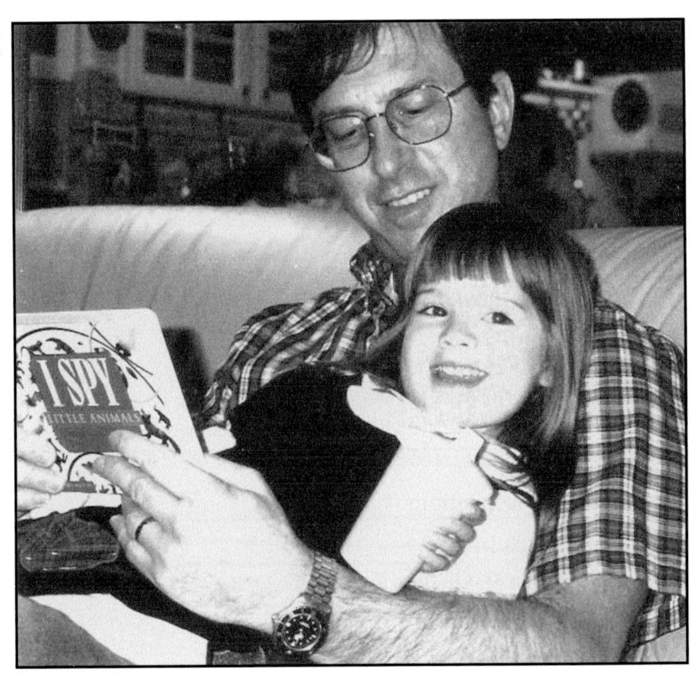

Figure 7-2. Grandpa's changing roles in retirement can include caring for grandchildren.

that links engagement in social activities and participation in social networks to decreased cognitive and physical decline . . . [and to] improved overall quality of life" (AOTA, 2009, p. 2).

For occupational therapists, enabling social participation is a key role with older individuals and populations.

At retirement, daily interaction with coworkers is lost, putting new retirees at risk for social isolation. Family connections, which may not have been nurtured while working, often cause stress rather than satisfaction, according to some studies. Some married retirees find their new-found togetherness 24/7 to be more intrusive than satisfying (Szinovacz & Davey, 2004). An important intervention for occupational therapy may involve identifying occupations that retired couples enjoy doing together, as well as a rebalancing of home maintenance, financial management, and social planning activities.

Retirees with grandchildren may want to change their grandparenting style with retirement (Figure 7-2). Neugarten and Weinstein (1964) identified five patterns of grand parenting: formal, fun-seeking, surrogate, distant, and conveyer of family wisdom. Younger grandparents more likely choose the distant and fun-seeking styles. Retirees may wish to spend more time with grandchildren and to add some wisdom and advice giving to the mix. However, grandparents who become surrogate parents may be risking their own health and well-being because of the disruption child care places on their own meaningful occupations (Ludwig, Hattjar, Russell, & Winston, 2007). In an unpublished study of meaningful activities for older adults in the U.S. and Costa Rica, family relationships and interactions with adult children and grandchildren was the number 1 priority for both cultures (Cole, 2001).

Rebalancing One's Time

Socio-emotional selectivity theory identifies a change in time perspective in older adulthood, adding the recognition that their "time left to live" is limited. Awareness of death gives a new importance to making each day count. With that in mind, occupational therapists can take a closer look at the way clients spend their time, with the following goals:

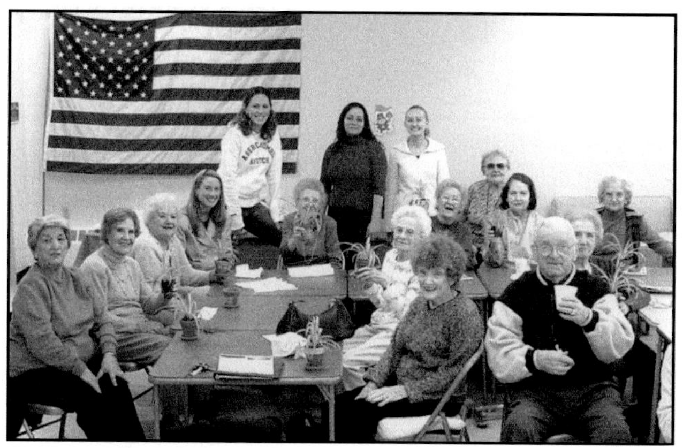

Figure 7-3. Occupational therapy group intervention: from outdoor gardening to caring for houseplants. (Reprinted with permission of Elm Terrace Senior Housing, Stratford, Connecticut.)

- Eliminate occupations that have little meaning, such as watching TV.
- Identify gaps in time that can be available for meaningful occupations such as volunteering, socializing, exercising, or creative pursuits (Figure 7-3).
- Recognizing or establishing routines for obligatory activities such as self-care, home maintenance, grocery shopping, and paying bills.
- Balancing occupational areas of avocation, leisure, self-care, and sleep to meet the older adult's changing physical and psychological needs.

A good occupational therapy evaluation for this area is the activity configuration, which asks clients to keep track of what are doing each hour of the day for 1 week. Filling this out with their family members may assist elderly clients who have memory difficulties (Table 7-2).

The outcome of an activity configuration is a discussion of one's process skills (AOTA, 2014). Occupational therapists need to help older adults to perform occupations more efficiently in order to pace themselves and conserve energy for their most meaningful tasks. Often this means the intentional learning and practice of routines until they become automatic, requiring less physical and mental energy. For example, forming the habit of assembling all ingredients and equipment for a specific meal before beginning the preparation saves on time and energy of making multiple trips to the refrigerator or pantry. Using routines for taking care of basic needs enables the client to spend more time and energy on enjoyment and socialization.

Recognizing Age- and Health-Related Adaptations

A recent study found that leisure participation in older adulthood was "generally preceded by engagement in the same activities earlier in life" (Agahi, Ahacic, & Parker, 2006). In other words, elders continued their lifelong interests when choosing leisure activities in retirement, and they did so in many cases despite functional declines. Occupational therapists assist clients who have health conditions in adapting the form and structure of occupations that have held meaning for them earlier in life. For example, an older client who once enjoyed mountain climbing might need to adapt hiking plans for more level terrain, wear supportive footgear, and limit the length and pace of exploratory walking.

The older adults in Figure 7-3 are not permitted to garden outside their small apartments, even if they felt energetic and flexible enough to do so. Occupational therapy students have helped them adapt their interest in gardening by potting and learning to care for houseplants.

Another occupational therapy approach that sheds light on the role of occupation in well-being is the concept of personal projects (Christiansen, Backman, Little, & Nguyen, 1999). In a study of

Table 7-2

Occupational Activity Configuration

	Mon.	Tue.	Wed.	Thurs.	Fri.	Sat.	Sun.
1 am							
2 am							
3 am							
4 am							
5 am							
6 am							
7 am							
8 am							
9 am							
10 am							
11 am							
Noon							
1 pm							
2 pm							
3 pm							
4 pm							
5 pm							
6 pm							
7 pm							
8 pm							
9 pm							
10 pm							
11 pm							
Midnight							

120 adults, perceived progress in completing personal projects that represented meaningful occupations for individuals was highly correlated with well-being. Engaging occupations, a related concept, was identified by Jonsson et al. (2001; Jonsson, 2011) as those that evoked a depth of passion or feeling, with a specific meaning for the retiree. The presence or absence of engaging occupations "appeared to be the main determinant of whether participants were able to achieve positive life experiences as retirees" (Jonsson et al., 2001, p. 428).

Redesigning One's Lifestyle

The Well Elderly study (Clark et al., 1998) mentioned earlier offers a good example of an occupational therapy intervention program with third age older adults. These researchers note that older adults often have "neither the knowledge nor the ability to determine health-relevant consequences of their occupations" (Clark et al., 1998, p. 329). Eight modules are identified, which guide small groups (of 8 to 10 members) of community-living older adults through an "occupational self-analysis" (Clark et al., 1998, p. 330). Each module forms a structure for several group meetings, which includes some form of didactic presentation, peer exchange, direct experience, and personal exploration. The format allows members to learn, discuss, problem-solve, and make choices according to their own interests and needs. The module content areas are as follows:

1. Introduction to the power of occupation: discussion of how occupational choices affect well-being and create daily structure and meaning.
2. Aging, health, and occupation: building healthy occupational habits and activities.
3. Transportation: alternative ways to access and participate in the community.
4. Safety: in the home and neighborhood, crime prevention strategies, body mechanics.
5. Social relationships: dealing with loss, maintaining friendships, and finding new friends.
6. Cultural awareness: learning and sharing diverse aspects of group members and appreciating how culture shapes our daily occupations and social expectations.
7. Finances: learning skills of budgeting, managing money, and engaging in affordable occupations.
8. Integrative summary: lifestyle redesign journal, and reviewing the collected occupational knowledge and experience of the group using writing and photographs to construct individual roadmaps for the road ahead.

Two replications of the original Well Elderly study have confirmed the effectiveness of this well-designed occupational therapy intervention with both individuals and groups of community-dwelling elders (Clark et al., 2012; Mountain & Craig, 2011). Occupational therapists have the skills to assist older adults in thinking about what needs changing, restructuring one's time to accommodate the changes, and balancing occupations to maintain or restore health, socialization, and personal fulfillment.

End-of-life Issues

Theories of Old Age

Jung and Erikson pioneered the extension adult development theory into later life. Jung (1933) observed the tendency for introversion in later years, focusing on more philosophical and spiritual issues. Of eight stages of focusing on psychosocial development, Erikson's final two stages apply to older adulthood: generativity vs. self-absorption and ego integrity vs. despair (Erikson, 1963; Schuster, 1992; Westermeyer, 2004). Although Erikson envisioned his eight stages as epigenetic, requiring resolution of conflicts in a defined hierarchy, the tasks are potentially reversible and do not necessarily follow a rigid sequence or specific timing (Vaillant, 1993). The primary focus of generativity is "the culmination of adulthood when the individual becomes a responsible guide or mentor for the next generation" (Jetten, Haslam, & Haslam, 2012). More recently, two aspects of generativity have been identified by McAdams, Hart, and Maruna (1998): a desire to play an active role in the next generation and empathy or compassion for others. The extension of generativity into old age was demonstrated by Shmotkin, Blumstein, and Modan (2003), who found that volunteer roles resulted in more positive psychological functioning and reduced mortality risk for the 75 to 94 age group. The primary focus of Erikson's integrity phase is the personal satisfaction with one's accomplishments and contributions, giving importance to the tasks of reminiscence and life review, the late-life resolution of unfinished issues, and reconciliation of past rifts with significant others.

Fourth Age and Other Contemporary Theories

While Laslett's theory represents a continued hierarchy of developmental stages, it acknowledges the relative health and vitality of the 60 to 80 age group as compared with octogenarians (80+), who may indeed exhibit the characteristics of disengagement found by Cumming and Henry (1961) so long ago. However, contemporary theorists view the voluntary withdrawal from selected social roles and obligations as a more positive developmental step (Carr & Manning, 2010; Tornstam, 2011). Johnson and Barer (1992) found that 50% of those older than 85 years could be considered disengaged. Signs of this were a redefinition of social boundaries, a change in time orientation, and a decrease in emotional intensity. This finding supports the theory of socioemotional selectivity described below.

Socioemotional Selectivity Theory

A fundamental change in future time perspective accounts for some of the voluntary narrowing of one's social circles with aging. The fourth age adult's time orientation changes to focus on the present, while future and past diminish. Future becomes less relevant as death approaches, while the past fades away along with the loss of contemporaries who remember them when they were younger. Emotional intensity appears to diminish in elders who have come to terms with mortality, perhaps because they have nothing left to fear. Those older than 85 spend more time sleeping and feel fairly comfortable with spending time alone (Larson, Czikszentmihalyi, & Graef, 1982).

Fourth age elders tend to change their goals from future orientation to goals that make the present more fulfilling, such as loss prevention, continued generativity, greater emotional rewards, and social selectivity (Penningroth & Scott, 2012). Longtime friendships and family relationships take on a deeper meaning, while more superficial relationships are dropped (Wright & Patterson, 2006). This voluntary disengagement allows older adults to conserve emotional energy, pace themselves, and reduce worry about others (Adams, 2004). Another study supporting socioemotional selectivity theory (Carstensen, 1992/1998; Carstensen, Isaacowitz, & Charles, 1999) suggests that social supports provided by new acquaintances within retirement communities are not as meaningful and do not replace the support of longtime friendships (Potts, 1997).

Gerotranscendence Theory

Gerotranscendence, another contemporary outgrowth of disengagement theory, focuses on the positive potential of cognitive changes that occur as the aging individual constructs a new reality, one that shifts from pragmatic and materialistic to a more cosmic and transcendent world view. This internal, contemplative way of life, which trades in meaningless socialization for solitude, appears to be accompanied by an increase in life satisfaction (Tornstam, 1997, 2000, 2011). The cosmic dimension, which conceptually unites the past and present, may symbolize for the older individual true wisdom. In this state, the individual feels free to select only activities that are meaningful and to ignore the necessity for social reciprocation or convention.

Joan Erikson, Erik Erikson's wife and frequent collaborator, wrote at age 93 about the need for solitude as a possible Erikson's ninth stage, a "deliberate retreat from the usual engagements of daily activity . . . a paradoxical state that does seem to exhibit a transcendent quality" (Erikson, 1997, p. 25)."

Baltes' Selection, Optimization, and Compensation Near the End of Life

Baltes and others focus on the balance of positive and negative factors throughout the lifespan, and they note that the scale tips toward the negative as the end of life approaches (Baltes, 1997; Baltes & Baltes, 1990; Baltes & Smith, 2001; Freund & Baltes, 2000). In late life, people compensate for lost capacities through the use of adaptive devices, community resources, or the assistance of caregivers. Ludwig (1998) illustrated this process by describing the "unpackaging" of routines in older women who changed their occupational priorities once child rearing and caregiving obligations ended.

Baltes (1997) built on Laslett's theory in several ways. If the degree of completeness can be defined as the balance between gains and losses in functioning, Baltes cited the fourth age as the most "radical form of incompleteness" (Baltes, 1997, p. 13). Although third agers, thanks to medical, technical, social, economic, and educational advances, have ensured their continued health and psychological functioning, fourth agers face dramatic age-related losses. According to the Berlin Aging Study (Mayer & Baltes, 1996), physical vitality and intelligence declined significantly after age 80, although social and personality factors remained stable. The fourth age may "test the limits of psychological resilience" with regard to maintaining the balance of positive and negative factors, and increasingly so when illnesses such as Alzheimer's are considered (Rapp, Krampe, & Baltes, 2006, p. 52).

Central to this theory is the concept of self-management. Older adults continue to exert control over aging by making individual choices (selection) about their goals and how they allocate limited resources (optimization) to reach them. Baltes uses the following example: "At 80, (noted pianist) Arthur Rubenstein was asked how he managed to still give such excellent concerts . . . He offered three reasons. First, he played fewer pieces—an example of selection. Second, he practiced these more often—an example of optimization. Finally, he played slow movements more slowly, to make it appear as though he were playing the piano faster in the fast movements than he was actually able to—an example of compensation" (Baltes, 2006, p. 35). This illustrates how the application of SOC theory helps older adults to retain their sense of identity and dignity.

Transition From Third to Fourth Ages

By definition, fourth agers have at least one disability that causes them to be dependent on others. Choices need to be made about who will provide needed services. Cultural beliefs vary widely concerning family caregiving, and it cannot be assumed that Grandma will move in with one of her adult children.

Mature Dependence: Making Choices for Needed Care

In a study of self-care with Norwegian retirees, Soderhamn, Skisland, and Harrman (2011) identified some important characteristics of the transition to the fourth age, which they called *mature dependence*. The term implies a dignified acceptance of dependence, which requires "a great capacity to ask for and receive help" in self-care activities elders find difficult or can no longer accomplish alone. Also central to mature dependence are feelings of connectedness and reciprocity, the continued self-concept as a competent and worthwhile adult who also contributes something back to family, friends, and those who provide the care (Soderhamn et al., 2011, p. 277).

Adams, Roberts, and Cole (2011) compared the changes in investment in activities and interests between the young-old (64 to 79) and the old-old (80+). Her findings support specific aspects of disengagement, socioemotional selectivity, and gerotranscendence theories and can guide occupational therapists in determining appropriate interventions for this population. Adams found that interest in some activities diminished significantly from the third to the fourth ages, while other interests remain keen. In summary, this study found that after age 80, interests shift away from active instrumental and social pursuits requiring physical or social effort and toward more social intellectual and spiritual pursuits (Adams, 2004; Adams et al., 2011). These researchers also found that a premature withdrawal from active social pursuits such as attending meetings and planning future events can occur in the presence of functional impairments or can indicate the onset of depression. For occupational therapists, it is important to identify the true developmental stage for clients with mental and physical health conditions. When illness interferes with typical third age

Table 7-3

Adams' Research on Changing Investment in Activities in Elders' Lives

Less Interested After 85	More Interested After 85
Making and creating things	Hearing from family and friends
Shopping and buying things	Spiritual life/prayer
Making plans for the future	Pleasure in small things
Keeping up with hobbies	Visit with family
Entertaining others in my home	Religious services
Social events with new people	Reading, puzzles, computer
Taking care of people and things	Getting together with old friends
Meeting new people	Keeping up with current events
Concern with others' opinions of me	Worrying about friends/family's problems
Feeling I should share opinions and advice	Being a good neighbor

Adapted from Adams, K. B. (2004). Changing investment in activities and interests in elders' lives: Theory and measurement. *International Journal of Aging and Human Development, 58*, 87-108.

pursuits, occupational therapists might help clients identify a need to re-establish social roles and activities such as those listed in Table 7-3, column 1.

Occupational therapists need to be aware of the signs of gerotranscendence and to avoid forcing unwelcome socialization upon fourth age older adults. Those activities in Table 7-3, column 2, can serve as a guide in planning meaningful activities for clients in this stage of life.

Choices for Contexts of Care

As Baltes warned, there comes a time when the negative effects of aging outbalance the positive and the older adult needs the care of others for survival. Currently there are a broad range of choices, depending on one's financial resources and the level of care needed. According to the U.S. Bureau of the Census, only 5% of those older than 65 years live in nursing homes, and about 50% of those older than 95 years live there (USBC, 2010). Researchers predict that the vast majority of older adults who need long-term care will receive it in the community or in their homes (Caffrey, Sengupta, Moss, Harris-Kojetin, & Valverde, 2011). Aging in place means staying in one's own home with adaptations for safety and function and regular visits by health care professionals. Alternately, a client might move in with a family member, invest in specialized housing such as a retirement community or an assisted living facility, or for more frequent care, enter a nursing home. Crist (1999) compared the quality of life among these choices for older adults with an average age of 87. She found that specialized housing offered the highest quality of life related to socialization, while nursing homes offered the lowest quality of life. In each of these choices, occupational therapists can adapt the environment to maximize occupational performance in self-care, self-management, and other activity choices, recognizing that changes in personal routines and habits are more difficult for the older age group. Elders who choose to live alone may need assistance in finding resources to take care of basic necessities. Occupational therapists need to be knowledgeable about community services including housekeeping, transportation, and socialization opportunities that are not beyond the abilities of the elder client.

Changes in residence and living conditions cause stress at any age but may be more stressful for the older adult who simultaneously faces a decline in health status. An older adult who has well-learned routines for self-care may be able to function fairly independently in a familiar environment, but that same individual may be totally dependent in unfamiliar one. Occupational therapists may need to work with the elder and caregivers to re-establish self-care routines in a new setting and to bring in familiar objects, such as quilts, pictures, books, or a wall clock with a familiar look and sound. One older adult who tended to get agitated found it a great comfort to sit and rock in a familiar rocking chair that was brought in by her daughter.

Choices for Scaling Down Belongings

The transition of moving to smaller living quarters involves making decisions about what to keep and what to give away, sell, or discard. Tasks such as these require a high level of cognition. When a fourth age client shows signs of mild dementia, the sorting of belongings may require the help of a family member. Some tasks for the occupational therapist, family, and client in this area are determining criteria for what to keep, what to discard, and who will be recipients of discarded items. Making these choices depends on what goals and occupations the client selects as priorities. Once that decision is made, the accompanying decisions about what will be kept become much easier. For the gardener, appropriate tools and outdoor clothing would be important to keep, for example. Adaptations to allow the older gardener to continue that work might also become the role of the occupational therapist.

Supporting Self-Management for Chronic Conditions

For occupational therapists, supporting client self-management refers to helping clients to care for themselves, including making good choices to preserve their own health, well-being, and life meaning. In the presence of illness, self-management means "ability to manage the symptoms, treatment, physical and psychosocial consequences, and lifestyle changes inherent in living with a chronic condition" (Barlow, Wright, Sheasby, Turner, & Hainsworth, 2002). Occupational therapists working in home and community health care suggest that self-management support be an important new role for occupational therapists (Vance & Siebert, 2009).

In 2007, the most common primary diagnoses for those using home health services were diabetes mellitus (10.1%), heart disease (8.8%), cancer (3.9%), chronic obstructive pulmonary disease (3/4%), and stroke (3/3%). Of these, 80% had at least one limitation in activities of daily living (ADL), 50% had four to five areas of limitation, and 40% to 50% did not receive professional help with ADLs (Caffrey et al., 2011). This study demonstrates the need for more occupational therapy services in home care for those with chronic diseases.

For occupational therapists, self-management support has been defined as a client-centered, collaborative process toward achieving functional independence and maintaining health and well-being (Vance & Siebert, 2009). These authors stress the importance of evaluating occupational performance in the context of routines, taking into account all of the client's daily activities, with a focus on energy conservation, balancing fitness and function, and measuring outcomes over the range of occupations performed. The two most frequent causes for rehospitalization for home health clients with chronic conditions are ineffective medication management and falling. Occupational therapists can enable clients to organize routines for taking multiple medications, and preventing falls, by explaining the connection between the medications and their resulting effects on symptoms that interfere with occupational performance. For example, taking "water pills" improves one's ability to breathe and prevents the dizziness that might cause a fall. Likewise, daily physical exercise increases endurance for doing the activities that give life meaning, such as going on an outing with grandchildren. Occupational therapist-facilitated groups in the community can also effectively support self-management of chronic conditions, as demonstrated by Lorig, Sobel, Gonzalez, and Minor (2006).

Facilitating Information Literacy

Finding information about any subject is as easy as connecting to the World Wide Web, as any student can tell you. This potentially makes the Internet a powerful self-management tool for those who use it wisely and with discretion. The problem is, many of today's seniors have not yet crossed the "digital divide" and remain "digital immigrants" (Prensky, 2008). Occupational therapists can help clients to explore ways to access the Internet and build their searching skills to keep abreast of the latest developments of concern to their own health conditions. According to Post (2010), occupational therapists "can empower clients to increase control over their own health and better manage disease and risk by helping them to access health information more efficiently" (p. 3).

Safety Issues in Physical, Cognitive, and Sensory Loss

An impairment that results in loss of function may trigger an occupational therapy referral to evaluate a clients' physical ability and competence to engage in daily activities within safe parameters. Occupational therapists must often walk a fine line between function and safety when making recommendations for older clients. For example, an occupational therapist evaluated Jacob's home setting after rehabilitation for a hip replacement. Jacob now used a rolling walker, which fit easily through doorways but got caught on the throw rugs in his bedroom. Following protocol, the occupational therapist recommended removing all the throw rugs. Jacob objected, because under the rugs was a hardwood floor, and when Jacob got up at night, he sometimes fell off the edge of the bed, and the rugs would cushion his fall. So instead of removing the rugs, the occupational therapist had a bed pole installed (a floor to ceiling pole positioned next to the bed), which Jacob could grip while sitting up in bed, allowing him stability to prevent falling and orienting him to his walker parked next to it.

Maintaining Physical Fitness

A recent conversation with older adults living in a senior housing project focused on their fear of falling. Many of these elders had health conditions that affected their mobility, including arthritis, hip or knee replacement surgery, multiple sclerosis, and low vision. Their fear of falling prevented them from performing health maintenance activities, like walking around the block or taking public transportation to community social activities and services. This exemplifies one of the many barriers to participation that could be addressed by occupational therapists. Adapted senior fitness programs provide needed exercise that gives clients the confidence to try other activities without the fear of falling. Occupational therapists can add a fun element to exercise, such as dancing to the oldies or organizing teams to compete for a prize. Once established, fitness teams may become self-sustaining, encouraging one another to keep going.

The Choice to Stop Driving

Driving safety is one of the special certification programs offered to occupational therapists by AOTA and offers training in evaluating and remediating the driving skills of all adults. This and other driving safety programs have provided many useful interventions for older drivers, including visual, motor, educational, passenger, and medical (Hunt & Arbesman, 2008). However, even with additional "refresher" training, many older adults will exhibit dysfunctions that render them unable to drive a car safely. This is an especially significant loss, because for many it means giving up a large part of their independence, especially in areas where public transportation is unavailable. One recent study notes that driving cessation "triggers a subjective shift in self-perception," signifying a move from the third to the fourth age (Jetten & Pachana, 2012). According to these authors, driving symbolically represents "competence, independence, freedom, and mobility" (p. 104). Giving up driving threatens an older adults' sense of well-being, igniting fears of abandonment, social isolation, and dependence on others and excluding them from mainstream society (Windsor et al., 2007). Occupational therapists must recognize the importance of this transition to prevent these fears from becoming a reality. Finding ways for clients to remain members of the social groups and organizations that contribute to their social identity and well-being will significantly reduce the stress that often accompanies loss of the ability to drive.

Compensating for Sensory Loss

Many products may be found on the market to compensate for sensory loss. Beyond the obvious hearing aids and spectacles, one finds devices such as talking alarm clocks, sound-enhanced telephones, lighted magnifiers, and large print books. However, the occupational therapist's role will often be to adapt these enhancers for use with specific activities and environments to enable desired occupational performance. For example, inserting textured tape on the numbered dial of the microwave enables the client with low vision to choose the correct number of minutes for heating up a frozen dinner independently. Discussion with older adults regarding other safety issues may include driving safety, walking safety, meal preparation safety, use of home appliances, reaching for items in high or low cabinets, home repair activities, and yard work or gardening. Communication devices and accessibility in case of emergency is another important consideration for occupational therapists working with elders living alone.

Preventing and Managing Cognitive Decline

Cognitive loss may be the most feared decline in older adulthood. Some researchers have found that lifestyle choices have a protective benefit, such as regular physical and mental exercise (Plassman, Williams, Burke, Hoslinger, & Benjamin, 2010) and engaging in mentally challenging occupations (Metz & Robnett, 2011).

Allen's cognitive disabilities reconsidered (Levy & Burns, 2011) model provides a scientific backdrop to guide occupational therapy interventions for cognitive decline. Allen's cognitive levels in reverse can parallel the major phases of dementia, as follows:

- Mild dementia represents Allen cognitive level (ACL) 5, highlighting a loss of the ability to plan ahead or anticipate consequences (e.g., cannot manage finances or host social events).
- Moderate dementia roughly corresponds to ACL 4, noting the inability to understand what cannot be seen (e.g., cannot safely use appliances or machinery).
- Severe dementia might represent ACLs 3, 2, and 1, conveying a downward sequence of losses beginning with the loss of ability to perform tasks that require more than one step. Most ADL activities require assistance at this level, unless the client has well-learned routines. This exemplifies why learning routines earlier in the process is important to preserve some level of functional independence in self-care.

The Allen cognitive level screening, the routine task inventory, and the Allen diagnostic module, provide the occupational therapist with an opportunity to observe a client's level of problem solving in ADL. Guidelines of environmental adaptations, caregiver education, appropriate adaptive equipment, and assistance required for maximum functional independence within safety parameters may be found in Allen, Blue, and Earhart (1995, 2001). Levy and Burns (2011) apply the Allen cognitive levels in rehabilitation of adults with dementia; they further define nine cognitive performance test (CPT) levels in working with older adults.

Another helpful approach for clients with dementia is reminiscence. Because long-term memory usually remains intact, even clients with moderate to severe dementia can benefit from reminiscence, but mostly when offered in groups (Haslam, Jetten, Haslam, & Knight, 2012). According to these authors, the sharing of distant memories of the self within a group provides a buffer against identity loss. When compared with individual reminiscence therapy and group games, the group reminiscence activity produced the most improvement in cognitive performance and general well-being for clients with moderate to severe dementia (p. 303). This finding supports the use of Mildred Ross' five stage groups, using reminiscence themes and socialization strategies, for this population (Cole, 2012; Ross, 2007).

Hospice Care: Occupational Therapy Roles

By definition, clients qualify for hospice care only within their last 6 months of life, through a doctor's certification of limited life expectancy. Hospice brings a more humane end to life, often avoiding costly and disruptive medical procedures to artificially prolong life. Some studies of hospice use in the U.S. and Canada revealed that use of hospice services has increased markedly, but the timing of referral remains poor, with one third enrolled within 7 days of death (Hospice Foundation of America, 2010). A broad range of health conditions may be the cause, the most common of which are cancer and heart disease (Caffrey et al., 2011). Hospice care may be provided at specialized facilities or in the client's own home, guided by the following five principles:

1. Pain and symptom control, for comfort, not cure
2. 24-hour care available in familiar and comfortable surroundings
3. Diagnostic honesty, full openness with client and family
4. Quality of life for client, respect for preferences and choices
5. Bereavement care for the family

According to AOTA, occupational therapy's role in hospice care is to contribute to a comprehensive plan involving the client and family in daily living activities of work, leisure, and self-care (AOTA, undated brochure). Occupational therapists work to enable occupations as follows:

- Enabling occupations that help clients tie up loose ends
    - Finishing or handing off work-related tasks if recently employed
    - Mounting and labeling photographs
    - Writing down experiences or family history
    - Writing letters or e-mailing estranged relatives or friends
    - Finishing personal projects
- Continuing routine occupations that maintain client sense of well being
    - Independence in self-care as desired
    - Care of pets, gardening
    - Sharing meals with significant others
    - Distance participation in meaningful group activities (computer, camera cellphone, conference calls)
- Enabling occupations that deepen spiritual experience
    - Participation in religious rituals, discussions, reading
    - Giving away belongings that symbolize connection with others
    - Craft projects that have symbolic meaning, memorial quilts, jewelry making
    - Remembering, thanking, or forgiving others through occupations, such as writing poems, stories, cards, artwork or music, giving gifts
    - Planning one's own funeral, with or without family input

In the hospice setting, occupational therapists need to advocate for conditions that help clients to make the most of their time left to live. Assessing client's roles, routines and occupational priorities become a basis for occupational therapy client advocacy with the health care team. Sometimes lowering medication may be preferred to enable client choice, and the distraction of occupation can serve to diminish the experience of pain. Terminally ill clients often prefer to endure some pain in order to continue valued social roles or deal with end-of-life issues through engagement in occupations. Energy conservation becomes an important strategy for occupational therapy, so that clients can engage in occupations that have the highest priority for them. For example, clients may choose to have self-care tasks done by others, so that they can save their energy for communication with significant others, event planning, or creative efforts (Jacques, 2002; Marcil, 2005).

Most hospice programs do not include occupational therapy services because they are unaware of the valuable services occupational therapists can provide (Tigges & Marcil, 1988). These authors suggest that occupational therapists approach hospice programs through volunteering, offering educational presentations, or doing pilot research projects to demonstrate occupational therapy's value for terminally ill clients.

VOLUNTEERING

Volunteering Defined

Volunteering refers to unpaid work. The word implies that persons participate in volunteer roles by choice, and that these roles have some purpose or usefulness for others, the community, or society. According to the U.S. Department of Labor, in 2011, 26.8% of adults volunteered at least once through or for an organization. Of these, persons aged 35 to 54 years were most likely to volunteer (approximately 30%), while persons in their early 20s were least likely (19.4%) (www.bls.gov, 2012). Those 55 years of age and older averaged 28.1%, with this declining as age increased. Those employed full or part time had a higher volunteer rate than those not in the work force (2011).

According to an Experience Corps study (AARP, 2003) the "next generation of retirees will be the healthiest, longest lived, best educated, and most affluent in history" (p. 1). Yet many healthy older Americans with no care giving responsibilities currently do not engage in any productive role, either paid or unpaid (Zedlewski & Butrica, 2007). This fact gives cause for concern, especially when one considers the overwhelming evidence that as people age, their engagement in volunteering provides multiple health benefits (Brown et al., 2011; Lum & Lightfoot, 2005; Yuen, 2007). In addition to the traditional volunteer for charity organizations, volunteering refers to community service learning, student internships, and court-ordered programs. These areas define the more formal volunteer roles. The more informal work activities people do without pay might include caregiving for children or aging relatives, home and yard maintenance, or providing occasional help to one's neighbors and friends. The domains of concern for occupational therapists outlined by the AOTA Framework are volunteer exploration and volunteer participation.

Volunteer exploration is defined as "determining community causes, organizations, or opportunities for unpaid 'work' in relationship to personal skills, interests, location, and time available" (AOTA, 2014, p. 21). In this aspect of volunteering, the tasks are similar to those required for seeking paid work. The client's knowledge, skills, and interests need to be evaluated and matched to available opportunities for local volunteer positions. For some clients, occupational therapists may need to take a closer look at the tasks and determine the activity demands required in the volunteer "jobs" being considered. AOTA (2014) defines activity demand as "the aspects of an activity, which include the objects and their properties, space, social demands, sequencing or timing, required actions and skills, and required underlying body functions and body structure needed to carry out the activity" (p. 638). A part of exploration also considers time availability. The occupational therapist may need to look at a client's overall use of time to determine how much time would be optimal for that individual to devote to volunteering.

Volunteer participation is defined by AOTA (2014, p. S21) as "performing unpaid work activities for the benefit of identified, selected causes, organizations, or facilities." Occupational therapists may assist clients in establishing needed skills, building or remediating required abilities for the tasks involved, and/or making the necessary adaptations to enable the client to participate in a volunteer experience safely.

Purpose of Volunteering

Giving back to the community, working for valued causes, making new friends, learning new skills, and finding expression for one's talents, skills, and creativity are some of the many reasons why people volunteer. It cannot be assumed that motivation for volunteering is always altruistic. Different reasons for volunteering have been associated with different age groups. For example, children and adolescents may volunteer for the purpose of increasing their understanding of, or empathy for, disadvantaged groups such as the homeless (Karafantis & Levy, 2004). Kuperminc, Holditch, and Allen (2001) suggest that adolescents who volunteer benefit from a greater sense of connection to their communities, a better work ethic, and a greater concern for the welfare of others. For adolescents, this finding may suggest that youths at risk for problem behaviors might volunteer as a preventive measure.

Young adult students may seek or be required to volunteer in unpaid internships with the purpose of learning and acquiring job-related skills. Internships form a part of the standard training of certain professions, occupational therapy among them. Volunteer roles for students in many different fields, including business, communications, journalism, and the law, may lead to future employment opportunities. New graduates and those temporarily unemployed may view volunteering as a continuation of their career path, or an opportunity for finding "the key to the boardroom door" (Graff, 1993). Six motivational factors were identified by Okun, Barr, and Herzog (1998): career, enhancement, protection, social, understanding, and values.

In midlife, parents who experience a diminished caregiving role as their children grow up may fill the void with volunteer activities. Full-time workers and breadwinners have little time to devote to volunteering, yet workers are more likely to volunteer than the unemployed, possibly due to corporations that encourage civic engagement in their communities. Those with chronic mental or physical illness may seek volunteer work as an alternative to competitive employment. This group is of special concern for occupational therapists, who may need to help clients overcome both internal and external barriers to volunteer participation.

For older adults, one indication of productive aging is volunteering. Some researchers consider volunteering a "very significant form of social participation for seniors" (Godbout, Filiatrault, & Plante, 2012, p. 23). One of the major motivators for this age group is altruism, accompanied by the need to feel useful and productive (Brown, et al., 2011). In considering both formal and informal roles, 26% of older adults volunteer for organizations, 29% informally help the sick or disabled, and 33% help to care for their grandchildren (Caro & Morris, 2001). For many older adults, volunteering replaces the lost worker role, fills gaps in increased leisure time, and provides meaning or purpose in daily activities (Mulcher, Burr, & Caro, 2003). However, Ewald (1999) points out that volunteering does not provide meaning if it is considered busy work. Good matches need to be made between a person's talents and a real need in the community for the elder "to mentor, educate, assist, and guide the next generation" (p. 325). Here again, occupational therapists need to develop knowledge of volunteer opportunities in order to use activity analysis and synthesis in matching volunteer roles with client abilities and priorities.

Benefits of Volunteering

The benefits of volunteering differ across age groups and are closely tied with the reasons for volunteering. For children and adolescents, service to the community and broadening understanding and empathy for diverse social groups are an important benefit. However, to enact this benefit, the volunteer experience must be combined with education and a facilitated discussion of the meaning of the service, a potential role for occupational therapists working with youth.

For students and young adults, career exploration and networking for future career development might be paramount. Volunteers in the public education, public service, or law enforcement are examples of areas that build volunteer skills and understanding of how the system works. Occupational therapy students regularly volunteer as a prerequisite for educational program admission. Additionally, occupational therapists themselves may find volunteering useful in paving the way for community-based employment or advocacy.

While volunteering can have mutual benefits for persons of any age, recent research tells us that those who benefit the most from volunteering are older adults. This age group has been widely studied, and the results demonstrate that volunteering prevents depression (Musick & Wilson, 2003), increases physical and psychological health (Greenfield & Marks, 2004; Lum & Lightfoot, 2005), increases well-being (Morrow-Howell, Hinterlong, Rozario, & Tang, 2003; Pavlova & Silbereisen, 2012; Wheeler, Gorey, & Greenblatt, 1998), and in many cases prolongs life (Musick, Herzog, & House, 1999). For this reason, occupational therapy interventions with this population should include volunteer exploration, placement, and ongoing problem solving in the volunteer workplace.

Volunteer Interventions: Occupational Therapist Roles

Guiding the Exploration Process

Evaluation of the client's skills and abilities, as well as limitations and barriers are the first concern of the occupational therapist. In many ways, preparing to volunteer resembles preparing a resumé for employment, and in fact some volunteer placement agencies require the potential volunteer to submit a resumé. Many community organizations depend on volunteers to supplement the work of paid employees. This requires a commitment of time and energy, and potential volunteers need to be willing to make such a commitment.

Assessing Client Reasons for Volunteering

The next step in searching for volunteer opportunities requires a clarification of the client's reasons for volunteering. Some common reasons are the following:

- Substitute work role, career exploration, learn new skills
- Altruistic, furthering a cause I believe in
- Socialization, make new friends
- Structure time, get out of the house and do something useful for others
- Egoistic, use talents, be creative, mentor others
- Leisure focus, do something I enjoy

Interventions that assist the client in clarifying their volunteer desires and specific interest areas will greatly facilitate the location of appropriate opportunities.

Table 7-4

Examples of Volunteer Clearinghouse Websites

Volunteer Group	Internet Address
Retired Senior Volunteer Program (RSVP)	www.seniorcorps.gov
Quintessential Careers (paid & unpaid)	www.quintcareers.com/volunteering.html
Service Corps of Retired Executives (SCORE)	www.score.org
Volunteers in Service to America (VISTA)	www.friendsofvista.org or www.recruit.cns.gov
AARP Community Service Website	www.aarp.org/about_aarp/community_service /index.html *or* www.aarp.org/community_service
Woman's Day volunteers	www.womansday.com/volunteer
End Childhood Hunger	www.strength.org
Volunteer Talent Bank (VTB)	www.serviceleader.org/old/advice/seniors/html
Foster Grandparents	www.seniorcorps.org/joining/fgp
Senior Companion Program	www.seniorcorps.org/joining/scp
National Retiree Volunteer Center (NRVC)	www.voa.org/tier3_cd.cfm
Volunteer Abroad	www.volunteerabroad.com
Volunteer Match	www.volunteermatch.org

Where to Find Volunteer Opportunities

One only needs to enter the word *volunteering* in any Internet search engine to find thousands of volunteer opportunities (Table 7-4). Most internet clearinghouses identify organizations within a few miles of one's local area and classified according to specific areas of interest. However, many clients, especially those with a lower socioeconomic status, may not have Internet access or the skills necessary to use these services. The occupational therapist should be prepared to search the Internet and narrow down options that are appropriate for the client. To do the job right, the occupational therapist needs to investigate the job descriptions for volunteers and to analyze the specific tasks required. Follow-up phone calls or on site visits may be required to assess the many task demand and contextual factors involved, especially for clients with a disability that must be accommodated.

Identifying Volunteer Roles

Once the client skills and priorities have been identified, client reasons for volunteering need to be matched with the types of volunteer jobs available. One volunteer clearinghouse (www.nottinghamcvs.co.uk) categorizes the types of volunteer roles as follows:

- Practical, immediate action: concrete tasks such as feeding the homeless
- Helping people solve their problems: advocacy, crisis intervention
- Getting the organization's job done: managing, office tasks, fund-raising
- Concern for people and relationships: providing caregiving, social support
- Influencing and promoting change: political action, lobbying for social change

This website offers a questionnaire to help identify which type applies to the individual.

Volunteering provides a sense of continuity, commitment, and connection for older adults, who make their unpaid work roles a part of their identity, according to Brown et al. (2011). Clients need to feel that the volunteer role they perform has both a personal and an organizational meaning, and this requires a good match between meeting client needs, such as socialization or an outlet for skills and creativity, and meeting the needs of recipients of service. According to Merrill (2000), for persons to view their volunteering positively and sustain their interest, there needs to be a balance between giving and receiving.

Common Barriers to Volunteer Participation

Many other factors contribute to this mutual satisfaction of needs. Some are adequate training and coordination of volunteers, clear expectations of the volunteer role, adequate supervision and positive reinforcement, flexibility in time constraints, and willingness to accommodate to physical and social contexts. Two common barriers from the client's perspective are time and financial constraints (Warburton, Paynter, & Petriwskyj, 2007). Older adults who enjoy the freedom of traveling frequently or planning spontaneously hesitate to commit themselves to specific days and times for volunteering on an ongoing basis. In a recent study of retired occupational therapists, Cole and Macdonald (2011) found that although "retirees are highly motivated by altruism and the wish to stay connected with others through volunteering, they often find the existing structure of the organizations unable or unwilling to provide the kinds of volunteer roles that meet their needs and goals" (p. 18). In a more general study, retirees had trouble finding volunteer opportunities that were appealing and flexible (Mutchler, Burr, & Caro, 2003). When problems arise, the occupational therapist may facilitate mutual problem solving in the volunteer workplace. Consulting with organizations that depend on volunteers to guide them in revisioning the way they define and organize volunteer roles might be an important new role for occupational therapists in the community.

Lack of Structure

Volunteer roles vary widely in the amount of structure they provide. Some, such as the AARP Driver Safety Program, are highly structured with specific job descriptions and a training program for each role (www.aarp.org/life/drive/drivervolunteer). Others, such as friendly visitor programs, depend on the volunteers to structure their own schedule and work. Studies of burnout and dropout show that volunteers are more likely to leave a volunteer job because of too little structure and role ambiguity (Ross, Greenfield, & Bennett, 1999). The occupational therapist can work with clients and volunteer supervisors to organize and structure the volunteer role according to the needs of both.

Inadequate Supervision

For direct service roles, such as adult literacy or soup kitchens, feedback in the form of appreciation or suggestions may come directly from the recipients. Volunteers in these types of settings report an increase in satisfaction with volunteering. However, there are many behind-the-scenes, fund-raising, or administrative roles that do not provide much feedback or appreciation. Volunteers need guidance and feedback in order to serve more effectively and to reap the benefits of volunteering, such as daily meaning and a sense of well-being. Some organizations have performed their own studies of volunteer retention and have developed strategies for giving needed feedback, such as recognition events or awards. However, occupational therapist's can advise volunteer organizations in providing the effective supervision to meet the needs of specific clients or client groups. For example, volunteers with mental health issues need a great deal of reassurance and direction with regard to appropriate social behaviors and boundaries. Knight (2004) identifies several keys to continued volunteer participation for those with mental health conditions, including peer support networks, utilization of home health aides, individual case management, and crisis intervention programs.

The Stigma of Disability

Perhaps the most disturbing barrier to volunteer participation is social stigma. The social attitudes of volunteer recruiters play an important part in the successful placement of those with mental or physical disabilities. A study by Lauber, Nordt, Falcato, and Rossler (2002) found two categories of social attitude toward volunteers in psychiatry: (1) antipathetic, including a negative view of mental illness and a desire for social distance, and (2) socially responsible, including a positive attitude and an interest in social issues. Advocacy is needed to overcome the barrier of stigma for all types of disability, and this may become the focus of occupational therapy for specific clients who wish to participate in specific community services.

Unreasonable Expectations

Some areas of volunteering involve greater levels of stress and emotional burden than others. In studying volunteer burnout with persons with AIDS, emotional overload was a common reason for dropout (Ross et al., 1999). Caregiving roles for many special populations have a similar risk, and this needs to be considered in the occupational therapy volunteer role analysis. Some volunteers have a greater capacity for emotional involvement than others. For example, those who volunteer in bereavement or hospice programs need a high tolerance for dealing with intense emotions of others (Mitchell & Shuff, 1995). Physical limitations also place volunteers at risk for burnout, such as too many hours or not enough coverage for specific roles. Older adults may need to consider energy limitations and fatigue when scheduling volunteer hours.

Time Constraints

In assisting clients with volunteer roles, the occupational therapist needs to be aware of the balance of activities that make up a client's lifestyle. Linda Fried, director of the Center for Aging and Health at Johns Hopkins University, suggests 15 hours a week of volunteering are needed for older adults to reap health benefits (Marek, 2005). However, the amount of time clients can devote to volunteer roles will vary widely, and occupational therapists need to consider each client's individual needs. Working with activity patterns, daily routines, and time management become the focus of occupational therapy in this area.

Physical and Social Contexts

Volunteers with disabilities will need a variety of physical and social adaptations to the contexts of volunteer roles. Physical adaptations will be similar to those needed for adapting work settings and work task demands. Social support has perhaps the greatest influence of volunteer satisfaction and well-being (Sadler & Marty, 1998). Positive relationships with volunteer coworkers is a powerful motivator in volunteer retention and sustained interest. Many older adults depend on volunteering to meet their needs for social contact, while others need to feel needed, useful, and appreciated. Building social environments that support volunteer participation must include opportunities for social interaction and positive reinforcement.

Enabling Client Opportunities for Community Involvement

The enduring truth that helping others also helps yourself cannot be questioned. Yet many organizations report severe shortages of volunteers, while many qualified and motivated people never consider volunteering. Community clearinghouses and listings do not go far enough in matching potential volunteers with the right placements. This would be an excellent role for future occupational therapy community efforts. Recent evidence provides some guidance for getting clients involved in volunteering. Currently, many older volunteers do so as a continuation of roles they began earlier in life, making it easier to transition from work to retirement. Retirees who did not volunteer while working may need to learn this new role, and they are more easily enticed through personal invitations to "help out" (Brown et al., 2011). Furthermore, intergenerational volunteering appeals because it gives elders the opportunity to pass on knowledge, wisdom, and lessons in life experience to future generations (Godbout et al., 2012).

Helping Others Like Yourself

Many human interest stories in the media showcase the therapeutic value of victims and survivors helping others like themselves. Most self-help organizations have come into existence this way, including Alcoholics Anonymous, Breast Cancer Support Service, American Society of Pain Management, Compassionate Friends, and Weight Watchers. The timing of one's involvement in public sharing of one's experiences is critical and different for each individual. In the continuum of adaptation to chronic illness, early stages of shock, denial, and anger do not lend themselves well to any interventions, peer or otherwise. Occupational therapists may create group interventions that focus on the transition from denial to acceptance of one's illness or injury and the limitations it imposes on continued participation in life. The success of occupational therapy interventions that remediate or compensate for disability may depend on client readiness to accept such help. Peer volunteers may be a valuable resource in creating such readiness for therapy. As occupational therapy becomes effective in enabling occupational performance, clients might be encouraged to join self-help groups that encourage sharing of experience and group problem solving.

Public Service at the Community Level: Advisory Boards, Senior Centers, and Consumer Groups

Occupational therapy roles with volunteers include encouragement of participation on appropriate advisory boards, community leadership groups, and advocacy groups. In the case example of Al later in this chapter, advisory board participation led to continued employment opportunities after an involuntary retirement due to illness. Clients need to be empowered to participate in their communities at whatever level they are able. As occupational therapists become more knowledgeable about public service opportunities, they will more easily find ways to involve clients who would benefit from such connections.

Advocacy for Self and Others

Several studies have reported the need for parents of children with disabilities to learn the role of advocacy for their children (Lawlor & Mattingly, 1998; Pearl, 1993). Volunteering with school systems, community service organizations, and health agencies are all good ways to learn how the system works, learn how to make it work for you, and find helpful connections for enacting social change. Adults with acquired illness also identify "the system" of health service delivery to be a major obstacle to accessing services such as occupational therapy that would enable their continued participation in important life roles (Macdonald, 1998). Advocacy groups for other causes such as Defenders of Wildlife and the American Society for the Prevention of Cruelty to Animals offer a variety of volunteer opportunities that can be easily found on their websites.

Religious, Ethnic, and Political Organizations

These organizations offer volunteer opportunities across the lifespan. As people age, connections with their religious and cultural background take on deeper meaning. Volunteering may be a good way for older adults to keep in contact with others who share similar values and beliefs.

Informal Caregiving as "Volunteer" Work

As a final word, family members and friends who regularly perform caregiving need to be recognized for the very important role that they play in the lives of clients. In client-centered care, family caregivers may be equal partners in choosing, planning, and carrying out therapeutic interventions. Especially for older women, caregiving often goes unrecognized as a positive productive (volunteer) role (Nestenuk & Price, 2011). The burden of caregiving should be considered when designing meaningful occupational therapy interventions, and support for the caregiver needs to be included in the process. Occupational therapists should treat this form of volunteering with the highest respect and admiration.

Baby Boomers and Volunteering

Baby boomers, born 1946 to 1964, form the next several waves of retirees to become available for volunteering, but population studies predict that they may not be as motivated to do so as older cohorts (Mercer, 2011). Boomers, dubbed selfish and self-absorbed, "haven't embraced civic engagement the way they have Botox and Viagra" (Mercer, 2011, p. 18). Their goal is not so much altruism or a sense of obligation to give back, but they very much want to "make a difference." Noting this, Erwin Tan, director of Senior Corps, has changed the name of Retired Senior Volunteer Program to Coming of Age, for greater appeal to boomers. Unlike traditionalists, whose main concern is feeling needed and connected, baby boomers want to use their talents, knowledge, and life experience to make a real social impact. Boomers need more freedom in their volunteer roles, so that they can change to form of giving and add their own ideas. They are comfortable working as members of teams, with the authority to solve problems creatively and if necessary redefine their job descriptions accordingly. This attitude change obviously requires occupational therapists and others to take a different approach when assisting boomer clients with volunteer exploration and participation (Cole & Macdonald, 2011).

Case Examples

Case 1: Al

Al is a 65-year-old heart transplant recipient who has been retired for the past 10 years. He is married to his wife of 44 years and the father of three adult sons and grandfather of three. Prior to his heart failure, Al enjoyed a successful career as an industrial engineer. Born with a heart defect, Al's leisure pursuits tended to be passive and public service–oriented. They including power boating and wine making, photography and painting, church treasurer, president of Civitan, treasurer of the local power squadron, and board of directors at a local marina.

Al's experience gives us some insights regarding the transition to retirement. Although his retirement was involuntary and unexpected, his active public service prior to his illness paved the way for volunteer and part-time employment in retirement. His appointment to the Waterfront Harbor Management Commission before his heart transplant led to his appointment as Stratford harbormaster, a part-time paid position, afterwards. He continues his roles in former community

Table 7-5

Al's Typical Week: 37 Hours Volunteering, 23 Hours Leisure, and 44 Hours Social Occupations

	Mon.	Tues.	Wed.	Thurs.	Fri.	Sat.	Sun.
1 am	Sleep	Sleep	Sleep	Sleep	Sleep	Sleep	Sleep
2 am	"	"	"	"	"	"	"
3 am	"	"	"	"	"	"	"
4 am	"	"	"	"	"	"	"
5 am	"	"	"	"	"	"	"
6 am	"	"	"	"	"	"	"
7 am	"	"	"	"	"	"	"
8 am	Coffee w/retirees	Coffee	Breakfast	Coffee w/retirees	Coffee at Bagel King	"	"
9 am		Volunteer newsletter prep	Volunteer budget prep			Volunteer meeting	Coffee at Bagel King
10 am	Computer			Photos on computer	Shop for wine-making supplies		
11 am	Pay bills		Purchase supplies for event			Fund raising event	Boating with wife & friends
Noon	Volunteer	Lunch					
1 pm	Volunteer	Volunteer	Lunch on boat	Lunch with Sikorsky retirees			
2 pm	Shopping	Banking					
3 pm		Read mail	Boat work		Make wine		
4 pm	Painting		Volunteer inventory	Update volunteer files			
5 pm		Dinner					
6 pm	Dinner	Condo board meeting	Dinner out with wife		Volunteer dinner in another town	Clean up	
7 pm	Dishes			Dinner		Dinner out with friends	Dinner out with family
8 pm	Board meeting		Read mail	Dishes			
9 pm			Computer e-mail	Read mail & paper			
10 pm		Wine/ snack				TV	
11 pm	TV	TV	TV	TV	TV		TV
Midnight	Sleep	Sleep	Sleep	Sleep	Sleep	Sleep	Sleep

groups and additionally has become a mentor to other heart transplant recipients, currently serving as chairman of the heart transplant advisory commission (Table 7-5).

Case 2: Debi

Debi led a very active lifestyle for 25 years, working as a cardio-pulmonary nurse. She was married and raising two boys, working as a ski instructor and sailing instructor during weekends and free time. For some reason, she suddenly developed a latex allergy that went undiagnosed until it almost killed her. At age 47, Debi suffered a stroke, which required her to spend several weeks in a semi-comatose state in the intensive care unit. Hospitals are very dangerous places for someone with a latex allergy because objects containing latex are everywhere, including blood pressure cuffs, stethoscopes, disposable gloves, oral and nasal airway tubes, tourniquets, syringes, electrode pads, and intravenous tubing, not to mention balloons and elastic bands. The allergy complicated her recovery in many undetermined ways, which led to her post-retirement vocation.

Occupational therapy issues for Debi included dressing and basic ADL strategies, neurodevelopmental treatment for her right-sided hemi-paresis, and communication interventions for aphasia. Debi's top-priority task was using her laptop computer to communicate. Unfortunately, occupational therapy did not help her with this task in her biomedically oriented rehabilitation program. Hopefully, that would be different today.

Debi's case demonstrates how clients can turn their own disability into a volunteer advocacy role. In the years following her stroke, Debi used her knowledge of nursing and her own experience to create and publish a latex allergy newsletter, which originated on her laptop computer and reached out to other latex allergy sufferers internationally. Debi has thoroughly researched the medical objects containing latex, alternative equipment, and procedures for filtering the toxic materials for patients and has presented this information at conferences for nurses and other medical personnel. She has written letters and testified at public hearings to influence public policy regarding latex labeling and usage. A network of fellow sufferers now regularly contribute to the informational website she has created.

Case 3: Matt

Matt climbed the corporate ladder the hard way, going to college at night while driving a truck to support a wife and three children until he earned a BS in marketing at age 30. Major events in his life include some major losses, including the untimely death of his younger brother and his father, a bitter divorce, and being fired from two corporate jobs. At age 53, after 20 years with the same corporation, he was "downsized," this time with a 2-year severance package. Matt reported that 90% of his personal identity is tied up in his work role. Remarried for 22 years, he had poor relationships with his three adult children but a close one with his sister's family. The same year Matt retired, he and his wife moved from a large home to a two-bedroom condo on the water. After a period of relief from stress and sleeping late, Matt's health began to decline. With no daily structure and bereft of a highly valued work role, Matt became preoccupied with symptoms of a stomach ulcer, acid reflux, and arthritis in his knees and shoulder. Signs of depression, insomnia, and generalized anxiety soon joined the rapidly expanding list of medical complaints. Occupational therapy assessment included the timeline in Table 7-6. Occupational therapy interventions included leisure exploration, volunteer exploration, and daily time structuring.

Re-establishing daily routines in a new location became the first priority. A dog that used to run freely outside now needed to be walked on a leash. Regular hours for arising, dressing, showering, dog walking, mealtimes, and bedtime addressed the depression and insomnia (combined with medication). Additionally, Matt took on some of the household tasks such as laundry and kitchen cleanup, because his wife still worked full time. Leisure choices from the past, scuba diving and downhill skiing, required travel to distant locations. Matt, now living on the water, decided to take up swimming and boating instead. Afternoons he swam in the condo pool, and he began attending boat shows and signed up for a local learn-to-sail course. Eventually, with regular walking, his arthritis symptoms subsided and he began meeting neighbors during walks with the dog. Volunteering had never interested Matt in the past. However, an opportunity presented itself when neighbors invited him to join the condo finance committee. He soon discovered that his corporate purchasing experience could assist the condo in getting the best prices for needed goods and services. A year later, Matt was elected to the condo board of directors.

Table 7-6
Matt's Timeline
• Born 1944 in New Yor City • '62 high school graduation • '63 first marriage • '64, ' 66, '68 children born • '66 brother died in Vietnam War • '70 BS degree • '70 first house • '70 employed as buyer • '71 began skiing • '76 divorce • '76 death of father • '76 moved back home • '77 fired from job • '77 new job in New York City • '79 fired from job • '79 depression, ulcer • '80 new job purchasing • '82 second marriage • '82 second home • '82 five teenage children • '82 marriage counseling • '84 Hawaii, scuba diving • '86 Cozumel, scuba trip • '87, ''0, '92, '95, '97 children's graduations and marriage • '97 death of mother • '98 retirement • '98 moved to condo • '99 depression, GERD • 2001 first boat • '02 elected to condo board

References

Adams, K. B. (2004). Changing investment in activities and interests in elders' lives: Theory and measurement. *International Journal of Aging and Human Development, 58*, 87-108.

Adams, K. B., Roberts, A., & Cole, M. (2011). Changes in activity and interest in the third and fourth age: Associations with health, functioning and depressive symptoms. *Occupational Therapy International, 18*, 4-17.

Agahi, N., Ahacic, K., & Parker, M. (2006). Continuity of leisure participation from middle to old age. *The Journals of Gerontology: Series B: Psychological sciences and Social Sciences, 61B*, S340-347.

Allen, C., Blue, T., & Earhart, C. (1995). *Understanding cognitive performance modes.* Ormond Beach, FL: Allen Conferences, Inc.

Allen, C., Blue, T., & Earhart, C. (2001). *Understanding cognitive performance modes*, Ormond Beach, FL: Allen Conferences.

AOTA. (2014). Occupational therapy practice framework: Domain and process, (3rd ed.), 68(Suppl. 1), S1-S48.

AOTA. (2010). Occupation and activity based interventions: Critically appraised topic: What is the evidence that participation in occupations and activities supports the health of community dwelling older adults? *AOTA Critically Appraised Topics and Papers Series*, www.aota.org, Retrieved August 8, 2010.

Atchley, R. C., & Barusch, A. (2004). *Social forces and aging: An introduction to social gerontology* (10th ed.). New York, NY: Wadsworth.

Atchley, R. C. (1989). Continuity theory of normal aging. *Gerontologist, 29*, 183-191.

Atchley, R. C. (1976). *The sociology of retirement.* New York, NY: Halsted.

Atchley, R. C. (1975). Adjustment to loss of job at retirement. *Int. J Aging Hum Dev., 6*, 17-27.

Azar, B. (2008). *Presidential initiatives: Aging redefined.* American Psychological Association. http://www.apa.org/monitor/2008/10/aging-society.aspx. Retrieved July 22, 2012.

Baker, D. W., Sudano, J. J., Albert, J. M., Borawski, E. A., & Dor, A. (2001). Lack of health insurance and decline in overall health in late middle age. *New England Journal of Medicine: 345*, 1106-12.

Baltes, P. B. (2005). *A psychological model of successful ageing.* Keynote Lecture, 2005 World Congress of Gerontology, Brazil. Retrieved November 5, 2006 from http://www.baltes-paul.de/SOC.html.

Baltes, P. B. (2006). Facing our limits: Human dignity in the very old. *Daedalus, 135*, 32-39.

Baltes, P. B., & Baltes, M. M. (Eds.), (1990). *Successful aging: Perspectives from the behavioral sciences.* New York, NY: Cambridge University Press.

Baltes, P. B., & Carstensen, L. L. (1996). The process of successful ageing. *Aging and Society, 16*, 397-422.

Baltes, P. B., & Smith, J. (1990). *The psychology of wisdom and its ontogenesis.* In Sternberg, Ed. *Wisdom: Its nature, origins, and development.* New York, NY: Cambridge University Press.

Baltes, P. B., & Smith, J. (2002). *New frontiers in the future of aging: From successful aging of the young old to the dilemmas of the fourth age.* Keynote paper retrieved April 22, 2005, from www.valenciaforum /Keynotes/pb.html.

Barlow, J., Wright, C., Sheasby, J., Turner, A.,& Hainsworth, J. (2002). Self-management approaches for people with chronic conditions: A review. *Patient education and counseling, 48*, 177-187.

Bonder, B. R. (2001). *The psychosocial meaning of activity.* In Bonder, B. R., & Wagner, M. B. (Eds.) *Functional performance in older adults*, (2nd ed.). Philadelphia, PA: F. A. Davis.

Bornstein, R. (1992) *Psychosocial development of the older adult.* In Schuster C. S., & Ashburn S. S., *The process of human development: A holistic life span approach* (pp. 893-896). Philadelphia, PA: Lippincott.

Brown, J. W., Chen, S., Mefford, L, Brown, A., Callen, B., & McArthur, P. (2011). Becoming an older volunteer: A grounded theory study. *Nursing Research and Practice, 2011*, Article ID 361250, 8 pages.

Cahill, K. E., Giandrea, M. D., & Quinn, J. F. (2012). Older workers and short-term jobs: Patterns and determinants. *Monthly Labor Review, 135*(5), 19-32.

Caro, F. G., & Morris, R. (2001). *Maximizing the contributions of older people as volunteers.* In Levekoff, S. E., Chee, Y. K., & Noguchi, S. (Eds.), *Successful and productive aging.* New York, NY: Springer.

Carstensen, L. L. (1992). Social and emotional patterns in adulthood. *Psychology and Aging: 7*, 331-338.

Carstensen, L. L. (1998). *A lifespan approach to social motivation.* In J. Heckhausen & C. S. Dweck (Eds.). *Motivation and self-regulation across the life span* (pp. 341-364). New York, NY: Cambridge University Press.

Carstensen, L. L., Isaacowitz, D. M., & Charles, S. T. (1999). Taking time seriously: A theory of socioemotional selectivity. *American Psychologist, 54*, 165-181.

Chop, W. (1999). *The social aspects of aging.* In Chop, W., & Robnett, R. *Gerontology for the health care professional.* Philadelphia, PA: FA Davis.

Christiansen, C. H., Backman, C., Little, B. R., & Nguyen, A. (1998). Occupations and well-being: A study of personal projects. *American Journal of Occupational Therapy, 53*, 91-100.

Clark F., Azen S., Zemke R., Jackson J., Carlson M., Mandel D. . . . .Lipson L. (1997). Occupational therapy for independent-living older adults: A randomized controlled trial. *Journal of the American Medical Association, 278*, 1321-1326.

Clark, F. A., Jackson, J. M., Carlson, M. E., Chou, C. P., Cherry, B. J., Jordan-Marsh, M., . . . Azen, S. P. (2011). Effectiveness of a lifestyle intervention in promoting the well-being of independently living older people: results of the Well Elderly 2 Randomized Controlled Trial. *Journal of Epidemiology and Community Health, 66,* 782-790.

Cohen, G. D. (1999). Human potential phases in the second half of life. American Journal of *Geriatric Psychiatry, 7,* 1-7.

Cole, M. B. (2012). *Group dynamics in occupational therapy,* (4th ed.). Thorofare, NJ: SLACK Incorporated.

Cole, M. B., & Macdonald, K. C. (2011). Retired occupational therapists' experiences in volunteer occupations. *Occupational Therapy International, 18,* 18-31.

Cole, M. B. (1998). Time mastery in business and occupational therapy. *Work: A Journal of Prevention, Assessment, & Rehabilitation, 10,* 119-127.

Cole, M. B. (2001). *Meaningful occupations of older adulthood across cultures.* Unpublished manuscript.

Cornwell, B., Laumann, E., & Schumm, P. (2008). The social connectedness of older adults: A national profile. *American Social Review, 73,* 185-203.

Crist, P. A. (1999). Does quality of life vary with different types of housing among older persons? A pilot study. In Taira, E. D., & Carlson, J. L. (Eds.), *Aging in place: Designing, adapting, and enhancing the home environment.* Binghamton, NY: Haworth Press.

Cumming, E., & Henry, W. (1961). *Growing old: The process of disengagement.* New York, NY: Basic Books.

Daly, M. C., & Bound, J. (1996). Worker adaptation and employer accommodation following the onset of a health impairment. *The Journal of Gerontology, 51,* S53-60.

De Boer, A. G., van Beek, J. C., Durinck, J., Verbeek, J. H., & van Dijk, F. J. (2004). An occupational health intervention programme for workers at risk for early retirement: A randomized controlled trial. *Occupational and Environmental Medicine, 61,* 924-9.

Di Mauro, S., Leotta, C., Giuffrida, F., Distafano, A., & Grasso, M. G. (2003). Suicides and the third age. *Archives of Gerontology & Geriatrics, 36,* 1-6.

Disney, R., Grundy, E., & Johnson, P. (1994). The Dynamics of retirement: analysis of the retirement surveys. Research report N. 72. Retrieved at www.dwp.gov.uk/asd/asd5/72summ.asp on April 22, 2005.

Erikson, E. H. (1963). *Childhood and society.* New York, NY: Norton.

Erikson, E. H., & Erikson, J. M. (1997). *The life cycle completed.* New York, NY: Norton.

Ewald, P. D. (1999). *Future concerns in an aging society.* In Chop, W. C., & Robnett, R. H. (Eds.), *Gerontology for the health care professional.* Philadelphia, PA: FA Davis.

Fletcher, W. I., & Hansson, R. O. (1991). Assessing the social components of retirement anxiety. *Psychological Aging, 6,* 76-85.

Formosa, M. (2000). Older adult education in a Maltese University of the Third Age: a critical perspective. *Education and Aging, 15,* 315-334.

Gallo, W. T., Bradley, E. H., Siegel, M., & Kasl, S. V. (2000). Health effects of involuntary job loss among older workers: Findings from the health and retirement survey. *The Journals of Gerontology Series B, 55,* 131-140.

Geerts, C., Ponjaert-Kristoffersen, I., Verbandt, C., & Verte, D. (1999). Women and their retirement: Adaptation as a dynamic assessment process. *Gerontology and Geriatrics. 30,* 6-11.

Godbout, E., Filiatrault, J., & Plante, M. (2012). The participation of seniors in volunteer activities: A systematic review. *Canadian Journal of Occupational Therapy, 79*(1), 23-33.

Graff, L. L. (1993). The key to the boardroom door: policies for volunteer programs. *The Journal of Volunteer Administration, 11,* 30-36.

Greenfield, E. A., & Marks, N. F. (2004). Formal volunteering as a protective factor for older adults' psychological well-being. *The Journals of Gerontology Series B, 59,* S258-264.

Gruber, J., & Wise, D. (1999). Social Security, retirement incentives, and retirement behavior: An international perspective. *EBRI Issue Brief, 209,* 1-22.

Hanson, K., & Wapner, S. (1994). Transition to retirement: Gender differences. *Int J Aging Hum Dev: 39,* 189-208.

Harkapaa, K. (1992). Psychosocial factors as predictors for early retirement in patients with chronic low back pain. *Journal of Psychosomatic Research, 36,* 553-9.

Haslam, C., Jetten, J., Haslam, S., & Knight, C. (2012). *The importance of remembering and deciding together: Enhancing the health and well-being of older adults in care* (pp. 297-315). In J. Jetten, C. Haslam, & S. Haslam (Eds.), *The Social Cure: Identify, Health & Well-being.* New York, NY: Taylor & Frances Psychology Press.

Havighurst, R. (1961). Successful aging. *The Gerontologist, 1,* 8-13.

Health and Retirement Study (2008). Retrieved at http://hrsonline.isr.umich.edu/sitedocs/surveydesign.pdf on August 4, 2012.

Hershey, D. A., & Mowen, J. C. (2000). Psychological determinants of financial preparedness for retirement. *Gerontologist, 40,* 687-697.

Holmes, T. (1978). Life situations, emotions, and disease. *Psychosomatic Medicine, 9,* 747.

Hospice Foundation of America (2010). Three studies examine end-of-life care in US and Canada. Retrieved at http://blog.hospicefoundation.org/2010/10/three-studies-examine-end-of-life-care.html on July 22, 2012.

Hunt, L., & Arbesman, M. (2008). Evidence-based and occupational perspective of effective interventions for older clients that remediate or support improved driving performance. *The American Journal of Occupational Therapy, 62,* 136-148.

Jackson J., Carlson M., Mandel D., Zemke R., & Clark, F. (1998). Occupation in lifestyle redesign: The well elderly study occupational therapy program. *American Journal of Occupational Therapy, 52,* 326-336.

Jacques, N. D. (2002). Working with the dying older patient. In Lewis, C. B. (Ed.), *Aging: The health-care challenge,* (4th ed). Philadelphia, PA: F. A. Davis.

Jetten, J., & Pachana, N. (2012). *Not wanting to grow old: A social identity model of identity change analysis of driving cessation among older adults* (97-113). In J. Jetten, C. Haslam, & S. Haslam (Eds.), *The Social Cure: Identify, Health & Well-being.* New York, NY: Taylor & Frances Psychology Press.

Johnson, C. L., & Barer, B. M. (1992). Patterns of engagement and disengagement among the oldest old. *Journal of Aging Studies, 6,* 351-364.

Jonsson, H. (2011). The first steps into the Third Age: The retirement process from a Swedish perspective. *Occupational Therapy International, 18,* 32-38.

Jonsson, H., Josephsson, S., & Kielhofner, G. (2001). Narratives and experience in an occupational transition: a longitudinal study of the retirement process. *American Journal of Occupational Therapy,* 55, 424-432.

Jung, C. G. (1933). *Modern man in search of a soul.* New York, NY: Harcourt, Brace & World.

Karafantis, D. M., & Levy, S. R. (2004). The role of children's lay theories about the malleability of human attributes in beliefs about and volunteering for disadvantaged groups. *Child Development, 75,* 236-250.

Karpansalo, M., Manninen, P., Kauhanen, J., Lakka, T. A., & Salonen, J. T. (2004). Perceived health as a predictor of early retirement. *Scandinavian Journal of Work, Environment & Health, 30,* 287-92.

Knight, E. L. (2004). Exemplary rural mental health services delivery. *Behavioral Healthcare Tomorrow, 13,* 20-24.

Knight, J., Ball, V., Corr, S., Turner, A., Lowis, M., & Ekberg, M. (2007). An empirical study to identify older adults' engagement in productivity occupations. *Journal of Occupational Science, 14,* 145-153.

Krause, N. (1986). Social support, stress, and well-being among older adults. *The Journals of Gerontology: Series A, 41,* 512-519.

Kuperminc, G. P., Holditch, P. T., & Allen, J. P. (2001). Volunteering and community service in adolescence. *Archives of Pediatrics & Adolescent Medicine, 12,* 445-457.

Larson, R., Czikszentmihalyi, M., & Graef, R. (1982). *Time alone in daily experience: Loneliness or renewal?* In Peplau, L. A., & Perlman, D. (Eds.), *Loneliness: A sourcebook of current theory, research, and therapy.* New York, NY: Wiley-Interscience.

Laslett, P. (1989). *A Fresh Map of Life: The Emergence of the Third Age.* Cambridge, MA: Harvard University Press.

Laslett, P. (1997). Interpreting the demographic changes. *Philosophical Transactions of the Royal Society B: Biological Sciences, 352*(1363), 1805-9.

Lauber, C., Nordt, C., Falcato, L., & Rossler, W. (2002). Determinants of attitude to volunteering in psychiatry: Results of a public opinion survey in Switzerland. *International Journal of Social Psychiatry, 48,* 209-219.

Lawlor, M., & Mattingly, C. (1998). The complexities embedded in family centered care. *American Journal of Occupational Therapy, 52,* 259-267.

Levy, L., & Burns, T. (2011). *Cognitive disabilities reconsidered model: Rehabilitation of adults with dementia.* In N. Katz (Ed.*), Cognition, Occupation and Participation Across the Life Span: Neuroscience, Neurorehabilitation, and Models for Intervention in Occupational Therapy* (pp.407-441). Bethesda, MD: AOTA.

Lin, J., Guerrieri, J., & Moore, A. (2011). Drinking patterns and the development of functional limitations in older adults: Longitudinal analysis of the health and retirement survey. *Journal of Aging Health, 23,* 806-821.

Lo, R., & Brown, R. (1999). Stress and adaptation: Preparation for successful retirement. *Australian and New Zealand Journal of Mental Health Nursing, 8,* 30-38.

Lorig, K., Sobel, D., Gonzalez, V., & Minor, M. (2006). *Living a healthy life with chronic conditions: Self management of heart disease, arthritis, diabetes, asthma, bronchitis, emphysema, and others.* Bounder, CO: Bull.

Ludwig, F. M. (1998). The unpackaging of routine in older women. *American Journal of Occupational Therapy, 52,* 168–178.

Ludwig, F. M., Hattjar, B., Russell, R., & Winston, K. (2007). How caregiving for grandchildren affects grandmothers' meaningful occupations. *Journal of Occupational Science, 14,* 40-51

Macdonald, K. C. (1998). *Adaptation to physical disability: The experiences of five women aged fifty to sixty.* New York University: Dissertation.

Mandel, B., & Roe, B. (2008). Job loss, retirement and the mental health of older Americans. *Journal of Mental Health Policy and Economics, 11,* 167-176.

Marcil, W. (2005). Hope without a future. *Advance for Occupational Therapy, 21*(6),18-19,

Marek, A. C. (2005). *48 Volunteer. In Fifty ways to fix your life,* p. 84. US News & World Report, Dec. 27, 2004-Jan. 3, 2005.

Mayring, P. (2000). Retirement as crisis or good fortune? Results of a quantitative-qualitative longitudinal study. *Zeitschrift für Gerontologie und Geriatrie, 33,* 124-133.

McAdams, D. P., Hart, H. M., & Maruna, A. S. (1998). *The anatomy of generativity.* In McAdams, D. P., & de St. Aubin, E. (Eds.), Generativity and adult development (pp.7-43). Washington, DC: American Psychological Association.

McAndrew, J. M. (2002). *Stress and aging.* In Lewis, C. B. (Ed.), *Aging: The health-care challenge,* (4th ed.). Philadelphia, PA: F. A. Davis

Mercer, M. (2011). *Boomers get their groove back.* AARP.org/bulletin, Jan-Feb 2011, 16-20.

Merrill, J. (2000). You don't do it for nothing: women's experiences of volunteering in two community well woman clinics. *Health & Social Care in the Community, 8,* 31-39.

MetLife Foundation (2005). *New face of work survey.* Retrieved at http://www.encore.org/find/resources/new-face-of-work-survey on December 1, 2011.

Metz, A., & Robnett, R. (2011). Engaging in mentally challenging occupations promotes cognitive health throughout life. *Gerontology Special Interest Section Newsletter* (AOTA), June, 1-4.

Mitchell, C. W., & Shuff, I. M. (1995). Personality characteristics of hospice volunteers as measured by Myers-Briggs Type Indicator. *Journal of Personality Assessment, 65,* 521-532.

Morris, J. K., Cook, J. G., & Shaper, A. G. (1994). Loss of employment and mortality. *British Medical Journal, 308,* 1135-9.

Morrow-Howell, N., Hinterlong, J., Rozario, P. A., & Tang, F. (2003). Effects of volunteering on the well-being of older adults. *The Journals of Gerontology Series B, 58,* S137-145.

Musick, M. A., Herzog, A. R., & House, J. S. (1999). Volunteering and mortality among older adults: findings from a national sample. *The Journals of Gerontology Series B, 54,* S173-180.

Musick, M. A., & Wilson, J. (2003). Volunteering and depression: The role of psychological and social resources in different age groups. *Social Science & Medicine, 56,* 259-269.

Mutcher, J. E., Burr, J. A., & Caro, F. G. (2003). From paid worker to volunteer: Leaving the paid workforce and volunteering in later life. *Social Forces, 81,* 1267-1293.

National Institutes of Health, (2009). Growing older in America. Retrieved http://www.nia.nih.gov/health/publication/growing-older-america-health-and-retirement-study/chapter-1-health on August 10, 2012.

Neugarten, B. L., & Weinstein, K. (1964). The changing American grandparent. *Journal of Marriage and the Family, 26,* 199-204.

Nuttman-Schwartz, O. (2004). Like a high wave: Adjustment to retirement. *Gerontologist, 44,* 229-36.

Okun, M. A., Barr, A., & Herzog, A. R. (1998). Motivation to volunteer by older adults: A test of competing measurement models. *Psychology and Aging, 13*, 608-621.
Parker, R. G. (1995). Reminiscence: A continuity theory framework. *Gerontologist, 35*, 515-25.
Parsons, P. A. (2003). From the stress theory of aging to energetic and evolutionary expectations for longevity. *Biogerontology, 4*, 63-73.
Pavlova, M. K., & Silbereisen, R. K. (2012). Participation in voluntary organizations and volunteer work as a compensation for the absence of work or partnership? Evidence from two German samples of younger and older adults. *The Journals of Gerontology Series B, 67*, 514-524.
Pearl, L. (1993). *Providing family centered intervention.* In W. Brown, S. Thurman, & Pearl, L. (Eds.), *Family-centered early intervention with infants and toddlers: Innovative cross-disciplinary approaches* (pp. 81-101). Baltimore, MD: Brookes.
Penningroth, S., & Scott, W. (2012). Age-related differences in goals: Testing predictions from selection, optimization, and compensation theory and socioemotional selectivity theory. *International Journal of Aging and Human Development, 74*, 87-111.
Perreira, K. M., & Sloan, F. A. (2001). Life events and alcohol consumption among mature adults: A longitudinal analysis. *Journal of Studies on Alcohol and Drugs, 62*, 501-8.
Plassman, B., Williams, J., Burke, J., Holsinger, T., & Benjamin, S. (2010). Systematic Review: Factors associated with risk for and possible prevention of cognitive decline in later life. *Annals of Internal Medicine, 153*, 182-193.
Post, K. (2010). Technology, information literacy, and evidence based practice. Technology *Special Interest Section Quarterly* (AOTA), September, 1-4.
Potts, M. K. (1997). Social support and depression among older adults living alone: The importance of friends within and outside of a retirement community. *Social Work, 42*, 348-362.
Prensky, M. (2001). *Digital natives, digital immigrants. On the Horizon* (NCB University Press, 9, 5, October).
Presis. (2012). *Working while sick.* Monthly Labor Review Online, May 2012. Retrieved at http://www.bls.gov/opub/mlr/2012/05/précis.htm on July 26, 2012.
Quick, H. E., & Moen, P. (1998). Gender, employment, and retirement quality: A life course approach to the differential experiences of men and women. *Journal of Occupational Health Psychology, 3*, 44-64.
Rapp, M. A., Krampe, R. T., & Baltes, P. B. (2006). Adaptive task prioritization in aging: Selective resource allocation to postural control is preserved in Alzheimer disease. *American Journal of Geriatric Psychiatry, 14*, 52–61.
Reitzes, D. C., & Mutran, E. J. (2004). The transition to retirement: stages and factors that influence retirement adjustment. *The International Journal of Aging and Human Development, 59*, 63-84.
Retirement Living Information Center (2004). Aging baby boomers shun the "R" word. Retrieved at www.retirementliving.com/RLart229.htm on November 12, 2004.
Riley, M., & Riley, J. (1994). Age integration and the lives of older people. *Gerontologist, 34*, 110-115.
Rosenkoetter, M. M., & Garris, J. M. (1998). Psychosocial changes following retirement. *J Adv Nursing, 27*, 966-976.
Ross, M. W., Greenfield, S. A., & Bennett, L. (1999). Predictors of dropout and burnout in AIDS volunteers: a longitudinal study. *AIDS Care, 11*, 723-731.
Rothenbacher, D., Arndt, V., Fraisse, E., Zschenderlein, B. Fliedner, T, & Brenner, H. (1998). Early retirement due to permanent disability in relation to smoking in workers of the construction industry. *Journal of Occupational & Environmental Medicine, 40*, 63-68.
Rowe, J. W., & Kahn, R. L. (1998). *Successful aging: The MacArthur Foundation Study shows you how the lifestyle choices you make now—more than heredity—determine your health and vitality.* New York, NY: Pantheon Books.
Sadler, C., & Marty, F. (1998). Socialization of hospice volunteers: members of the family. *American Journal of Hospice & Palliative Medicine, 13*, 49-68.
Salokangas, R. K., & Joukamaa, M. (1991). Physical and mental health changes in retirement age. *Psychother Psychosom. 55*, 100-107.
Schuster, C. S. (1992). *Development frameworks of selected stage theorists.* In Schuster, C. S., & Ashburn, S. S., *The process of human development: A holistic life span approach* (pp. 893-896). Philadelphia, PA: Lippincott.
Sharpley, C. F. (1997). Psychometric properties of the Self-perceived Stress in Retirement Scale. *Psychol Rep., 81*(1), 319-322.

Shmotkin, D., Blumstein, T., & Modan, B. (2003). Beyond keeping active: concomitants of being a volunteer in old-old age. *Psychological Aging, 18*, 602-607.

Soderhamn, O, Skisland, A., & Herrman, M. (2011). Self-care and anticipated transition into retirement and later life in a Nordic welfare context. *Journal of Multidisciplinary Healthcare, 4*, 273-279.

Stav, W., Hallenen, T., Lane, J., & Arbesman, M. (2012). Systematic review of occupational engagement and health outcomes among community dwelling older adults. *American Journal of Occupational Therapy, 66*, 301-310.

Szinovacz, M. E., & Davey, A. (2004). Honeymoons and joint lunches: effects of retirement and spouse's employment on depressive symptoms. *The Journals of Gerontology Series B, 59*, 233-45.

Tigges, K. N., & Marcil, W. M. (1988). *Terminal and life-threatening illness: An occupational behavior perspective.* Thorofare, NJ: SLACK Incorporated.

Tornstam, L. (2011). Maturing into gerotranscendence. *Journal of Transpersonal Psychology, 43*, 166-180.

Tornstam, L. (1997). Gerotranscendence: The contemplative dimension of aging. *Journal of Aging Studies, 11*, 143-154.

Tornstam, L. (2000). Transcendence in later life. *Generations, 23*(4), 10-14.

US Bureau of Census. (2010). *Comprehensive analysis of fast-growing 90 and older population.* Newsroom: Aging Population. Retrieved at http://www.census.gov/newsroom/releases/archives/aging_population/cb11-194.html on August 27, 2012.

US Dept. of Labor (2011). *Volunteer rate rises in 2011.* Retrieved at www.bls.gov/opub/ted/2012/ted_20120223.htm on July 26, 2012.

Vaillant, G. E. (1993). *Wisdom of the ego.* Cambridge, MA: Harvard University Press.

Vance, K., & Siebert, C. (2009). Supporting self-management in home health and the community. *Home and Community Health Special Interest Section Newsletter*, September, 1-4.

Velde, B., & Fidler, G. (2002). *Lifestyle performance: A model for engaging the power of occupation.* Thorofare, NJ: SLACK Incorporated.

Warburton, D., J., Paynter, C. A., & Petriewskyj, A. (2007). Volunteering as a productive aging activity: Incentives and barriers to volunteering by Australian seniors. *Journal of Applied Gerontology, 26*, 333-354.

Warner, D., Hayward, M., & Hardy, M. (2010) The retirement life course in America at the dawn of the twenty-first century. *Population Research and Policy Review, 29*, 893-919. (NIH Public Access Author Manuscript).

Warr, P., Butcher, V., & Robertson, I. (2004). Activity and psychological well-being in older people. *Aging Mental Health, 8*, 172-183.

Westermeyer, J. F. (2004). Predictors and characteristics of Erikson's life cycle model among men: A 32 year longitudinal study. *International Journal of Aging and Human Development, 58*, 29-48.

Wheeler, J. A., Gorey, K. M., & Greenblatt, B. (1998). The beneficial effects of volunteering for older volunteers and the people they serve: a meta-analysis. *The International Journal of Aging and Human Development, 47*, 69-79.

Wilson, S. E. (2001) Socioeconomic status and the prevalence of health problems among married couples in late life. *American Journal of Public Health, 91*, 131-135.

Withnall, A. (2002). Three decades of educational gerontology: Achievements and challenges. *Education and Aging, 17*, 87-102.

Windsor, T. D., Ansley, K. J., Butterworth, P., Luszcz, M. A., & Andrews, G. R. (2007). The role of perceived control in explaining depressive symptoms associated with driving cessation in a longitudinal study. *The Gerontologist, 2*, 215-223.

Wright, K., & Patterson, B. (2006). Socioemotional selectivity theory and the macrodynamics of friendship: The role of friendship style and communication in friendship across the lifespan. *Communication Research Reports, 23*, 163-170.

Wyant, S., & Brooks, P. (1993). *The changing role of volunteerism.* Pap Ser United Hospital Fund, NY. April (23), 1-37.

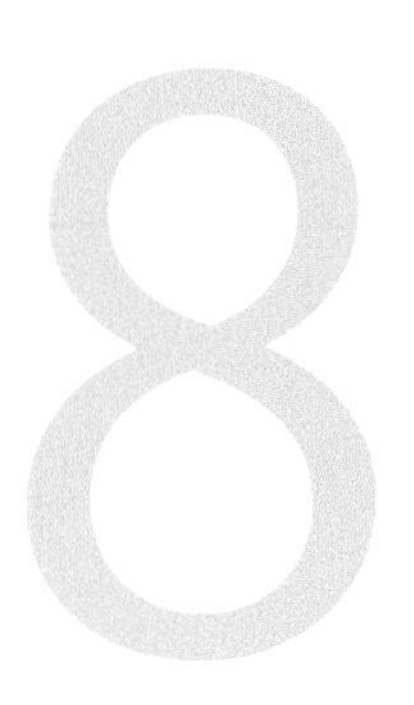

Leisure

Margo Ruth Gross, EdD, LMFT, LMT, OTR/L
Peter Tascione, OTR/L

Chapter Objectives

By the end of this chapter, the student will be able to do the following:

- Define leisure as it pertains to the Occupational Therapy Practice Framework (AOTA, 2014).
- Describe specific models/frames of reference that address leisure for assessment and intervention.
- Comprehend and be educated about safety issues when addressing leisure needs.
- Delineate between the roles of the occupational therapist and the occupational therapy assistant as they pertain to the occupation of leisure.
- Comprehend and identify physical and psychological implications as related to decreased independence in leisure.
- Comprehend issues related to leisure in specific settings
- Comprehend issues related to leisure when using objects or equipment.
- Describe the impact of contextual and environmental factors upon leisure.
- Identify appropriate leisure intervention strategies based on various performance skills and client factors.
- Identify specific leisure compensation/adaptation strategies.
- Identify general leisure remediation strategies.
- Identify leisure compensation/adaptation intervention strategies related to vision, perception, and cognition.
- Identify general leisure maintenance strategies.

Meriano C, Latella D.
Occupational Therapy Interventions: Function and Occupations, Second Edition (pp 403-431).

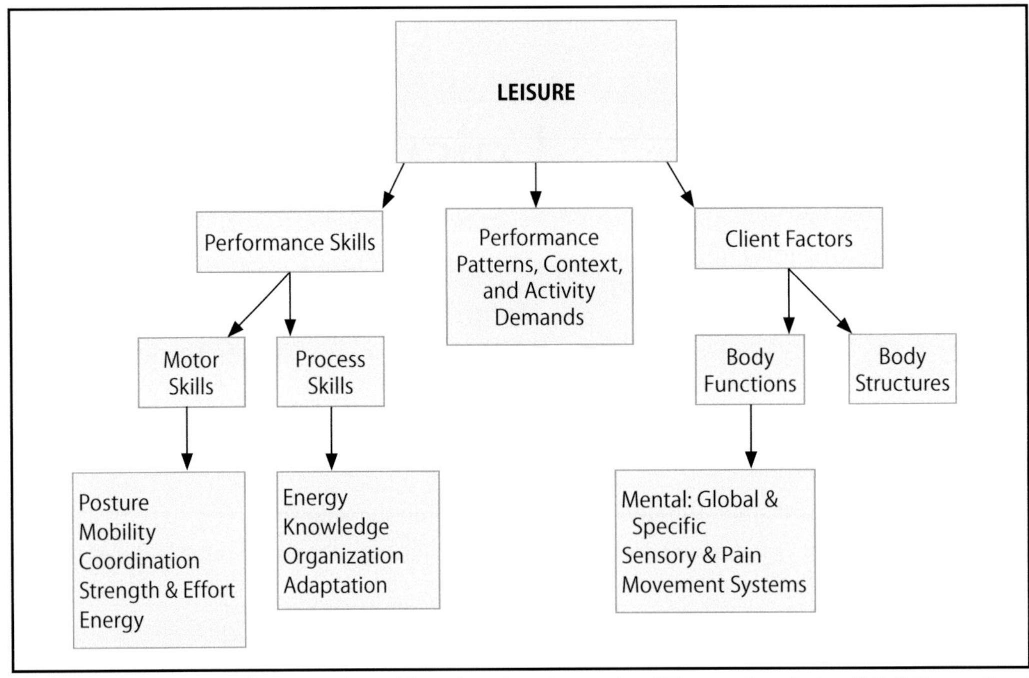

Figure 8-1. Components of leisure. (Adapted from American Occupational Therapy Association. [2014]. Occupational therapy practice framework. *American Journal of Occupational Therapy, 68*[Suppl. 1], S1-S48.)

Introduction

Leisure time has different meanings for individuals from different cultures, ethnic identities, gender identities, and social classes, affecting the way in which occupational therapists utilize the concept for intervention. According to the *Random House Dictionary*, leisure is "time free from the demands of work or duty, when one can rest, enjoy hobbies or sports, etc." (1987, p. 1100). The Occupational Therapy Practice Framework further defines leisure as "a nonobligatory activity which is intrinsically motivated and engaged in during discretionary time, that is, time not committed to obligatory occupations such as work, self-care, or sleep" (AOTA, 2014, p. S21; Parham & Fazio, 1997, p. 250). The AOTA framework document further defines the components of leisure as described in Figure 8-1.

"Free" time spent outside of paid work has both an objective and subjective understanding for each individual. This phenomenological point of view may be elucidated by engaging clients in a discussion about what leisure time means to them personally. Professionals need to be aware of their own biases, beliefs, and assumptions about leisure, as well as to be as open-minded as possible during such an interview.

In order to develop satisfactory performance skills for participation in leisure activities that are client-centered, questions involving the client's freedom of choice, level of motivation, and desired amount of relaxation or enjoyment need to be proposed. Leisure time, in balance with work and rest, is central to a person's well-being and is validated by a sense of perceived satisfaction and fulfillment in the activity. The perception of leisure or recreational activities as "leisurely" may or may not be held by a particular client; instead, free time may be seen as providing opportunities for novelty, excitement, interaction with others, or even escape from involvement with the larger community (Edginton, Jordan, DeGraaf, & Edginton, 1995). The needs met by a particular leisure activity may be simplistic, as in the case of providing relaxation, or multifaceted, including offering avenues for emotional expression, creative expression, physical exercise, relationship building, respite from interaction, cognitive stimulation, entertainment, or self-improvement.

The occupational therapy assessment process, using semistructured and open-ended questioning, ought to sufficiently uncover areas that could provide satisfaction in a variety of contexts for leisure fulfillment. Eliciting the clients' story in such a way as to encourage the development of analogies or metaphors can help explain their experiences with some cohesiveness. Assessment tools need to be chosen to match the factors that are consonant to clients' culture, age, and level of physical as well as psychological involvement. Another semi-structured assessment would be to use a calendar for 1 week, and ask the client to write down every activity he or she engages in, from waking up to going to bed. Asking questions informally while the client is completing the form will reveal subjective feelings about the activities, or clients can rate them as positive and fun (+) vs boring and laborious (–).

In addition, this will reveal a balance, or lack thereof, in work/productivity, leisure/recreation, and self-care/rest. A list of possible leisure time pursuits is included at the end of this chapter to serve as a guide for an interview.

Healthy communication and social skills, impulsive control, relaxation techniques, and self-esteem are just a few factors that can be enhanced through leisure pursuits. The occupational therapist, however, must be aware of the coexisting mental health functioning of the client along with the physical disability, as well as the client's leisure interests. The humanistic nature of occupational therapy addresses the "whole person," not just the simple components such as bilateral grip strength and functional mobility, and with a thorough occupational profile and analysis of occupational performance, a complete "picture" of the client can be achieved.

Leisure Exploration

Assessments and Evaluations

Occupational therapy practitioners promote and educate clients about the importance of living a balanced life composed of time for self-care, work, school, leisure, and social participation. One of the imperative tasks of occupational therapists is to determine the interests and values of clients, a task that helps to include the clients in intervention, develop rapport between client and therapist, and assist with client motivation. The frame of reference or model used might determine the choice of evaluation and assessment tools. An excellent resource by I. E. Asher (2014) is listed in the References section. Each frame of reference has a different perspective on leisure exploration, and it can be useful to blend approaches for a well-rounded initial assessment.

Several assessment tools exist to further explore a client's ability to engage in leisure; the most commonly used standardized assessments include the Allen cognitive level (ACL) test, the Kohlman evaluation of living skills (KELS), and the performance assessment of self-care skills (PASS). From Canada, the Canadian occupational performance measure (COPM) is available.

Commonly used evaluation tools utilized by occupational therapists to assess a person's ability to engage in leisure tasks are described below, although the resources are available in American Occupational Therapy Association (AOTA) publication texts and are worth exploring to be kept current.

Canadian Occupational Performance Measure

This tool was created for assessment of children and adults who can cognitively prioritize and rate their preferences in leisure, work/play, and self-care categories. This model ensures a client-centered and a collaborative approach to goal setting, necessary to ensure client compliance and motivation. The COPM and its underlying theory emphasizes the cooperation and collaboration between the occupational therapist and the client to formulate the final intervention plan (Law et al., 2005). Without compliance, the outcomes would probably not be motivating. The combination of subjective prioritizing of tasks combined with the objective rating system takes the steps to combine cognitive and emotional/mental aspects of the client in formulating the desired outcomes.

One of the benefits of the COPM is it can be utilized with any population. An example of the clinical use for spinal cord injury was studied, and it was determined the tool was useful for goal setting (Gustafsson, Mitchell, Fleming, & Price, 2012). While goal setting may not include only leisure, as this is oftentimes a younger population, leisure will play an important role in returning to daily occupations.

The Allen Cognitive Level Test

The ACL is a cognitive screening tool designed by Claudia Allen, OTR, and sold by S & S Worldwide in Colchester, Connecticut. This leather-lacing task is administered to clients to provide the occupational therapist with a measure of how a person learns according to 6 levels of cognitive functioning described by Allen (Allen, Earhart, & Blue, 1992). The strengths of this assessment include a relatively speedy format for administration and scoring, an excellent opportunity to observe problem-solving skills and frustration levels, and offering recommendations on how to best facilitate a client's capacity to learn. The authors' experience has identified weaknesses in this tool to include scoring discrepancies based on a client's past experience with stitching and difficulties in administration to clients without adequate bilateral upper extremity (UE) functioning. A larger version of the task is available for clients with low vision.

The Kohlman Evaluation of Living Skills

The KELS is a task-based, interview-style living skills evaluation developed by Linda Kohlman-Thomson and is often used by occupational therapists to create discharge recommendations and assist the treatment team when planning for a client's transition into the community. The evaluation is divided into the following five subsections: self-care, money management, work/leisure, transportation, and telephone (Thomson, 1992). The leisure section of the KELS inquires as to whether the client engages in leisure activities alone and with others as well as when the client last engaged in leisure activities.

The Performance Assessment of Self-Care Skills

The PASS is an evaluation designed by Rogers and Holm (1994). This evaluation is a testing tool developed to assess a person's ability to perform living skills. The PASS is primarily task-based with 26 testing sections. Skill performance can be tested by administering task 22, playing bingo. The client is first instructed in the rules of the bingo game and then asked to mark the numbers called and identify when bingo occurs; the occupational therapist assesses whether the client marked the numbers heard correctly and whether he or she was aware when bingo had occurred.

Informal Leisure Checklists

Occupational therapists often administer informal leisure checklists, as this type of testing can be an easy and effective way of determining a client's past, present, and future interests in leisure. An informal leisure checklist also may seem less threatening to a client than a formal evaluation. The checklist often provides numerous examples of types of leisure activities such as bowling, jogging, art, and playing a musical instrument, which can serve as "tickler" ideas for clients needing to explore new options. When a newspaper is available listing social events, movies, and other club or group supports are available in the surrounding area, use it to display a smorgasbord of options to adapt for the client.

The therapist can gather information in less formal assessments using published leisure checklists, role checklists (see the MOHO frame of reference from University of Chicago), and worksheets for self-awareness in recovery such as those developed by Gross and DeMatteo (1998). These can be used individually or in groups to identify values, habits, and preferences for leisure activities.

Intervention Implications

If formal and informal testing yields deficiency in leisure engagement, then the occupational therapist designs an intervention plan with the client to address leisure needs. Each intervention plan will be inherently different given individual client interests and the type of clinical care setting in which the intervention will take place.

Other factors to consider when designing an intervention plan to address leisure skills include issues in context and accessibility, such as cultural barriers, physical barriers, financial barriers, transportation barriers, and temporal barriers. An example of an inventive plan for a client with a more passive involvement in a leisure activity is provided below.

A 35-year-old female client with a wheelchair as her only transportation would like to attempt international travel and she is currently in a financially disadvantaged situation. The occupational therapist may assist the client in developing this interest by introducing her to the travel section of the library and bookstore or to magazines published abroad. The occupational therapist can also assist the client in locating (in newspapers, bulletin boards, and on the Internet) local lectures by people who have engaged in foreign travel, creatively satisfying her urge to be exposed to novel cultures. While this does not allow her to travel, it engages her in an area of interest.

Additional factors to consider when designing occupational therapy intervention for leisure skills are the activity demands, such as appropriateness of activity, supplies, funds, staff time, and location of activity. In order to uphold the dignity of the client, every attempt should be made by the occupational therapist to make interventions as age-appropriate as possible.

In relation to these additional factors, a list of questions and concerns has been provided below. These should be reviewed prior to the initiation of an activity.

Additional Factors to Consider

- Will the planned leisure activity be meaningful and of interest to the client?
- Is the activity age-appropriate?
- What supplies are needed to plan for the desired leisure intervention?
- Does the facility have the budget to allow for the desired leisure intervention?
- Is there enough staff available to assist with the intervention?
- Will the desired leisure intervention fit within the time frame of the planned session?
- Where will the intervention occur, on the facility grounds or in the community?
- If in the community, how will transportation be arranged and which staff members are able to assist?
- Will the client need a pass or doctor's order if the leisure activity is off the unit?
- Does the client need medical clearance from the doctor to engage in the leisure activity?
- Is this a leisure activity the client can pursue in the community once discharged from occupational therapy? Does the leisure intervention have carry-over?

Adapting Leisure

Occupational therapists often must adapt a leisure activity to the individual needs of the client. For example, planning for a leisure intervention involving dance movements for adult clients who have experienced a traumatic brain injury (TBI) would be quite different from planning the same intervention for adult clients who have experienced a myocardial infarction (MI), or heart attack.

For the group of clients who have experienced a TBI, some factors to consider include the following:

- Are the clients able to initiate movement?
- Do any of the clients have a seizure history?
- Do perseverative movements or thoughts impede task function?
- Is sexual impulsivity a problem for any of the clients in the group?
- What is the range of motion (ROM) and grade of muscle tone of the affected limb(s) among the participants? Are the participants on any restrictions of movement?
- How do the cognitive deficits, if applicable, from the TBI impede the participants' ability to learn?
- Will the participants be seated in wheelchairs?

In comparison, some factors to consider if planning a similar intervention for a group of clients who have had an MI include the following:

- Are there any activity restrictions, such as lifting?
- How much endurance do the participants have? Can they tolerate a regular session or would two short sessions be more appropriate?
- Do any of the participants require closely monitored vital signs, such as blood pressure and oxygen saturation?
- Should the group include education regarding stress reduction and potential risk factors to be aware of during physical activities?

The fact that the group for individuals with TBI has a markedly higher number of considerations than the group for individuals with MI highlights the point that some group activities require much more adaptation than others depending on the composition of the group.

Leisure Activity Adaptations

Nearly any leisure activity can be adapted with the cooperative effort of problem solving that occurs between the occupational therapist and the client. Often a creative, problem-solving approach, with a healthy dose of humor, needs to be applied in order to persist until an adaptation is considered satisfactory by the client.

The following are just a few of the many ways in which leisure activities can be adapted. These suggestions have been grouped by client factors and processing skills.

Client Factors: ROM, Strength, and Coordination

- Clients with UE deficits can join in a game of cards with the use of a plastic card holder.
- Card sorters can be used in place of shuffling bilaterally for clients with decreased coordination.
- Bowling ramps can be used with a client who may be unable to lift the ball. With this device, the bowling partner can line up the bowling ramp according to the direction of the bowler prior to the push of the ball.

- For clients with decreased UE strength or decreased coordination, throwing the bowling ball "granny style" can be attempted. The client bends both knees and throws the ball toward the pins with both hands.
- For clients with more significant deficits in strength, be sure to use lighter weight bowling balls, or instead attempt duckpin bowling, which uses lighter balls.
- For clients with decreased hand strength, a table clamp can be used to hold the pages open for reading.
- For clients with decreased grip strength, use larger-handled paintbrushes, markers, and pencils. Other options are to make a universal cuff or cut cylindrical foam tubing to be placed over art utensils.
- Tape large strips of sheet paper on the wall when engaging a client in mural art while also working on increasing UE strength.
- Use tape to hold paper in place during art activities if the client only has unilateral UE functioning.

Client Factors: Sensory Functions

- For clients who have decreased grip strength due to a sensory loss, use larger-handled paintbrushes, markers, and pencils.
- Making a universal cuff or cutting cylindrical foam tubing to be placed over art utensils can enable gross grasp positions for utilizing tools more efficiently.
- Keeping all materials within the clients' visual parameters will allow them to check on the impact of tool use and prevent injuries.

Client Factors: Endurance

- The amount of endurance and need for rest must be determined by the evaluation and reassessed with client feedback and input during this collaborative process.
- A pattern of gain can be documented with relation to time involvement, amount of focused concentration, and requests for break times.

Specific Mental Functions: Cognition and Perception

- Upon evaluation, the level of cognitive ability can establish parameters for single- or multistep tasks that will guide the choices for intervention activities.
- Establishing the purpose and motivational factors will also guide the depth of intellectual challenge or lack of challenge required from the client.
- The visual motor and perceptual motor abilities can potentially limit the complexity and speed of required tasks within each recreational activity.
- For bowling, create a line down the center of the lane using brightly colored, removable electrical tape.
- Use brightly colored adhesive tape to make a border around the paper for a client with neglect or hemianopsia.

Sensory Functions: Low Vision

- Clients with low vision can play cards by using a deck of cards with enlarged numbers and face cards.

- For bowling, create a line down the center of the lane using brightly colored, removable electrical tape.
- Use books with large print and be sure there is ample reading light. A clip-on book light would be helpful.
- The Society for the Blind can offer magnifier machines to read books on tape and CD for clients with significant visual impairments.

Leisure by Intervention Setting Change: Context and Environment

Economic realities, physical conditions, or physical access to leisure or recreational pursuits can be potential barriers for a person dealing with a temporary or permanent disability. Community agencies offering recreational facilities, while in compliance with the Americans with Disabilities Act (1990, P.L.101-336), may not be easily accessible to some populations with disabilities, and some clients' inability to advocate for increasing the availability of services can serve to limit opportunities. Communication or language deficiencies on the part of the staff, or lack of knowledge related to adaptive devices used to assist physically challenged individuals, can lead to organizational barriers.

There is a role for occupational therapy in creating outreach programs within community programs to reduce the lack of understanding, ignorance, or fear on the part of management or staff. Creation of new service delivery options in library settings, indoor bowling, skating arenas, gyms, or swimming clubs would help to deliver multiple avenues for leisure and recreational activities for varied populations.

When the occupational therapist creates a plan for developing a person's leisure skill intervention, he or she must consider the setting in which the intervention will occur. For example, typical settings can include hospital rooms, rehabilitation rooms, inpatient psychiatric units, community settings, or homes. If the client is in a hospital room and has a strong interest in playing basketball, it is understandable that the client will not be able to run up and down the halls of the hospital dribbling the ball. How can his or her interest in basketball be adapted? Perhaps by using a suction-cup basketball net and foam ball certain clients would be more successful executing the skills necessary for a successful recreational experience. Discovering what the client's leisure interests are at the time of administering formal and/or informal occupational therapy testing is essential for guiding the client and will help to foster a better rapport.

The following are examples of leisure activities that can be adapted for use in occupational therapy interventions among the more common client care settings.

Hospital Room (for Client on Bed Rest)

- Computer or tablet use for Internet or games
- Card decorating and card writing
- Artwork
- Board games and cards
- Making tissue flowers
- Origami
- Exercise
- Painting fingernails
- Decorating flower pots
- Making potpourri sachets

- Collage
- Crossword and perceptual puzzles
- Knitting, sewing, and crochet
- Reading the "funnies"/comics

Rehabilitation Room or Clinic Setting (for Individual or Group Sessions)

- Foam basketball with suction cup net
- Suction cup or safety darts
- Video and computer games
- Board and card games
- Exercise
- Word search and crossword puzzles
- Dancing
- Singing and karaoke
- Cooking
- Letter writing
- Listening to music
- Playing piano or keyboard

Inpatient Psychiatric Unit (for Individual or Group Sessions)

- Artwork: painting, drawing, clay, papier-mâché, collage
- Making jewelry
- Card design
- Indoor gardening
- Decorating T-shirts
- Painting ceramic figurines
- Stained glass (plastic)
- Dance
- Exercise
- Pet therapy
- Writing in journal
- Writing poetry
- Reading portions of plays aloud
- Cooking
- Creating weekly newsletter with articles written and illustrated by clients
- Bingo
- Crafts

Community Psychiatric Setting

- Planning and participating in an ice cream social
- Creating art, planning and participating in an art exhibit
- Creating parade float and walking with float during parade
- Baking and hosting a bake sale
- Trips to local community leisure resources such as libraries, museums, art galleries, animal shelters, parks, and farms
- Starting a bowling or softball team
- Creating crafts throughout the year and having an annual craft sale
- Involving clients in making plans to go to events such as basketball and baseball games, theater, movies, or political rallies
- Initiating a community garden

Leisure and Safety

With participation in leisure activities, there are varying levels of potential injury that are evident throughout the continuum of life. Examples include a 17-year-old female who fractures her radius while playing high school field hockey; the 40-year-old male who acquires a torn meniscus while skiing down the black diamond trail; or the 70-year-old male who nicks his hand during a woodworking project. Analysis of acceptable risk and those leisure activities that need to be adapted modified, or as the last resort restricted, is part of the interrelated process of evaluation, intervention, and therapeutic outcomes. The occupational therapist is aware of safety concerns associated with body structure/function as well as activity demands (objects, social demands, space demands, and sequencing). Of course, the general therapeutic goal is for the individual to take part in leisure activities in the safest manner possible. While leisure exploration and evaluation of leisure has already been discussed in this chapter, the leisure planning activity sheet (Figure 8-2) will address safety concerns as an individual researches areas of interest.

Client Factors (Body Structure/Function) Related to Activity Demands/Medical Contraindications and Precautions

Before a client can take part in any leisure activity, body functioning as related to safety of activity demands must be determined. This information can be obtained through the medical chart and by consulting with the treating physician and health care team. A fall risk assessment is a common safety factor. Another would be cardiac precautions. Can the individual who is 75 years old and has experienced an MI 2 months prior take part in the team-building group parachute activity? An immediate question would be, what metabolic equivalents are required to perform the specific leisure activity? Are isometric fitness activities safe? It is also important to not assume only older adults have cardiovascular precautions. Individuals of all ages can have physical activity restrictions for a multitude of medical issues.

Understanding precautions related to the impact of medication on body functions is also vital. Many medications may be sedative in nature and cause hypostatic changes. Other medications could be activating, and others still may cause sensitivity to certain foods, temperature, and/or direct sunlight. Imagine the impact this information could have on an occupational therapy community outing if a group of clients wanted to arrange a picnic in a local park on a sunny day. Medication, the effects from food, and the natural environment could be easily overlooked.

Client Leisure Planning Activity Sheet

1) Name the leisure activity that you want to enjoy:

____

2) Identify the date of the activity:______________________________

3) Identify the specific location and address: ______________________________

____

____

4) What will be the travel time to the location as well as the return time?

____

5) What mode of transportation will be needed?

____

6) Is the site accessible for your functional mobility needs (i.e., ramp, elevator)?

____

7) How much time do you plan to devote to the activity?

____

8) What will be the financial cost of the entire activity including transportation?

____

9) Do you plan to go alone or will there be others with you? Describe:

____

10) Describe safety concerns: ______________________________

11) List three numbers you would call for assistance in case of an emergency:

____

____

____

12) Describe your expectations for this community activity. What do you want to experience?

____

____

Figure 8-2. Sample form created by Robert DeMatteo, OTR/L.

Physiological factors must always be considered. An example would be the use of a product containing latex, such as balloons; a client could have an allergic reaction if he or she is predisposed to that type of sensitivity. Does the client have a pacemaker or any type of vitals monitor, and will a specific electronic leisure item interfere with physiological functioning?

Another consideration is being aware of the client's special dietary restrictions. Some clients may have food allergies, such as peanuts, dairy products, certain fruits, or shellfish. Again, this information can be obtained by asking the client, checking the medical chart, and consulting with caregivers and medical staff. It is critical to know the ingredients being used for the task of food preparation, such as with cooking groups.

General health and wellness should also be promoted. Obesity, diabetes, and heart disease are common health problems in the adult population. Certain medications have side effects that can cause increased appetite and weight gain. Common occupational therapy leisure group activities have included such things as baking cakes, brownies, and sweets. It would not be appropriate to have a leisure cooking or baking activity with high-sugar or high-fat items with clients who have the above-mentioned concerns. Alternative healthy food choices should be presented as part of general care such as with low-fat and low- or no-sugar products.

As part of any activity involving eating and drinking, body structure and body function is analyzed. The occupational therapist would inquire about issues of dysphasia and other feeding issues. Are there contraindications for certain foods due to aspiration risk? Can the client safely chew, swallow, and digest the food planned for the activity? Speech and language pathologists and dietitians can work together with occupational therapists regarding these issues. For more information regarding eating/dysphagia, see Chapter 3.

General precautions related to body structures and functions must also be considered for fitness and sports-related leisure activities. The potential for injury increases with these types of activities. Consider what would be required if a client wanted to snowboard, kickbox, skateboard, play lacrosse, or lift weights. A thorough task analysis is essential. An occupational therapist can research a specific fitness activity through consulting with sports coaches, fitness trainers, local gyms, clubs, and websites. Clinicians associated with sports medicine and physical therapy may also be resources.

Activity Demands

Activity demands, according to the Framework (AOTA, 2014), include the objects/materials used during leisure tasks, the space demands or physical environment where the task is completed, the social demands of the task, such as rules of a game, as well as the required body functions/structures discussed above. Each of these activity demands has safety concerns that need to be addressed.

Objects Used and Their Properties: General Information for All Settings

Whether it is an inpatient hospital setting, partial-hospital program, skilled nursing facility, a group home, a community clubhouse, or a home care environment, the following precautions apply:

- The occupational therapist must be aware of the chemical contents, temperature, stress indications, and general safety precautions related to leisure materials. This is especially evident with arts and craft materials. Certain glues, inks, wood stains, and oil paints contain toxins, and skin contact is contraindicated. Special ventilation may also be required to utilize some of these products. Some materials could be flammable or harmful if ingested.
- The occupational therapist must determine whether use of the materials matches the age and cognitive/behavioral skills of the client. Consider the scenario of an individual with an Allen cognitive level of 4.0 who wanted to engage in oil painting as a hobby. At first, the activity appears to be a safe and healthy pastime, but with further analysis the potential for harm is discovered. The client lives in a one-room apartment with limited ventilation and plans to use turpentine in open coffee cans as a medium for the oil paint. The activity does not match the space demands or physical environmental requirements for safe participation. The client also smokes. Decreased insight into how the vapors from the solvent could be harmful as well as the risk of fire is noted. After researching painting supplies, the occupational therapist learns

that acrylic paint can mix with water and there is decreased risk of harmful fumes and combustion. The acrylic is substituted for the oil paint and the activity is modified so the client can still partake in her desired leisure interest.

The occupational therapist can obtain product information by reading chemical content and caution labels. Certain inpatient settings, such as hospitals and skilled nursing facilities, have material data sheets. The occupational therapist can also consult with craft and hardware stores or even the manufacturer regarding product safety.

Other leisure products such as modes of transportation, safety gear, and electronics also have various safety precautions. For example, an occupational therapist would consider the activity demands of operating a bicycle as related to the general functioning of the rider. Imagine if the client wanted to participate in four-wheeling with a recreational quad-bike, water-skiing, or using a snowmobile. Safety concerns are evident for such tasks. Similar safety concerns are also present for more common activities such as driving to see a movie. The basic safety questions for all forms of locomotion would be the following: Could the individual drive in an appropriate manner? Is there a need for a driving evaluation? Is the client aware of safety precautions?

The occupational therapist should be aware of the proper way for a client to wear such items as a safety helmet, knee/elbow pads, a chest protector, a groin cup, and safety goggles. Roller skating, playing football, and welding a metal sculpture are just a few activities that utilize safety gear. It is important to remember that using protective gear does not mean the risk of injury is totally eliminated. For example, a safety helmet in batting practice can reduce the force of a ball hitting an individual's head, but the person's face and neck are still vulnerable to harm. Many safety items have force, impact, and weight limitations. The baseball helmet may be effective to a certain amount of foot-pounds of pressure per square inch before cracking. Awareness of the manufacturer's product precautions and guidelines for safety items is a critical part of proper task analysis.

Knowledge of the proper electrical plugs and outlets as related to such devices as radios, electric musical instruments, electronic games, and computers is important. A safety concern would be whether the power strip is overloaded with various plug-ins. The occupational therapist would also be aware of any signs of malfunctioning, worn, or damaged leisure materials. When possible, the client should also be encouraged to check for item defects.

Many social and leisure activities involve food. An occupational therapist may facilitate a leisure cooking group, such as a holiday lunch party or a community client picnic. Often, the clients may bring in food items from home as part of the activity. The general precautions for all food include the following:

- Is the food fresh?
- Is it thoroughly cooked?
- Was it refrigerated properly?
- Was it handled properly (i.e., did the client wash his or her hands during preparation)?
- Are the utensils clean?

Objects: Physical Disabilities With the Comorbidity of Behavioral Health Issues (Objects in Relation to Mental Functions)

Part of leisure task analysis is knowledge of the materials associated with the activity and the safety precautions. The safety precautions are closely related to the global and specific mental functions of the client. This is especially evident among populations with behavioral health issues in inpatient psychiatric settings, group homes, skilled nursing facilities, and TBI programs. While arts and crafts task activities are common occupational therapy modalities in these settings, proper selection and storage of the materials is critical because suicidal and self-harming behavior

Date:	Item:	Quantity:	Time-Out:	Time-In:
	Scissors	10		
	Latch-hooks	7		
	Glue gun	3		
	Cans of wood stain	5		
	Spools of twine	2		
	Long-handled paint brushes	13		
Signature:				

Figure 8-3. Example of an occupational therapy leisure material safety sheet. (Created by Robert DeMatteo, OTR/L.)

is a factor with some clients. Examples of materials that warrant concern include items referred to as "sharps," such as latch-hooks, scissors, and knitting needles. Other items include yarn and ribbon, which can be doubled up to make a noose; a paintbrush or a sharpened colored pencil, which has the potential to puncture; a simple plastic bag used to carry craft materials, which can cause asphyxiation; and even a common paperclip or a staple from the binding of a magazine, which can be bent and used to scratch or lacerate. Unfortunately, when performing a task analysis, the occupational therapist must think in terms of the protection of the client and the staff. Awareness of the client's psychiatric history and behavioral status is always the first step. Again, checking the chart and consulting with the team/staff and the physician are critical.

An example of a safety scenario is when a client who can safely take part in a task leisure activity on the unit has materials that another client may try to take in order to cause self-harm. The occupational therapist must be vigilant regarding who is allowed to have the materials and who is not. Consider the example of clients in an inpatient neurorehabilitation unit making wooden ornaments for the holiday during an occupational therapy task/leisure group. The clients want to keep their crafts, although the occupational therapist understands the balsa wood can be snapped to make a jagged point. The clients who made the ornaments do not have aggressive or self-harming behavior, and they ask to keep their projects in their rooms on the unit. The occupational therapist needs to take the ornaments and put them in a locked storage area because of another client who was not in the group but is still in the facility and has a history of decreased impulse control and violent outbursts. As a result, it would be highly unsafe for the ornaments to be lying around. The occupational therapist consults with the clients and assures them that they may have their ornaments back when they are discharged to go home.

The following list regarding the storage of leisure materials is valid for both inpatient and outpatient settings:

- A written inventory of all the items is highly recommended.
- A count should be made both before materials go out to be used by the clients and when they are returned (e.g., how many scissors were given to the group and how many were collected at the end).
- On the inventory list, there should also be an indication of the storage site area (e.g., locked ventilated storage cabinet or third locked drawer in occupational therapy office).
- A sign-out/sign-in time along with staff signatures is beneficial in tracking items (Figure 8-3).

Activity Demands/Social Demands

Many leisure activities involve such components as physical touch, socializing with peers and members of the opposite sex, competition, and the encouragement of humor and laughter. With these components, there could be related safety issues. Consider a client who sustained a TBI and now has frontal-lobe syndrome or a client who experienced a right-hemisphere cerebral vascular accident. Decreased impulse control, difficulties modulating frustration and anger, impairment of abstract thinking and higher-level judgment, and misinterpretation of social cues are just a few elements of the symptomology. What might happen if a client with the above-mentioned issues took part in a group hug as part of a team-building leisure activity? Decreased control related to sexual impulses and inappropriate touching could be a risk factor. Leisure pursuits that involve competition, from a simple board game to more intense activities such as a tennis or basketball game, could be triggers for angry outbursts. The client may have difficulty tolerating the outcome of losing. An example of this is how the client with impulse control issues could react if spiked at the net while playing volleyball. Humor, jokes, and lighthearted teasing can also be misconstrued as insulting. Often in team sports, a coach may try to motivate a person by verbally "pushing" the individual to do better. Comments like, "Go! Go!" and "You're too slow! Pick up the pace!" may at first seem like appropriate encouragement, but again due to impairment of higher-level cognition, the client could have an adverse emotional reaction. A pat on the shoulder may cause a client to retaliate with a physical outburst. Some clients with physical disabilities may have other types of coexisting cognitive or behavioral health issues such as anxiety disorders, social phobias, and histories of post-traumatic stress disorder. Consider the example of a client with paraplegia who also has severe panic attacks and is asked to introduce herself for the first time in an occupational therapy leisure group. While promoting socialization and the enhancement of quality of life is the therapeutic goal, the client instead may be experiencing a spike in stress and highly uncomfortable psychological and physiological responses. The intervention choice of a group at this stage in her recovery is too challenging, and the flight/fight response takes over her body, limiting her successful participation. Establishing a therapeutic relationship comes first, then understanding the clients' goals, followed finally by using clinical reasoning to individualize the interventions.

Another example could be a client with multiple sclerosis who has a history of physical and sexual abuse. Intimacy issues and difficulties with physical touch are noted. Holding hands in a team building exercise or interacting with other male group members may be viewed by this client as adverse, thus increasing the likelihood of their nonparticipation.

Concerning all the above-mentioned cognitive and behavioral issues, participation in leisure pursuits is still facilitated, although with implementation of modification, adaptation, prevention, relearning, and new learning. Encouraging the client to take part in a leisure role offers an opportunity to address cognitive impairments, inappropriate social conduct, impoverished and dominating habits, as well as pathologies related to psychosocial issues.

Articles that described use of novel modalities for occupational therapy intervention with veterans with post-traumatic stress disorder symptomatology include one that describes, for example, surfing as a means of meeting the occupational therapist goals of developing social and leisure habits and routines for wellness (Rogers, Mallinson, & Peppers, 2014). The intensity of this sport meets the need to engage in "high-risk" situations and to learn to trust your own body to ride the wave. The study sample started with 14 participants, 11 of whom completed the study. A noncontrolled study but the first of its kind to focus on lowering depression and providing the satisfaction of the same adrenaline rush achieved in combat yet in a more constructive way. This small sample may limit the generalizability of the results, although the outcome was better than expected by the authors (Rogers, Mallinson, & Peppers, 2014). The authors were pleased that the compliance with a 5-week therapy regime increased, and they attributed this potentially to interest in being outdoors and engaging physical, physiological, and mental capacities, similar to prior military training and experience.

Activity Demands, Space Demands, Sequencing

These factors will be covered when the client leisure activity planning sheet is completed, with discussion and exploration to assess the necessary adaptations required for successful execution of the activity by the client. Certain occupational therapy settings may create limitations until the full community re-involvement phase is under way.

General Precautions for Community Leisure Activities

One of the many client-centered goals of occupational therapy is for the individual to partake in and enjoy healthy leisure activities out in society. Community outings such as client picnics, visiting a bookstore, going to a restaurant, or viewing a play can be highly therapeutic experiences to promote learning, adaptation, individual satisfaction, and enhancement of general quality of life. However, along with the value of community integration activities, there are added safety concerns. For example, there is no longer the support of a controlled environment such as a hospital or a rehabilitation facility. In implementing a community-based leisure activity, objects and their properties, space demands related to physical context, social demands, sequence and timing, required actions, and client factors need to be analyzed. The basic question would be whether the client can safely tolerate the event. The following are examples of safety factors for consideration:

- The number of staff needed to facilitate and supervise the outing as related to the acuity of the client and/or number of clients in a group
- The type of transportation needed and the accessibility to the client, such as a van with a lift vs a public bus
- The accessibility of the site to the client (e.g., wheelchair ramps, elevators, level walkways, and bathrooms)
- Knowledge of the site as related to additional safety hazards (e.g., near a lake, near a road with traffic, or near a heavy crime area)
- Knowledge of the closest hospital in case of emergency
- Having access to communication lines in case of an emergency (e.g., more than one cellphone, or access to a landline if cellphone service is not available)
- Knowledge of accurate directions to the site and an alternative route in case of traffic issues
- Knowledge of accurate travel time and the duration of the leisure event
- Awareness of the client's medication schedules and other time-based procedures, such as breathing interventions, colostomy, and catheter routines
- Safety implications related to weather (e.g., whether the client can tolerate direct sunlight, heat, humidity, or cold)
- Having a back-up plan for temporary shelter if there are weather or temperature changes
- Bringing umbrellas and extra warm clothing in case of weather changes
- Staff being trained in CPR and first aid
- Occupational therapist and staff having an established, written emergency protocol for community outings

Precautions Related to Utilization of the Internet and Computers

Computers and the Internet enable wide participation in leisure activities within the virtual context. The massive popularity of video games, music downloading, chat rooms for socialization, and the various types of virtual activities available present related risk factors. One precaution is to consider whether the video game or website is age-appropriate for the client. Concerning an adult client, the question would be: Does the client have the global mental functions to access a particular type of media with no adverse effects? It is common for an Internet subscriber to be bombarded with junk e-mail advertising adult websites, cheap prescription medication, and stock investments. There is also the potential to acquire addictions to pornography or mail-order prescriptions. The easy access of buying online could also lead to shopping addiction. In addition, there is the widespread danger of identify theft. The Internet can be an effective leisure outlet for many individuals, but activity demands must correspond with client factors. Consider the scenario of a client with an ACL of 5.0 who has a history of cerebral palsy and has decreased self-esteem due to difficulties with body image. The client's left UE has a manual muscle testing rating of "poor" due to neurological pathology. Muscle wasting is evident, and the limb hangs unusably by his side. The client often states he is "ugly" because of his arm. Past hospitalizations for major, recurrent, severe depression are noted. The client lives alone in an apartment building for individuals with disabilities. He reports difficulty with socialization and expresses to the occupational therapist that he is often lonely. After saving up for a computer as part of an intervention goal, he begins to utilize the Internet and is soon bombarded with e-mails offering various chat services for a monthly fee. The client has access to a credit card and starts to give out his personal information online, including his Social Security number. The client reports, "I made a bunch of new girlfriends." The potential for the client to be taken advantage of is high. The occupational therapist intervenes and provides safety education as part of leisure planning. The client agrees to utilize a spam-blocking feature offered by his Internet service. Money management and proper use of a credit card are addressed, as are alternative social leisure outlets.

The right of access and privacy is an additional issue concerning an adult client's use of the Internet or other types of media. If the individual can utilize websites, chat rooms, or purchase items online with no adverse effects, then there is no need for a therapeutic intervention. The occupational therapist must not try to restrict an adult client's right to access information, read particular material, listen to certain types of music, or communicate with another individual just because it may seem offensive. It is important to realize that the occupational therapist's moral or religious values must not impede the client-centered approach.

Community Leisure for the Adult With Physical Disabilities

In analyzing therapeutic outcomes, a common indicator for improvement in function and independence is to be active and involved in one's own society. This is evident with participation in leisure. With an emphasis on a client-centered approach balanced with considerations for safety, the occupational therapist should encourage the client to partake in leisure activities out in the community.

A study conducted in England with clients in the community who had experienced stroke sought to encourage the frequency of their outings. The randomized control study included 200 clients. The control group only received information via mail postings regarding ways to access community public transportation, and the intervention group received occupational therapist education sessions including assistance in utilizing the public transportation in seven sessions. Pre- and post-information surveys were mailed to all clients, and a significant number of the intervention group participants reported an increase of community involvement in outings as compared to the control group (Logan et al., 2004).

In order for the client and occupational therapist to work collaboratively to determine whether community leisure is appropriate, the following aspects in assessment must be considered:

1. Identification of client's leisure interests and leisure goals
2. Analysis of activity demands related to client factors
3. Adhering to safety issues
4. Access/transportation to community leisure sites
5. Verifying that the community leisure site is accommodating to the client
6. The leisure intervention plan allows for modification, adaptation, learning, and relearning
7. Quality of life is always promoted

Additionally, for the occupational therapist to facilitate effective leisure participation, it is paramount to have a working knowledge of what the client's community has to offer (refer to the adult community leisure list later in this chapter). This is further analyzed on a continuum according to which activities have no cost, a minimal charge, are moderately expensive, or are expensive. Cost, however, is all relative to the individual's income. A specific client may be on Social Security disability and only receive $500 dollars per month to pay rent for a subsidized apartment and to buy food. Paying $10 for admission to a movie and $7 for popcorn and a soda would seem extravagant. Another client with a different financial situation may be able to hire personal aides and dine at upscale restaurants. With this point understood, a real-world generalization is that most clients tend to have some financial limitations. The occupational therapist, in collaboration with the individual, has to be creative in leisure planning while adhering to a budget.

Despite financial restrictions, another common obstacle to community leisure is transportation. A common statement made by some clients is: "I want to get out more but I have no way to get there. I can get a medical cab to my office visit but that is it. I'm stuck if I want to do anything fun." The lack of transportation is due to many factors. A few examples are: (1) the client does not drive or has stopped driving; (2) the client lives in a location were there is no bus service or other types of mass transit; and (3) the transportation available does not accommodate the client's mobility needs (e.g., the wheelchair cannot fit in the back of the family's car). The occupational therapist can assist the client in problem-solving these obstacles by being aware of what supports are available in the community. Transportation factors such as driver retraining and acquisition of modified vans and cars are separate interventions. Consider identification of the following:

- Area bus routes, time schedules, and rates related to the client's location
- Area train and subway routes, time schedules, and rates related to the client's location
- Taxi services and rates
- Discount transit pass programs for clients with disabilities
- Van services offered by community mental health clubhouse programs
- Community senior shuttles
- Religious/church organizations that offer rides
- Safe transportation can be offered by family and friends
- Knowledge of transportation options that are accessible

Related to financial and transportation factors, another recommendation for effective leisure planning is for the occupational therapist to venture out into the client's community and see what leisure pursuits are available. Taking a drive around after work to conduct some "reconnaissance" will truly help in understanding the environment, activity demands, safety issues, and leisure sites.

Leisure Psychosocial Issues: Addiction

In the various populations in which occupational therapy is implemented, there is often the diagnosis of substance abuse or substance dependency. This includes clients with physical disabilities and not just those with coexisting mental health issues. In certain scenarios, these issues are openly identified, while at other times they can be far from evident. For example, there can be a teen with paraplegia who is starting to experiment with cannabis; a client with a history of TBI who is taking part in an outpatient partial hospital program and is addicted to cocaine; a 40-year-old male machine operator who is receiving a splint for carpal tunnel syndrome at a hand therapy clinic and reports having chronic pain issues but is also addicted to oxycodone and exhibits medication-seeking behavior; and the 75 year old who has experienced a cerebral vascular accident and is receiving occupational therapy on a home-care basis, has a history of alcoholism, and is now addicted to lorazepam.

One of the core principles of occupational therapy is to promote quality of life through working with the client to extinguish maladaptive habits and acquire alternative healthy roles and routines. One of the many areas of functioning that is adversely affected by substance abuse and addiction is participation in healthy leisure activities. Occupational therapy can assist in a client's recovery by enhancing sober leisure pursuits. Usually, this is one of the major occupational therapy intervention goals in both inpatient and outpatient mental health settings. Clients with addiction issues often report that their leisure activities revolve around "using." Bars, dance clubs, keg and dorm parties, sporting events, and concerts are just a few examples of places where alcohol and street drugs are common. These events and activities can also be outlets for socialization. A common dilemma for clients in recovery is making decisions regarding keeping or ending friendships with individuals who also have drug and alcohol issues. Many clients in early rehabilitation often express that they feel lonely and bored with the prospect of no longer being able to "party" or to hang out with certain people. A key slogan in 12-step recovery programs is "changing people, places, and things" (Alcoholics Anonymous, 1984). Occupational therapy can assist with this concept by facilitating involvement in new leisure activities and social outlets that are drug- and alcohol-free. The following are a few examples that clients could consider:

- Connecting with a local gym or YMCA
- Going out to eat with sober friends rather than going to a bar
- Seeing a movie
- Going to coffee houses and hearing live music
- Attending Alcoholics Anonymous (AA) or Narcotics Anonymous (NA) social events such as sober dances and picnics

The occupational therapist should also consult with the client and analyze what sober leisure interests he or she has had in the past. A major goal of recovery is to regain previous healthy habits and roles. It is important to identify whether the client has specific talents that can be fostered into sober leisure pursuits. It may be discovered in an occupational therapy session that the client has talent for such things as drawing, sculpture, playing an instrument, softball, creative writing, repairing vintage cars, singing, etc. The occupational therapist would encourage the client to restart a specific leisure interest as long as it did not trigger a relapse. The additional therapeutic benefit of fostering personal creative talents is the enhancement of self-worth and self-esteem.

Another addiction that is not always initially identified is gambling. There has been a surge of gambling addiction in the United States, as evidenced by an 800% increase in gambling losses from 1982 to 2007 (Stuart, 2011). This increase can be attributed to the development of new casinos, online Internet betting, state lotteries, and televised poker tournaments. Gambling addiction can be a devastating illness in which an individual can lose everything, such as their life savings, automobile, home, relationship with family, and sense of self-worth. A particular profile for the illness is the "escape gambler" (Gamblers Anonymous, 2005). This type of behavior involves gambling not for the purpose of acquiring money or for the excitement of winning but rather to distract and "numb" the individual from emotional pain. Some older adults can be prone to this condition due to psychosocial and physical stressors such as the following:

- Death of a spouse
- Decreased contact with family and friends
- Boredom
- Decline in physical health and independence

Additionally, weekly bingo and senior bus trips to casinos can be contraindicated for some clients. Even facilitating an occupational therapy leisure group in which the activity has win/lose competitive components can be a trigger to gambling.

Alcohol, street drugs, pain medication, benzodiazepines, and gambling are common addictions, although shopping, sex, and overeating all have the potential to be addictive. These activities are often related to adult leisure. When an occupational therapist is facilitating leisure planning with a client, it is important to be vigilant about potential addiction issues. This is valid for working with children, teens, adults, and the geriatric population. It is also valid for clients with physical disabilities. A goal of occupational therapy is to promote participation in sober, healthy leisure pursuits.

Potential Leisure Activities List

The following is a list of additional activities to assist with leisure planning and implementation. Potential safety and budget issues have been mentioned when appropriate. These options could be reviewed by occupational therapists with clients to determine which leisure interests are appropriate. In some cases clients can then investigate options independently, and in other cases clients may require additional assistance from the occupational therapist. Resources to locate leisure activities include the following:

- Leisure sections of area newspapers
- Events offered by the public library
- Events offered at area community colleges (some programs allow clients to audit classes for free)
- Senior center programs
- Mental health community clubhouse programs
- Church social programs
- Parks and recreation programs (Figure 8-4)

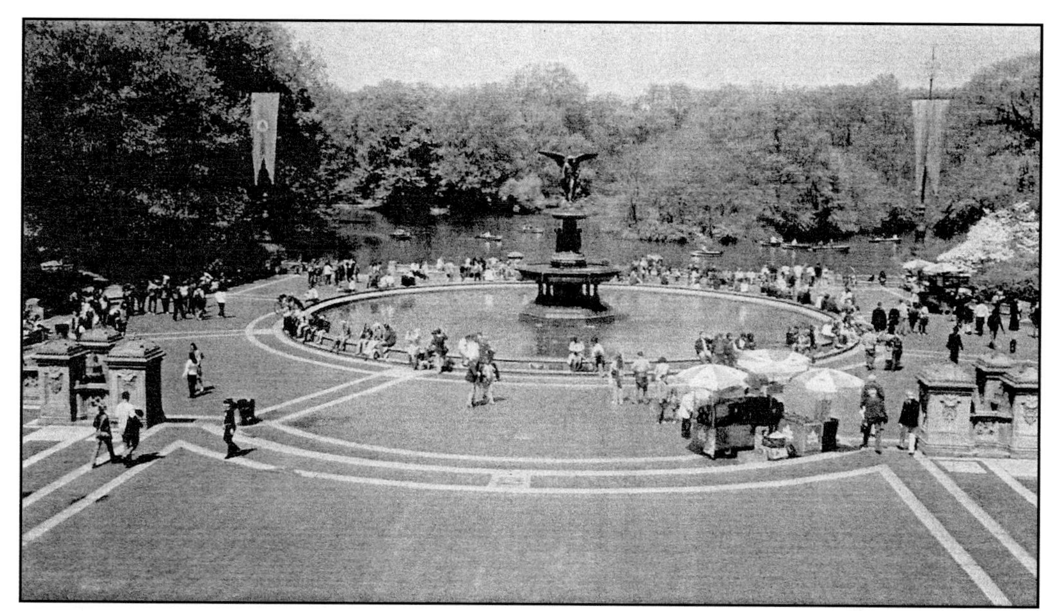

Figure 8-4. Clients should be encouraged to utilize available parks among other resources. (Photo of Central Park by Robert DeMatteo.)

- Adult continuing education programs (e.g., Learning Annex)
- Leisure events sponsored by AA/NA (e.g., picnics and sober dances)

Movies

- Multicinema complexes
- Art-house theaters
- Second-run movie theaters that offer reduced admission
- Bargain matinee specials/senior discounts
- Film programs offered at local libraries and colleges
- Movie theaters that offer accommodations for the hearing impaired
- Film study classes and discussion groups at area colleges

Places to Eat in the Community

- Listings of area restaurants (including prices)
- Obtaining discount coupons for restaurants offered in local newspapers
- Identify restaurants that offer early bird specials
- Calendar of potluck dinners offered by area community organizations or church groups
- Lunch and dinner programs offered by community mental health clubhouses
- Identify restaurant sites that are contraindicated for clients with obesity or special dietary needs (e.g., an all-you-can-eat buffet); identifying sites that offer healthy cuisine would be a therapeutic goal

- Identify eating establishments that do not offer alcohol (for clients with substance abuse issues)

Bars, Dance Clubs, Live Music Venues, Singles Clubs, Comedy Clubs

- Area listings as well as cover charge prices
- Identify times and days when there is no cover charge
- Obtain free admission passes on establishment websites

These types of community leisure outlets are only appropriate for adult clients who have the mental functions to safety interact within these types of environments. It is contraindicated for clients with substance abuse or addiction issues to take part in outings to the above-mentioned sites. Sober dance parties sponsored by AA/NA are a safer alternative.

Coffee Houses

- Can be a safe, alternative adult social setting without the element of alcohol
- Identify coffee houses that offer nightly live music or poetry readings
- Listings of bookstores that have an in-house café (e.g., Barnes and Noble)
- Internet cafés
- Safety concerns regarding client's ability to tolerate caffeine is noted

Fitness/Sports Outlets

- List of area gyms
- YMCA (identify whether local branch offers scholarships and reduced rates for clients with financial constraints)
- Martial arts clubs/schools
- Yoga classes
- Tai chi classes
- Local running tracks
- Mall walking programs
- Public tennis courts
- Public and private golf courses
- Water aerobics programs
- Community swimming pool programs
- Community marathon programs
- Wheelchair basketball leagues
- Area softball leagues (can be sponsored by various community programs, such as parks and recreation, community mental health, and AA/NA)
- Skiing/snowboarding outlets
- Hunting, shooting ranges, archery clubs
- Fishing events

- Bicycle clubs or events
- Roller skating tracks
- Indoor rock-climbing gyms
- Viewing community sporting events: high school, college, professional
- Parks and recreation and adult continuing education programs offering various adult fitness and sports options

Nature Leisure Outlets

- Listing of area parks
- Walking and hiking trails (client should understand difficulty ratings related to specific routes)
- Hiking clubs
- Area beaches, lakes, ponds
- Nature walks or organized education programs
- Bird watching groups
- Area zoos and aquariums

Art/Creative Expression Outlets

Fine art and craft classes are offered at area art schools, colleges, parks and recreation programs, adult continuing education programs, and senior centers (some colleges allow individuals with disabilities, especially seniors, to audit or take classes for reduced rates) (Figure 8-5).

- Local art shows, craft bazaars
- Art exhibits, galleries, museums
- Music lessons of all types
- Local chorus or choir
- Concerts, musical events of all types
- Plays, musicals, local theater events
- Acting classes
- Community theater
- Poetry or creative writing groups
- Book clubs

Case Study 1: Tom, Traumatic Brain Injury

Tom is a 34-year-old man who sustained a TBI due to a motorcycle accident. He was in a coma for 3 days. Multiple bilateral lower extremity (LE) fractures were noted. After hospitalization and 2 months of inpatient rehabilitation, he was transferred to an outpatient neurorehabilitation program. Occupational therapy, physical therapy, and speech therapy were implemented as part of the intervention protocol. Tom presented with periodic lability, impulsivity, and decreased frustration tolerance due to damage to the frontal and prefrontal cortex. His ACL score was 5.0. Partly

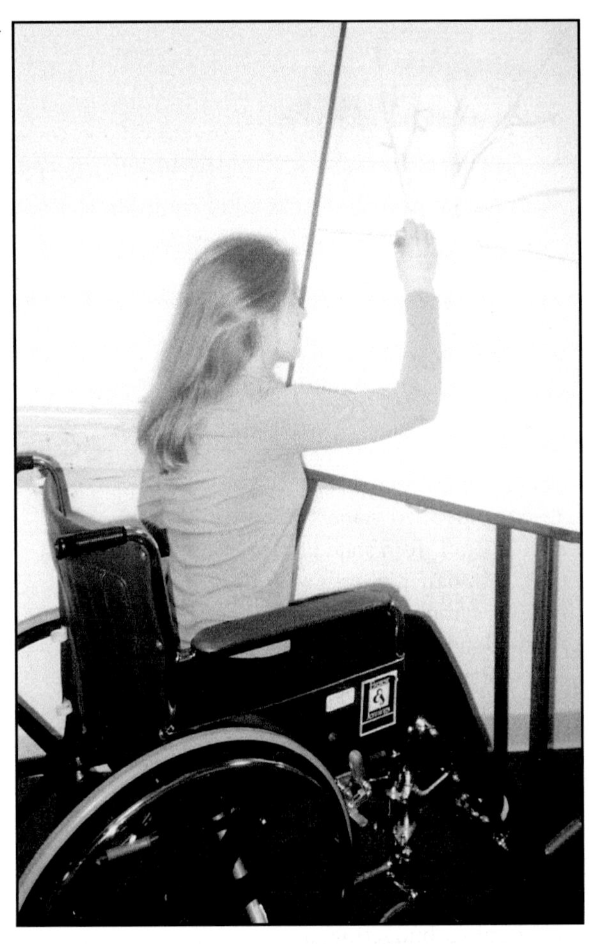

Figure 8-5. Clients should be encouraged to investigate and pursue leisure interests such as art.

through analysis of occupational performance, it was determined that his higher-level judgment was impaired as related to accessing his needs and safety. Tom reported that he wanted to ride his motorcycle again, despite having periodic difficulties with spatial relations, visual tracking, sustained and divided attention, and topographical orientation. A labored gait was noted due to 5 cm of bone being removed from his left femur and the insertion of internal fix-caters and rods. Bilateral UE structure, muscle strength, and sensation were within functional limits; however, there was periodic decreased gross motor coordination.

Prior to the accident, Tom was a successful builder and general contractor. He had an associate's degree in business from an area community college. It was accepted that the client had functioned at an ACL rating of 6.0. He had never married and had recently ended a long-term relationship with a girlfriend. No children were noted. Tom expressed his only family contact was with his elderly aunt, who was his caregiver when he was a child. The team social worker noted in the psychosocial report that Tom's father died when he was 5, and his mother was unable to parent due a long history of major chronic depression and substance abuse issues. No specific religious affiliation was reported. Tom stated, "I don't go to church or anything like that, but I do believe in God." His major social support was with two close male friends he described as his "riding buddies." Reportedly, the two friends were in weekly contact with the client.

The neurologist deemed it unsafe for Tom to drive any vehicle at this time due to neurovisual impairment and difficulties with attention. There was also a single episode of a seizure during

Narcotics Anonymous. (1982). *Narcotics anonymous.* Van Nuys, CA: World Service Office.

Online Casino. (2004). 13% increase in gambling addiction help line in 2004. Retrieved at www.onlinecasino.org/news/13-increase-in-gambling-addiction-help-line-in-2004.php on June 9, 2004.

Parr, M. G., & Lashua, B. D. (2004). What is leisure? The perceptions of recreation practitioners and others. *Leisure Sciences, 26*, 1-17.

Random House Dictionary (2nd ed.). (1987). New York, NY: Random House.

Rogers, C. M., Mallinson, T., & Peppers, D. (2014). High-intensity sports for posttraumatic stress disorder and depression: feasibility study of ocean therapy with veterans of Operation Enduring Freedom and Operation Iraqi Freedom. *American Journal of Occupational Therapy, 68*(4), 395.

Rogers, J. C., & Holm, M. B. (1994). PASS: Performance assessment of self-care skills. Version 3.0. Pittsburgh, PA: WPIC.

Rossman, J. R., & Schlatter, B. E. (2000). *Recreational programming: Designing leisure experiences.* Champaign, IL: Sagamore.

Stuart, E. (2011). Gambling on the rise: Is America becoming addicted? Retrieved at http://www.deseretnews.com/article/700169522/Gambling-on-the-rise-Is-America-becoming- addicted.html?pg=all on November 30, 2014.

Thomson, L. K. (1992). *The Kohlman evaluation of living skills* (3rd ed.). Bethesda, MD: AOTA.

Wilcock, A. A., Chelin, M., Hall, M., Hamley, N., Morrison, B., Scrivener, L., Townsend, M., & Treen, K. (1997) The relationship between occupational balance and health: A pilot study. *Occupational Therapy International, 4*(1), 17-30.

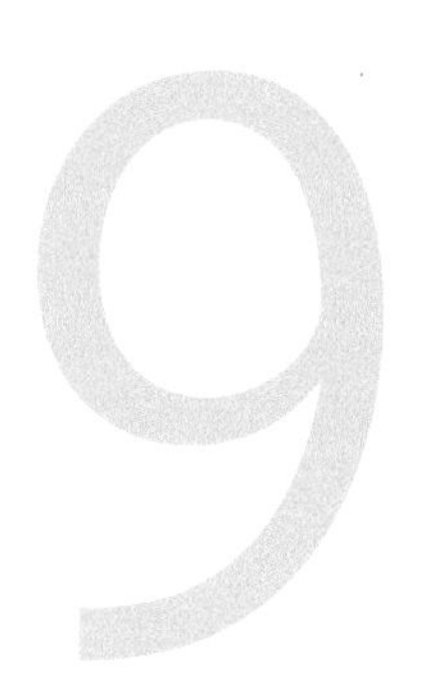

Social Participation

Roseanna Tufano, LMFT, OTR/L

Chapter Objectives

By the end of this chapter, the student will be able to do the following:

- Define social participation as it pertains to the Occupational Therapy Practice Framework.
- Describe specific models/frames of reference as related to social participation.
- Delineate between the role of the occupational therapist and the occupational therapy assistant (OTA) as they pertain to the occupation of social participation.
- Define the role of the occupational therapist as it pertains to peer/friend interactions for adults, older adults, and adults with disabilities.
- Comprehend and identify related physical implications as related to decreased independence in social participation.
- Describe barriers for adults with disabilities in developing and sustaining meaningful peer/friend and intimate relationships.
- Describe the impact of contextual factors upon social participation.
- Identify appropriate social participation intervention strategies based on various performance skills and client factors.
- Identify specific social participation compensation/adaptation strategies.
- Identify general social participation remediation strategies.
- Identify social participation compensation/adaptation intervention strategies related to vision, perception, and cognition.
- Identify general social participation maintenance strategies.

Meriano C, Latella D.
Occupational Therapy Interventions: Function and Occupations, Second Edition (pp 433–477).

Introduction

Occupational therapy practitioners service a broad range of human occupations and activities that make up people's lives (American Occupational Therapy Association [AOTA], 2014). Social participation is a significant occupation and performance area of concern within the practice of occupational therapy. Social participation activities are those associated with organized patterns of behavior that are characteristic of an individual interacting with others within a given social system (adapted from Mosey, 1996, p. 340). Throughout an individual's life, involvement in various groups, organizations, clubs, and social systems overlaps and changes across the lifespan. Social participation activities are multidimensional, complex, and best understood in a top-down approach. The AOTA Framework (2014) specifically guides occupational therapy practitioners to assess social participation and role functioning within community, family, and peer/friend interactions. Humans develop aspects of their own social identity by inclusion in various groups and affiliations. For example, a person may select social activities based on religious or spiritual beliefs, racial empowerment, political parties, civic activities, and personal interests. Significant relationships, such as those with parents, an intimate partner, a spouse, sibling, grandparents, and coworkers, all have the potential to influence an individual's social identity and self-concept throughout the lifespan. According to the National Institutes of Health (NIH), these social and cultural factors play a central role in illness prevention, maintenance of good health, and treating disease, noting that an individual's social ties, the quality of social relationships, and social resources can "mediate the effect of stress on health" (Consortium of Social Science Associations, 2000). Faced with an onset of illness or disease, an individual's role performance in society may be altered, although his or her perception of self-identity and established habits and roles may remain the same. As a result, individuals with disabilities are five times more likely than able-bodied individuals to indicate that they are dissatisfied with their lives due to social isolation and lack of a full social life. Sixty-four percent of adults with disabilities report they are not able to get around town, attend cultural or sporting events, or socialize with friends as much as they would like (Kaye, 1997).

Occupational therapy offers a unique understanding and skill set to this life-preserving occupation called *social participation*. In this chapter, social participation will be explored using a top-down perspective that starts at a client's roles within community, family, and peer/friend relationships. Figure 9-1 will serve as the base model for understanding the components of social participation as defined by the Framework document (AOTA, 2014). Examples to illustrate therapeutic interventions will focus on typical adult development and adults with a physical disability as commonly seen in occupational therapy practice.

In order to effectively promote social participation, occupational therapists must incorporate their own therapeutic use of self. By definition, social participation consists of individuals engaging with one another. Every client meeting offers the therapist a unique opportunity to model effective information exchange, strategies, interpersonal boundaries, and the building blocks of therapeutic social relationships. Methods of social participation interventions can be occupation-based and/or purposeful activities that may be preparatory, educational, and/or consultative in nature (AOTA, 2014).

Client-centered practice is a natural fit for promoting social participation within the therapeutic relationship. Occupational therapists must show sensitivity to a person's cultural, physical, social, personal, temporal, and virtual contexts and environments, which influence the individual's performance in social participation (AOTA, 2014). These contexts are unique to the client, are often interrelated, and influence how the client creates his or her own personal identity. In this chapter, specific examples of social participation including these unique conditions are further examined. Within the occupation of social participation, performance patterns such as habits, roles, routines, and rituals all represent a client's preferences regarding meaningful social relationships

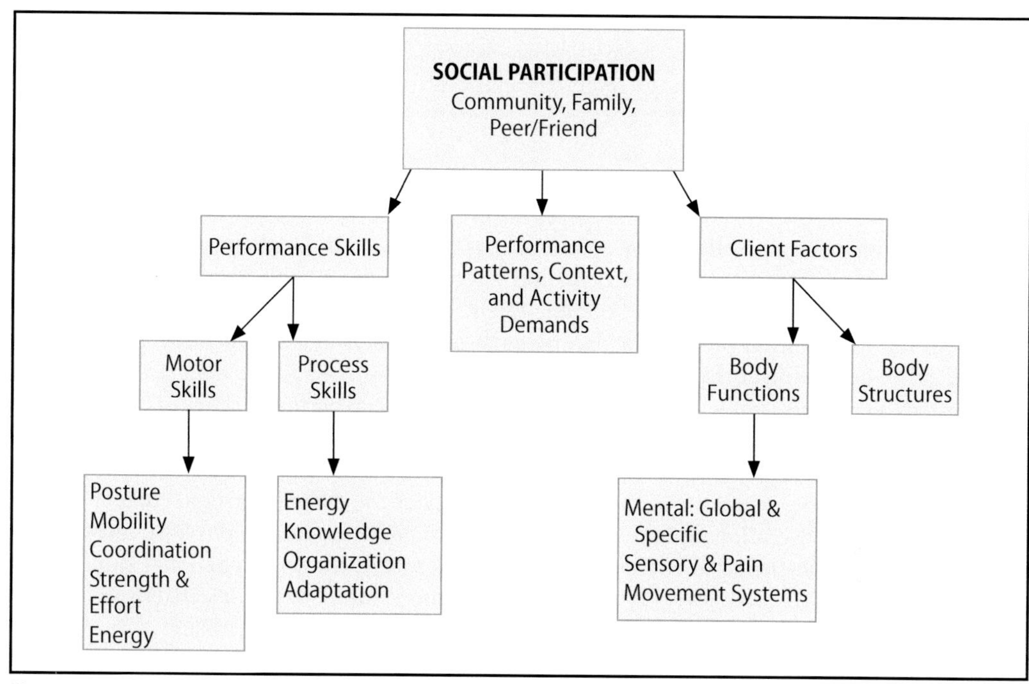

Figure 9-1. Components of social participation. (Adapted from American Occupational Therapy Association. [2002]. Occupational therapy practice framework: Domain and process. *American Journal of Occupational Therapy, 56*[6], 609-639.)

and activities (AOTA, 2014). The complex interaction of these components and the impact on a client's development as a social being are discussed in this chapter. Considerations on the activity and occupational demands of social activities, including the various aspects required to perform meaningful social behaviors, will also be discussed. The role of the occupational therapy assistant as a contributor to the intervention process of social participation will also be examined.

Theory guides all occupational therapy practice. The authors of this chapter discuss how four common occupational therapy models promote social participation as a means to an end. The psychosocial aspects of a disability as it relates to social participation will also be addressed through case examples and a review of the literature. Occupational therapy interventions specific to promoting social participation for persons with a physical or neurological impairment are given throughout the chapter. An emphasis on both physical and emotional safety is also discussed. Lastly, common interpersonal themes for persons with a disability are highlighted with discussion of the occupational therapist's role in promoting health and well-being.

Intervention Process

The World Health Organization (WHO, 2001) defined social participation for the lifespan as "the nature and the extent of an individual's involvement in life situations." The extent to which an individual becomes involved in daily social activities may be limited by disability. Hence, the challenge of developing meaningful interventions lies in the accurate assessment of the client's abilities and learning styles, and by choosing the best combination of interventions for the individual's unique occupational performance. Occupational therapists must complete three substeps in a comprehensive intervention process that includes the following: (1) the design of the intervention plan, (2) the implementation of the intervention itself, and (3) an intervention review to assess effectiveness in meeting desired outcomes. Inclusion of an occupational therapist's therapeutic use of self entails establishing a meaningful and reciprocal approach to care. Data gathering often begins with the client's occupational profile and assessment of current functioning. The Framework (2014) groups all occupational therapy interventions according to the following categorization:

- Direct service
- Education and training
- Consultation

The role of the occupational therapy practitioner is multifaceted. Identifying goals and collaboratively implementing client social participation interventions is complex and involves different types of clinical reasoning. The Framework document, as depicted in Figure 9-8, guides the practitioner in the intervention process for occupational engagement relative to social participation (AOTA, 2014). Beginning at the top, the occupational therapist must gather data to understand a client's social roles. This is followed by the an assessment of social performance skills and patterns that are needed within the client's different contexts. Social activities are analyzed to understand the specific demands of the activity and how they match the individual client's factors and performance abilities. The occupational therapist must consider the client's personal context such as chronological age and spatiotemporal stage, among other contexts such as physical, mental, and social. Because the challenge of occupational therapy is to maximize occupational (functional) performance in everyday activities, varying methods of intervention may be selected to ensure that carry-over of intervention strategies is transferable into one's natural environment.

Therapeutic Use of Self

Defined as an increased awareness of one's own values, beliefs, and attitudes (AOTA, 2014), this powerful phenomenon highlights the importance of a healthy interpersonal connection between the occupational therapist and the client. For example, a young adult with a developmental disability who has difficulty maintaining physical boundaries in social situations may require concrete and tangible cuing by the therapist in one-to-one and small group activities. This may begin with practicing with the occupational therapist. Targeted, remedial behaviors are graded in difficulty by the practitioner to build on success. The occupational therapist may begin with practicing proper eye contact and a greeting handshake only to advance to other activities such as verbal greeting and reciprocal dialogue while keeping a socially accepted personal space. Complex social skills may require not only verbal instruction but also role-playing, videotaping, and other visual mechanisms for feedback. In this instance, it will be the role of the occupational therapist or occupational therapy assistant to determine the client's cognitive abilities and capacities for learning in order to later choose the appropriate level and type of intervention for successful performance. The true testament of successful intervention would be the exhibition of appropriate social skills not only in role-playing sessions, but in one's natural environment. Successful intervention is measured by the quality and duration of carry-over regarding learned techniques in all situations faced by the client.

Direct Service

Although direct, face-to-face interventions with clients are just one type of service delivery, they are the cornerstone of intervention. Composed of multilevel approaches, direct service has as an overall goal to improve occupational performance of the individual client (Scheinholz, 2001). Direct service begins with the screening process to determine the need for occupational therapy service, followed by formal assessments, intervention plan development, discharge planning, education, and the implementation of a maintenance plan that matches a client's assessment data and overall purpose. By tailoring the intervention plan to the individual, the occupational therapy professional hopes to remediate and maximize functional performance. Social participation goals may include the establishment of an intervention plan as well as activities that allow for the client to achieve organized patterns of behavior expected of an individual in community settings and in peer/friend or family relationships (AOTA, 2014). Examples of direct service interventions using remedial, compensatory, and adaptive approaches will be explored later in this chapter.

Education and Training

The type and level of education and training that are appropriate and most beneficial for clients depend on one's cognitive reasoning. The ability to process new information and adapt behaviors to all environments is called *transfer of learning* (Allen et al., 2007). The role of the occupational therapy practitioner in the establishment of social performance goals is twofold. It includes the ability to determine how best the client learns and to educate and assist the client using approaches that generate successful outcomes.

For example, John, a 21-year-old man with a mild developmental intellectual disorder, is seeking meaningful recreational activities that will allow him the ability to meet people in his community. John has had occupational therapy throughout his high school years. A year-end individualized education plan (IEP) goal for John is to join a community organization. Based on data acquired from the client interview, initial observation, and assessment, the occupational therapy practitioner determines that to increase John's successful carry-over of learned social techniques, he needs assistance in the form of verbal cues when meeting an individual for the first time. In addition to the verbal cuing process, he also can benefit from simulated social skill practice and therapist modeling. Thus, with this two-tiered approach, John is more likely to demonstrate successful new learning. The methodology chosen by the occupational therapist will have a direct effect on carry-over of learned skills to multiple social situations. Educating a client about the socialization process can be enhanced through repetitive and structured training sessions that include rehearsal and practice of various targeted skills.

Identifying an individual's learning style to enhance the educational process of learning new skills is best understood from both observation and interview. Additionally, limitations such as an individual's lack of social awareness regarding acceptable behavior must first be addressed for successful interaction within the individual's social system (Mosey, 1996). From an occupational therapy perspective, education about social norms and roles and social skills training are prescriptive for lifelong adaptation and success in social participation.

Consultation

Often the expert skills of an occupational therapist are sought to enhance the performance of a client or organization. In this type of intervention, the occupational therapist may provide either direct or indirect service functions for the purpose of enhancing favorable occupational outcomes. Referring back to John, the occupational therapist may further identify areas of concern that are environmental or systems-based. Let us say that John continues to attend a bingo game at a local church hall but frequently interrupts the group with questions about the last number called. An occupational therapist consultant may be asked to attend a bingo group session in the community and offer advice to the church leaders who are sponsoring the event. An expert consultant may suggest that John's issue may be resolved by a change in seating location that enables him to not only hear but see the letter and number being called. This occupational therapy consultant integrates clinical reasoning that includes John's cognitive abilities and learning style from previous sessions. A consultative recommendation is therefore given to the team to carry out. Consultation requires a competent experience level of the practitioner. In this indirect type of service delivery, occupational therapy can not only enhance the individual's social participation but also promote healthy social group functions within a community setting.

Occupation-Based Models and Social Participation

This section will briefly highlight how occupational therapy practice models can be used as theoretical foundations to promote social participation. The four models are the model of human occupation (MOHO), occupational adaptation (OA), ecology of human performance (EHP), and person-environment-occupation-performance (PEOP). The reader is encouraged to learn more about each model and further understand theoretical assumptions and intervention guidelines that may be directly applied to enhance occupational engagement and social participation.

Model of Human Occupation

MOHO is a client-centered model that provides a framework for understanding the complexities of human occupation. MOHO is based on a systems view of how an individual interacts with the environment to "create a network of conditions which influence an individual's motivation, actions, and performance" (Barrett & Kielhofner, 2003, p. 213). It is an excellent theory to use for the enhancement of social participation. The following are some highlights from this theory.

The therapist needs to specifically address how internal components of a person such as volition, habituation, and performance capacity impact social participation (output). The external environment is a direct source of feedback that can positively or negatively influence participation. This open system cycle must be considered for assessment and intervention planning.

Let us consider the following example. An older woman who has experienced a cerebral vascular accident (CVA) is struggling with the loss of ability to cook holiday meals for her extended family, a role she has held for many years and from which she derived a sense of pride. She tells the occupational therapist that she is very motivated to increase her ability to cook once again.

An occupational therapist can investigate social role disruption of the client by gathering data from the client. Some relevant questions may include the following: What social activities are most important and meaningful to you? What are the expectations of your social role functioning by your family? The occupational therapist considers whether the client can re-establish these roles or if new roles need to be acquired (Barrett & Kielhofner, 2003).

The volition of a client can be considered by asking: How much do you value cooking for your family on holidays? What is your interest in continuing this activity? How motivated are you to return to this social role?

Habits and routines of the client may be considered by asking: What habits or social routines did you have prior to the onset of illness, and what routines do you currently have? What habits and routines do you wish to restore in your life?

Performance capacity can be assessed by asking about and observing the client as she performs a cooking task: What are the skills you need to make a holiday meal successfully?

MOHO emphasizes the impact of feedback to the change process. The occupational therapist must also investigate how the client's environment and direct feedback will impact occupational performance by asking: What do you think will be the response from your family if you were to cook a holiday meal? What impact will their feedback have on your occupational goal to return to cooking holiday meals once again?

Occupational Adaptation

This complex and neuroscience-based occupational therapy model, developed by Schkade and Schultz, "provides an additional dimension to the understanding of occupation and adaptation and their relationship to health" (Reitz & Scaffa, 2001, p. 65). For persons who may have a neurological impairment or brain dysfunction, this model is a relevant theory for the promotion of social participation because it focuses on the interactive and adaptive process between a person and his or her occupational environment.

The therapist works in collaboration with the client to focus on the process of adaptation in response to occupational challenges. An occupational therapist begins by assessing a person's ability to perform a task and considers his or her physical, sensorimotor, cognitive, and psychosocial skills. It is best to observe the client performing tasks in a specific, desired environment. The client's adaptive capacity is assessed by observing him or her completing a task in a specific context. The occupational therapist is particularly observant of the client's ability to complete tasks successfully according to the demands of self and society. The inability to complete tasks in a productive, acceptable manner is viewed as a problem with adaptation. Mastery in occupational performance involves a congruent match in a client's abilities to perform tasks successfully within the context of a specific environment. An intervention plan is developed to address occupational readiness and desired occupational activities futuristically.

For example, a client with rheumatoid arthritis enjoys the social role of hosting and entertaining friends. Her health condition has impacted her physical capacity to carry food trays and remain on her feet for hours at a party. An occupational therapist can promote the client's adaptive capacity to fulfill the tasks of this social role by the inclusion of energy conservation and proper positioning techniques. These interventions are examples of adaptive strategies to manage her physical limitations in a productive way. The client will hopefully report that she feels satisfied to complete the tasks of a good hostess and happy that she can meet the social expectations of her friends at a house party.

"From an occupational adaptation standpoint, occupation plays a significant role as a facilitator in social participation" (Barrett & Kielhofner, 2003, p. 222). This model has been used for research studies including the examining of community integration following CVA. The reader is encouraged to further explore how this model can be applied to restore social participation following illness by enhancing adaptation.

Ecology of Human Performance

Developed at the University of Kansas by W. Dunn and colleagues (Dunn, Brown, & McBuigan, 1994), the ecology of human performance model emphasizes the importance of the transaction effect among person, occupation, and context. With its focus on ecology, it targets the role of context in task performance. Based on social justice principles, this model supports the inclusion of persons of all abilities and their human right to engage in society. Therefore, this occupational therapy model is a natural fit for promoting social participation for clients of all ages across the developmental continuum.

The EHP model proposes the following five types of therapeutic intervention approaches: (1) establish/restore skills, (2) alter a task to match the capacity of a client, (3) adapt/modify the environment or context to enhance successful interaction, (4) prevent further impairment or minimize risks in performance, and (5) create inclusive environments that promote occupational engagement for all.

This model promotes both direct and indirect service for occupational therapists and the clients that are served. From a consultant and indirect delivery focus, occupational therapists often create or design programs to enhance social participation within a natural context. One such example is the development of community-based wellness programs (Dunn, Brown, & McGuigan, 1994; Reitz & Scaffa, 2001, p. 65). Wellness programs promote health and well-being by offering people a healthy activity within a supportive context. Such programs often provide a secondary gain of increased community exploration and social interaction. Examples include the creation of a walking club for seniors or an intergenerational program involving school-aged children. Among other benefits, both programs would increase opportunities for socialization and engagement.

Person-Environment-Occupation-Performance

The person-environment-occupation-performance (PEOP) model is an interdisciplinary model that incorporates the Canadian Association of Occupational Therapists (CAOT) guidelines and client-centered practice. It was devised by C. Baum and C. Christiansen and first published in 1991. "The PEOP process model guides the client and practitioner to focus on the specific goals, contexts, interventions, resources, and anticipated outcomes needed to enhance occupational performance" and "was designed to encourage a balanced approach to care," which encourages occupational therapists to use a client-centered approach (Christiansen, Baum, & Bass, 2015, p. 40).

The PEOP model is very applicable to understanding social role functioning and social participation. The model builds on a person's innate desire to explore his environment and demonstrate mastery (human agency) while emphasizing the transactional nature of the person-environment-occupation-performance relationship. As originally described by Maslow, social belonging and inclusion is a basic human need; therefore, every client has some degree of desire to engage in social participation.

Social Participation, Health, and Well-Being

"Psychological and social well-being contribute to mental health and to successful engagement in meaningful occupations and roles" (AOTA, 2010, p. 1). A client's psychological well-being must remain a priority for the occupational therapy practitioner while promoting the occupation of social participation. As previously stated, involvement in various social and family relationships, roles, and community activities contributes to an individual's sense of self and helps to form one's social identity. As a result, a therapist must consistently pay close attention to how the client is responding to social reintegration strategies. "Clients who exhibit self-efficacy, hopefulness, and motivation are able to successfully adapt to change and engage appropriately in desired socially constructed activities and situations. In contrast, clients struggling to successfully engage in their daily occupations may be experiencing psychosocial difficulties" (AOTA, 2010, p. 2).

During an initial evaluation, practitioners need to thoroughly assess a client's self-functions. According to the Framework, this category includes body image, self-esteem, self-concept, social interaction skills, energy, and drive functions, as well as motivation, impulse control, interests, and values (AOTA, 2014). Throughout the intervention process, these functions should continue to be monitored during interactions with the client, and changes should be recognized and addressed. In most cases, changes in these aspects of psychosocial functioning may not be overtly shown by the client. For example, the client may not say to a therapist that he is not feeling good about himself today but instead state, "I am feeling lazy," or refer negatively to himself by stating, "I'm stupid. I can't do anything right. I hate myself." In addition, there may be subtle changes in body language and posture as well as decreased eye contact. As another example, an adult client with a recent left upper extremity (UE) amputation, initially appearing eager to get back into the community, may suddenly feel uncomfortable and extremely self-conscious while at a town council meeting. Later in therapy sessions, he may appear withdrawn and disconnected during interactions with the therapist, commenting that he is "a useless man with a stump."

Throughout the intervention process, clients must be encouraged to verbalize their concerns about perceived inadequacies in self-concept and social barriers. Significantly, the therapist must realize that persons with disabilities face many social obstacles and stigma.

The practitioner must maintain open lines of communication and promote an honest dialogue regarding social activities and sensitive topics such as dating, sexuality, and physical intimacy. In most cases, questions or concerns about intimacy or sexuality can be stress-provoking for a client. The impact of a physical disability or illness often leads to a period of adjustment regarding one's self-functions such as personal identity, self-esteem, and self-concept (Livneh & Antonak, 1997, 2001, 2005). Beginning with the initial session, a practitioner sets the stage to promote effective communication between him- or herself and the client, based on the building of trust and mutuality (Tickle-Degnen, 1995). Thus, to build a healthy helping relationship, it is paramount that therapists possess strong self-knowledge of their own needs, perceptual biases, and capabilities (Hopkins & Tiffany, 1988). Per Hopkins amd Tiffany (1988), the therapist's own self-confidence and ability to be honest and open in this type of relationship as well as the extent to which he or she is able to communicate "unconditional positive regard" and empathy for the client will ultimately affect the client's ability to invest trust in the relationship (p. 109).

It is also important for the therapist to take into account the client's psychological history. Does the client have a preexisting diagnosis of anxiety and/or depression?

Adjustment to a physical disability includes reactions such as anxiety, anger, and depression (Livneh & Antonak, 1997). For example, anxiety after a stroke is a common emotional reaction that may be caused by a psychological fear of abandonment, feelings of helplessness, an inability to externalize concerns or misinterpretations in social interactions due to cognitive impairments (Versluys, 1995). In addition, occupational therapy practitioners must realize there is a high prevalence of psychiatric disorders and distress in individuals with chronic physical illness (Wells, Golding, & Burnham, 1988a). For example, clients living with multiple sclerosis are at risk for anxiety and depression, as they cope with what is described as "riding a roller coaster in the dark; its unpredictability can cause an individual to plummet from joy to despair" (President & Fellows of Harvard College, 1997, p. 4). Since multiple sclerosis attacks different areas of the central nervous system, the disease may be as individualized as the individual it affects (1997). As a result, depression can often manifest when an adult with multiple sclerosis, or any chronic illness, undergoes a struggle with issues of dependency and independence. The adult needs to maintain as much autonomy and role identity as possible, while accepting an inescapable reliance on others (Cavallo, 1989).

Given the potential risks of psychological implications following an acquired physical disability, occupational therapists should actively address psychological and social issues as part of the adjustment process. Suicide is a real risk for a depressed client with a life-altering physical disability or disease. It is estimated that persons with spinal cord injuries commit suicide three times more frequently than do the general population (Cao, Massaro, Krause, Chen, & Devivo, 2014). Every practitioner must assess the psychological and physical safety of clients.

Social Participation and Safety Considerations

Interventions in social participation often take place in the community setting or home environment. Several key elements regarding safety must be considered by the practitioner, including the client's mental functions, personal safety awareness, environmental/community demands and barriers, and health and wellness habits and routines.

When examining a client's overall safety in the community, the occupational therapist must always consider the client's abilities and limitations relative to mental functions including perceptual, thought, language, and higher-level cognitive reasoning. Safety awareness is a concept that involves reasoning and judgment. Practitioners need to evaluate how a client's personal factors may impact his or her ability to maintain safety during social activities. For example, an older adult with a history of CVA and subsequent cognitive impairment may demonstrate difficulty sustaining attention as he attempts to cross the street. The practitioner notices that he is easily distracted by noise and activity from the environment. An occupational therapist intervention plan might include increasing awareness of safety precautions in both familiar and new social environments. In another example, a young adult with a brain injury may show intolerance to close physical contact. He is observed to push people out of his personal space when he feels "crowded upon." In this situation, an occupational therapy intervention plan might include a session to increase socially appropriate ways to express his discomfort about personal space that are nonintrusive and noninvasive to others.

Ensuring a client's personal safety in the community includes educating the client on potentially dangerous interpersonal situations, appropriate social boundaries when engaging with others including those unfamiliar to the client, and methods of seeking out help in emergency situations. In some instances, clients may also be encouraged to seek additional educational opportunities on self-defense strategies to further promote a sense of personal empowerment in the community.

Environmental and community safety considerations ensure the client's physical and psychological well-being. Occupational therapy practitioners conduct assessments of environmental demands and barriers including potential fall risk factors. Environmental demands and barriers in homes and public buildings are often obscure to a client and may include uneven travel surfaces, stairs or slopes, static or moving obstacles such as furniture or pedestrians, traffic crossings, weather conditions, and even poor lighting (Clemson, Cumming, & Roland, 1996; Patla, 2001). The therapist and client should collaboratively determine the severity and potential safety hazards of each environmental demand and barrier based on the client's own abilities and limitations. The therapist should realize that although some environmental demands such as traffic crossings or pedestrians cannot be avoided, others situations such as uneven travel paths can be avoided and directions to end locations revised (Patla, 2001).

Given the complexity of assessing the community setting for safety hazards, occupational therapists must also thoroughly assess a client's community mobility (see Chapter 4), including the client's risk of falling. Falls are the leading cause of accidental death in the home because one in three adults over the age of 65 will fall each year, putting a social and economic strain on the clients and society as a whole (DiFabio & Seay, 1997; Frith & Davidson, 2013). Individual factors that may cause an increased risk of falling include being of female gender and an older adult, medication use, comorbidities that impact strength or balance, physical and mobility limitations, limited vision, dizziness, incontinence, and cognitive impairments (Braun, 1998; Nazarko, 2012).

While determining potential fall risk factors and subsequent reduction strategies with a client, therapists can discuss the client's own perceptions or fears of falling, which may further impact his or her motivation level and interest to engage in community-related activities. Not surprisingly, many elderly people appear to reduce their activity levels due to these fears (Braun, 1998). The opposite correlation has also been found, where the reduction in social participation decreases an individual's balance skills. In fact, the decrease in social participation has a greater impact on balance skills than the fear of falling (Allison, Painter, Emory, Whitehurst, & Raby, 2013).

Lastly, another important component to managing client safety is the maintenance of general health and wellness habits and routines. For most clients, engaging in social activities means more personal freedom and consequent opportunities to make choices regarding one's own health care. Occupational therapy practitioners can provide factual knowledge and education to clients on basic nutrition or dietary needs based on comorbidities, healthy sleep habits, disease prevention strategies, and possibly safe sex practices. As a health care practitioner, it is important to note that people 50 years and older compose the fastest-growing HIV-infected group, increasing 138% since 1993 (Moore & Amburgey, 2000). Further discussion of sexuality and intimacy as a component of social participation can be found later in this chapter.

Table 9-1

Examples of Context in Social Participation

Context	Social Participation Example
Cultural	A young mother with depression participating in the tradition of Sunday dinner with the extended family.
Physical	A wheelchair-bound individual finding accessible restaurants where he or she can enjoy eating out with friends.
Social	Expectations of family and friends that an elderly widow with chronic obstructive pulmonary disease should join a senior center to avoid isolation.
Personal	A single parent with the financial means to hire a babysitter and buy movie tickets or attend a concert with peers.
Spiritual	A retired social worker volunteering to run a youth group at the local church as a way to give back to the community and set a positive example.
Temporal	An individual with arthritis choosing an afternoon rather than a morning coffee date so she can have adequate time to prepare.
Virtual	An adolescent making plans with friends or gathering information about upcoming events by means of e-mail, chat rooms, or telephone.

Adapted from American Occupational Therapy Association. (2002). Occupational therapy practice framework: Domain and process. *American Journal of Occupational Therapy, 56*(6), 609-639.

Social Participation and Contexts

The Framework identifies six contexts, also referred to as the environment, to be considered in the occupational therapy evaluation process. In this section, each context and/or environment will be briefly described and examples given to help the reader understand its relationship to social participation. Coster (1998) defined social participation as "the extent to which a child is able to orchestrate engagement or participation in an occupation in a context which is positive, personally satisfying and acceptable to the responsible adults in society" (p. 340). This statement is important in considering that our adult routines and preferences are influenced by childhood experiences within familiar contexts. Please refer to Table 9-1 for further examples of how contexts and environments relate to social participation.

The cultural context includes "customs, beliefs, activity patterns, behavioral standards, and expectations accepted by the society of which a client is a member (AOTA, 2014, p. 9). Stigma and negative attitudes of society have long been documented as having impact on social participation (Law & Dunn, 1993b). A common social issue seen in practice includes how to greet persons of diverse cultures. In Western culture, eye contact and a firm handshake are socially acceptable. Occupational therapists must be sensitive to not impose their own internal values and beliefs onto a client. This seemingly gracious social greeting may be offensive for a client who is not part of Western culture. A culturally sensitive practitioner will actively seek to learn about the social participation habits and routines of the client when creating a meaningful intervention plan. Family beliefs and traditions regarding social activities are very important to a person. Practitioners should assess the social roles and obligations of each unique individual.

The physical environment refers to the "natural (e.g., geographic terrain, plants) and built (e.g., buildings, furniture) surroundings in which daily life occupations occur" (AOTA, 2014, p. 8). The physical environment can either facilitate or act as a barrier to social participation for persons of all abilities (Law & Dunn, 1993b). Occupational therapists are well-trained in assessing both the physical demands of an environment and client factors. As described in the previous section, consideration of a client's physical environment is a part of a comprehensive intervention plan. For example, a client with moderate to severe arthritis in her hips may insist on shopping at her favorite grocery store despite her own physical limitations and the crowded aisles of the small market. A practitioner would assess the client's physical abilities and consider the impact posed by environmental barriers in her preferred physical context. Common environmental barriers that can impact social participation include crowded, excessively noisy, or inaccessible places.

The social environment consists of the presence of relationships with, and expectations of, persons, groups, and populations with whom clients have contact (e.g., availability and expectations of significant individuals, such as a spouse, friends, and caregivers). Studies show the significance of a support system to recovery (Livneh & Antonak, 2005). While most social networks and relationships provide emotional support, some can hinder a person's ability to progress (Radomski, 2008). For older adults who have lost a significant other, increased social participation serves as an active coping strategy to deal with the negative effects of widowhood (Utz, Carr, Ness, & Wortman, 2002). This social seeking may be due in part to the social context of friends and relatives rallying around and lending support (Lopata, 1996).

Personal context refers to demographic features of the individual, such as age, gender, socioeconomic status, and educational level, that are not part of a health condition (WHO, 2001). This context area is commonly addressed in an occupational profile. It is also good medical practice to have this personal information about every client who seeks a health care service. Practitioners must consider personal variables when selecting appropriate intervention strategies. For example, an older adult who has a playful nature may take offense to playing childhood games during a social activity group.

Temporal context is defined as "stage of life, time of day or year, duration or rhythm of activity and history" (AOTA, 2014, p. 9). Temporal considerations would include whether the time of day of an occupational therapy session is compatible with the client's energy level, time management capabilities, ability to access transportation, and pain management/medication needs. In addition, practitioners should consider the client's stage of life, as well as the ability to access opportunities for social participation that are appropriate and relevant to this stage. For example, a support group for persons with multiple sclerosis would be relevant for a young, newly diagnosed mother, while a retired individual might choose a yoga class sponsored by the local senior center.

Virtual context refers to interactions that occur in simulated, real-time, or near-time situations absent of physical contact. This particular context is becoming more important for both clients and practitioners (AOTA, 2014, p. 9). Virtual considerations would include assessing whether the use of technology, such as telephones, computers, and the Internet, is a helpful link to socializing with others or if it keeps the client isolated by acting as a substitute for face-to-face contact. According to Letts, Rigby, and Stewart (2003), electronic aids to daily living can allow individuals with disabilities enhanced communication and increased community access. In a case study that included the use of a computer as an environmental facilitator to promote social role resumption after a head injury, a client was able to re-establish his roles as a brother and son and re-establish contacts with extended family when given computer-related interventions (Gutman, 2000).

Social Participation and Performance Skills

"Performance skills are goal directed actions that are observable as small units of engagement in daily life occupations" (AOTA, 2014, p. S7). Fisher and Griswold (2014) categorized performance skills into three broad categories: motor skills, process skills, and social interaction skills. Each of these skill sets occurs within a client's different contexts and/or environment and is learned over time (AOTA, 2014, p. S7). The Framework (AOTA, 2014) further delineates each category of performance skills, and the reader is advised to review this document for further knowledge.

Social interaction skills are defined as "occupational performance skills observed during the ongoing stream of a social exchange" (Boyt Schell et al., 2014a, p. 1241). It is easy to imagine that the skills within this broad category are precursor steps to achieving the occupation of social participation. Having said this, skills are outward actions or behaviors that exemplify a common form of engagement; it would be too simplistic to assume that mastery of these social interaction skills yields healthy and fulfilling relationships. Interpersonal relationships are a complex phenomenon that includes social interaction skills as only one component of a larger picture. To list a few examples, social interaction skills include gestures, spoken words, taking turns when speaking, tone of voice, and empathy (AOTA, 2014). Occupational therapists can promote learning of social skills to enhance quality social participation. Physical impairments such as an acquired brain injury can result in the disruption of social interaction skills. A common goal for intervention may include social skill training to restore prior learned skills.

Motor skill impairments may impact the cluster of social skills related to body language and communication. For example, a 70-year-old man with Parkinson's disease may appear expressionless; however, this is a manifestation of motor impairment rather than a true depiction of his internal mood. An occupational therapist can educate family members about the body changes that occur with Parkinson's disease to support communication with their loved one.

Process skills have a direct effect on social participation. Thinking and reasoning impact everything that we do in life. Impairment in cognition and processing alters one's ability to perceive social cues, associate meaning, and to express oneself in socially acceptable ways. Cognitive impairments may not be visible to the general public. It is common for persons to misunderstand the intentions and behaviors of a person with a cognitive disability. For example, a person who is aphasic following a brain injury is unable to express his thoughts in spoken language. This does not mean, however, that the client cannot understand when others speak to him or that the client is void of feeling and thinking. As part of a comprehensive intervention plan, practitioners may educate caregivers about the impact of aphasia and suggest alternate ways to communicate.

Social Participation and Performance Patterns

Performance patterns are the habits, routine, rituals, and roles used in the process of engaging in occupations or activities that can support or hinder occupational performance. Social habits, routines, rituals, and roles need to be considered when completing an intervention plan with a person, group, or population (AOTA, 2014).

The Framework document divides habits into three types: useful, impoverished, and dominating (AOTA, 2014). A useful habit promotes healthy social participation, such as productively conversing with classmates on a daily basis within one's student role. An impoverished habit diminishes healthy social participation and often results from the inability to cope effectively. An example of an impoverished habit includes social avoidance of public activities because one fears being stigmatized or criticized in public. A dominating habit is one that is primary and influencing to other habits; an example includes drinking alcohol before going to a social event to decrease social anxiety.

Routines are established sequences of occupations or activities that provide a structure for daily life; routines also can promote or damage health (Fiese, 2007; Koome, Hocking, & Sutton, 2012; Segal, 2004). A client's routine may be thought of as a process to meet an end goal. Routines include a series of habits and are broader in scope than habits. For example, a social routine may be "date night" every Saturday evening. Consider this example. A client who was recently injured in a car accident tells the occupational therapist that he wants to resume his Saturday night social activities with his wife, a routine that they have engaged in for many years. The occupational therapist needs to understand the meaningfulness and steps or habits of this routine from the client's perspective. An occupational therapist can effectively maintain the client's familiar structure and routine process of "date night" while providing education about ways to modify social task demands and navigate public places in a safe manner.

"Roles are sets of behaviors expected by society and shaped by culture and context; they may be further conceptualized and defined by a client (person, group, or population). Roles can provide guidance in selecting occupations or can be used to identify activities connected with certain occupations in which a client engages" (AOTA, 2014, p. S8). Upon review of this definition, it is understandable why occupational therapy scholars such as Christiansen and Baum (PEOP) and Trombly (occupational functional model) have used the term *top-down* when referencing the initial starting place for an occupational therapy evaluation process. Every role in life has a set of obligations and inherent social norms and behaviors (habits). These roles influence our individual routines and help to define relationship dynamics. An occupational therapist who completes an occupational profile is interested to learn about a client's preferred roles: past, present and future. Within this client-centered approach to collaborative intervention planning, the practitioner can further understand what will motivate a person to change. For example, a 40-year-old single woman, CEO of a well-known corporation, is diagnosed with breast cancer. She shares her anxiety about her body image and impact on her worker role. As the occupational therapist explores more about the client's perception, it is understood that the company markets itself as a "perfect," model business. The client wants to maintain her CEO worker position with its inherent social image and recover at the same time. Integrating each individual person's internal and external dynamics serves as a challenge to effective intervention planning and implementation.

Rituals are symbolic actions with spiritual, cultural, or social meaning. Rituals contribute to a client's identity and reinforce the client's values and beliefs (Fiese, 2007; Segal, 2004). It is respectful to ask a client about their rituals in life and how illness or disability has impacted their ability to carry these out. For example, when working with a client who is at the end stage of life, it is good practice to assist with preparation for death. An occupational therapist must consider the inclusion of rituals when designing intervention planning and implementation for chronic illnesses and terminal disease. Often, it is our own anxiety that prevents us from assisting our clients with this transitional stage of development.

Social Participation and Activity and Occupational Demands

Previously, it was noted that client-centered intervention is a multitiered process. So far, we have discussed the significance of contexts, skills, and patterns to social participation. In this section we will discuss how the demands of an activity can impact social participation. According to the Framework (2014), activity demands are a group of components within an activity that include objects, space, social demands, sequencing or timing, required actions, and required underlying body functions and body structure needed to carry out the activity. Persons with developmental and physical disabilities are commonly faced with barriers to successful performance such as fear of injury or re-injury, presence of pain, reduced level of energy, lack of appropriate transportation, and lack of support for participation (Oman & Reed, 1998). These common concerns may have direct impact on the client's ability to meet the demands of social activity and participation. Table 9-2 lists examples of activity demands as they relate to social participation.

Table 9-2

Examples of Activity Demands in Social Participation

Activity Demands	Definitions (AOTA, 2002, p. 624)	Social Participation Examples
Objects and their properties	The tools, equipment and materials used in the process of carrying out an activity	• Tools: games • Materials: clothing • Equipment: tables, chairs • Inherent properties: room temperature and setup
Space demands (physical context)	The physical environmental requirements of the activity	• Large community room for a church social function
Social demands (social and cultural contexts)	The social structure and demands that may be required by the activity	• Social rules or etiquette at a function • Expectations of other persons participating in the activity
Sequence and timing	The process used to carry out the activity	• Steps: how a social function follows a schedule • Sequence: understanding process of the bingo game
Required actions	Motor, process, and communication/interaction skills required of a individual to carry out an activity	• Motor: grasping bingo chips • Process: multiple card scanning • Communication: knowing when to announce a winning card
Required body functions	Physiological functions to support the actions of an activity	• ROM of UEs for manipulation of chips • Ability to sustain attention to caller of the game
Required body structures	Anatomical parts required to perform the activity	• Number of hands • Number of eyes

Adapted from American Occupational Therapy Association. (2002). Occupational therapy practice framework: Domain and process. *American Journal of Occupational Therapy, 56*(6), 609-639.

Role of the Occupational Therapy Assistant

The primary role of the occupational therapy assistant is to carry out the intervention as planned and supervised by the occupational therapist following completion of the evaluation (Scheinholz, 2001). The occupational therapy assistant, although routinely supervised by the occupational therapist, must also demonstrate sound clinical judgment for efficacy in the intervention process. The level and frequency of supervision is determined by years of experience of the occupational therapy assistant, the requirements of the regulatory agencies governing practice, and the level of need of the client(s) within the caseload (AOTA, 2013). As community-based occupational therapy services evolve, the role of the occupational therapy assistant continues to expand. It is imperative that intervention approaches be discussed collaboratively according to the occupational therapy assistant guidelines for continuity of care and role delineation between occupational therapist and occupational therapy assistant.

Social participation goals and interventions include engagement in community, peer/friend, and family relationships. Quite often, this means interventions are performed in a community setting or in the presence of significant others. Because of this, the competency of the occupational therapy assistant and the amount of supervision provided are vital. The occupational therapy assistant in a community setting must recognize what resources are available to the client and use a systems perspective to fully understand interactive environmental influence on behaviors. The occupational therapy assistant must also seek the appropriate supervision necessary to insure the intervention plan is achievable or, if not, adapt it for successful client performance in collaboration with the supervising occupational therapist.

Community Aspects of Social Participation

Community participation is characterized by the Framework (2014) as activities that result in successful interaction at the community level (e.g., neighborhoods, organizations, work, or school).

All human beings seek to be members of their individual communities. Examples include work activities such as meetings and events, a volunteer group such as gathering food sources for the local soup kitchen, a social club such as for senior citizens, or a civic organization such as one promoting human rights. For those with acquired disabilities, reintegration into the community is a relevant and challenging goal for occupational therapy practice. Adaptation to social skill performance, activity demands, and the modification of one's environment is often needed to accommodate changes in one's health condition. Each of these forays has its own set of challenges, but it is the ultimate challenge of the occupational therapist to assist the client in finding the just-right path, thus overcoming the barriers to independent and meaningful functioning. Uniquely, not only do cognitive, physical, and psychosocial barriers exist through this challenge, but the ways in which to participate in community activities also differ from culture to culture (Baum & Law, 1997).

The area of occupation known as social participation is defined as "activities associated with organized patterns of behavior which are characteristic and expected of an individual or an individual interacting with others within a given social system" (Mosey, 1996, p. 340). The act of participating in social situations includes integration into the community, with family and with peers or friends. Importantly, the role of the occupational therapist and the intervention strategies may vary depending on the client's place along the life continuum. For purposes of this text, the discussion will focus on the adult, older adult, and adults with disabilities.

Adult Community Social Participation Roles

Social participation for an adult may include a variety of activities, and successful integration will depend greatly on the individual's desired outcomes. Socioeconomic factors may impact the adult's ability to choose meaningful activities. Community access and activity opportunities may be limited as well. Other personal factors to be considered when assisting the client with social participation goals are the client's marital status, religion, social skill levels, and communication and interaction skills. An adult will typically seek groups or organizations with matching interest levels. Men and women may also choose group activities and social settings based on gender differences. Further, throughout the lifespan, an individual's roles change depending on his or her occupation and peer group. Thus, the level of community participation often reflects one's adult development and temporal context. For example, the young adult recently graduated from college may seek entirely different social participation activities than a married adult with children and an established career.

Older Adult Social Participation Roles

Older adults quite often demonstrate a dichotomous tract with respect to their level of interaction in their community. The well elderly may consider many options and choose a multitude of opportunities in order to stay connected with friends, families, and community. The frail older adult or the individual with significant health concerns may be at great risk for social isolation (Iecovich & Biderman, 2012).

Older adults with poor health habits and routines are often the most in need of services but the least likely to seek access to them. The healthy older adult values being an active member of the community. WHO (2001) objectives of healthy aging clearly identify the significance of occupational therapy's role in community-based practice. Practitioners must assist clients to access activities within their preferred community to promote their overall sense of well-being along the life continuum.

Adults With Disabilities and Social Participation Roles

For adults with disabilities, the physical environment, the attitudes of society, and policies can either facilitate or act as barriers to social participation (Law & Dunn, 1993b). All too often, occupational therapy can make the difference between successful community reintegration for clients and impending social isolation. When an adult with a disability faces challenges to participate in a community setting, both the medical model and social models of intervention are equally explored. Occupational therapy interventions are based on assessment of a client's social and personal factors, the demands of the occupation or activity that he wishes to engage in, and the external factors of the environment (Rogers & Holm, 2003).

Family Aspects of Social Participation

Family social participation is defined as activities that result in successful interaction in specific required and/or desired familial roles (Mosey, 1996, p. 340). These activities can range from in-house celebrations, holidays, and traditions to community activities that family members participate in together. Frequency may vary from weekly dinners, ongoing religious activities, or occasional functions such as family weddings or reunions involving a larger network of extended family. In addition, social participation can encompass talking to relatives on the phone or communicating via email. Virtual contexts promote social participation for families who often have conflicting schedules, limited access to transportation, or live far away from one another.

Family Composition

The role of each family member and overall family composition is affected by culture, family finances, general economic issues, the environment, and legislation. Family roles can include, but are not limited to, the following: mother, father, grandparent, child, sibling, spouse, partner, and widow. When considering family roles, the therapist should be aware that the scope of a family unit has evolved and expanded in recent years for a variety of reasons. "There are more extended families, single-parent families, teenage parents, grandparents as primary caretakers, joint custody situations, and foster parents" (Wooster, Gray, & Gifford, 2001, p. 240). Divorce is more accepted by society and therefore more prevalent. In addition, it is common for divorced individuals to remarry and create blended families. Same-sex relationships are also more common, with recent legislation allowing for same-sex marriages. All of these social norms will continue to have an impact on family dynamics. Occupational therapy must be sensitive to the ever-changing constellation of the family unit and its significance to a client's recovery.

Adult Family Roles

Socioeconomic trends impact adult roles and occupations. For example, more women are college educated, and consequently more women are joining the workforce and juggling household responsibilities along with work responsibilities. In addition, more adult children are moving back into their parents' home after college to save money and defray the high cost of college loans. These adult children are marrying later and having children later in life. This trend of adult children living at home causes parents to experience the "empty nest" transition later in life, described in the peer/friend section of this chapter.

In addition to the roles designated by position in the family, there are also the occupations adults take on that are associated with their responsibilities in the family structure, occupational roles such as wage earner, homemaker, student, cook, driver, and child care provider.

Older Adult Family Roles

Life expectancy has increased, thus impacting the nature of family. Many older adults are taking on increased responsibilities for care of their loved ones. For example, many adults remain active in their communities after retirement by taking on part-time jobs for financial reasons or by volunteering as a way to stay socially connected to others. Many older adults help their family members with child care responsibilities. The older adult population is the fastest growing. According to the U.S. Census Bureau population projections, America's elderly are expected to make up more than 20% of the population by 2050. This is a projected increase of 147% for those aged 65 years and older, while the projected increase for the population as a whole is only 49% (U.S. Census Bureau, 2005).

Occupational therapists must have a foundational understanding of human development and role acquisition throughout the aging process to remain current with population trends. Practitioners are instrumental with helping clients and their families to cope with change while maintaining healthy social routines throughout the lifespan.

Dealing With Disability and Social Integration

An individual dealing with the onset of illness or disability has to learn to ask for and accept help. The development of health conditions requires a client to deal with the loss of meaningful roles, and the loss of autonomy and independence. These issues can be overwhelming and often result in depression and a decrease in social participation (Brown, Hasson, Thyselius, & Almborg, 2012). The motherhood model compares family care to a type of social phenomenon in which adults with disabilities are treated as children. While society encourages family caring and kinship, adult dependence is often disapproved of (Jongbloed, Stanton, & Fousek, 1993).

Individual adjustment to disability may include concurrent feelings of loneliness and social isolation. These feelings can be exacerbated by societal attitudes, stereotypes, and lack of understanding or education on the part of one's social contexts. Becker defines the term *master status*, which preempts all other levels in a social hierarchy (Conneeley, 2002). For example, if a client feels stigmatized by the attitudes of others, he or she may adopt a new social role or "status" of a disabled individual as a way to cope.

Another social role phenomenon is called *stranger status*. This term describes an individual who is part of a group yet feels that he or she is outside of it (Conneeley, 2002). This perceived outsider position can also have a negative impact on social roles and self-esteem.

Impact on Family Roles and Social Participation

When changes in roles become necessary secondary to disability, the person's entire family may be affected. For example, if a homemaker can no longer cook meals and care for her children, the missing functions of this role will need to be assumed by another person. As a result, her husband, extended family, and even the children will have to compensate for the change in social role functioning. "Occupational therapists and occupational therapy assistants bring broad expertise to intervene with family caregivers to facilitate caregiving and promote better health because of their knowledge and skills in addressing the physical, psychosocial, cognitive, sensory, and contextual elements that affect participation and engagement in everyday life activities" (AOTA, 2013).

Disability can also have a major impact on marriage and couple relationships. Changes in one's health status provide a challenge to both partners' communication skills, established habits, patterns of intimacy, and beliefs. With major advances in medical technology and improved standards of living, couples are living much longer with chronic illness and disabling conditions (Rolland, 1994a). The couple must address changing boundary issues, traditional divisions of labor, the undercurrent themes of loss, and the need to redefine their relationship.

For example, the partner with a disability may consider him- or herself a burden, while the partner who is taking on more responsibilities may feel resentment. In addition, these new feelings may trigger guilt in one or both partners. Physical limitations may also pose a challenge to the relationship. For example, physical limitations secondary to stroke or spinal cord injury have an ongoing impact on intimacy and social participation, while conditions such as multiple sclerosis or rheumatoid arthritis may have unpredictable exacerbations and remissions that partners need to further manage.

It is important to note that some families become more resilient and experience strengthened relationships following a serious illness or disability. As described by Conneeley (2002), positive relationships evolving after such events may result in spiritual growth, increased awareness of the importance of family, and the establishment of new values.

Disability of parents causes a role reversal when adult children who have depended on their parents for many years now have to take on the responsibility of caring for one or both of their parents, grandparents, or an aging relative. At times, these adult children are still caring for their own children. The growth of this dual responsibility has been coined "sandwich generation," referring to the individual being sandwiched between two very different needs at opposite ends of the developmental spectrum. These caregivers are caught between what their children need and what their parents need and often have little or no time to engage in their own meaningful social activities outside of the family.

Women are currently assuming a primary role when a family member needs care; however, men are increasing their roles as family caregivers, and the number of men assuming the role of primary caregiver is on the rise (Robinson, Bottorff, Pesut, Oliffe, & Tomlinson, 2014). Therapeutic issues regarding family caregivers and meeting their needs constitute good care, a topic that will be addressed in more detail later in this chapter.

Changes in an individual's health status may result in a new "family" context to assist with care of the individual. Extended family filling in or an increase in level of involvement with families of origin are common scenarios. For adults with developmental disabilities, peers and staff members at group homes, foster homes, and halfway houses often take on the roles of extended family. This may include celebrating holidays with residents as well as accompanying them out into the community. For these adults, social participation is most often arranged by others, and they are usually part of a structured group of peers.

With the increase in average lifespan, more elders are coping with disability and needing assistance to carry out daily routines. Occupational therapists often evaluate elderly clients at critical life stages such as nursing home placement or early onset of a progressive illness. Nursing homes, adult day programs, and assisted living programs are typical settings that foster transition with life changes that impact a client's roles and increased dependence on others. While social opportunities in the community are often limited for these elders, in-house activities are provided within easy access and in a more structured and safe environment.

Family Reactions to Illness/Disability

Reactions to the onset of illness or disability by family members vary but may include shock, denial and disbelief, anger, hostility, unrealistic expectations, or disengagement from the client (Livneh & Antonak, 1997).

While some families pull together, support the client, and accept the illness, others may minimize or fully deny any problems or need for a change in their routines. This presents a problem for the therapist trying to gain support for the client. For example, a lack of family cooperation may hinder follow-through on interventions such as home exercise programs. It is best for the therapist to gently approach families in shock by presenting plans as options or contingencies and then providing educational materials as well as resources when appropriate.

When family members react with anger and hostility, the therapist needs to empathize without personalizing the feelings and without feeding into unrealistic expectations. The occupational therapist should assess the level of family involvement the client and family are accustomed to and support it. When family members are very involved, it may be beneficial to educate them regarding the role of occupational therapy and to routinely incorporate use of counseling skills during intervention sessions. When families have unrealistic expectations, the therapist may need to share goals and set limits while maintaining a therapeutic relationship.

At times, families may disengage for a variety of reasons, which may include frustration, feeling overwhelmed, harboring guilt, feeling burnout, or concealing resentment from previous unresolved conflicts with the family member who is now ill.

Family Caregiver Issues

Many older adults living in the community require long-term care, and this care is often provided by family caregivers. Caregivers face a variety of stressors on a daily basis, including fear something will happen to their loved one, difficulties juggling work and home responsibilities, social isolation, role changes, and limited income/loss of income due to time constraints.

Social isolation is a leading contributor to stress among family caregivers. This is a common problem, especially for clients with dementia and their caregivers (Rosenthal, 2014; Szekais, 1991). Socialization becomes more difficult for the individual as the illness progresses, and he or she may often require more assistance from the family to socialize and interact with others successfully. As socialization becomes more difficult and more assistance is required in maintaining self-care and other daily routines, socialization tends to decrease for both the caregiver and the patient. Family caregivers need ongoing support and encouragement to continue to socialize in order to maintain their own mental and emotional wellness as well as energy level. Also, it is necessary to provide opportunities for the individual with dementia to socialize in order to maintain cognitive and affective functioning (Rosenthal, 2014; Szekais, 1991).

Family caregivers also lose important roles and take on new roles secondary to dealing with chronic illness. Lost roles may include those of leisure such as gardening, dancing, and civic duties. These roles are often no longer possible due to time constraints and energy demands. Former social role functioning is replaced with being a caregiver and case manager, which often include the added responsibilities of researching options for the loved one, dealing with finances, making arrangements for transportation and equipment, and assisting with medications.

When discharging a client home to a family caregiver, the age and physical status of the caregiver must be taken into consideration. Family educational training should address goals and specific procedures in a format that the caregiver can understand. If multiple family members will be assisting the client, they should be educated about the need for consistent and reliable care. This will be addressed further in the intervention section of this chapter.

Meeting the Needs of the Family

The family will need information about the illness, intervention, and prognosis in order to know what is expected, as well as information about the role of occupational therapy. Likewise, the family will need to develop skills in order to cope with the effects of illness and the changes that will occur as a result. In addition, families will need to learn how to interact effectively with health care providers.

Lastly, the family will need support. The therapist can provide support by just listening and empathizing. Common scenarios include allowing a family to vent, deal with change, and mourn the loss of past roles and functioning. The therapist can assist the family and client with decision making by outlining options within the scope of occupational therapy services. For example, the therapist can let the family know that social participation is an important occupation and within the realm of occupational therapy practice (AOTA, 2014).

The therapist can also help the client and family locate appropriate resources or groups that will provide additional and ongoing support, and when indicated, may help the family access respite care. Respite care can be provided inside the home or at facilities in the community. Many assisted living facilities, nursing homes, and adult day care centers provide respite care services for family members to take a much-needed vacation or attend to personal matters without worrying about the safety of their loved one (Paulson, 1991).

In addition, local hospitals usually run a variety of support groups and community-based health programs at no or low cost. Examples range from arthritis exercise groups and cardiac rehabilitation to groups providing support to caregivers and groups for families dealing with grief and loss. These venues provide support as well as an opportunity to meet and socialize with others dealing with some of the same issues.

Involving Family

When working with families, the therapist needs to demonstrate a variety of skills and coping strategies in order to establish and maintain rapport to set the stage for appropriate interventions. The following is a list of considerations for the practitioner:

- Be tolerant, respectful, flexible, knowledgeable, and compassionate.
- Further consider context, habits, and patterns of the client and family (see the occupational profile in Chapter 1).
- Be respectful of family culture and dynamics.
- Be flexible, as change takes time and requires the use of creativity and clinical reasoning skills.
- Be knowledgeable: teach skills at client's level of understanding to convey knowledge appropriately.
- Grade and adapt activities and home care routines as needed for success.
- Use lay terms when talking with family members, and provide written instructions for them to refer to whenever possible.
- Work with interdisciplinary team members to provide structure and continuity.

The partnership model, proposed by Crabtree (1991), describes a joint decision-making process among family members with an older adult to promote their expertise in caregiving and incorporate knowledge of the family member's wishes. Involving the family early on when the older adult can partner with them in decision making will lead to more informed and less overwhelmed experiences if they need to take over and advocate on behalf of their family member. The client will need to consent if able and give durable power of attorney to a family member if this situation occurs.

The family can become an ally in partnering with the client to maximize independence and promote community integration. In addition, the family can help the client follow through on programs to get lasting benefits from therapy. The therapist must gather information from the client and family to determine role patterns of the family, the degree to which the environment has influenced roles, and how the disability has affected occupational performance (Jongbloed, Stanton, & Fousek, 1993). Specifically, the therapist needs to find out what roles each member of the family fulfills, how these roles have changed, and most importantly if there is role flexibility when needed. Further, the therapist needs to determine how involved family members wish to be and how the support received from family influences role maintenance for the client.

Peer/Friend Aspects of Social Participation

Social participation as it relates to peer/friend interactions consists of activities at different levels of intimacy, including engaging in desired sexual activity (AOTA, 2014). Relationships with friends or cohorts can provide meaningful experiences for individuals and are interrelated to their overall sense of wellness. In addition, the individual's gender, age, and disability status can further indicate how these social interactions, or lack thereof, can impact an individual's health and involvement in his or her community.

Friendships are significant human experiences for several reasons. Friends support each other emotionally, are willing to see things from the other's point of view, and provide assistance and feedback when needed (Lutfiyya, 1997). These types of relationships also involve enjoyment, acceptance, trust, respect, mutual assistance, confiding, understanding, and spontaneity (Brintnall-Peterson, 2004). In a crisis situation or personal tragedy, an individual's close friends, outside of his or her own family of origin, can even serve as a protective factor when faced with life-changing experiences and psychosocial stressors (Simmons Longitudinal Study, 2004).

Peer Versus Friend

Peer relationships are not the same as friendships. Although friendships and peer groups occur in the social context of an individual's environment, the latter may be based solely on existing common characteristics that are influential in establishing norms, role expectations, and social routines (AOTA, 2014; Kindermann & Sage, 1999). Generally, peers are individuals that a person identifies or compares themselves with who are usually, but not always, of the same age group. Acceptance by the peer group is often desirable and based on recognition of similarity (Bourne, 1998; Cook & Semmel, 1999). In addition, peer groups influence an individual's belief structure and system of rules, values, and goals based on commonality of its group members (Bourne, 1998).

Through the lifespan, an individual's peer group changes based on the individual's roles and occupations. In adulthood, a career woman's peers may be her female coworkers. In older adulthood, a retired man's peers may be members of his fishing club. For an adult male with a recent spinal cord injury (SCI), his peer group may consist of other SCI survivors from a local sports group. Often, these common peer bonds can be the basis of friendship development.

Adult Friendships

The term *social convoy* describes the network of close relationships we maintain throughout life. In general, an individual's social convoy consists of two to five close friendships and does not necessarily change during adulthood, although the actual members may change (Brintnall-Peterson, 2004). During emerging adulthood, between the ages of 18 to 30, individuals often begin to establish themselves outside of their families of origin and create a social support network of friends, colleagues, and intimate partnerships, which becomes extremely important in defining a sense of self (Simmons Longitudinal Study, 2004). Some close friendships in adulthood may actually be those first established during childhood or adolescence. Through middle adulthood, from the ages of 40 to 65, friendships and social circles are further seen as support systems that help in the adjustment of midlife transitions. During these so-called midlife crises, individuals may view themselves in terms of how many years they have to live versus how many years they have lived (Rathus, 1988).

Older Adult Friendships

Late or older adulthood begins at age 65. As we age, friendships change because of declining individual physical and mental capacities and life cycle transitions including retirement and the death of a spouse. Per Rathus (1988), the basic challenge for individuals in older adulthood is to maintain the belief that life is meaningful and worthwhile in the face of the inevitability of death. Within this psychosocial development theory, an individual's support network aids in the adjustment of these life changes.

Social Isolation With Older Adults

Older individuals are more likely to lose family members and friends due to illness and death and are more vulnerable to loneliness and social isolation (Yeh & Lo, 2004). Studies suggest that feelings of loneliness for older adults contribute to increasing functional disability, especially greater activities of daily living (ADL) dependency (2004). As a result, social relations are often still regarded as an important criterion of quality of life in old age and a key environmental factor enhancing health, participation, and psychosocial security (Bukov, Maas, & Lampert, 2002; Yeh & Lo, 2004).

Gender Differences in Friendships

According to Bell (1981), gender is the most important factor with regard to friendship variations. Interestingly, women tend to define friendship in terms of closeness and emotional attachment, whereas men often have less intense, more action-oriented friends. This concept is further described by Block (1980) as "convenience or activity friends," which are segmented or centered around particular activities (Traustadottir, 1993). In addition, researchers have argued that men tend to have significantly fewer close or best friends than women throughout the lifespan. Specifically, throughout the adult years, women seem to have larger social convoys than men and also maintain these relationships longer (Brintnall-Peterson, 2004). Although male friendships may be less intimate and fewer than their female counterparts, these relationships still serve to buffer stress and reduce depression in the same way women's friendships do (Traustadottir, 1993).

In older adulthood, similar gender trends in friendship continue. Interestingly, as women tend to have larger groups of friends, they are more susceptible to emotional stress when negative experiences happen to their cohorts. In addition, women are generally faced with a more significant psychological life adjustment after the death of a spouse, as they tend to live longer than men (Brintnall-Peterson, 2004).

Dating and Partnerships

According to Levinson, the ages of 33 to 40 are characterized by an individual's desire to settle down. Often during this transitional period, men seek independence and autonomy in their interpersonal relationships. Women may have a newfound interest in childbearing and are more likely to undergo a transformation in role functioning from being cared for to caring for others (Rathus, 1988). In a survey of college men and women, it was determined that several psychological traits including fidelity, warmth, sensitivity, and honesty were relatively more important in long-term relationships than physical attractiveness (1988). Additionally, for mate selection, women often place greater emphasis on characteristics such as dependability, kindness, professional status, and fondness for children than men do, and men place relatively greater importance on physical attractiveness than do women (Rathus, 1988). Commonly, individuals are likely to meet their partners in work environments, social situations, and leisure time (Brown, 1996). A recent study of the complexities associated with the traits of choosing a mate determined this complexity required a multicontextual view of the traits. While a long list of common traits was cited from the literature, the "value of considering both individual variation and population-level measures when addressing questions of sexual selection" is of importance (Lee, Dubbs, Von Hippel, Brooks, Zietsch, 2014).

There are potentially several advantages of partnerships and marriage. Such companionship offers each individual various opportunities to share a wide range of experiences and promote social learning and adaptation, which further promotes motivation and emotional development (Brown, 1996). It is also well known that partnership and marriage lead to greater longevity, thus married individuals enjoy better health than those of other marital statuses (Brown, 1996; Christiansen, 1990). Specifically, in a comparison study between married and unmarried men and women, it was concluded that divorced, single, and separated individuals experienced much higher rates of disease, morbidity, disability, mental neuroses, and mortality than their married counterparts (Christiansen, 1990; Roelfs, Shor, Kalish, & Yoguv, 2011).

Intimacy and Sexuality

The complexity of human sexuality includes body image, self-concept, gender identity, beliefs and feelings about sex, capacities for love and friendship, social behavior, and overt physical expression of love or sexual desire (Gourley, 2002). Humans are considered sexual beings; therefore, sexual identity and fulfillment of sexual roles and expression are intrinsic components of the overall human experience.

An individual's ethical, religious, and spiritual beliefs, cultural traditions, and moral concerns further influence patterns of sexual behavior, as well as levels of intimacy with others (Gourley, 2002; Rathus, 1988). Intimacy can be described as feelings of closeness and affection between interacting partners, the state of having revealed one's innermost thoughts and feelings to another individual, relatively intense forms of nonverbal engagement (notably touch, eye contact, and close physical proximity), particular types of relationships (especially marriage), and sexual activity (Mackey, Diemer, & O'Brien, 2000). Additionally, intimacy from a psychosocial perspective can be considered a sense that one can be open and honest in talking with a partner about personal thoughts and feelings not usually expressed in any other relationship (Mackey et al., 2000).

In general, humans crave intimacy, to love, and to be loved (Barbor, 2001). In a study of same- and opposite-gender couples, participants described intimacy as the verbal sharing of inner thoughts and feelings between partners along with mutual acceptance of those thoughts and feelings (Mackey et al., 2000). Sexuality, as a form of intimacy, is also associated with happiness, overall well-being, and also longevity; studies have shown that frequency and enjoyment of sexual intercourse are significant predictors of longevity (Nusbaum & Hamilton, 2002).

Notably, sexual function and intimacy with others should be considered relevant throughout the lifespan, as an elderly widow may be as concerned about her sexuality as a young adult (Nusbaum & Hamilton, 2002). Society views older adults as asexual beings, incapable of healthy sexual relationships. This stereotype is also predominantly significant for postmenopausal women (Gourley, 2002). In contrast, researchers discuss studies that show older adults are interested in sexual intercourse and enjoy sexual activities (Moore & Amburgey, 2000; Syme, 2014).

As previously mentioned in this chapter, it is significant to note that individuals 50 years of age and older are the fastest growing HIV-infected group, increasing 138% since 1993, and they constitute 11% of people in the United States diagnosed with AIDS (Moore & Amburgey, 2000). Health care workers often lack awareness of this prevalence, probably due to societal stereotypes of this age group and limited educational focus. In addition, older adults in general often lack knowledge of risk-taking behaviors and are often hesitant to discuss their sexual activities with others (Moore & Amburgey, 2000).

Adults With Disabilities and Friendships

The development of any friendship depends on the opportunity to interact with others, appropriate social and interpersonal skills, and the ability to initiate and sustain a relationship; some or all of these components are often challenging for the adult with a disability (Gordon, Tantillo, Feldman, & Perrone, 2004). Problematically, people with cognitive or mental limitations do not always understand how to interpret what others are thinking and expressing nonverbally, further impacting their ability to develop and maintain social relations (Greenfield, 2005).

As previously described in this section, many friendships maintained in young adulthood are formed during childhood and adolescence. As a result, students with disabilities who are offered mainstream educational opportunities generally have an advantage in participating more fully in society than children or adolescents who are segregated into special schools or classes (Kaye, 1997).

Most young adults with a disability have limited out-of-school contacts, negligible participation with organized social activities, and a predisposition toward sedentary activities (Ng, Dinesh, Tay, & Lee, 2003). Even for previously mainstreamed students with disabilities, this cycle of social alienation unfortunately worsens when young adults leave the structure of a school setting. For example, young adults with cerebral palsy tend to become less socially active and more isolated after leaving school (Ng et al., 2003).

Additionally, adults with chronic disabilities have fewer opportunities to form meaningful relationships unless social bonds were developed prior to the onset of the disability. Also, many disabled individuals primarily interact with family members, caregivers, or health care providers and others in the programs in which they participate. Notably, outside of family relations, individuals with disabilities may have no freely given and chosen relationships, thus becoming further alienated from the community and isolated from others (Lutfiyya, 1997).

Social Isolation and Disability

Social isolation is a major reason for dissatisfaction with one's life. Fifty-one percent of adults with disabilities surveyed by Harris in 1994 reported a problem with their social life (Kaye, 1997). A more recent study found low levels of social support among individuals with physical disabilities (Forouzan et al., 2013). Studies also indicate that high levels of loneliness negatively affect mental and physical health, because depression, anxiety, and low self-esteem appear to be related to loneliness (Hopps, Pepin, Arseneau, Freschette, & Begin, 2001).

Although social integration for persons with a disability is a significant component of the Americans with Disabilities Act, comparable surveys from the Harris group in 1986 and 1994, respectively, indicate little evidence of progress (Kaye, 1997). Researchers further argue that social isolation can also be a result of living alone, because people with disabilities are more than twice as likely to live alone as those without disabilities, according to data from the 1990 National Health Interview Survey (1997). Significantly, as the adult person with a disability ages, social participation will become a major area of concern. It is estimated that over one-third (33.9%) of those over the age of 65 with disabilities live by themselves (1997).

Barriers to Social Relationships

Friendships and interpersonal connections are significant experiences in the lives of all people, including those with a disability (Chen, Brodwin, Cardoso, & Chan, 2002; Gordon, Tantillo, Feldman, & Perrone, 2004). As previously described, adults with disabilities may have fewer opportunities to create these bonds due to several factors, including longstanding negative social attitudes and stigma, often described as invisible community barriers (Gordon, Tantillo, Feldman, & Perrone, 2004). Researchers have found that societal attitudes toward fully integrated individuals in the community have become more positive in the vocational and educational arenas but not within personal and social relations (Chen et al., 2002). In the United States, attitudes toward disability vary dramatically according to social contexts, with more positive attitudes held toward people with disabilities in work situations than in dating and marriage (Chen et al., 2002). This social rejection is evident in other cultures and is somewhat hierarchical in nature, depending on the type of disability. In a study of students in Hong Kong and Taiwan, for example, individuals with physical disabilities were viewed more positively than individuals with developmental delays and mental disorders, questionably due in part to Chinese culture, in which persons with severe intellectual disorders and mental illness are often viewed as a source of shame by their parents and kept at home out of public attention (Chen et al., 2002). Historically, mental illness and intellectual cognitive disorder have been noted to be the least socially accepted. Intellectual cognitive disorders have specifically been described as "the most socially invisible of all people with disabilities" (Gordon et al., 2004, p. 101).

In additional research studies, adults with disabilities have been viewed by their nondisabled counterparts as nonequals and in most cases not perceived as potential friends. Able-bodied individuals also tend to view those with disabilities as different across several social dimensions. For example, individuals who are more socially anxious, uneasy about dating, and less likely to date may experience an "interaction strain" between the two parties (Gordon et al., 2004).

Women in particular may have more of a challenge in social settings than do their male counterparts. In a recent studies, women with physical disabilities reported significantly lower levels of self-esteem and perceptions of how others see them compared to women without disabilities. Hence, they face serious social isolation and dissatisfaction with their relationships, which also puts them at a distinct disadvantage for quality-of-life experiences compared to women in general (Brown, 2014; Nosek & Hughes, 2001). Per Matheson (2003), "to be a disabled woman is to be, in the eyes of many, somehow less of a woman, less of an individual than the nondisabled people around you" (p. 44).

Dating and Partnerships for Adults With Disabilities

Adults with disabilities are often deprived of ordinary social stimulation and the possibility of developing friendships and intimate, long-term partnerships, which are essential tools for adulthood (Brown, 1996). The concept of dating and potentially developing an intimate bond with someone else is a common desire for many.

Past research noted that people who acquire their disabilities early in life are more likely to delay marriage or remain single. Specifically, 40.7% of 25 to 44 year olds with disabilities lack a live-in spouse or partner, compared to only 29.7% of the nondisabled population in that age group (Kaye, 1997). Small qualitative studies also suggest that disability limits the ability of women especially to find romantic partners and thus to form families (1997). In addition, emerging disabilities may also dissolve pre-disability relationships. In one study, half of the women who had relationships prior to their SCI endured the break-up of those relationships following the injury (1997).

Persons with a developmental disability, similar to their counterparts, also have the desire to maximize their self-fulfillment and to participate fully in mainstream life by forming intimate connections (Lerner, 2005). An adult with Down's syndrome is more likely to partner with someone else with a disability, since the majority of people with Down's syndrome mostly meet other people with disabilities (Brown, 1996). These relationships, including marriage, can increase the quality of life and self-esteem for both spouses (Lerner, 2005). However, there are multiple challenges that these individuals face due to their social, emotional, and adaptive limitations. Challenges include difficulties accessing necessary community resources and inappropriate involvement by significant others. Ultimately, the success of marriage and intimate partnerships depends greatly on the type of support the couple receives and how they respond overall to these challenges (Lerner, 2005).

Intimacy and Sexuality for Adults With Disabilities

Sexuality and intimacy are essential parts of an individual's self-identity and self-esteem, regardless of one's abilities (Versluys, 1995a). Significantly, acute or chronic disability or illness may disrupt sexual activity because it interferes with cognition, motor skills, coordination, sensory skills and the individual's sense of self, thus impacting the individual's ability to fulfill his or her identified sexual roles and habits (Dahl, 1988; Gourley, 2002). In addition, disfiguring conditions such as amputation or mastectomy or conditions such as incontinence can raise anxiety about attractiveness and may undermine an individual's self-image, inducing concern about a loss of desirability and lowered self-worth (Glass & Soni, 1999; Rolland, 1994). As described in Hendley (1996): "a disability shatters our image of ourselves. Changes in how the body looks, loss of independence, diminishment of a traditional role—all of these can impact on our image of ourselves as sexual beings" (p. 17).

Notably, the onset of impairments early in life often produces low social and sexual confidence about one's future, whereas individuals who acquire a disability in adulthood are much more focused on the past (Livneh & Antonak, 1997). The process of adjustment varies for each person. How people view their disability and who they see as responsible for managing the effects of the condition strongly influence their ability to cope (Glass & Soni, 1999). Defining sexuality as more than just a physical function is particularly important for people with disabilities (1999).

Although an individual's disability may vary, society has placed an added challenge by minimizing a realistic and positive identity as a sexual being and the opportunity for sexual expression and fulfilling sexual relationships (Bidgood, Boyle, & Ballan, 2004). Societal attitudes may imply that persons with disabilities are not fully human, meaning that they do not have sexual desires. An individual who is not able to use part of his or her body still has an equal right to full sexual expression; cognitive or mental limitations do not preclude an individual's participation in sexual activity (Glass & Soni, 1999; Gourley, 2002). The National Women's Health Information Center reports that many medical professionals are often misinformed about the sexual potential of women of any age with disabilities and as a result do not encourage them to resume normal sexual activities. In addition, older women also reported they often do not receive adequate education on sexual function related to disability (Gourley, 2002).

The sexuality of individuals with developmental disabilities has also been historically misunderstood in society. For example, allegations of individuals with developmental delays being asexual, oversexed, sexually uncontrollable, sexually animalistic, subhuman, dependent and childlike, as well as breeders of disability have been discussed in the literature (Bidgood, Boyle, & Ballan, 2004; Gourley, 2002).

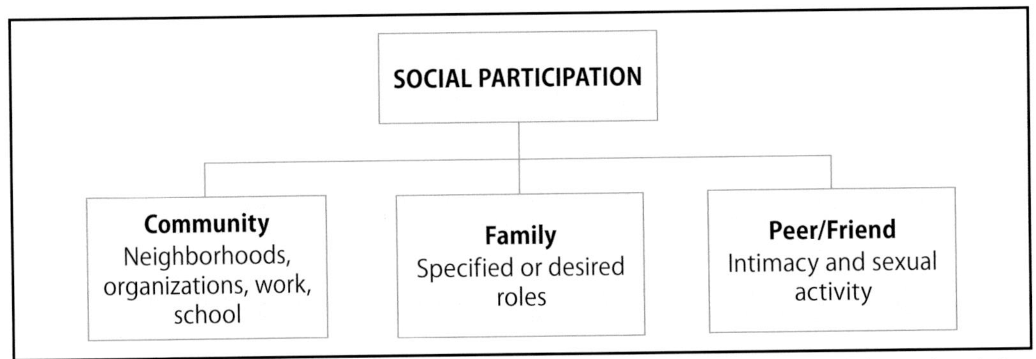

Figure 9-2. Components of social participation activities. (Adapted from American Occupational Therapy Association. [2002]. Occupational therapy practice framework: Domain and process. *American Journal of Occupational Therapy, 56*(6), 609-639.)

In general, individuals with developmental disabilities do not always receive adequate or accurate education on sexuality or sexual relationships (Greenfield, 2005). For adults with a severe disability, the greatest barrier that impacts sexuality are the attitudes and knowledge base of staff with whom they are involved, as well as parents who have been responsible for their upbringing (Brown, 1996). As a result, these individuals may have difficulty conceptualizing appropriate physical interactions with others and understanding sexual feelings. The Association for Retarded Citizens (ARC) states that persons with intellectual disorders have the fundamental right to learn about sexual functions and relationships and should be able to make informed decisions regarding their own sexuality (Gourley, 2002).

Various intervention strategies addressing issues on sexuality, intimacy, and peer/friend interactions will be discussed later in this chapter.

Remediation/Compensation/Adaptation Intervention Strategies for Social Participation

Practitioners use a holistic intervention model to assist clients with social participation. Taking into account such factors as age, disability, and social skills, the therapist can assist with the transition to community activities. Across the lifespan, the challenge to be a purposeful being is at the core of an individual's identity. Occupational therapy practice (AOTA, 2014) includes a three-tiered approach: (1) remediation, (2) compensation/adaptation of the task, and (3) maintenance of successful performance through caregiver education and environmental modifications. The overall approach to intervention will depend primarily on the client's abilities to engage in occupations and the disruptions that are caused by disabilities at the performance skill level.

Occupational therapists and occupational therapy assistants work collaboratively with clients to promote desired participation in activities at home, school, the workplace, and other community life situations (Figure 9-2). This also includes successful role performance in each of these areas (AOTA, 2014). Because disease and disability may negatively impact successful role performance, the practice of occupational therapy is vital to engagement in occupation and social participation. It is important to understand the impact of each person's individual diagnosis and prognosis when generating an intervention plan. This section will look at Framework-proposed intervention guidelines applied to social participation. A case example of a woman with a CVA is presented next. We will begin with her story, followed by five intervention guidelines.

Case Study 1: Mary, Cerebral Vascular Accident

Mary is a 70-year-old widow who lives with her daughter, son-in-law, and two granddaughters in a two-level home. She drives, is completely independent with her ADLs and instrumental ADLs, and is an active social participant in her church's ladies auxiliary and religious education program, in which she serves as an instructor. Medically, she also has a history of diabetes and hypertension. While driving to church on a Sunday, Mary begins to feel dizzy and has a sudden onset of blurred vision. She loses control of her car and hits a barrier wall on the side of the road. Upon the arrival of an emergency crew and with first aid administered, she is rushed to a local hospital's emergency department. A battery of tests reveals that Mary has had a left-sided CVA with resulting visual/perceptual deficits, mild aphasia, and right-sided flaccidity of her UEs and LEs. After a brief acute hospital stay, Mary is admitted to a rehabilitation facility for continued therapy intervention. The following are some initial clinical reasoning thoughts by the occupational therapist:

- An occupational therapy evaluation of Mary will need to take many factors into account when determining functional outcome levels.
- Goals aimed at remediation must include Mary's desire to return to her daughter's home with residual motor, perceptual, process, and interaction skills restored to functionally independent levels.
- A comprehensive intervention plan must also include Mary's desire to return to teaching religious education and remaining an active member of the church auxiliary.

Performance skills to be assessed include the following:

- Sensory perceptual skills
- Motor and praxis
- Emotional regulation skills
- Cognitive skills
- Communication and social skills

Remediation

Remediation is the act of treating a "condition" and allowing an individual to regain lost skills and function. In simplest terms, a client enters intervention with goals aimed at restoration of a prior level of functional capacity. Occupational therapy determines what skills are restorative in the above-stated goals (Figures 9-3, 9-4, and 9-5). Occupational therapy will begin by restoring as many skills as possible based on Mary's health condition.

Compensation/Adaptation Interventions for Clients With Decreased Performance Skills/Client Factors

Coordination Deficits

The compensatory approach to intervention allows for functional task independence with variations of the components of task performance. This intervention approach assumes the client will not immediately be able to restore task abilities and provides an opportunity for independent performance with an alternative approach or with the use of adaptive equipment. The occupational therapist has the ability to assist the client in achieving independence through changing the task or changing the tools for the client to achieve independence. Compensatory interventions to increase

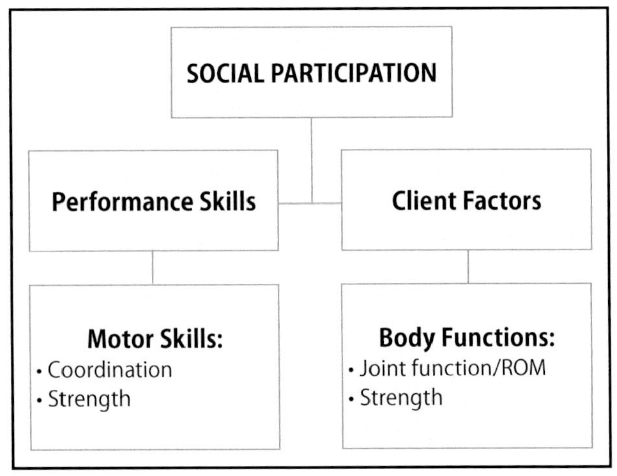

Figure 9-3. Relationship of ROM, strength, and coordination to social participation. (Adapted from American Occupational Therapy Association. [2002]. Occupational therapy practice framework: Domain and process. *American Journal of Occupational Therapy, 56*(6), 609-639.)

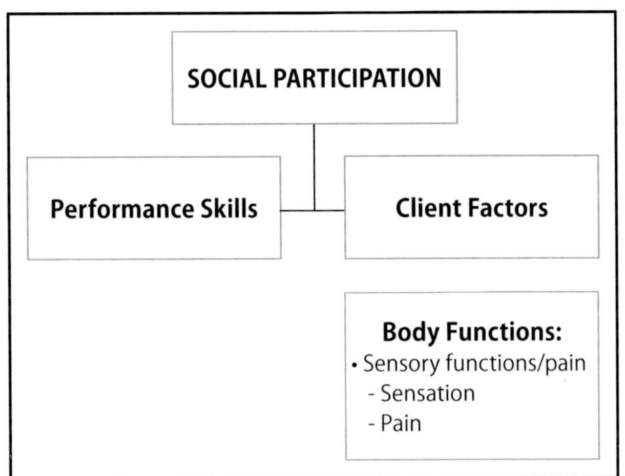

Figure 9-4. Relationship of sensation/pain to social participation. (Adapted from American Occupational Therapy Association. [2002]. Occupational therapy practice framework: Domain and process. *American Journal of Occupational Therapy, 56*(6), 609-639.)

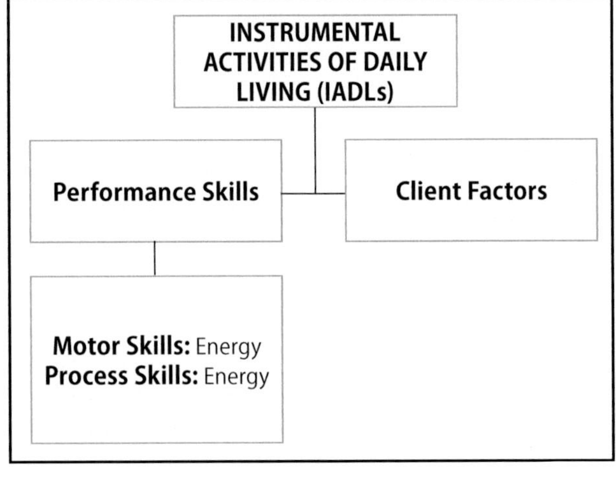

Figure 9-5. Relationship of energy/endurance to social participation. (Adapted from American Occupational Therapy Association. [2002]. Occupational therapy practice framework: Domain and process. *American Journal of Occupational Therapy, 56*(6), 609-639.)

Table 9-3

Examples of Compensation/Adaptation Strategies for Range of Motion, Strength, and Coordination Deficits

Performance Skill Deficit	Examples of Compensatory/Adaptation Intervention
ROM	• The client is instructed in hemi-dressing techniques until she can perform the tasks independently with or without adaptive equipment. • Social participation goals would include Mary's ability to self-toilet while at all functions. • Incorporating the family into intervention for caregiver education on an active assistive range of motion (AAROM) program may be vital to Mary's future success.
Strength	• The client is instructed to perform techniques in sitting and supine or gravity-eliminated planes to compensate for UE strength deficits. • Mary would then be able to meet the goal of active participation in her church group functions either at standing or seated (compensatory) levels.
Coordination	• The client is provided with elastic shoelaces and a button-hook secondary to impaired fine motor coordination of the digits. • Socially, Mary would be able to gain independence of her abilities to perform clothing management and manage barriers to access in her physical environment.

social participation for clients with motor skill deficits are included in Table 9-3, using Mary as the example.

With social participation in mind, the compensatory intervention approach may shift to the community environment that Mary is seeking to re-enter. Mary's goal is to be able to socially participate in the annual holiday dinner sponsored by the ladies' auxiliary. For the past 15 years, Mary has served as the chief menu planner and hostess for the gala event. In order for her to achieve this goal, she must be able to communicate her thoughts and ideas. With her handwriting ability limited by her CVA, a compensatory approach to intervention in this example may include Mary using a tape recorder to dictate the menu to a friend or purchasing an assistive computer technology package that recognizes voice input and converts it to script. Both the tools used to perform the task and the task itself have been modified for successful independent performance. The occupational therapist or occupational therapy assistant would provide the intervention opportunities for Mary to become proficient with the tools provided.

Cognitive, Perceptual, and Visual Limitations

Cognitive, perceptual, and/or visual limitations (Figure 9-6) are arguably the most challenging of barriers to overcome for successful community social participation re-entry. A client with cognitive deficits may demonstrate a range of social abilities and, despite a need for assistance, may make it difficult for caregivers and peers to advise and assist the client (Pollard, 2000). Social skills necessary for advanced participation goals may be impaired, leaving an individual and his or her caregiver socially isolated.

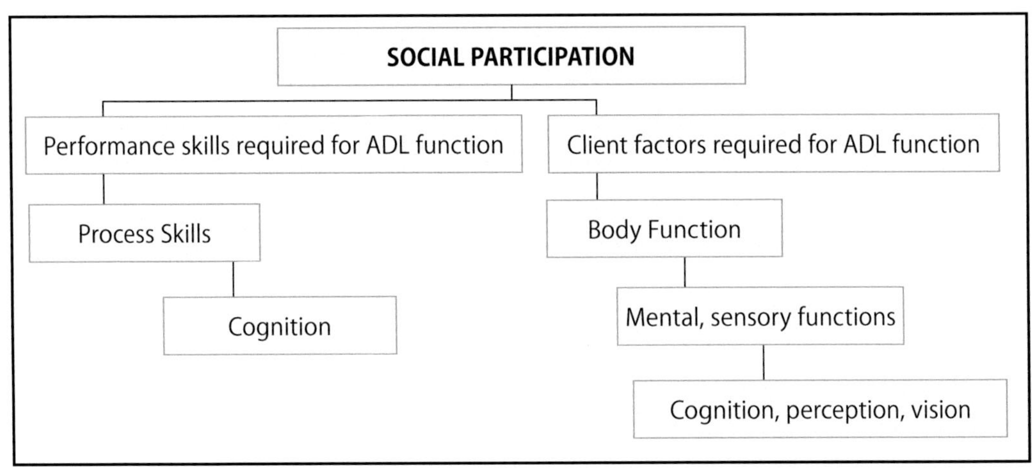

Figure 9-6. Components of performance skills/client factors related to social participation. (Adapted from American Occupational Therapy Association. [2002]. Occupational therapy practice framework: Domain and process. *American Journal of Occupational Therapy,* 56(6), 609-639.)

Table 9-4

Examples of Compensation/Adaptation Strategies for Cognition Deficits

Performance Skill Deficit (Process Skills)	Examples of Compensatory/Adaptive Interventions
Knowledge/memory	• The client is instructed in the use of a daily planner for social activities.
Temporal organization	• The client is instructed in the use of "to do" lists in order to initiate tasks.
Organizing space and objects	• The client is visually cued through the use of lists or verbally cued for the setup of a room for social activities. This may include the assistance of family members or peers to guide and assist the client as necessary.
Adaptation	• The client is instructed in various techniques aimed at providing alternative approaches for successful independent functioning in the social environment.

Cognitive Limitations

The performance skills in Table 9-4 are vital to successful performance in the social environment. One of the performance skills is cognition (Figure 9-7) which impacts everything that we do. Memory impairment is a common symptom of a CVA and impacts the ability for new learning. It may interfere with the ability to resume independent functioning in a social setting. The establishment of routine and structure is imperative in these cases, yet the client is often faced with challenges that require external assistance. Compensatory approaches for community reintegration may focus on the client's ability to seek assistance effectively when challenged with a situation that causes anxiety (Allen, 1996).

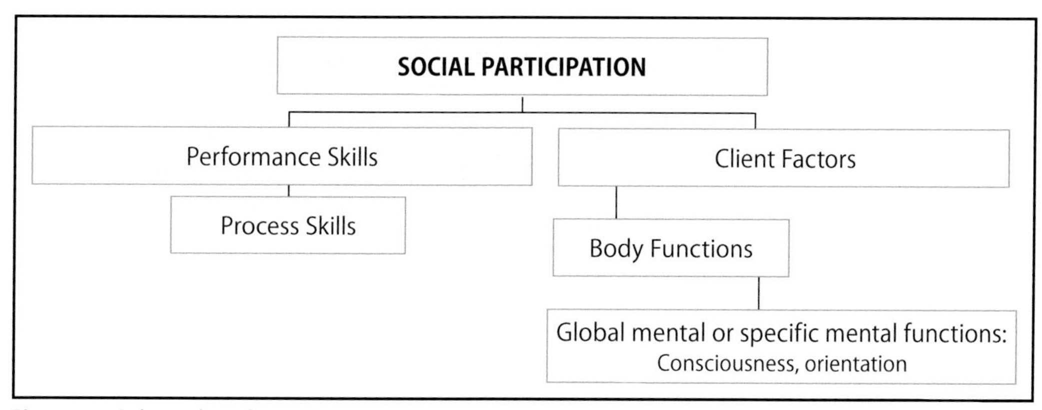

Figure 9-7. Relationship of cognition to IADLs. (Adapted from American Occupational Therapy Association. [2002]. Occupational therapy practice framework: Domain and process. *American Journal of Occupational Therapy, 56*(6), 609-639.)

In addition to the process skills noted in Table 9-4, the AOTA Framework (2014) identifies body function categories that are cognitive and perceptual in nature. These functions may be further divided into two specific categories: global mental functions and specific mental functions (AOTA, 2014).

- Global mental functions include arousal and orientation. The quality of social participation is, indeed, highly connected to the individual's ability to maintain a level of arousal throughout the activity, as well as to be able to participate in the "here and now" with others in the setting. Social isolation of the client and caregiver is common in situations in which the client may exhibit negative behaviors and lack the ability to identify meaningful social cues.
- Specific mental functions include attention, memory, perception, higher-order thought processes, and mental functioning (process skills, such as motor planning). While clients may be instructed to use appropriate adaptive techniques for successful performance in a social setting, quite often deficits in higher-order/executive functioning lead to diminished participation in familiar settings due to social embarrassment. The occupational therapist or occupational therapy assistant may perform an environmental assessment of the social context to integrate with the client's mental functioning. An occupational therapist must use sound clinical reasoning when analyzing Mary's role functions and capacity for social reintegration to desired social activities. Should Mary's executive function deficits as a result of her CVA impact her ability to act as the finance chair of the dinner event (past role), an alternative suggestion may be proposed for Mary to take on the role of menu planner and preparation supervisor with assistance. This altered role with its respective modification of activity demands will still meet Mary's goal of social engagement in her community. She is more likely to succeed at this new role because it better matches her cognitive functioning.

Perceptual Limitations

The occupational therapist may further provide task modifications for perceptual limitations (Figure 9-8) such as a written itinerary for Mary of the chronological events of the dinner so she is able to be oriented to the program at all times. Mary can be instructed to use a date book for visual reminders and dates. The occupational therapist or occupational therapy assistant can hold a simulated rehearsal of the meeting in the actual environment prior to the actual date. This preparatory method can ease Mary's anxiety, integrate task modifications, and familiarize the client with environmental supports and barriers (Table 9-5).

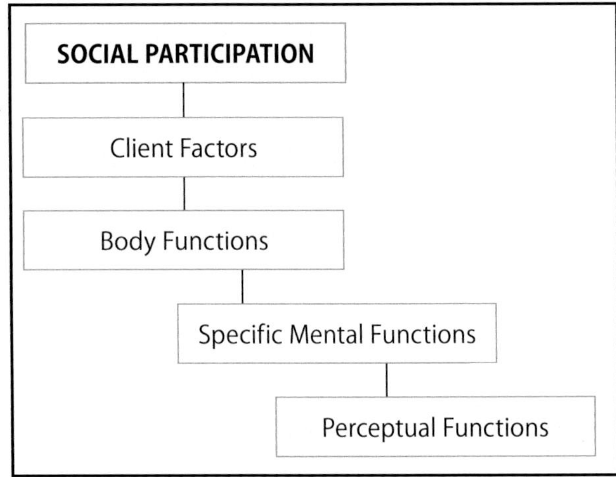

Figure 9-8. Relationship of perception to social participation. (Adapted from American Occupational Therapy Association. [2002]. Occupational therapy practice framework: Domain and process. *American Journal of Occupational Therapy, 56*(6), 609-639.)

Table 9-5

Examples of Compensation/Adaptation Strategies for Perception Deficits

Performance Skill Deficit	Examples of Compensatory/Adaptive Interventions
Motor planning/ apraxia	• Instruct the client using the best learning method for him or her and provide external cuing as needed for successful task performance. • The ability to succeed in social activities may depend on the ability to motor plan; therefore, family or peer training for safety may be necessary.
Visual fixation/ scanning	• Instruct the client in the ability to scan all environments, objects, and people in the same methodology.
Visual inattention/ neglect	• Instruct the client in head-turning strategies when meeting new people or navigating the environment so as not to miss environmental and social cues.
Body scheme	• Instruct the client to use a mirror or seek the counsel of a family member or friend prior to attending a community event to ensure that dressing, grooming, and hygiene tasks are successfully performed.
Visual discrimination	• Instruct the client in various compensatory visual techniques aimed at providing visual feedback to the client until (if) visual or perceptual issues resolve.

Visual Limitations

The physical aspect of sight is explored in this section (Figure 9-9). Nearly 80% of our social cueing is derived from visual feedback (Warren, 1995). If an individual has a visual impairment, intervention is especially warranted to provide safe opportunities for successful community reintegration. Impaired vision is defined as a change in or loss of a visual field. The term *low vision* will also be used to refer to this category of impairment, and the reader is encouraged to see Chapter 5 for a more thorough understanding of this condition.

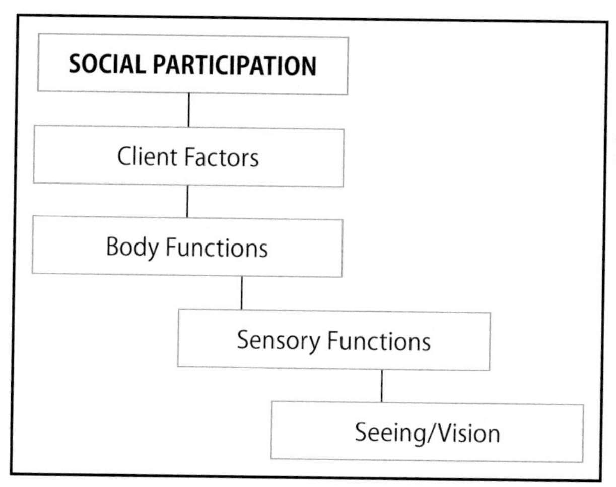

Figure 9-9. Relationship of vision to social participation. (Adapted from American Occupational Therapy Association. [2002]. Occupational therapy practice framework: Domain and process. *American Journal of Occupational Therapy, 56*(6), 609-639.)

Table 9-6

Examples of Compensation/Adaptation Strategies for Vision Deficits

Performance Skill Deficit	Examples of Compensatory/Adaptive Interventions
Visual field loss/cut	• Instruct the client in head-turning and scanning techniques. • Arrange a neuro-opthalmology consult to assess for prism glasses.
Low vision	• Instruct the client in the use of visual assistive technology aids and lighting changes so that he or she has successfully navigated the community environment.

The most common loss of vision as it relates to aging is the loss of visual acuity. However, neurological disease processes such as CVA, brain injury, and multiple sclerosis may also lead to visual changes. These changes may include the loss of a partial field of vision, also called a field cut. Other diseases such as glaucoma and macular degeneration lead to a syndrome known as low vision. Because lighting varies tremendously in all community environments, an individual with low vision may find the social context to be a challenge. For example, an individual with low vision who might have enjoyed going to lunch with friends at a particular restaurant may be less inclined to participate socially if unable to see well in this environment. The occupational therapist may suggest compensatory strategies for the client to promote safe, social engagement. These strategies may include instruction in the use of magnifiers and providing contrasting color backgrounds to minimize the loss of visual discrimination. Because there is no cure for low vision, all interventions aimed at this disease will be adaptive and compensatory in nature (Table 9-6).

Strategies to Enhance Communication and Social Skills

Clearly, promoting social interaction skills is a primary focus for occupational therapy practitioners. The Framework defines social interaction as "conveying intentions and needs and coordinating social behavior to act together with other people" (AOTA, 2014, p. S26).

This performance skill includes a physical component, information exchange, and interpersonal relations. All of these components are ultimately vital elements to an individual's ability to communicate and interact with others in an interactive environment (AOTA, 2014). The practitioner's therapeutic use of self is the foundation of all intervention strategies addressing social interactions (AOTA, 2014). The occupational therapist may be described as an interpersonal coach who guides various social intervention strategies during individual or group experiences.

Modeling

Modeling may be described as the "silent influence." It actually occurs every time a therapist interacts with a client and not just when the therapist is consciously attempting to teach specific behaviors or actions (Denton, 1987). Individuals learn by observing the behaviors and actions of a role model and then by imitating and practicing the behavior (Versluys, 1995a). Modeling activities not only provide verbal experiences through information exchange but also give nonverbal, social cues regarding the physical components of social interactions. For example, the way the therapist maintains eye contact and gestures with his or her hands provides modeling for the client on socially acceptable nonverbal communication strategies. Each therapy session provides a unique opportunity to further promote and practice appropriate social interactions that can then be integrated into the client's social contexts.

Within a social group setting, models for social behavior include not only the therapist but other clients as well. Group participants provide another dimension of social reinforcement to the individual (Versluys, 1995). Additionally, when out in the community, family members and peers can serve as role models to encourage carry-over of appropriate communication strategies learned in therapy sessions. For example, family members and caregivers can model appropriate information exchange by introducing friends to the client and asking questions to initiate and stimulate ongoing conversations.

Role-Play

Role-playing is a particularly helpful purposeful activity used in occupational therapy sessions. It offers a client the opportunity to practice or test new verbal and nonverbal skills. Rehearsal of social situations can enhance the individual's awareness of feelings, attitudes, and behaviors of others; this self-awareness is needed to manage effective social performance in the community (Denton, 1987; Gutman, Raphael-Greenfield, & Salvant, 2012). Role-playing and rehearsal as an intervention strategy offer an opportunity for the client to act out new interpersonal scenarios that he or she may potentially encounter in the community within a safe, nonthreatening environment. Scenarios can be constructed in one-to-one sessions or within a group setting. Role-playing activities are often organized around a simulated situation such as being appropriately assertive or demonstrating personal boundaries in a social activity. As a result of this type of interpersonal intervention, the client may be able to further identify problems he or she may anticipate once out in the community (Gutman et al., 2012; Versluys, 1995).

To further illustrate these intervention techniques, we will examine the previous example of a client named John with a developmental intellectual disorder. John identifies that social participation is a major goal for therapy. He verbalizes to the occupational therapist that he is apprehensive about going to the movies with a new friend. He is clearly nervous and somewhat pressured to have his new friend "like him." He wonders what they will talk about. How will he start off a conversation? Based on John's concerns, the occupational therapist selects role-playing as a preparatory method and purposeful activity for intervention. Role-playing and rehearsal can best prepare John ahead of time for possible social interactions and provide awareness of potential interpersonal roadblocks. John and the occupational therapist can practice how to initiate and maintain conversation about personal interests while also guiding him to avoid sensitive topics. Additionally, role-playing can offer an opportunity for John to practice nonverbal communication techniques including body language and physical boundaries. John and the occupational therapist can simulate various degrees of physical proximity and discuss what are socially acceptable boundaries regarding body positioning. This intervention allows the therapist and client to collaboratively address the upcoming social event, giving John strategies and increasing his self-confidence.

Videotaping

Audiovisual tools such as videotaping provide a real-time feedback mechanism for educating a client about communication/interaction skills. This visual learning tool provides an individual with the opportunity to review his or her own performance. Newly acquired skills or practiced behaviors may need to be changed or altered several times to reach the most desired outcome (Denton, 1987; Sibley et al., 2012). Watching one's own performance on video allows a person to increase self-awareness regarding his or her skills and abilities. A potential drawback to this technique is that the client's overall presentation may change if he or she is uncomfortable with being recorded. The practitioner would need to assess the client's readiness for media use as an intervention prior to implementing this strategy.

Community Outings

Field trips are occupation-based intervention activities that offer an opportunity for the individual to apply communication/interaction skills within the real-world setting (Denton, 1987).

Community-based interventions also provide a unique way to incorporate context and environmental feedback. Practitioners and other trusted members can offer feedback to the client during the actual social event or field trip. This feedback should be tempered to fit the needs of the situation and the client's ability to accept feedback while in a social context. Another approach might be for the practitioner and the client to further discuss and process the social event afterwards in a therapy session. The use of "real data" that emerged from the in vivo social context is a powerful tool for shaping a client's social interaction skills.

Common Barriers Impacting Social Participation

Personal Hygiene and Grooming Intervention Strategies

ADLs, including personal hygiene and grooming, are activities that are oriented toward taking care of one's own body (previously described in Chapter 3). These activities are also essential components to effective social participation because they impact how others will perceive and respond to an individual during communal interactions. These social perceptions, then, are ways in which we form and modify impressions of others (Rathus, 1988). Fundamentally, these preconceived notions are considered to be basic human nature and can be formulated solely based on an individual's outward physical appearance, including his or her hygiene and grooming practices.

Adults with various disabilities may face several challenges when completing their ADLs. Often, the occupational therapy practitioner will introduce various strategies to optimize an individual's occupational performance in this area, including the use of assistive devices and/or adaptive equipment. It is important to assist a client to carry over these techniques into his or her own environment. If the client lives with family, it is helpful for the therapist to schedule a family training session to familiarize caregivers with the adaptive equipment. Practitioners can help the client and caregivers maintain strategies for safety and independence gained during therapy sessions. Please see Chapter 3 for more information on ADLs.

Within the focus of self-care, the occupational therapist needs to also educate the client about social norms relating to hygiene and grooming practices. Intervention plans should be based on the client's abilities and limitations, including financial means. As previously described in this chapter, adults with disabilities are often faced with significant social stigma and invisible barriers that impact their ability to fully integrate into all aspects of the community. Limited knowledge and understanding of social norms, including those regarding personal appearance, may be an additional hindrance for clients who are trying to reintegrate into their community.

Occupational therapy practitioners may find initial discussions on personal hygiene and grooming practices to be sensitive topics for the client. Often there is an element of embarrassment or modesty for the client, as if they know they need to improve some aspect of their self-care but are not quite sure how to go about it. Sometimes, the topic may be too personal for the client and he or she may not feel comfortable talking about these issues with a therapist of another gender. There may be other times when the client may be relieved that he or she is given the opportunity to talk with an expert about topics that are usually avoided in social conversation. It is important for the therapist to acknowledge and validate these feelings and respond to the client in a caring and direct manner. Verbal feedback to the client should be basic and nonjudgmental. The art of delivering constructive feedback involves the ability to focus on behaviors separately from sense of self or identity. For example, telling someone that his or her ADL habits are poor is a different message than telling someone that he or she is sloppy or stinks.

When beginning such conversations, the therapist may ask the client how he or she feels about his or her physical appearance. Does the client have specific concerns or questions about how he or she appears to others? The therapist should also inquire about the client's typical self-care routine. Education about social aspects of personal care may include self-care/hygiene frequency, coordination of dress, coiffing, halitosis, and use of deodorant/antiperspirant, body sprays, and colognes. Verbal and/or written information is helpful, and therapists need to provide adequate explanation about how these issues are important from a social perspective. For example, John with a developmental intellectual disorder joins the neighborhood social club, which he will be attending three times per week. During therapy, the occupational therapy practitioner asks John how often he takes a shower and changes his clothes. He explains that he showers once a week on Sundays and does his laundry on the same day. Although he demonstrates an understanding that if his clothes are stained or soiled he needs to change them before embarking out into the community, he continues to wear the same undergarments each day, is malodorous, and has unruly hair during most therapy sessions. The therapist also notes that during a community outing several passersby stared and pointed at him. Additionally, John had a difficult time getting the bank teller's attention in line, and it appeared that he was being avoided.

The therapist realizes that John is unable to pick up on subtle social cues about how he is perceived by others in public. Further, the occupational therapist anticipates that given his current appearance, he will not be able to optimally perform and get his social needs met in the community. The occupational therapist decides to approach the subject tactfully, providing basic concrete information to the client. He explains in simplistic terms about good hygiene practices and body functions, educating the client on how glands produce secretions, causing smells, and how these smells can be modified by various hygiene products. The therapist further describes the need for clean undergarments and appropriate seasonal fabrics that can act as protective agents during inclement weather or allow the body to breathe. The concept of halitosis and appropriate oral hygiene is explored. Adequate hair management and basic coiffing techniques are discussed.

The therapist notes that John appears interested in the discussion and poses several questions to him: What is the difference between deodorant and body spray? Can dry mouth from medications make someone's breath smell badly? As therapy progresses during weekly intervention sessions, the occupational therapist notices improvements not only in the client's grooming but in his overall presence. His posture and eye contact have improved, and his affect appears brighter.

The therapist can determine how much further to explore self-care issues with John based on his interest and motivation to further enhance his appearance. Significantly, if the client continually dismisses feedback on his hygiene and grooming practices and is frequently not engaged in therapist-initiated conversations on such topics, the therapist probably needs to limit his or her focus on the issue. Ultimately, the client must be motivated to participate in such aspects of therapy and be willing to pursue behavioral changes in order to further impact social participation performance.

Strategies to Enhance Sexual Activity

Like any other meaningful occupation in an individual's life, an individual's sexuality is a relevant issue for the occupational therapy intervention process (Gourley, 2002). As stated by the Sexuality Information and Education Council of the United States, individuals with disabilities have the same right to education on sexuality, sexual health care, and opportunities for sexual expression as their nondisabled counterparts (Gourley, 2002).

Unfortunately, sexual expression is an important but often overlooked ADL (Estes, 2002). It is common for clients, as well as therapists, to be potentially embarrassed or unsure about how to initiate discussions about sexual activity. Prior to discussing sexuality with a client, the therapist should have a sense of his or her own bias, attitudes, and feelings on the topic of concern. Clients may trigger feelings of discomfort unintentionally (Gourley, 2002). Quality health care includes holding sexual health at equal status with physical, spiritual, social, and emotional care (Nusbaum & Hamilton, 2002).

Although several health care specialties, as well as clients, agree that addressing sexual health should be an integral component of intervention, there are complex factors that interfere with addressing rehabilitation clients' sexual expression needs (Estes, 2002). Research indicates that there is limited knowledge, training, and experience in the area of sexuality by occupational therapists (Estes, 2002). In some cases, therapists may generally assume that the client has discussed such topics with other members of the health care team or that it may not be a priority for him or her at the present time. A client may legitimately feel uncomfortable talking about such topics due to his or her generational or cultural background, gender (or the gender of the therapist), or lack of self-confidence following the onset of an injury or disability (Estes, 2002). Additionally, if the practitioner avoids the topic, the client may assume the subject is inappropriate to discuss (Gourley, 2002). Subsequently, some therapists fear that if they initiate conversations on sexuality, the client will misinterpret their intentions, which could result in accusations of sexual harassment (Estes, 2002). Ultimately, if therapists do not feel comfortable discussing or providing education on sexuality to the client, it is their professional responsibility to adequately refer the client to additional health care specialists.

When addressing sexuality, occupational therapists need to provide concrete, simple information in a nonjudgmental manner that is consistent with the client's level of mental functioning (Gourley, 2002; Nusbaum & Hamilton, 2002). The therapist should also use professional judgment in determining how far to pursue the conversation with the client and minimize anxiety or embarrassment. Frequently, practitioners can help ease the potentially uncomfortable client by acknowledging and validating his or her concerns and apprehensions.

When working with clients with developmental disabilities, it is important to keep in mind that their exposure to education on this topic is probably limited. As previously mentioned, education provided to the client with a developmental delay should originate from his or her needs and mental functions, realizing information is better processed in small doses with much repetition (Greenfield, 2005). Often, these clients may be confused or unsure as to what constitutes "normal" sexual behaviors, aspects of attractiveness to others, and levels of sexual desire. It is often advantageous for occupational therapy practitioners to reassure individuals that "normal" covers a wide range of degrees of interest in sexual relationships and behaviors (Gourley, 2002). Hence, a vital component of an educational approach is to eliminate myths and misinformation (Versluys, 1995).

Therapists can offer education and information on sexual activity in a variety of ways. Again, the client's needs, comfort level, abilities, and limitations will guide the appropriate manner of teaching. In some instances, individual counseling sessions and or group discussions may be appropriate. Techniques often include both verbal and written education and may or may not include the partner of the client, based on the client's request. Role-play scenarios can also offer the occupational therapy practitioner a starting point when working with clients with limited mental functioning to find out what they know about intimate relationships in a nonthreatening way (Greenfield, 2005). For educating and teaching individuals who have a developmental disorder, other creative intervention methods may include dolls, pictures, videos, games, and slides on topics of sexuality (Greenfield, 2005).

Since sexual activity is a lifelong element of an individual's identity, the occupational therapy practitioner must also initiate discussion with older adult clients. Education may focus on the multiple physiological and psychological changes that impact an individual's sexual roles and habits during this life stage. Information on the impact of aging on sexuality, including medication side effects, can be presented (Gourley, 2002). In addition, as previously described in this chapter, the number of older people infected with HIV is growing. Thus, therapists must consider these clients as an at-risk population for infection. Therefore, the therapist can offer open-ended discussions either individually or in a group setting, while providing basic verbal and written information about the risks of HIV transmission.

Sexuality and interventions for sexual behavior can also be found in Chapter 3 of this text.

Maintenance Intervention Strategies

Maintenance level interventions attempt to ensure carry-over of social skill performance and future planning. Maintenance of skill performance is typically offered once remedial and adaptive techniques have been successfully introduced and deemed to be effective. Client and caregiver education is monumental in this process. In addition to education models, clients may also be provided with lists of community resources, including support groups for peer and social interaction. In the ever-changing world of health care and the lessening of funding sources, occupational therapy practitioners find themselves in the role of educator from the onset to the termination of the intervention session. Even with the best intentions to remediate the problems identified, the occupational therapist is often forced to quickly move to adaptive and maintenance intervention strategies secondary to reimbursement demands and time restrictions. A client facing the challenge of social participation in a community setting must not only have the motivation to succeed but also the willingness to explore alternative options along the road to success.

Summary Questions

1. Define and discuss examples of three aspects of social participation.
2. Discuss unique issues that family/caregivers face in relation to a client's social participation.
3. Discuss strategies for the occupational therapist to involve family members in the intervention process related to social participation.
4. Explain the significance of peer/friend and intimate relationships in various stages of life as related to social participation.

References

Allen, C. K., Austin, S. L., David, S. K., Earhart, C. A., McCraith, D. B., & Riska-Williams, L. (2007). *Manual for the Allen cognitive level screen-5 and large Allen cognitive level screen-5*. Colchester, CT: S&S Worldwide.

Allen, C. K., Earhart, C. A., & Blue, T. (1992). *Occupational therapy treatment goals for the physically and cognitively disabled*. Rockville, MD: American Occupational Therapy Association.

Allison, L. K., Painter, J. A., Emory, A., Whitehurst, P., & Raby, A. (2013). Participation restriction, not fear of falling, predicts actual balance and mobility abilities in rural community-dwelling older adults. *Journal of Geriatric Physical Therapy, 36*(1), 13-23.

American Occupational Therapy Association. (2007). AOTA's Societal Statement on Family Caregivers. *American Journal of Occupational Therapy, 61*, 710.

American Occupational Therapy Association. (2008). Position paper occupational therapy services in the promotion of psychological and social aspects of mental health. Rockville, MD; American Occupational Therapy Association.

American Occupational Therapy Association. (2013). *The reference manual of the official documents of the American occupational therapy association* (18th ed.). Bethesda, MD: AOTA.

American Occupational Therapy Association. (2014). Occupational therapy practice: Domain and process. *American Journal of Occupational Therapy, 68*(Suppl. 1), S1-S48.

Barbor, C. (2001, January/February). Finding real love—intimacy and alienation. *Psychology Today, 34*, 42-49.

Barrett, L., & Kielhofner, G. (2003). Theories derived from occupational behavior perspectives. In E. B. Crepeau, E. S. Cohn, & B. A. B. Schell (Eds.), *Willard and Spackman's occupational therapy* (10th ed., pp. 209-233). Philadelphia, PA: Lippincott, Williams & Wilkins.

Baum, C. M., & Law, M. (1997). Occupational therapy practice: Focusing on occupational performance. *American Journal of Occupational Therapy, 51*(4), 277-288.

Bell, R. R. (1981). *Worlds of friendships*. Beverly Hills, CA: Sage Publications.

Bidgood, F. E., Boyle, P. S., & Ballan, M. (2004). Forty years of knowledge-SIECUS on sexuality and disability. *Sex Information and Education Council of the United States Report, 32*(2), 28.

Block, J. D. (1980). *Friendship: How to give it, how to get it*. New York, NY: Collier Books.

Bourne, H. (1998). Peer pressure. In J. Kagan (Ed.), *Gale encyclopedia of childhood and adolescence* (pp. 493-495). Detroit, MI: Gale Research.

Boyt Schell, B. A., Gillen, G., & Scaffa, M. (2014). Glossary. In B. A. Boyt Schell, G. Gillen, & M. Scaffa (Eds.). *Willard and Spackman's occupational therapy (12th ed.)* (p. 1241). Philadelphia, PA: Lippincott Williams & Wilkins.

Bradford, E. L. (2001). The importance of friendship. Retrieved at http://www.mhaoc.com/lack.html on May 14, 2005.

Braun, B. J. (1998). Knowledge and perception of fall-related risk factors and fall-reduction techniques among community-dwelling elderly individuals. *Physical Therapy, 78*, 1262-1276.

Brintnall-Peterson, M. (2004, March-May). Friendships are important across the years. Happenings: Dane County Association for Home and Community Education Cooperative Extension-University of Wisconsin, 9-10.

Brown, C., Hasson, H. Thyselius, V., & Almborg A. H. (2012). Post-stroke depression and functional independence: a conundrum. *Acta Neurologica Scandinavica, 126*(1), 45-51.

Brown, R. I. (1996). Partnerships and marriage in Down syndrome. *Down Syndrome Research and Practice, 4*(3), 96-99.

Brown, R. L. (2014). Psychological distress and the intersection of gender and physical disability: Considering gender and disability-related risk factors. *Sex Roles, 71*(3-4), 171-181.

Bruce, M. A., & Borg, B. (2002). *Psychosocial frames of reference: Core for occupation-based practice* (3rd ed.). Thorofare, NJ: SLACK Incorporated.

Bukov, A., Maas, I., & Lampert, T. (2002). Social participation in very old age: Cross-sectional and longitudinal findings from BASE. *Journals of Gerontology Series B: Psychological Sciences and Social Sciences, 57*, 510-517.

Cao, Y., Massaro, J. F., Krause, J. S., Chen, Y., & Devivo, M. (2014). Suicide mortality after spinal cord injury in the United States: Injury cohort analysis. *Archives of Physical Medicine and Rehabilitation, 95*(2), 230-235.

Cavallo, P. (1989). Teens, guilt and MS: Some guidelines to coping—multiple sclerosis. *Inside MS, 7*(3), 19.

Chen, R. K., Brodwin, M. G., Cardoso, E., & Chan, F. (2002). Attitudes toward people with disabilities in the social context of dating and marriage: A comparison of American, Taiwanese, and Singaporean college students' attitudes toward disability. *Journal of Rehabilitation, 68*, 5-11.

Christiansen, B. J. (1990). The costly retreat from marriage—married individuals deemed healthier. *Saturday Evening Post, 262*, 32-35.

Clemson, L., Cumming, R. G., & Roland, M. (1996). Case-control study of hazards in the home and risk of falls and hip fractures. *Age and Ageing, 25*, 97-101.

Conneeley, A. C. (2002). Social integration following traumatic brain injury and rehabilitation. *British Journal of Occupational Therapy, 65*(8), 356-362.

Consortium of Social Science Associations. (2000). National institutes of health conference highlights importance of social and behavioral influences on health. Retrieved at http://www.cossa.org/july102k.html on May 14, 2005.

Cook, B. G., & Semmel, M. I. (1999). Peer acceptance of included students with disabilities as a function of severity of disability and classroom composition. *Journal of Special Education, 33*, 50-61.

Coster, W. (1998). Occupation-centered assessment of children. *American Journal of Occupational Therapy, 52*(5), 337-344.

Crabtree, J. L. (1991). Ethical dilemmas and the older adult. In J. M. Kiernat (Ed.), *Occupational therapy and the older adult: A clinical manual* (pp. 338-350). Gaithersburg, MD: Aspen.

Dahl, M. R. (1988). Human sexuality. In H. L. Hopkins & H. D. Smith (Eds.), *Willard and Spackmans's occupational therapy* (7th ed.) (pp. 354-358). Philadelphia, PA: J.B. Lippincott.

Denton, P. L. (1987). *Psychiatric occupational therapy: A workbook of practical skills*. Boston: Little, Brown & Co.

DiFabio, R. P., & Seay, R. (1997). Use of the "fast evaluation of mobility, balance and fear" in elderly community dwellers: Validity and reliability. *Physical Therapy, 77*, 904-917.

Dunn, W., Brown, C., & McGuigan, A. (1994). The ecology of human performance: A framework for considering the effect of context. *American Journal of Occupational Therapy, 48*, 595-607.

Estes, J. P. (2002). Beyond basic ADLs- Sexual expression is an important but often overlooked activity of daily living. Retrieved at http://www.rehabpub. com/features/42002/7.asp on April 23, 2005.

Forouzan, A. S., Mahmoodi, A., Shushtari, Z. J., Salimi, Y., Sajjadi, H., & Mahmoodi, Z. (2013). Perceived social support among people with physical disability. *Iranian Red Crescent Medical Journal, 15*(8), 663-667.

Frith, J., & Davidson, J. (2013). Falls. *Reviews in Clinical Gerontology, 23*, 101-107.

Glass, C., & Soni, B. (1999). ABC of sexual health: Sexual problems of disabled patients. British Medical Journal, 318, 518-21.

Gordon, P. A, Tantillo, J. C., Feldman, D., & Perrone, K. (2004). Attitudes regarding interpersonal relationships with persons with mental illness and mental retardation. *Journal of Rehabilitation, 70*(1), 50-56.

Gourley, M. M. (2002). Sexuality and disability. In K. Krapp (Ed.), *Gale encyclopedia of nursing and allied health*. Vol. 4. (pp. 2203-2206). Farmington Hills, MI: Thomson Gale Group.

Greenfield, M. (2005). Talking about sexuality with individuals with intellectual disabilities: Notes from the field. Planned Parenthood Federation of America, Inc. *Educator's Update, 9*(5), 1-6.

Gutman, S. A. (2000). Using a computer as an environmental facilitator to promote post head injury role resumption: A case report. *Occupational Therapy in Mental Health, 15*, 71-90.

Gutman, S. A. (2012). The effect of an occupational therapy role-playing intervention on the social skills of adolescents with Asperger's syndrome: A pilot study. *Occupational Therapy in Mental Health, 28*(1), 20-35

Hanschu, B. (2004). Using a sensory approach for adults with developmental disabilities. In M. Ross & S. Bachner (Eds.), *Adults with developmental disabilities: Current approaches in occupational therapy.* Rockville, MD: AOTA.

Hendley, J. (1996). Sexual problems your doctor may not have mentioned to you—intimacy and multiple sclerosis. *Inside MS, 14*(1), 14-17.

Hopkins, H. L., & Tiffany, E. G. (1988). Occupational therapy—A problem solving process. In H. L. Hopkins & H. D. Smith (Eds.), *Willard and Spackmans's occupational therapy* (7th ed., pp. 102-111). Philadelphia, PA: J.B. Lippincott.

Hopps, S. L., Pepin, M, Arseneau, I., Frechette, M., & Begin, G. (2001). Disability related variables associated with loneliness among people with disabilities. *Journal of Rehabilitation, 67,* 42-49.

Iecovich, E., & Biderman, A.(2012). Attendance in adult day care centers and its relation to loneliness among frail older adults. *International Psychogeriatrics, 24*(3), 439-448.

Jongbloed, L., Stanton, S., & Fousek, B. (1993). Family adaptation to altered roles following a stroke. *Canadian Journal of Occupational Therapy, 60*(2), 70-77.

Kaye, H. S. (1997). *Disability watch: The status of people with disabilities in the United States.* Volcano, CA: Volcano Press.

Kindermann, T. A., & Sage, N. A. (1999). Peer networks, behavior contingencies, and children's engagement in the classroom. *Merrill-Palmer-Quarterly, 45,* 143-171.

Law, M., & Dunn, W. (1993a). Challenges and strategies in applying an occupational performance measurement approach. *American Journal of Occupational Therapy, 47*(5), 431-436.

Law, M., & Dunn, W. (1993b). Perspectives for understanding and changing the environment for children with disabilities. *Physical and Occupational Therapy in Pediatrics, 13,* 1-17.

Lee, A. J., Dubbs, S. L., Von Hippel, W., Brooks, R. C., & Zietsch, B. P. (2014). A multivariate approach to human mate preferences. *Evolution and Human Behavior, 35*(3), 193-203.

Lerner, P. (2005). Marriage for the developmentally disabled. *Spirit Magazine, 1*(4), 70-74.

Letts, L., Rigby, P., & Stewart, D. (2003). *Using environments to enable occupational performance.* Thorofare, NJ: SLACK Incorporated.

Livneh, H., & Antonak, R. (1997). *Psychosocial adaptation to chronic illness and disability.* New York, NY: Aspen.

Livneh, H., & Antonak, R.(2001) Psychosocial adaptation to chronic illness and disability: A conceptual framework. *Rehabilitation Counseling Bulletin, 44*(3), 151-160.

Livneh, H., & Antonak, R.(2005) Psychosocial adaptation to chronic illness and disability: A primer for counselors. *Journal of Counseling and Development, 83,* 12-20.

Lopata, H. Z. (1996). *Current widowhood: Myths and realities.* Thousand Oaks, CA: Sage Publications.

Lutfiyya, Z. M. (1997). The importance of friendships between people with and without mental retardation. In M. L. Hardman, *Persons with severe disabilities: educational and social issues* (pp. 101-129). New York, NY: Allyn and Bacon.

Mackey, R. A., Diemer, M. A., & O'Brien, B. A. (2000). Psychological intimacy in the lasting relationships of heterosexual and same-gender couples. *Sex Roles: A Journal of Research, 43*(3/4), 201-227.

Matheson, L. (2003). Defined by disability. *Off Our Backs, 3*(1/2), 44-45.

Moore, L. W., & Amburgey, L. B. (2000). Older adults and HIV. *Association of Perioperative Registered Nurses Journal, 71*(Elderly Care), 873.

Mosey, A. C. (1996). *Applied scientific inquiry in the health professions: A epistemological orientation* (2nd ed.). Bethesda, MD: AOTA.

Nazarko, L. (2012). Falls: Individual risk factors. *British Journal of Healthcare Assistants* 6(1), 8-12.

Ng, S. Y., Dinesh, S. K., Tay, S. H., & Lee, E. H. (2003). Decreased access to health care and social isolation among young adults with cerebral palsy after leaving school. *Journal of Orthopaedic Surgery, 11*(1), 80-89.

Nosek, M. A., & Hughes, R. B. (2001). Psychosocial aspects of sense of self in women with physical disabilities. *Journal of Rehabilitation, 67*(1), 20-25.

Nusbaum, M. R., & Hamilton, C. D. (2002). The proactive sexual health history. *American Family Physician, 66,* 1705-1712.

Oman, D., & Reed, D. (1998). Religion and mortality among the community dwelling elderly. *American Journal of Public Health, 88*(10), 1469-1475.

Patla, A. E. (2001). Mobility in complex environments: Implications for clinical assessment and rehabilitation. *Journal of Neurologic Physical Therapy, 25*(30), 82.

Paulson, C. P. (1991). Home care programs. In J. M. Kiernat (Ed.), *Occupational therapy and the older adult: A clinical manual* (pp. 220-239). Gaithersburg, MD: Aspen.

Pollard, N. (2000). *Allen cognitive levels: Differing social abilities.* Bethesda, MD: AOTA.

President & Fellows of Harvard College. (1997). Living well with multiple sclerosis. *Harvard Health Letter, 22*(10), 4-6.

Radomski, M. V. (2008) Assessing context: personal, social, and cultural. In Radomski, M. V., & Latham, C. A. T. (Eds.), *Occupational therapy for physical dysfunction* (6th ed. pp. 285-295) Philadelphia, PA: Lippincott, Williams & Wilkins.

Rathus, S. A. (1988). *Psychology* (4th ed.). Chicago, IL: Holt, Rinehart, and Winston.

Reitz, S. M., & Scaffa, M. E. (2001). Theoretical frameworks for community-based practice. In M. E. Scaffa, (Ed.), *Occupational therapy in community-based practice settings* (pp. 51-84). Philadelphia, PA: F.A. Davis.

Robinson, C. A., Bottorff, J. L., Pesut, B., Oliffe, J. L., & Tomlinson, J. (2014). The male fact of caregiving. *American Journal of Men's Health, 8*(5), 409-426.

Roelfs, D. J., Shor, E., Kalish, R., & Yoguv, T. (2011). The rising relative risk of mortality for singles: Meta-analysis and meta-regression. *American Journal of Epidemiology, 174*(4), 379-389.

Rogers, J. C., & Holm, M. B. (2003). Evaluation of areas of occupation activities and daily living and instrumental activities of daily living. In E. B. Crepeau, E. S. Cohn, & B. A. B. Schell (Eds.), *Willard and Spackman's occupational therapy* (10th ed., pp. 789-795). Philadelphia, PA: Lippincott, Williams & Wilkins.

Rolland, J. S. (1994a). *Families, illness and disability: An integrative treatment model.* New York, NY: Basic Books.

Rolland, J. S. (1994b). In sickness and in health: The impact of illness on couples' relationships. *Journal of Marital and Family Therapy, 20*(4), 327-347.

Rosenthal, M. S. (2014) Caregiver-centered care. *JAMA, 311*(10), 1015-1016.

Scheinholz, M. K. (2001). Community-based mental health services. In M. E. Scaffa (Ed.), *Occupational therapy in community-based practice settings* (pp. 291-317). Philadelphia, PA: F.A. Davis.

Sibley, M. H., Pelham, W. E., Mazur, A., Gnagy, E. M., Ross, J. M., & Kuriyan, A. B. (2012). The effect of video feedback on the social Behavior of an adolescent with ADHD. *Journal of Attention Disorders, 16*(7), 579-588.

Simmons Longitudinal Study (2004). *Parental Newsletter,* 1-6.

Syme, M. L. (2014). The evolving concept of older adult sexual behavior and its benefits. *Generations-Journal of the American Society on Aging, 38*(1), 35-41.

Szekais, B. (1991). Treatment approaches for patients with dementing illness. In J. M. Kiernat (Ed.), *Occupational therapy and the older adult: A clinical manual* (pp. 192-219). Gaithersburg, MD: Aspen.

Taylor, R. R. (2008). *The intentional relationship: Occupational therapy and use of self.* Philadelphia, PA: F.A. Davis.

Tickle-Degnen, L. (1995). Therapeutic rapport. In C. A. Trombly (Ed.), *Occupational therapy for physical dysfunction* (4th ed., pp. 277-285). Boston, MA: Williams & Wilkins.

Traustadottir, R. (1993). The gendered context of friendships. In A. N. Amado (Ed.), *Friendships and community connections between people with and without developmental disabilities* (pp. 109-127). Baltimore, MD: Paul H. Brookes Publishing.

United States Census Bureau. (2005). Facts for features: Older Americans month celebrated in May. Retrieved at http://www.census.gov/press-release/www/releases/archives/facts for features special editions/004210 .html on May 24, 2005.

Utz, R. L., Carr, D., Ness, R., & Wortman, C. B. (2002). The effect of widowhood on older adult social participation: An evaluation of activity, disengagement and continuity theories. *Gerontologist, 12*(4), 522-533.

Versluys, H. P. (1995a). Evaluation of emotional adjustment to disabilities. In C. A. Trombly (Ed.), *Occupational therapy for physical dysfunction* (4th ed.) (pp. 225-233). Boston, MA: Williams & Wilkins.

Versluys, H. P. (1995b). Facilitation psychosocial adjustment to disability. In C. A. Trombly (Ed.), *Occupational therapy for physical dysfunction* (4th ed.) (pp. 377-389). Boston, MA: Williams & Wilkins.

Warren, M. (1995). Providing low vision rehabilitation services with occupational therapy and ophthalmology: A program description. *American Journal of Occupational Therapy, 49*(9), 877-883.

Wells, K., Golding, J., & Burnham, M. (1988). Psychiatric disorder in a sample of the general population with and without chronic medical conditions. *American Journal of Psychiatry, 145*, 976-981.

Wilbarger, P. (1995). The sensory diet: Activity programs based on sensory processing theory. *American Journal of Occupational Therapy, Sensory Integration Special Interest Section Quarterly, 18*, 1-4.

Wooster, D. A., Gray, L., & Gifford, K. E. (2001). Specialized practice in home health. In M. E. Scaffa (Ed.), *Occupational therapy in community-based practice settings* (pp. 223-252). Philadelphia, PA: F.A. Davis.

World Health Organization. (2001). Mental health: New understanding, new hope. World Health Report, XVIII, 178.

Yeh, S. J., & Lo, S. K. (2004). Living alone, social support and feeling lonely among the elderly. *Social Behavior and Personality, 32*(2), 129-138.

10 Health and Wellness

Francine M. Seruya, PhD, OTR/L

Chapter Objectives

By the end of this chapter, the student will be able to do the following:

- Define health and wellness as it relates to the Occupational Therapy Practice Framework.
- Comprehend the "create, promote" (health promotion), "maintain," or "prevent" (disability prevention) approaches to occupational therapy intervention and the relationship to health and wellness.
- Describe the impact of contextual and environmental factors on wellness.
- Describe specific models/frames of reference as related to wellness.
- Identify teaching/learning principles related to wellness.
- Identify how an occupational therapy practitioner may be involved in wellness education.

Introduction

The Occupational Therapy Practice Framework (3rd ed., American Occupational Therapy Association [AOTA], 2014) is a document rich in detail and guidance for occupational therapy practice with individuals who have disabilities; however, the same document can guide practice in wellness and prevention. In the ideal world, disabilities would not exist and prevention techniques would keep all individuals well. Ours, however, is not an ideal world, so the work of occupational therapists must be to assist our clients in developing strategies to promote their maximum health and wellness. The Framework (AOTA, 2014) identifies the intricate relationship between health, well-being, and participation as paramount in facilitating an individuals' ability to participate in meaningful occupations.

Health and wellness are essential components for the ability to actively partake in the activities, roles, habits, routines, and rituals that contribute to an individual's identity and self-efficacy. Although frequently used interchangeably, health and wellness are separate and distinct concepts. The World Health Organization (WHO) defines health as "a state of complete physical, mental, and social well-being, and not merely the absence of disease or infirmity" (WHO, 2006, p. 1). Utilizing

Meriano C, Latella D.
Occupational Therapy Interventions: Function and Occupations, Second Edition (pp 479-492).

this definition of health directs practitioners to move away from the dominant, medical model presumption of health being exclusively dependent on the lack of illness or disease and expand their understanding of health to incorporate other dimensions of an individual, including their mental and social well-being. This definition also acknowledges that health is intricately related to the concept of wellness.

A positive state of health in the physical, mental, and social domains provides a foundation to achieve wellness. Wellness, as defined by the National Wellness Institute (NWI), "is a conscious, self-directed and evolving process of achieving full potential . . . an active process through which people become aware of, and make choices toward, a more successful existence" (NWI, n.d., para. 1). The concept of wellness also embodies the notion that wellness is related to a satisfactory quality of life. Healthy People 2020 (United States Department of Health and Human Services, 2010) identifies health-related quality of life as being an interconnected and measurable component of well-being. Here, well-being is understood to be linked to concepts such as life fulfillment and satisfaction as a direct corollary of health status. Occupational therapy has long embraced the notion that participation in occupation is inexorably related to an individuals' state of health and wellness (World Federation of Occupational Therapists, 2010).

Domain of Occupational Therapy as Related to Health and Wellness

Occupation

Occupation as outlined in the Framework includes activities of daily living (ADL), instrumental activities of daily living (IADL), rest and sleep, education, work, play, leisure, and social participation (AOTA, 2014). Optimal health and wellness allow for engagement and participation in these occupations. Although, each area of occupation is individualized, various general themes can be identified. For example, a well adult is typically independent in ADL, and while IADL levels may vary due to the individual's context, generally well adults manage independently. An individual who has sufficient sleep is more likely to fully participate in daily tasks. Education and/or work depend on the adult's developmental stage, although typically a well adult has managed these occupations at least most of his or her life. Lastly, engagement in play, leisure, and social participation are also important components to life balance and integral aspects of a being a well adult.

Client Factors, Performance Skills, and Performance Patterns

If individual client factors, performance skills and performance patterns are maximized, then wellness in the areas of occupation is likely to be supported. Being well does not require all factors, skills, and patterns to be at optimal levels but implies that the individual has developed adaptations that support health. The use of the establish, restore (remediation, restoration), and modify (compensation, adaptation) intervention approaches to address problems in the areas of client factors and performance skills as a result of injury or illness are typical in traditional, rehabilitation-type models of occupational therapy intervention. Using these approaches, the occupational therapist seeks to create or restore skills or provide assistance to the client in developing new approaches to complete activities. In a wellness model, the practitioner's intervention approach is geared toward using the create, promote (health promotion), maintain, or prevent (disability prevention) model. Here the intention is to utilize the individual's current skills to promote healthy living rather than developing or remediating underlying body or skill components. For example, wellness activities utilizing a create intervention approach could consist of developing a class to be provided in a local senior center to teach simple home modifications for older adults. Likewise, using a prevention approach, the occupational therapist might work with a client to develop a morning stretching routine to prevent stiffness to allow for prolonged independence in the completion of morning ADLs. Client factors, performance skills, and performance patterns are highly individualized, and it is the practitioner's role to help identify the occupations and activities that the client finds meaningful and relevant. This will allow the practitioner to facilitate the client's ability to participate in those occupations to the extent possible based on the individual's current physical and social emotional status in order to promote overall health and wellness.

Contexts and Environments

Health and wellness are influenced and must be understood through the individual's personal context and environment. Context and environment are complicated by the different boundaries of the individual or society. For example, cultural traditions or values will be different from person to person. What may be an appropriate mealtime ritual in one culture may not be acceptable in another. What is considered appropriate face-to-face communication may be considered insulting virtually. Wellness of any given individual cannot be understood until all areas of context and environment are assessed. The occupational therapist must be sure to ascertain as part of the occupational therapy profile the current context and environment in which the client will need to be able to perform his or her occupations. The context must be analyzed to determine whether there are any barriers or existing supports that will hinder or facilitate participation. Understanding the contextual and environmental components will be essential in implementing successful wellness interventions. The occupational therapist must account for the feasibility to utilize wellness strategies in the client's current context. For example, the occupational therapist may have to address the cultural and social context when working with a client to change mealtime rituals to account for new medication regimes due to conflict with certain religious practices.

Theoretical Paradigms Associated With Health and Wellness

In determining how to address health and wellness, the occupational therapy practitioner has to consider a clients' occupational profile as well as stated goals. Critical analysis of the consumers' needs will guide the practitioner to choose an appropriate theoretical model to guide the intervention. The use of theoretical models to guide practice provides a sound foundation to base interventions and allows the practitioner to select appropriate assessment and outcome measures. As engagement in occupation is critical in promoting health and wellness, occupation-based theoretical models are an appropriate source of guidance for building assessment and intervention plans. Within occupational therapy there are several occupation-based models that can be utilized. In addition to occupational therapy–specific models, multidisciplinary models that are appropriate to health and wellness should also be considered. Finally the mind-body connection should be considered when addressing health and wellness as a part of intervention.

Occupational Therapy Models

The Model of Human Occupation

The model of human occupation (MOHO) (Kielhofner, 1995, 2002; Kielhofner & Burke, 1980) is an occupation-based model that was developed and primarily constructed on the theories of occupational behavior articulated by Mary Reilly and general systems theory posited by von Bertalannfy. This model theorizes that people are occupational beings by nature and they are driven to participate in meaningful activities. Keilhofner conceptualized the individual as an "open system" in which change and adaption are made based on feedback from the social and environmental contexts in which they exist. MOHO places great emphasis on the interaction between the person, task, and environment because they are all part of a dynamic, interconnected system in which impact on one component will have an effect on the others. Occupational function is exemplified by the person's ability to select and complete preferred occupations to allow for a basic quality of life. The practitioner's role when implementing this model would be one of support and assistance in facilitating a client's ability to participate in selected occupations.

Person-Environment-Occupation-Performance

Another occupation-based model that addresses health and wellness is the person-environment-occupation-performance (PEOP) model (Christiansen & Baum, 1991; Christiansen, Baum, & Bass, 2015). Like MOHO, PEOP views the interaction between the person, environment, and occupation as central to the therapeutic process. Christiansen et al. (2015) suggest that this model is applicable to individuals, organizations, communities, and larger populations. The model is specifically used in health promotion programs. As a part of its theoretical base, PEOP theorizes that individuals are driven to explore and control their environments to achieve a level of mastery that in turn provides the basis for self-efficacy and well-being (Christiansen et al., 2015). Through the interaction with their environment, individuals are able to explore and find personally relevant activities. The ability to participate in occupational activities that are personally meaningful leads to the development of life roles. Function from the perspective of this model is exemplified by an individual's ability to satisfy personal and societal expectations. PEOP acknowledges that the ability to fulfill occupations is an essential component to a state of personal health and wellness.

Other models that embrace the interconnectedness of the person, environment, and occupation in facilitating personal engagement include the Canadian model of occupational performance (CAOT, 1997), occupational adaptation (Schkade & Schultz, 1992), and the ecology of human performance (Dunn, Brown, & McGuigan, 1994). All of these models share the perspective that an individual is an occupational being by nature and by participating in those activities that are deemed meaningful to the individual to facilitate a positive quality of life, health, and well-being.

Multidisciplinary Models

The topic of health is of concern to many disciplines in addition to occupational therapy and has been the focus of theory development and research, particularly in the last 50 years. Several models for understanding health and wellness are shared by health care professionals across many disciplines and are briefly described here.

Biopsychosocial Model

This model presents a psychological and medical model of understanding wellness. The body's physical systems, such as nervous, endocrine, digestive, cardiovascular, and immune, work in harmony to maintain wellness. Stresses from external forces impact the balance of these systems and cause sickness. Stress can be from numerous sources. Biological stress might be pollution. Psychological stress might be work performance. Interpersonal stress might include relationship issues. Physiological stress includes addictions. Any combination of stresses may cause sickness depending on the human's ability to cope (Sarafino, 2002; Taylor, 1999).

Health Behavior Theories

Bandura's work on self-efficacy (1997) and Becker's examination of locus of control (1974) help explain how individuals stay well. Locus of control shows that individuals approach healthy behaviors whether or not they believe there is control over the situation. Individuals with an internal locus of control believe their actions contribute to their health. Individuals with an external locus of control believe health is caused by fate or things outside of their control. Health care providers must assess the individual's locus of control before providing advice. Pender (1982) adds demographic, biological, social, and environmental factors to locus of control to explain how individuals receive cues from outside factors to influence their locus of control.

Health Belief Model

The health belief model examines why individuals fail to be healthy. Key to this model is the perception of the risk of unhealthy behaviors. Susceptibility, severity, benefits of behaviors, and costs/barriers are weighed by each individual before making changes in unhealthy behaviors (Rotter, 1966). An individual may make nonscientific assessments of the risks, such as "my grandmother ate a high-fat diet and never had a stroke." An individual's behavior has little to do with the message being sent by the health care worker.

Transtheoretical Model

This model examines healthy behaviors as a progression through stages (Prochaska & DiClemente, 1982). Precontemplation, contemplation, preparation, action, and maintenance map the changes in health behaviors. This model states that individuals do not necessarily go through these stages in order and often repeat stages or fail to move out of a stage toward health. Health care practitioners should consider the individual's current stage when providing guidance.

Mind-Body Connection to Health and Wellness

Both those who reimburse as well as consumers are demanding that services be evidence-based. In addition, consumers want choices in health care, including alternative intervention methods that have been shown to be effective. The occupational therapist must be well-read in the literature and able to translate meaningful options to the consumer. Theories that address the mind-body connection and awareness of the impact of social connectedness and spirituality should be considered when assessing and providing intervention in the areas of health and wellness (Table 10-1).

There is a great variety of opinion regarding the effect of the mind on the body's health and wellness. Some research has demonstrated that as high as 90% of all diseases have an emotional root (Hafen, Karren, Frandsen, & Smith, 1996). Emotions have been demonstrated to be triggers to physical illness such as heart disease, digestive problems, and accidents. The immune system in human beings is known to have chemical relationships with emotions. Physiological changes at the individual's cellular level may produce long-term effects causing disease or disability. While emotional issues such as stress, anger, and depression may play important roles in triggering an illness or accident, there are also emotional factors that may support wellness (WHO, 2005). Social supports and spirituality are examples of components thought to impact emotional state in a positive manner, as described below.

Social Supports

Long-term research has shown that good health and long life are tied to the amount of social support an individual enjoys (Hafen et al., 1996). The theory presented to explain this phenomenon is that social support (1) enhances positive feelings and self-esteem, (2) encourages stability and mastery of the environment, and (3) acts as a buffer against stress, therefore protecting the individual from stress-induced disease and accidents (Sheldon, Cohen, & Syme, 1985). This social support provides appraisal support (helping the individual assess stressful events), tangible support (such as financial resources), informational support (such as advice), and emotional support (including

Table 10-1 Emotions and Their Relation to Illness	
Accidents	Inattention due to emotional distractions makes us prone to accidents. An individual worried about falls is likely to become inactive and therefore at a great risk for falls.
Allergies and asthma	Stress causes allergy antibodies to increase and therefore trigger greater immune responses to the allergen. A child worried about his skill on the baseball team may internalize the stress and increase the chance to develop an asthma attack.
Arthritis	Several research studies have found a connection between emotional stress and the development of rheumatoid arthritis. Timing of emotional events such as divorce may indicate a relationship to the outbreak of the disease.
Back pain	Heavy lifting may not be the major factor in back pain. Back muscles may tense to emotional issues and therefore be at risk for injury.
Cancer	Cancer cells are thought to be in all individuals, but our immune system effectively controls them. Stressors such as emotions or other causes may reduce the effectiveness of the immune system to fight the cancer cells, leading to the need for medical assistance.
Diabetes	Individuals with depression seem to be more at risk of developing diabetes than those without; however, other issues may be trigger the depression such as environmental situations.
Heart disease and hypertension	Hypertension is a known factor in heart disease. Adrenaline released during anger speeds the heart and constricts the blood vessels, resulting in hypertension. Chronic anger may further the progress of heart disease.
Insomnia	Every individual has experienced a sleepless night due to rehashing of emotional thoughts at bedtime. Chronic insomnia interferes with the body's ability to retool.
Irritable bowel and stomach issues	An overreaction to environmental cues may trigger digestion problems for those who are hyper-alert.
Adapted from Hafen, B. Q., Karren, K. J. Frandsen, K. J., & Smith, N. L. (1996). *Mind/body health: The effects of attitudes, emotions, and relationships.* Boston, MA: Allyn and Bacon.	

reassurance) (Taylor, 1999). Coping skills in individuals with solid social support systems appear stronger. A social support system does not mean only a traditional family system but may include any individual support such as from a friend or service circle.

Spirituality and Health

Spirituality is often confused with religion, although it should be seen as separate (Seigel, 1993; Smith, 1993). For many individuals, religion supports their spirituality, but for many others religion is not a focus of their spirituality. It is important that the occupational therapy practitioner accurately assess the role of spirituality in the client's health.

Spirituality is more difficult to define than quantitative signs such as range of motion or assessment scores. Experts in medicine and spirituality (Seigel, 1993; Smith, 1993) define spiritual health as including the concepts of a state of well-being; self-forgiveness; self-love and freedom; peace with oneself; a sense of connectedness and wholeness; a feeling of meaning, purpose, and challenge; and positive expectations and hope.

Spirituality, as a client factor (AOTA, 2014), is often revitalized when a crisis becomes a growth experience. Often individuals report that their perspective on life changes dramatically when faced with a personal or family health crisis. Spiritual experiences are highly individualized and client-centered. Some clients report the power of prayer, while others prefer relaxation exercises. Some clients find meaning by attending formal church meetings, while others enjoy volunteer work. Myths, shrines, customs, and healers all represent different mediums that may support an individual's connectedness to their spirituality. Spirituality is a personal faith or hope that may or may not be connected to a formal religion.

Practice Guidelines That Support Wellness

In addition to guidance from theoretical models and scholarly evidence, practitioners are also guided by the mandates and positions of the national association. The American Occupational Therapy Association (AOTA) has identified health and wellness as a practice area for occupational therapy practitioners. Several documents have been generated to guide the practitioner in implementing health and wellness models. AOTA has indicated that intervention in chronic care management is an essential component to occupational therapy intervention (AOTA, n.d.). Chronic diseases such as diabetes, heart disease, arthritis, and obesity expend the largest amount of resources from the U.S. health care system (Centers for Disease Control, n.d.). Interventions targeted at managing chronic conditions as well as developing healthy lifestyle changes can potentially decrease health care costs and improve overall quality of life.

AOTA has put forth position statements regarding the role of occupational therapy in the management of obesity (2013a), the use of environment to support engagement in health (2009), and the promotion of health and well-being (2013b). These documents all share the common thread that occupational therapy practitioners possess the knowledge and skills to facilitate the development of new, healthy lifestyles to allow for engagement in occupations that give meaning and purpose to an individual's life. Specific interventions indicated include the development of fall prevention programs for seniors, education and training regarding healthy eating and meal preparation for weight management, and the establishment of support groups for caregivers of individuals who have experienced significant illness or injury.

Just as no single occupational therapy theory can guide all occupational therapy practice, no one health theory can answer all health and wellness concerns. Theory does, however, guide our practice, providing direction and focus to the occupational therapy practitioner in developing effective intervention plans. Theory, in combination with the current scholarship from peer-reviewed research will provide the most effective intervention approach specific to each client (Table 10-2).

Intervention in Wellness

Intervention Approaches

Working toward a state of health and wellness, occupational therapy practitioners are able to utilize intervention models outlined in the Framework (AOTA, 2014) to guide service delivery. Specifically the "create, promote" approach is geared toward health promotion because it identifies the target population for this intervention to be those free of illness or disability. The "maintain"

Table 10-2

Evidence for Wellness Programs

Wellness Program	Learning Activities	Evidence
Depression	Moderate exercise and mood	Dimeo et al., 2001; Lawlor & Hopker, 2001; Lovejoy & Lane, 2000; Netz & Lidor, 2003; Russell et al., 2003; Turnbull & Wolfson, 2002
	Social support	Oman & Oman, 2003
	Cognitive reframing	Hewston et al., 2005; McHugh & Wierzbicki, 1998; McKay & Fanning, 2000; Odone, 1996; Totterdell, 1999
Eating healthy	Mood and food	Cools et al., 1992; Guinn, 1991; Heatherton et al., 1992; Ward & Mann, 2000
	Societal issues	Schotte et al., 1990
	Stress	Cartwright et al., 2003; Denisoff & Endler, 2000; Greeno & Wing, 1994; Ng & Jeffery, 2003
Fitness	Attitude	Blamey & Mutrie, 2004; Chatzisarantis et al., 2005; Dixon, Mauzey, & Hall, 2003; Mack & Shaddox, 2004
	Health	Larson & Zaichowsky, 1995; McKay et al., 2003; Thomas, Baker, & Davies, 2003
	Social support	Mathias et al., 1997; Phillips, 2005
	Cognitive reframing	Prestwich, Lawton, & Conner, 2003
Pain reduction	Back pain prevention	American Academy of Pediatrics et al., 2004; Wilson, 1998; Wortman, 2003
	Mind body connection	Atli & Loeser, 2004; McCaffrey, Frock, & Garguilo, 2003
	Massage or physical activity	Shealy, 2005; Teitelbaum, 2005
Sleep preparation	Sleep hygiene	Brown, Buboltz, & Soper, 2002; Sadeh, Keinan, & Daon, 2004
	Restorative benefits	Blissitt, 2001; Bower, 2004; Heuer & Klien, 2003; Trockel, Barnes, & Egget, 2000; Ward, 2004;
Smoking cessation	Relaxation exercises	Kassel & Shiffman, 1997
	Stress	Britt et al., 2001; Juliano & Brandon, 2002; Kassel, 2000; Parrott, 2000; Piasecki & Baker, 2000; Shiffman & Waters, 2004; Todd, 2004
	Cognitive reframing	Chassin et al., 2002; Ong & Walsh, 2001
	Weight gain	Ludman et al., 2002

(continued)

Table 10-2 (continued)

Evidence for Wellness Programs

Wellness Program	Learning Activities	Evidence
Stress reduction	Physical health	Edwards et al., 2001; Fontana & McLaughlin, 1998; Leitner & Resch, 2005
	Mental health	Dantz et al., 2003; Fletcher & Fletcher, 2005; Lumley & Provenzano, 2003
	Mind-body connection	Deckro et al., 2002
	Hardiness and motivation	Judkins, 2004; LePine, LePine, & Jackson, 2004; Peterson & Wilson, 2004
	Leisure	Misra & McKean, 2000
	Social support	Misra, Crist, & Burant, 2003

approach focuses on an individuals' ability to retain skills and as a result continue to participate in meaningful occupations to allow for satisfactory quality of life. Finally, the "prevent" (disability prevention) approach also provides intervention strategies targeted at averting a decrease in occupational performance (AOTA, 2014, p. S33). These intervention approaches direct occupational therapy practitioners to understand how the physical, emotional, and social contexts interact to impact on a clients' state of health and well-being.

The intervention approaches also acknowledge that deficits in physical, emotional or social domains can have a significant impact on an individuals' ability to participate in those occupations they find most meaningful and that provide them with a sense of well-being. Engagement in meaningful occupation is a cornerstone of the underlying philosophy of occupational therapy (Meyer, 1977). Facilitating individuals' ability to actively participate in those activities that allow them to live lifestyles that support their personal and social contexts leads to a positive state of health and wellness (Wilcock, 2006). Providing intervention in wellness is unique in that it often occurs in conjunction with more traditional rehabilitation programs. For example, the occupational therapy practitioner may as part of the intervention discuss with a client how he or she is able to manage typical habits and routines in light of recent injury. Then intervention will focus on working with the client to determine how to incorporate more healthy lifestyle choices to manage temporary or chronic conditions. Regardless of the intervention model utilized to provide treatment, interventions related to wellness typically incorporate a teaching paradigm.

Intervention Implementation

The Framework (AOTA, 2014) identifies "education and training" as a type of occupational therapy intervention. The occupational therapy practitioner needs to be cognizant that teaching adult learners differs from traditional pedagogical approaches. Numerous books have been written about educational theories (Sladyk, 2005). Pedagogy is the educational foundation of schooling through high school, based on pediatric theories. This section will look at theories specific to adults, commonly called *andragogy*.

Adults learn differently from children. Sometimes teachers or health care practitioners who use pedagogical techniques with adults actually insult the adult learner. Although some adults may prefer to learn the way they did in primary or secondary school, others appreciate different approaches that take into consideration the life experiences they have had. The key to teaching adults is flexibility and continual assessment of meeting their learning needs (Sheckley, 1984).

Adult learners are a widely diverse group who encompass many different styles, goals, and experiences (Cross, 1988). Understanding some of the major characteristics of this group can lead to more effective application of knowledge and transfer of learning to life situations. Adults are independent thinkers with a variety of thoughts and experiences that accompany them when embarking on new learning. Addressing this diversity of experience and needs will help the educator or therapist succeed.

Adults come to each learning experience with an integration of all prior learning experience (Kolb, 1984). For example, if a teenager had negative experiences in high school physical education class, as an adult he or she is likely to come to a wellness program based on physical exercise with negative feelings. If a client has had positive experiences all during the rehabilitation program, he or she is likely to be open to new experiences in an outpatient clinic. The role of an adult's life experience in forming new learning cannot be minimized. Formal and informal experiences (Bandura, 1978) are included in this integration of experiences; therefore, academic success in the past may predict openness to wellness ideas in the future. As the adult gets older, work experiences are added to this integration.

Brookfield (1990) noted that adults learn best in situations of mutual respect. Fostering the growth of the learner along a path to an ideal wellness goal is the job of the occupational therapy practitioner. Brookfield advocates that teachers help adult learners do the following: (1) identify and challenge assumptions and context, (2) imagine and explore alternatives, and (3) view knowledge with reflective skepticism. Simply providing the learner with information does not foster the transfer of knowledge (Brookfield, 1990).

Chaffee (1998) states that the key to successful adult thinking is in the following eight steps: (1) think critically, (2) live creatively, (3) choose freely, (4) solve problems effectively, (5) communicate effectively, (6) analyze complex issues, (7) develop enlightened values, and (8) think through relationships. He encourages adults to transform themselves though thinking and to create a life philosophy to follow. This requires a strong commitment to self-analysis, which many adults cannot call upon because of other factors. Wellness or lack of wellness is illustrated in this model when other factors interfere with the adult's ability to live freely.

Adult behavior is an interaction of person and environment (Bandura, 1978). Although most individuals believe the learner's responsibility is to learn, learners will act on their learning within the structure of their environment. As an example, in some cultures, women are not expected to be learners. Teaching an individual from this environment may be difficult but can be effective if the wellness educator considers the environment when developing interventions. When implementing educational programs with this type of population, the occupational therapist should consider working within the accepted cultural norms and, for example, might include the older women of the community as "teachers" in implementing wellness education for new mothers. Consideration of the context of the individual or group is essential in developing successful health and wellness initiatives.

In general, when addressing the unique learning needs of adults, several themes emerge. Adults bring with them an educational history that may or may not be positive. Adults learn through their experiences (experiential learning). Considering the life experiences of the adult learner in relation to the new information being learned is essential in developing new habits and routines to assist in healthier lifestyles. Personal context is important to developing successful interventions. Finally, mutual respect between the practitioner and the individual or group plays an important role in adult learning. All of these factors can influence the transfer of training to life situations. The goal of the wellness educator is to manage these factors in a way that is positive to the adult learner (Sladyk, 2005).

Utilizing this implementation approach in conjunction with guiding theoretical principles regarding health and wellness will allow the practitioner to develop interventions that are

Table 10-3

Sample Wellness Activities

Activities to Promote Sleep	
ADLs	Limit bed to sleeping or sexual activity. Do not nap, Take a warm bath 1 hour before bed. Avoid any liquid drink before bed, especially liquor or caffeine.
IADLs	Set up the bedroom to reduce distractions. If awake for more than a half hour, get up and do some other quiet activity. Get some bright light during the afternoon. Make lists of things to be accomplished tomorrow well before bedtime.
Education	Learn about other medical problems affecting sleep, such as back pain. Check medications to make sure there are no interactions affecting sleep. Consult a medical doctor or dentist for medical issues affecting sleep.
Work	Keep to a regular schedule. Learn assertiveness techniques to manage office stress. When racing thoughts occupy the mind at night, quietly tell them to stop by repeating the word *stop*. Replace racing thoughts with a peaceful mantra.
Play/leisure	Exercise regularly but never in the evening. Play, with fun as the goal each day. Do gentle, relaxing back stretches before bed.
Social participation	Find quiet time before bed to clear the mind. Socialize with positive individuals who bring joy, not stress.

individualized and meaningful. Developing and supporting the implementation of lifestyle changes that improve the overall health and wellness of the clients aligns well with the overarching themes of the profession. Facilitating the ability to engage in personally relevant occupations allows individuals to maintain health and wellness despite lingering challenges or chronic conditions.

Examples of Wellness Programs

There are many potential wellness programs that could be led by occupational therapy practitioners. Typically, a wellness program is developed out of an urgent need or a new understanding of a need not recognized before. Examples of potential wellness programs that can be developed for members of the community either as part of a formal health care system or in alternative delivery systems include adult education in accident prevention and home safety, Americans with Disabilities Act consulting, assistive living support, community redesign, diabetes self-management, pain self-management, and sleep readiness (Table 10-3).

Conclusion

The ability to participate in occupations and activities that are personally meaningful is key to an individual's health and wellness. The concepts of health and wellness can no longer be understood from a disability model but need to be explored with clients from one of prevention and lifestyle reconfiguration. Occupational therapy practitioners are well-suited to assess an individual's personal context and existing habits and routines and provide interventions to support the incorporation of new or adapted means to allow for people to participate in occupations.

Occupational models and other theories regarding health and wellness assist the occupational therapy practitioner in understanding and designing interventions that account for the interaction between the person, environment, and the desired occupational performance. AOTA (2010, 2013b) has identified health and wellness as an area practitioners need to consider when providing services. The management of chronic diseases such as diabetes, arthritis, and heart conditions has been recognized as a prime area for occupational therapy intervention. In addition to the management of chronic disease, prevention and lifestyle redesign has also been acknowledged as an area that is well-suited to the philosophical underpinnings of occupational therapy.

Utilizing intervention approaches that seek to assist individuals in creating new habits, rituals and routines; maintaining current levels and abilities to allow for continued participation in meaningful occupations; or preventing new or further illness or injury that would preclude them from participating in those tasks and occupations that support wellness are all well within the scope of occupational therapy practice. By using implementation approaches that acknowledge an adult's unique learning style and incorporating those concepts along with the distinct values of the individual, practitioners can facilitate change to allow for healthier lifestyles. In addition to working with individuals, occupational therapy practitioners can implement wellness programs in their facilities or within community settings that likewise support the ability to participate in those activities that promote overall health and wellness in the community at large. As occupational therapy continues to evolve, practitioners have wonderful opportunities to effect change in the health of our citizens.

Case Study 1: Julie

Julie is an occupational therapist employed by the mental health services department of a community hospital. Her department serves clients in both inpatient and outpatient programs with referrals to a variety of community support systems. Her department allows great flexibility in choosing frames of reference for her clients, and the hospital respects the services provided by occupational therapy.

After the birth of Julie's first child, she became aware that the mental health department did little to support new mothers. Julie believed occupational therapy could provide assistance with skill building for new moms, especially those dealing with postpartum depression. Julie began discussing the topic with peers and investigating needs. She connected with the maternal health department of the hospital and found they were eager to network with the staff in mental health. Julie explained occupational therapy services to the staff in maternal health and was encouraged to develop a program for new mothers with a focus on mental health. Julie developed a program that would see new mothers individually and help them network with friends and family for support as they adjusted to a new occupation.

Case Study 2

A small group of occupational therapy level II fieldwork students were completing their mental health fieldwork in a community clubhouse model for individuals with chronic and persistent mental health disorders. The students, under the supervision of an occupational therapist, were to develop a wellness program of their choice based on a needs assessment completed with clubhouse members and staff. The staff were very concerned with the smoking of members. Members were required to smoke outside and often were so busy smoking that they missed meetings or group activities. The students remembered from pathology class that individuals with schizophrenia had the highest smoking rate of all disabilities. The members of the clubhouse thought smoking was an issue. The students developed a smoking cessation group that met daily. The frames of reference selected were cognitive-behavioral with a health promotion influence. Activities included journaling, using the Internet for support information, psycho-educational tips for quitting, and peer support when members experienced the urge to smoke. On the first day, several members attended. They made a list of coping strategies based on experience and information from the American Cancer Society, including delaying a cigarette for as long as possible, making a plan, finding support, remembering the benefits of quitting, and performing relaxation exercises. Despite having the students as personal coaches, none of the members were able to reduce their smoking. The students met with the members and occupational therapy to evaluate the program. The occupational therapist reminded the students about the timing in Prochaska and DiClemente's health model (1982). Precontemplation, contemplation, preparation, action, and maintenance map the changes in health behaviors, although the staff and students jumped right to action and the members were not ready for change.

References

American Occupational Therapy Association. (2010). Occupational therapy's perspective on the use of environments and contexts to support health and participation in occupations. *American Journal of Occupational Therapy, 64* (Suppl.6), S57-S69.

American Occupational Therapy Association. (2013a). Obesity and occupational therapy. *American Journal of Occupational Therapy, 67* (Suppl.6), S39-S46.

American Occupational Therapy Association. (2013b). Occupational therapy for the promotion of health and well-being. *American Journal of Occupational Therapy, 67* (Suppl.6), S47-S59.

American Occupational Therapy Association. (2014). Occupational therapy practice framework: Domain and process (3rd ed.). *American Journal of Occupational Therapy, 68* (Suppl.1), S1-S48.

American Occupational Therapy Association. (n.d.a.). *The role of occupational therapy in chronic disease management* [Fact Sheet]. Bethesda, MD: Author. Retrieved at http://www.aota.org/-/media/Corporate/Files/AboutOT/Professionals/WhatIsOT/HW/Facts/FactSheet_ChronicDiseaseManagement.pdf.

American Occupational Therapy Association. (n.d.b.). *Occupational therapy's role in health promotion* [Fact Sheet]. Bethesda, MD: Author. Retrieved at http://www.aota.org/-/media/Corporate/Files/AboutOT/Professionals/WhatIsOT/MH/Facts/FactSheet_HealthPromotion.pdf.

Canadian Association of Occupational Therapists. (1997). *Enabling occupation: An occupational therapy perspective.* Ottawa, ON: CAOT Publications.

Center for Disease Control. (n.d.) Retrieved at http://www.cdc.gov/chronicdisease/overview/index.htm.

Christiansen, C., & Baum, C. M. (1991). *Occupational therapy: Overcoming human performance deficits.* Thorofare, NJ: SLACK Incorporated.

Christiansen, C., Baum, C. M., & Bass, J. (2015). *Occupational therapy: Enabling function and well-being* (4th ed.). Thorofare, NJ: SLACK Incorporated.

Dunn, W., Brown, C., & McGuigan, A. (1994). The ecology of human performance: A framework for considering the effect of context. *American Journal of Occupational Therapy, 48*, 595-607.

Kielhofner, G. (1995). *A model of human occupation: Theory and application* (2nd ed.). Baltimore, MD: Williams & Wilkins.

Kielhofner, G. (2002). *A model of human occupation: Theory and application* (3rd ed.). Baltimore, MD: Williams & Wilkins.

Kielhofner, G., & Burke, J. (1980). A model of human occupation, Part 1, Conceptual framework and content. *American Journal of Occupational Therapy, 34*, 572-581.

Meyer, A. (1977). The philosophy of occupational therapy, *American Journal of Occupational Therapy, 31*, 639-642. (Original work published in 1922)

National Wellness Institute. (n.d.). Retrieved at http://www.nationalwellness.org/?page=Six_Dimensions.

Schkade, J. K., & Schultz, S. (1992). Occupational adaptation: Toward a holistic approach to contemporary practice (Part 1). *American Journal of Occupational Therapy, 46*, 829-837.

United States Department of Health and Human Services. (2010). *Healthy People 2020, Foundation Health Measure Report, Health-Related Quality of Life and Well-Being.* Retrieved at http://www.healthypeople.gov/2020/about/HRQoLWBFullReport.pdf.

Wilcock, A. (2006). *An occupational perspective of health* (2nd ed.). Thorofare, NJ: SLACK Incorporated.

World Federation of Occupational Therapists. (2010). *Statement on Occupational Therapy.* Retrieved at http://www.wfot.org/Portals/0/PDF/STATEMENT%20ON%20OCCUPATIONAL%20THERAPY%20300811.pdf.

World Health Organization. (2006). *Constitution of the World Health Organization* (45th ed.). Retrieved at http://www.who.int/governance/eb/who_constitution_en.pdf?ua=1.

Appendix A
Resources

Resources have been supplied in chapters throughout the text. There is some overlap here because some suppliers provide equipment for various areas of intervention. This appendix is a general resource and is not intended to be all-inclusive but rather an introductory tool to expose the reader to resources for additional information. The authors and publisher do not specifically endorse any of these products; the list is provided for educational purposes only.

Aquatic Rehabilitation

Aquatic Resources Network

Phone: 715-248-7258

Fax: 715-248-3065

Website: http://www.aquaticnet.com

Website provides valuable and comprehensive resources including training opportunities, educational products, membership, and a provider/facility directory.

Recent textbooks as general resources to supplement continuing education in the area of aquatics include the following:

Comprehensive Aquatic Rehabilitation (3rd ed.) (2011) by Bruce E. Becker and Andrew J. Cole

The Use of Aquatics in Orthopedics and Sports Medicine Rehabilitation and Physical Conditioning (2013) by Kevin E. Wilk and David Joyner

Assistive Technology and Education-Related Resources

About Learning contains products and supports related to education of those with disabilities: 441 West Bonner Road; Wauconda, IL 60084; 800-822-4628; www.aboutlearning.com.

ABLEDATA is a project that maintains a database of information about more than 27,000 products for people with disabilities: 8630 Fenton Street, Suite 930; Silver Spring, MD 20910; 800-227-0216; www.abledata.com.

Meriano C, Latella D.
Occupational Therapy Interventions: Function and Occupations, Second Edition (pp 493-500).

Alliance for Technology Access is a national organization dedicated to providing access to technology for people with disabilities: www.ataccess.org.

Assistive Technology Access Partnership (ATAP) is a Rhode Island website with a list of statewide organizations and agencies, each with a targeted assistive technology focus, who work together to provide information and improve access to assistive technology for individuals with disabilities: www.atap.ri.gov.

Association for Higher Education and Disability (AHEAD) contains links regarding assistive technology as well as many other adult student options: www.ahead.org.

ATIA, the Assistive Technology Industry Association, is a not-for-profit membership organization for manufacturers, sellers, or providers of technology-based assistive devices and/or services: http://www.atia.org/i4a/pages/index.cfm?pageid=1.

CAST Universal Design for Learning is an organization committed to the research and development of innovative, technology-based educational resources and strategies: www.cast.org.

Equal Access to Software and Information is a project of the Teaching, Learning, and Technology (TLT) Group that serves as a resource to the education community by providing information and guidance on access to information technologies for individuals with disabilities. EASI disseminates information on developments and advancements within the adaptive computer technology field to colleges, universities, K-12 schools, libraries, and the workplace: http://easi.cc.

Job Accommodation Network is an international information network and consulting resource that provides information about employment issues, the Americans with Disabilities Act (ADA), and possible employment-related accommodations to employers, rehabilitation professionals, and persons with disabilities. Callers should be prepared to explain their specific problem and job circumstances. Sponsored by the President's Committee on Employment of People with Disabilities, the Network is operated by West Virginia University's Rehabilitation Research and Training Center. Brochures and printed materials are available at no cost: West Virginia University; 918 Chestnut Ridge Road, P.O. Box 6080; Morgantown, WV 26506-6080; Voice/TTY: 800-232-9675; www.jan.wvu.edu.

Independent Living Aids, Inc, is a supplier of a variety of different assistive technology options: P.O. Box 9022; Hicksville, NY 11802-9022; 800-537-2118; www.independentliving.com.

MaxiAids is a supplier of a variety of different assistive technology options: 42 Executive Blvd.; Farmingdale, NY 11735; 800-522-6294; www.maxiAids.com.

EnableMart is a catalog of a variety of different assistive technology options: 400 Columbus Street, Suite 100; Vancouver, WA 98669-3413; 800-640-1999; www.EnableMart.com.

Optelec U.S. offers a variety of solutions for those who are blind or visually impaired: 6 Lyberty Way; Westford, MA 01886; 800-828-1956; www.optelec.com.

RehabTool.com offers leading-edge assistive technology products and services for children and adults with disabilities. They can help you choose the right equipment for your needs with their popular product search and referral service: http://www.rehabtool.com.

Patterson Medical (Sammons-Preston Rolyan) is a supplier of various items for those with disabilities, with accessibility and assistive technology options: www.pattersonmedical.com.

Apple Computer Accessibility Center is committed to helping people with disabilities attain an unparalleled level of independence through a personal computer. Apple's commitment to accessibility is evident throughout the Mac OS X operating system, which is by design easy to use, but also includes a wide variety of features and technologies specifically designed to provide accessibility to users with disabilities. Apple refers to these features collectively as *Universal Access* and has integrated them right into the operating system so they can be used in conjunction with a variety of applications from Apple and other developers: www.apple.com/accessibility.

The Boulevard is a disability resource directory of products and services for the physically challenged, elderly, caregivers, and health care professionals: www.blvd.com.

gh Braille offers a full range of accessible media formats and software applications, including digital talking books, an accessible testing system, Braille, and tactile graphics, that enable people with visual disabilities to improve their educational experience, become more competitive in the workplace, and lead more enjoyable lives: www.ghbraille.com.

IBM Accessibility Center responds to requests for information on how IBM products can help people with a wide range of disabilities use personal computers. While the center is unable to diagnose or prescribe an assistive device or software, free information is provided on what is available and where users can go for more details: 11400 Burnet Road, Mailstop 9150; Alston, TX 78758; 800-426-4832; www.IBM.com/able.

Microsoft is committed to their mission of helping customers scale new heights and achieve goals they never thought possible. Delivering on this mission means Microsoft strives to build products that are accessible to everyone—including people with disabilities and impairments: http://www.microsoft.com/enable.

PACER Center, Parent Advocacy Coalition for Educational Rights, is an organization whose mission is to expand opportunities and enhance the quality of life of children and young adults with disabilities and their families, based on the concept of parents helping parents. The links and resources section has information related to accessibility and assistive technology as well as other resource centers for students with disabilities: http://www.pacer.org/about.

PEPNet, the Postsecondary Education Programs Network, is the national collaboration of the four regional postsecondary education centers for individuals who are deaf: http://www.pepnet.org/.

Recoding for the Blind and Dyslexic, National Headquarters; 20 Roszel Road; Princeton, NJ 08540; 866-732-3585; www.rfbd.org.

University of Washington—DO-IT: Disabilities, Opportunities, Internetworking, and Technology is a resource for students with disabilities. Links for assistive technology, universal design, and other items pertinent to adults with disabilities in postsecondary education are provided: www.washington.edu/doit.

Rehabilitation Engineering and Assistive Technology Society of North America is an interdisciplinary association of people whose purpose is to improve the potential of individuals with disabilities through the use of technology. RESNA serves as an information center to address research, development, dissemination, integration, and utilization of knowledge in rehabilitation and assistive technology settings: http://www.resna.org.

Other useful information about products that can assist individuals with mobility impairments can be found at the following websites:

Don Johnston, Inc: www.donjohnston.com

Infogrip: www.infogrip.com

Interlink Electronics: www.interlinkelec.com

Origin Instruments: www.orin.com

Penny & Giles: www.pgcontrols.com

Prentke Romich: www.prentrom.com

Craniosacral Therapy

The International Association of Healthcare Practitioners

Phone: 561-622-4334

Toll-free: 800-311-9204

Fax: 561-622-4771

Website: www.iahp.com

Website offers certification courses, provider directory, educational products, and membership opportunities.

Milne Institute, Inc.

Phone: 831-667-2323

Fax: 831-667-2525

www.milneinstitute.com

Website lists certification and continuing education courses available as well as educational products including texts, tapes, and DVDs.

Driver Rehabilitation

AOTA "Driving and Community Mobility": www.AOTA.org/olderdriver

The Association for Driver Rehabilitation Specialists (ADED)

Phone: 318-257-5055

Toll-free: 800-290-2344 (U.S. only)

Fax: 318-255-4175

Website: www.driver-ed.org

Adaptive Mobility

Phone: 407-426-8020

Website: http://www.adaptivemobility.com

Educational Opportunities

American Society of Hand Therapists: Educational workshops and webinars regarding hand function. http://www.asht.org/education/home-study

AOTA Continuing educational opportunities: http://www.aota.org under the link entitled *continuing education*

Links are provided for current online courses, workshops, courses, as well as downloadable continuing education articles.

In addition, the AOTA continuing education website provides information on opportunities available through not only the AOTA, but also AOTA-approved continuing education providers.

Ergonomics/Work Hardening

Human Factors and Ergonomics Society: www.hfes.org

Cornell University Ergonomics: http://ergo.human.cornell.edu/ergoguide.html

Ergo Web: www.ergoweb.com

Occupational Safety and Health Administration: www.osha.gov

The Baltimore Therapeutic Equipment (BTE) Work Simulator

Designed by the Baltimore Therapeutic Equipment Company, who merged with Hanoun Medical Systems in 2004 to form BTE Technologies, Inc: www.btetech.com.

The ERGOS Work Simulators: www.simwork.com

Valpar International Corp Work Assessments: www.valparint.com

Leisure

Gamblers Anonymous: www.gamblersanonymous.org

YMCA: www.YMCA.net

Low Vision Resources

The Internet Low Vision Society: www.lowvision.org

ABLEDATA

Phone: 800-227-0216

TTY: 301-608-8912

Website: www.abledata.com

American Federation for the Blind (AFB)

Phone: 800-232-5463

Website: www.afb.org

Other low vision resources:

www.allaboutvision.com/lowvision

www.magnifyingaids.com

www.lowvisioninfo.org

www.lighthouse.org

Lymphedema

National Lymphedema Network

Phone: 510-208-3200

Toll-free: 800-541-3259

Fax: 510-208-3110

Website: www.lymphnet.org

Offers an array of resources available to clinicians including membership opportunities and educational materials.

Academy of Lymphatic Studies

Phone: 800-863-5935 (U.S., & Canada)

Fax: 772-589-0306

Website: www.acols.com

Website lists current certification and training courses available.

Sample Manufacturer Contacts for Low-Load, Prolonged Stretch Devices or Dynamic Splinting Devices

Dynasplint Systems, Inc

Phone: 800-638-6771

Website: www.dynasplint.com

Empi

DJO, LLC

1430 Decision Street

Vista, CA 92081

Phone: 760-727-1280

Website: www.empi.com

Saebo: www.saebo.com

Mental Health/Psychosocial Support

Alcoholics Anonymous World Services, Inc: www.aa.org

N.A.M.I. (National Alliance for the Mentally Ill)

Founded in 1979 as the National Alliance for the Mentally Ill, it is a well-known nonprofit, self-help, support, and advocacy organization and a good resource for families, consumers and friends: www.nami.org

Brain Injury Association of America: www.biausa.org

National Family Caregiver Support Program

National Family Caregiver Support Program, developed by the U.S. Administration on Aging, part of the Department of Health and Human Services: www.aoa.acl.gov/AoA_Programs/HCLTC/Caregiver/index.aspx.

Myofascial Release

Myofascial Release Treatment Centers and Seminars

Phone: 610-644-0136

Toll-free: 800-FASCIAL (800-327-2425)

Fax: 610-644-1662

Website: www.myofascialrelease.com

Website lists certification and continuing education opportunities, articles and reviews, educational resources, and a provider directory.

Physical Agent Modalities (PAMs) Certification Programs/Education

AOTA continuing education on PAMS:

http://myaota.aota.org/shop_aota/prodview.aspx?TYPE=D&SKU=4861

Saginaw Valley State University distance education program: www.svsu.edu/cbed/ocepd/medical/physicalagentmodalitycredentialing/

Rehab Education 30-hour program:

www.rehabed.com/advanced-physical-agent-modalities-principles-and-practical-application/

Rehabilitative Equipment Distributors/Suppliers

Patterson Medical (Sammons Preston Rolyan)

Phone: 800-323-5547

Fax: 800-547-4333

Website: http://www.pattersonmedical.com

North Coast Medical, Inc

Phone: 800-821-9319

Website: www.ncmedical.com

AliMed, Inc

Phone: 800-225-2610

Website: www.alimed.com

Pro-Med Products
Phone: 800-542-9297
Website: www.promedproducts.com

Strain Counterstrain Techniques

Jones Institute (originators of the strain counterstrain technique): http://jiscs.com

Appendix B
Assessment Grid

Amy P. Burns, JD, MOT, OTR/L

While the primary focus of this text is adult intervention, evaluation is addressed briefly in multiple chapters. The function of the grid that appears in the following pages is to provide information regarding adult evaluations mentioned in these chapters, as well as other appropriate evaluations. Due to the large number of evaluations available, this grid is intended as a sampling, not a complete list of evaluations on each topic. The last column of the grid provides a location where the reader may look for further information. Again, this is not the only location, as some evaluations are available through multiple vendors. This list is for general educational and reference purposes only and is not intended to promote sale of any products. The information provided was accurate as of publication; however, some websites may change after the production of this text and may no longer be available.

Meriano C, Latella D.
Occupational Therapy Interventions: Function and Occupations, Second Edition (pp 501-522).

ASSESSMENT GRID

Name	Standardization	Validity/ Reliability	Setting Used	Areas Assessed	Information/Purchase
Posture/Balance/Mobility					
Berg Balance Scale (BBS) Berg, Wood-Dauphinee, Williams, & Maki, 1992 Measures 14 balance items. Includes sitting and standing unsupported, sit-to-stand, transfers, picking up objects from floor, and turning.	No	Valid and reliable.	Home or clinic setting.	Transfers, sitting, standing, balance.	Berg, K., Wood-Dauphinee, S., Williams, J. I., & Maki, B. (1992). Measuring balance in the elderly: Validation of an instrument. *Canadian Journal of Public Health*, 7-11.
Functional Reach Test Duncan, Weiner, Chandler, & Studenski, 1992 Simple way to measure standing balance. Measures the difference between arm's length and maximal forward reach.	Yes	Valid and reliable.	Wall and tape measure needed.	Reaching and balance. A quick screen.	Duncan, P. W., Weiner, D. K., Chandler, J., & Studenski, S. (1992). Functional reach: A new clinical measure of balance. *Journal of Gerontology, 45*(6): M192-7. Duncan, P. W., Studenski, S., Chandler, J., & Prescott, B. (1990). Functional reach: Predictive validity in a sample of elderly male veterans. *Journal of Gerontology, 47*(3), M93-M98.
Modified Gait Abnormality Rating Scale (GARS-M) Van Sweringen, Paschal, Bonino, & Yang, 1996 Seven-item assessment of gait, stepping and arm movements, staggering foot contact, hip ROM, shoulder extension, etc.	No	Valid and reliable.	Room to walk.	Hip ROM, foot contact, staggering, arm/leg symmetry, guarding.	VanSweringen, J. M., Paschal, K. A., Bonino, P., & Yang, J. F. (1996). The modified gait abnormality rating scale for recognizing the risk of recurrent falls in community-dwelling elderly adults. *Physical Therapy, 76*(9), 944-1002.

(continued)

ASSESSMENT GRID (continued)

Name	Standardization	Validity/ Reliability	Setting Used	Areas Assessed	Information/Purchase
Posture/Balance/Mobility					
Timed Get Up and Go (TGUG) Podsiadlo & Richardson, 1991 Measures the overall time to complete a series of functionally important tasks. Helps to identify clients with balance deficits.	No	Valid and reliable.	Room to walk 10 feet; chair.	Balance, posture, mobility. Static and dynamic balance tested.	Podsiadlo, D., & Richardson, S. (1991). The timed "up & go": A test of basic functional mobility for frail elderly persons. *Journal of the American Geriatrics Society, 39*(2), 142-148.
Tinetti, 1986 Measures a client's gait and balance.	No	Inter-rater reliability.	Room to walk 10 feet; chair.	Balance and gait.	Tinetti, M. E., Williams, T. F., & Mayewski, R. (1986). Fall Risk Index for elderly patients based on number of chronic disabilities. *American Journal of Medicine, 80*:429-434.
Cognition					
Bay Area Functional Performance Evaluation (BaFPE) Bloomer and Lang, 1987 Assesses how a client might function in task-oriented settings and settings with social interaction. Uses sea shells, design blocks, and associated items.	Yes	Valid and reliable.	Seated at table.	Memory, organization, attention span.	www.pattersonmedical.com
Behavioral Inattention Test Wilson, Cockburn, & Halligan, 1987 Assesses unilateral visual neglect. Includes card sorting, article reading, figure/ shape copying, etc.	Yes	Valid and reliable.	Quiet environment with minimal distractions.	Unilateral visual neglect, picture recalling, line crossing, article reading, phone dialing.	www.pearsonclinical.com

(continued)

ASSESSMENT GRID (continued)

Name	Standardization	Validity/ Reliability	Setting Used	Areas Assessed	Information/Purchase
Cognition					
Cognitive Assessment of Minnesota (CAM) Rustad et al., 1993 Assesses the cognitive ability-ties of adults with neurological impairments.	Yes	Valid and reliable.	Quiet room.	Attention, memory, visual neglect.	www.pearsonclinical.com
Contextual Memory Test Toglia, 1993 Assesses awareness of memory capacity, strategy use, and recall in adults with memory dysfunction.	Yes	Valid and reliable.	Quiet room with minimal distraction.	Memory, awareness of memory capacity, recall of line drawings.	www.pearsonclinical.com
Glasgow Coma Scale Teasdale, 1974 Measures response of eyes, verbal response, and motor response in numerical levels.	No	Reliable.	In hospital.	Alertness, awareness, verbal response, motor response.	www.mdcalc.com/glasgow-coma-scale-score/
Lowenstein Occupational Therapy Cognitive Assessment (LOTCA) (also LOTCA-Geriatric and Dynamic-LOTCA) Itzkovich, Averbuch, Elazar, Katz, 2000 Assesses clients with neurological deficits and mental health issues. Tests orientation, visual/ spatial perception, praxis, visuomotor. Includes cards, blocks, pegboard.	Yes	Valid and reliable.	Quiet environment with minimal distractions.	Orientation, perception, praxis, visuomotor, organization, thinking operations.	www.therapro.com

(continued)

ASSESSMENT GRID (continued)

Name	Standardization	Validity/ Reliability	Setting Used	Areas Assessed	Information/Purchase
Cognition					
Luria-Nebraska Neuropsychological Battery Golden, 1991 Reading numbers, writing words, differentiate hard/soft touch, sounds. Provides a pat- tern analysis of strengths and weakness across areas of brain function.	Yes	Valid and reliable.	Quiet environment with minimal distractions.	Numbers, reading, writing, touching.	www.wpspublish.com
Mini-Mental Status Evaluation (MMSE) (MMSE-2, 2013) Folstein, Folstein, & McHugh, 1975 Used to assess cognitive function.	Yes	Valid and reliable.	Seated at table.	Brain injury, writing, reading, drawing.	www.minimental.com Now has a mobile app—instant and automatic scores
Ranchos Los Amigos Developed at the Rancho Los Amigos Hospital in California by the Head Injury Treatment Team Medical scale, assesses the level of recovery of a client with a brain injury and those recovering from a coma.	No	Reliable.	In hospital.	Alertness, awareness.	Original Scale coauthored by Chris Hagen, PhD, Danese-Malkmus, MA, & Patricia Durham, MA. Communication Disorders Service, Ranchos Los Amigos Hospital, 1972. Revised 11/15/74 by Danese Malkmus, MA and Kathryn Stenderup, OTR
Rivermead Behavioral Memory Test (RBMT-3) Wilson et al., 2008 Assessment of gross memory impairments encountered by clients in their everyday lives. Identifies everyday memory problems and monitors change over time.	Yes	Valid and reliable.	Quiet environment with minimal distractions.	Memory: immediate and recall.	www.pearsonclinical.com

(continued)

ASSESSMENT GRID (continued)

Name	Standardization	Validity/ Reliability	Setting Used	Areas Assessed	Information/Purchase
Cognition					
Severe Impairment Battery (SIB) Saxton, McGonigle, Swihart, & Boller, 1993 Evaluates cognitive abilities at the lower end of the range (severely impaired dementia client). Allows for non-verbal and partially correct responses.	Yes	Valid and reliable.	Quiet room.	Memory, completing simple actions.	www.pearsonclinical.com
Autobiographical Memory Interview (AMI) Kopelman, Wilson, & Baddeley, 1990 Interview recalling events from the clients' past including school, wedding, children, etc.	Yes	Valid and reliable.	Quiet environment with minimal distractions.	Memory, retrograde amnesia.	www.pearsonclinical.com
Test of Everyday Attention Robertson, Ward, Ridgeway, Nimmo-Smith, 1994 Measures selective attention, sustained attention, and attentional switching. Includes map search, telephone search,elevator counting, etc.	Yes	Valid and reliable.	Quiet room; table and chairs.	Everyday materials (map searching, phone skills, etc.).	www.harcourt-uk.com/product.aspx?n=1315&s=2037&cat=2064&skey=2886

(continued)

ASSESSMENT GRID (continued)

Name	Standardization	Validity/ Reliability	Setting Used	Areas Assessed	Information/Purchase
Dexterity					
Disabilities of the Arm, Shoulder and Hand (3rd ed.) Solway, Beaton, McConnell, & Bombardier, 2006 Quantifies upper extremity limitations	No	Valid and reliable.	Questionnaire. Also, QuickDASH	Upper extremity disability.	Institute for Work & Health: www.dash.iwh.on.ca
Jebsen-Taylor Hand Function Test Jebsen, Taylor, et al., 1969 Assesses a broad range of hand functions used in daily activities. A 7-part test that uses common items such as paper clips, cans, pencils, etc.	Yes	Reliable.	Seated, requires adequate lighting.	Writing, page turning, lifting small/large objects, simulated feeding.	www.pattersonmedical.com
Manipulative Aptitude Test Roeder Measures hand/arm/finger dexterity and speed through sorting and assembling.	Yes	Valid and reliable.	Seated at a table or desk.	Dexterity, manipulative aptitude, dominant hand.	www.wisdomking.com/product140188c220087.html
Minnesota Rate of Manipulation University of Minnesota Employment Stabilization Research Institute, 1969 Assesses unilateral and bilateral manual dexterity along with eye-hand coordination. Provides information on standing tolerance, sustained neck flexion, weight-bearing, and repetitive reach.	Yes	Valid and reliable.	Table and chair.	Manual dexterity, turning, dis-placing.	www.amazon.com

(continued)

ASSESSMENT GRID (continued)

Name	Standardization	Validity/ Reliability	Setting Used	Areas Assessed	Information/Purchase
Dexterity					
Nine Hole Peg Mathiowetz, Weber, Kashman, & Volland, 1985 Client places 9 dowels in 9 holes while being timed.	Yes	Valid and reliable.	Table and chair.	Finger dexterity.	Mathiowetz, V., Volland, G., Kashman, N., & Weber, K. (1992). Nine-hole peg test. In Wade, D. T., *Measurement in neurological rehabilitation*. New York: Oxford University Press, 171. www.rehabmeasures.org
O'Connor Finger Dexterity Test O'Connor Requires hand placement of 3 pins per hole.	Yes		Table and chair.	Predictor of rapid manipulation of small objects.	www.rehaboutlet.com
O'Connor Tweezer Dexterity Test O'Connor Measures the speed with which a client can pick up pins with a tweezers, one at a time, and place the pin into a small hole.	Yes		Table and chair.	Finger dexterity, fine motor coordination, speed, eye hand coordination.	www.rehaboutlet.com
Purdue Pegboard Tiffin, 1948 Assesses gross movement of hands/fingers/arms, as well as fingertip dexterity.	Yes	Valid and reliable.	Table and chair.	Gross movement of hands, fingers, and arms; fingertip dexterity.	www.rehaboutlet.com

(continued)

ASSESSMENT GRID (continued)

Name	Standardization	Validity/ Reliability	Setting Used	Areas Assessed	Information/Purchase
Dexterity					
Range of Motion The measurement of the achievable distance between the flexed position and the extended position of a particular joint or muscle group.	Yes	Valid, not 100% reliable.	Comfortable for client, chair/ mat.	Biomechanical.	Multiple sources including: Latella, D., & Meriano, C. (2003). *Occupational Therapy Manual for the Evaluation of Range of Motion and Muscle Strength*. Clifton Park, NY: Thomson Delmar Learning.
Strength Testing The strength of each muscle group is measured on a scale of 0/5 to 5/5.	Yes	Valid, not 100% reliable.	Comfortable for client, chair/ mat.	Biomechanical.	Multiple sources including: Latella, D., & Meriano, C. (2003). *Occupational Therapy Manual for the Evaluation of Range of Motion and Muscle Strength*. Clifton Park, NY: Thomson Delmar Learning.
Sensation/Edema/Tone					
Ashworth Scale Ashworth, B. Modified Ashworth Scale Bohannon, Smith, 1987 Scale to define muscle tone.	No	Not tested.	Any	Muscle tone.	Ashworth, B. (1964) Preliminary trial of carisoprodol in multiple sclerosis. *Practitioner*, 192, 540. www.rehabmeasures.org
Touch Test Monofilaments; evaluates both diminishing and returning sensation.	No	Not tested.	Any	Sensation hand and foot.	www.rehaboutlet.com

(continued)

ASSESSMENT GRID (continued)

Name	Standardization	Validity/ Reliability	Setting Used	Areas Assessed	Information/Purchase
Sensation/Edema/Tone					
Volumeter Fill container with water, mea- sure the displaced water of both hands.	No	Not tested.	Countertop or table; need access to water faucet.	Edema, swelling of UE.	www.rehabmart.com
Vision/Visual Perception					
Benton Visual Form Discrimination Test Hamsher, Varney, & Spreen, 1983 Assesses the ability to discriminate between complex visual configurations. Book of line drawings.	No	Valid.	Seated at table, test at midline.	Neglect, neurological and psychological.	www4.parinc.com/products/product.aspx?productid=BENTON
Hooper Visual Organization Test (VOT) Hooper, 1983 Ability to visually integrate information into whole perceptions through the use of line drawings arranged in puzzles.	Yes	Valid and reliable.	Quiet environment with minimal distractions.	Organization of visual stimuli.	www.wpspublish.com
Motor Free Visual Perception Test (MVPT-3) Colarusso & Hammill, 2003 Assesses overall visual perceptual ability.	Yes	Valid and reliable.	Seated at table. Adequate light and free from distraction.	Visual perceptual.	www.wpspublish.com

(continued)

ASSESSMENT GRID (continued)

Name	Standardization	Validity/ Reliability	Setting Used	Areas Assessed	Information/Purchase
Vision/Visual Perception					
STROOP Color and Word Test Golden & Freshwater, 2002 Reading aloud colored words. The words themselves are names of colors, but the actual color is different than the name.	Yes	Valid and reliable.	Quiet environment with minimal distractions.	Brain function and planning.	www.wpspublish.com
Test of Visual Motor Skills (TVMS-3) Martin, 2009 Measures visual motor functioning using 16 geometric figures.	Yes	Valid and reliable.	Seated at table. Adequate light and free from distraction.	Visual motor.	www.wpspublish.com
Warren's Brain Injury Visual Assessment Battery for Adults (biVABA) Warren, 1998 Assessment of visual processing ability after a brain injury.	Yes	Valid and reliable.	Comfortable for client.	Visual perceptual processing, oculomotor function, how function is affected.	www.visabilities.com/bivaba.html
ADLs/IADLs					
Allen Cognitive Level Test (ACL) Allen, 1996 Leather lacing test.	Yes	Valid and reliable.	Environment with minimal distractions and good lighting.	Problem solving, sequencing.	www.allen-cognitive-network.org/

(continued)

ASSESSMENT GRID (continued)

Name	Standardization	Validity/ Reliability	Setting Used	Areas Assessed	Information/Purchase
ADLs/IADLs					
Arnadottir Occupational Therapy Neurobehavioral Evaluation (A-one) Arnadottir, 1990 Determines the impact of neurobehavioral impairments on activities of daily living and mobility tasks using a 5-point scale.	Yes	Valid and reliable.	Clinical.	ADLs, severity of neurobehavioral impairment, occupational performance.	http://strokengine.ca/assess/module_a_2d_one_indepth-en.html
Assessment of Motor and Process Skills (AMPS) Fisher, 1993 Observational assessment, measures the quality of a person's ADLs. Rates the effort, efficiency, safety, and independence of ADL motor/process skills. (*Training required.)	Yes	Valid and reliable.	Various conditions.	IADLs, motor skills and processing skills. Also, school version (School AMPS)	www.innovativeotsolutions.com/content/ Special training required. Once trained, materials are supplied.
Assessment of Occupational Functioning (AOF) Watts, Kielhofner, & Bauer, 1996 Assesses the functional capacity of residents in long-term treatment settings who have physical and/or psychiatric problems.	Yes	Valid and reliable.	Comfortable for the client.	IADLs, MOHO, volition, habituation, performance. Also, AOF-CV (collaborative version)	http://mh4ot.files.wordpress.com/2012/05/assessment-of-occupational-functioning-collaborative-version.pdf Contact: Janet Watts, PhD, OTR/L jhwatts@hsc.vcu.edu
Barthel Index Mahoney & Barthel, 1965 Assesses self-care functions in older adults.	No	Predictive validity.	Individual or group evaluation.	Self-care.	www.strokecenter.org/wp-content/uploads/2011/08/barthel.pdf

(continued)

ASSESSMENT GRID (continued)

Name	Standardization	Validity/ Reliability	Setting Used	Areas Assessed	Information/Purchase
ADLs/IADLs					
Canadian Occupational Performance Measure (COPM) Law, Baptiste, Carswell, McColl, Polatajko, & Pollock, 2005 Individualized outcome measure designed to detect changes in self-perception of occupational performance over time.	Yes, but not norm-referenced.	Valid and reliable.	Comfortable for client.	Occupational performances and perception.	www.caot.ca/copm/index.htm
Comprehensive Occupational Therapy Evaluation (COTE) Brayman, Kirby, Meisenheimer & Short Developed in an acute psychiatric setting. Identifies 25 OT-related behaviors within 3 categories (general behavior, interpersonal behavior, and task behavior).	Yes	Valid and reliable.	Where ever the task is performed.	Behavior.	Brayman, S. J., Kirby, T. F., Meisenheimer, A. M., & Short, M. J. (1976). The comprehensive occupational therapy evaluation scale. *Am J Occup Ther, 30*(2),94-100. http://www.oota.org/website/COTE.pdf
Direct Assessment of Functional Abilities (DAFA) Loewenstein, D., Amigo, E., Duara, R., et al. (1989) Direct measurement of the instrumental activities of daily living. Used to determine functional deficits in clients with mild cognitive impairment.	Yes	Valid and reliable.	Clinical setting, cafeteria, gift shop, and exam room.	IADLs.	Loewenstein, D., Amigo, E., Duara, R., et al. (1989). A new scale for the assessment of functional status in Alzheimer's disease and related disorders. *J Gerontol Psychol Sci, 44*, 114-121 http://gerontologist.oxfordjournals.org/content/38/1/113.full.pdf

(continued)

ASSESSMENT GRID (continued)

Name	Standardization	Validity/ Reliability	Setting Used	Areas Assessed	Information/Purchase
ADLs/IADLs					
Functional Independent Measure (FIM) UDSMR, 1993 Scale (range from 1-7) that measures a client's ability to function with independence. Collected upon admission to rehabilitation unit, upon discharge, and after discharge.	Yes	Valid and reliable.	Clinic or home setting.	ADLs, self-care, communication, cognitive function.	www.udsmr.org/WebModules/FIM/Fim_About.aspx Training required.
Independent Living Scales (ILS) Loeb, 2003 Offers assessment, daily living skills, self-advocacy training, and support with an issues that challenge the independence of a client.	Yes	Valid and reliable.	Table and chairs; can be bedside.	IADL, memory, orientation, money management, health, safety, etc.	www.pearsonclinical.com
Index of Activities of Daily Living (Katz ADL) Katz, 1963 Assesses functional status as a measurement of the client's ability to perform activities of daily living independently. (No longer in print, may still be seen in some clinics.)	Yes	Valid and reliable.	Inpatient observations.	ADL, biological and psychological function.	Katz, S., Ford, A. B., Moskowitz, R. W., Jackson, B. A., & Jaffe, M. W. (1963). Studies of illness in the aged: The index of ADL: A standardized mea- sure of biological and psychosocial function. *JAMA,185*, 94-9.
Kitchen Task Assessment (KTA) Baum & Edwards, 1993 Measures organization, planning, and judgment skills through common kitchen tasks.	Yes	Valid and reliable.	Kitchen/ cooking environment.	IADL, initiation, organization, sequencing, judgment, safety.	Baum, C., & Edwards, D. F. (1993). Cognitive performance in senile dementia of the Alzheimer's type: the Kitchen Task Assessment. *Am J Occup Ther, 47*(5), 431-436.

(continued)

ASSESSMENT GRID (continued)

Name	Standardization	Validity/ Reliability	Setting Used	Areas Assessed	Information/Purchase
ADLs/IADLs					
Klein-Bell Activities of Daily Living Scale Klein & Bell, 1982 Assesses age-related changes in activities of daily living ability. (No longer in print, may still be seen in some clinics.)	Yes	Valid and reliable.	General Rehabilitation setting.	ADLs.	Klein, R. M., & Bell, B. (1982). Self-care skills: behavioral measurement with Klein-Bell ADL scale. *Arch Phys Med Rehab, 63*(7), 335-8.
Kohlman Evaluation of Living Skills (KELS) Thompson, 1992 Ability to function in 17 basic living skills. Assesses skills in 5 areas: self-care, safety and health, money management, transportation/telephone, and work/leisure.	Yes	Valid and reliable.	Table and Chairs.	Self-care, safety and health, money management, transportation, telephone, work, leisure.	www.amazon.com
Level of Rehabilitation Scale (LORS-II) Carey & Posavac, 1982 Evaluates the success of inpatient rehabilitation programs.	Yes	Valid and reliable.	Hospital rehabilitation units.	ADLs.	Carey, R. G., & Posavac ,E. J. (1982). Rehabilitation program evaluation using a revised level of rehabilitation scale (LORS-II). *Arch Phys Med Rehabil, 63*(8), 367-370.
Milwaukee Evaluation of Daily Living Skills (MEDLS) Leonardelli, 1988 Information from clients and families; establishes baseline behaviors necessary to develop treatment plans and guide intervention in regard to daily living skills.	No	Valid and reliable.	Home environment.	ADLs, including communication, personal care, clothing care, etc.	www.amazon.com

(continued)

ASSESSMENT GRID (continued)

Name	Standardization	Validity/ Reliability	Setting Used	Areas Assessed	Information/Purchase
ADLs/IADLs					
Occupational Circumstances Assessment and Interview Rating Scale (OCAIRS) Version 4.0 Forsyth et al., 2005 A 40-minute interview that analyzes the extent and nature of a client's occupational adaptation and participation.	No	Valid and reliable.	Comfortable for the client.	MOHO, volitional, habituation, performance.	www.cade.uic.edu/moho/productDetails.aspx?aid=35
Occupational Performance History Interview (OPHI-II) Kielhofner et al., 2004 Interview that gathers the appreciation of a client's life history, the direction in which they want to take their life, as well as the impact of a disability on their life.	Yes	Valid and reliable.	Comfortable for the client.	Occupational roles, daily routine, critical life events.	www.cade.uic.edu/moho/productDetails.aspx?aid=31
Occupational Self Assessment Baron, Kielhofner, Ienger, Goldhammer, & Wolenski, 2006 This is a self-assessment of perceptions of strengths and weaknesses relative to occupational functioning.	Yes	Valid and reliable.	Comfortable for the client.	MOHO, volitional, habituation, performance.	www.cade.uic.edu/moho/productDetails.aspx?aid=2

(continued)

ASSESSMENT GRID (continued)

Name	Standardization	Validity/Reliability	Setting Used	Areas Assessed	Information/Purchase
ADLs/IADLs					
Performance Assessment of Self-care Skills (PASS) Holm & Rogers, 1994 Performance based observation tool covering functional mobility, personal care, and IADLs. Measures short term functional change in elderly after hospitalization. (Requires 2-day training workshop.)	Criterion referenced.	Valid and reliable.	Clinic and home version.	IADLs.	http://70.61.86.133/clinical/Clinical%20Programming/ADL/PASS.pdf Special training required. Once trained, materials are supplied.
The Role Checklist Version 2: Quality of Performance Scott et al., 2014 Assesses the values that clients place on their occupational roles.	Yes	Valid and reliable.	Comfortable for client.	MOHO, habituation subsystem.	www.rcv2qp.com/ Based on Oakley's 1986 Role Checklist.
Routine Task Inventory (RTI-II) Allen et al., 1992 Measures the level of performance in activities of daily living through observation and questioning.	No	Valid and reliable.	Clinic or home setting.	ADLs, effect of cognitive impairment on task performance.	www.allen-cognitive-network.org/index.htm
Environmental Evaluations					
Enabler Iwarsson & Slaug, 2001 Norm-based environment assessment, developed to assess the accessibility of housing and its close surroundings.	Yes	Valid and reliable.	Home environment and close surroundings.	IADLs, neurological, musculoskeletal, psychological, movement, cognition, physical.	Iwarsson, S., & Isacsson, A. (1996). Development of a novel instrument for occupational therapy assessment of the physical environment in the home methodological study on the Enabler. *Occup Ther J Res, 16*(4), 227-244. www.enabler.nu/index.html

(continued)

ASSESSMENT GRID (continued)

Name	Standardization	Validity/ Reliability	Setting Used	Areas Assessed	Information/Purchase
Environmental Evaluations					
HOME FAST Mackenzie, Byles, & Higginbotham, 2000 Screen to identify home hazards contributing to falls	No	Valid and reliable.	Home environment.	Client's function within environment.	Mackenzie, L., Byles, J., & Higginbotham, N. (2000). Designing the home falls and accidents screening tool (HOME FAST): Selecting the items. *Br J Occup Ther, 63*,260-269. http://www.bhps.org.uk/falls/documents/HomeFast.pdf
SAFER/SAFER-HOME Chui, Oliver, Marshall, & Letts. Client interview/observation	No norms, but manual available.	Valid and reliable.	Home environment.	Client's function within environment.	COTA comprehensive Rehabilitation and Mental Health Services. http://www.caot.ca/cjot_pdfs/cjot60/60.2oliver.pdf
Westmead Home Safety Assessment Clemson, 2006 Client interview/observation	No	Minimal evidence for validity & reliability.	Home environment.	Client's function within environment.	www.therapybookshop.com/coordinates/ Co-ordinates therapy services.
Communication and Social Interaction					
Worker Assessment of Communication and Interaction Skill (ACIS) Forsyth et al., 1998 Identity areas of strength and habits interfering with effective interaction	No	Valid and reliable.	During occupation and/or within a social group.	Observational assessment, communication and interaction skills.	www.cade.uic.edu/moho/productDetails.aspx?aid=1

(continued)

ASSESSMENT GRID (continued)

Name	Standardization	Validity/ Reliability	Setting Used	Areas Assessed	Information/Purchase
Communication and Social Interaction					
The Evaluation of Social Interaction (ESI) Fisher & Griswold, 2008 Performance of social interaction skills; quantitative assessment.	No	Valid and reliable.	During occupation.	Social interaction performance in the natural context of a person's desired occupation.	www.innovativeotsolutions.com/content/
Work and Retirement					
Transition to Work Inventory 3rd Edition, 2012	No	Valid and reliable.	Work-related questionnaire.	Determine worker-job fit.	http://jist.emcp.com/transition-to-work-inventory-third-edition-1832.html
Worker Environment Impact Scale (WEIS) Moore-Corner, Kielhofner, Olson, 1998 Assesses environmental characteristics that facilitate successful employment experiences. Goal is to maximize the 'fit' of the worker and their skill to the job environment.	No	Fair validity and reliability.	Comfortable for the client.	Space related issues, fit of environment.	www.cade.uic.edu/moho/productDetails.aspx?aid=12
Worker Role Interview (WRI) Version 10.0 Braveman et al., 2005 Identifies psychosocial and environmental factors that influence a client's ability to return to work.	Yes	Valid and reliable.	Work, comfortable for client.	Physical evaluation, essential job functions, psychosocial capacity to return to work.	www.cade.uic.edu/moho/productDetails.aspx?aid=11

(continued)

ASSESSMENT GRID (continued)

Name	Standardization	Validity/ Reliability	Setting Used	Areas Assessed	Information/Purchase
Leisure					
Activity Card Sort (2nd Ed.) Baum & Edwards, 2008 Measure of activity participation	No	Valid and reliable.	Institutional, recovering, and community versions.	IADLs and leisure.	http://store.aota.org
Adolescent Leisure Interest Profile (ALIP) Henry, 1998 Used to evaluate the leisure activities that clients enjoy.	No	Reliable.	Comfortable for client.	Sports, outdoor/indoor activities, creativity.	Henry S. D. (1998). Development of a measure of adolescent leisure interests. *AJOT, 52*, 531-539.
Adolescent Role Assessment (ARA) Black, 1976 Used to assess and identify deficiencies in the occupation choice process of adolescents.	No	Scores lack internal consistency.	Comfortable for client.	Childhood play, adult work, adolescent socialization.	Huebner, Emery, Shordike (2002). The Adolescent Role Assessment: Psychometric Properties and Theoretical Usefulness. *AJOT, March/April 2002, Vol. 56, 202-209*
Social Participation					
Coping Inventory Zeitlin, 1985 Profiles coping styles, as well as behaviors, that facilitate or interfere with adaptive coping. Self-administered and profiled.	No	Self-report and observation.	Comfortable for the client.	Sensorimotor, reactive behavior, self-initiated behavior, adaptive coping.	http://ststesting.com/CPOI.html

(continued)

ASSESSMENT GRID (continued)

Name	Standardization	Validity/ Reliability	Setting Used	Areas Assessed	Information/Purchase
Social Participation					
Life Satisfaction Index Neugarten, Havighurst, & Tobin, 1961 Looking at 5 factors that make up total life satisfaction (plea- sure, meaningfulness, feeling of success, self-image, happiness)	Yes	Valid and reliable.	Comfortable for the client.	Activity, developmental theory, internal satisfaction.	Neugarten, B., Havinghurts, R., & Tobin S. (1961). The measurement of life satisfaction. *J Gerontol*, 16, 134-143. https://instruct.uwo.ca/kinesiology/9641/Assessments/Psychological/LSI.html
Occupational Questionnaire (OQ) Kielhofner, 2002 Self-report assessment. Client documents the main activity which he or she engages in for each half-hour throughout the morning/day/evening and identifies each activity as work, ADL, recreation, or rest. Explores the meaning of leisure from the client's perspective.	Yes	Valid and reliable.	Clinic or home setting.	IADLs, volition, activity pattern, life satisfaction, interests, values, personal causation.	www.cade.uic.edu/moho/productDetails.aspx?aid=41
Volitional Questionnaire Version 4.0 de las Heras, Geist, Kielhofner, Li, 2003 Observational assessment, gathers information on a client's volition.	Yes	Valid.	Observations are context specific: leisure, work, ADL environments.	MOHO, volition subsystem, work, leisure, intrinsic motivation, values, interests.	www.cade.uic.edu/moho/productDetails.aspx?aid=8

(continued)

ASSESSMENT GRID (continued)

Name	Standardization	Validity/ Reliability	Setting Used	Areas Assessed	Information/Purchase
Wellness					
Coping Inventory: Self-Rated Form Zeitlin Client evaluates adaptive behavior for coping	No	Not tested.	Any.	Habits, skills, behaviors related to coping.	www.ststesting.com
Engagement in Meaningful Activities Survey (EMAS) Goldberg & Brintnell, 2002 Clients read statements about activities, put an 'X' in the box that best describes them (never to always).	Yes, for research purposes only.	Valid and reliable.	Comfortable for the client.	Activities.	www.caot.ca/conference/2009/presentations/Psychometric%20Properties.pdf
Stress Management Questionnaire (SMQ) Stein, 2003 Identification of symptoms linked to stress and coping strategies that aid in the reduction of stress.	Yes	Valid and reliable.	Comfortable for the client.	Coping, stressors, behavioral theory.	www.emergingmediainc.com/stressmaster/pdf/smq_bro.pdf

Financial Disclosures

Dr. Amy P. Burns has no financial or proprietary interest in the materials presented herein.

Marilyn B. Cole has no financial or proprietary interest in the materials presented herein.

Dr. Margo Ruth Gross has no financial or proprietary interest in the materials presented herein.

Dr. Kimberly D. Hartmann has no financial or proprietary interest in the materials presented herein.

Dr. Donna Latella has no financial or proprietary interest in the materials presented herein.

Dr. Catherine Meriano has no financial or proprietary interest in the materials presented herein.

Deanna Proulx-Sepelak has no financial or proprietary interest in the materials presented herein.

Dr. Martha J. Sanders has no financial or proprietary interest in the materials presented herein.

Dr. Francine M. Seruya has no financial or proprietary interest in the materials presented herein.

Peter Tascione has no financial or proprietary interest in the materials presented herein.

Roseanna Tufano has no financial or proprietary interest in the materials presented herein.

Tracy Van Oss has no financial or proprietary interest in the materials presented herein.

Robert Wright has no financial or proprietary interest in the materials presented herein.

Index

Printed in the United States
by Baker & Taylor Publisher Services